Review of Rheumatology

Nona T. Colburn

Review of Rheumatology

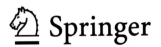 Springer

Dr. Nona T. Colburn
National Institutes of Health
NHGRI
Bethesda, Montgomery
MD, USA

ISBN 978-1-84882-092-0   e-ISBN 978-1-84882-093-7
DOI 10.1007/978-1-84882-093-7
Springer London Dordrecht Heidelberg New York

British Library Cataloguing in Publication Data
A catalogue record for this book is available from the British Library

Library of Congress Control Number: 2011939771

Springer is part of Springer Science+Business Media (www.springer.com)

To my husband Rouis, a cancer survivor
For your love, understanding, and support
And for teaching me, by example, to be
"tough"

Preface

The aim of this rheumatology review is to provide a concise source of information, written in an *outline form*, that will be a quick and easily accessible reference for not only those preparing for the rheumatology board exams, but will also serve as a succinct reference for all health care workers interested in the field of rheumatology. The outline style has been used successfully in review books of numerous medical disciplines. As the size of most current rheumatology review books approaches that of a textbook, it is becoming more difficult to find "just the facts".

Material covers chapters organized into 30 major topics, which will review basic musculoskeletal anatomy, immunology, genetics, major rheumatic diseases and their pathophysiology, and major rheumatic therapeutics. A synopsis of key areas of interest makes for an indispensable "quick reference".

Every effort has been made to ensure the accuracy of this work. However, the contents are to be used as a guide only. Health care professional should use sound clinical judgment and individualize therapy to each particular patient care situation. The information in *Rheumatology Review* is compiled from sources listed in the "Suggested Readings" section at the end of the book.

Nona T. Colburn, M.D.

Acknowledgement

I would like to thank the following individuals who took on the challenge of either reviewing various portions of this book or providing sage counsel during my education as a Rheumatology Fellow.

Dr. Daniel Kastner
Scientific Director
NHGRI/NIH
Bethesda, MD

Dr. Frank Pucino
Pharmacist
CC/NIH
Bethesda, MD

Dr. Elaine Remmers
Staff Scientist
NHGRI/NIH
Bethesda, MD

Dr. Michael Ward
Staff Clinician and Researcher
NIAMS/NIH
Bethesda, MD

I would also like to thank all those at Springer who made this publication possible, particularly Nadine Firth and Melissa Morton.

Contents

The Musculoskeletal System

Section A: Joints

1. Joints classifications
   a. Synarthrosis
      i. "Suture lines" of the skull where adjoining cranial plates are separated by thin fibrous tissue
   b. Amphiarthroses
      i. Adjacent bones are bound by flexible fibrocartilage that permits limited motion
      ii. Examples include the pubic symphysis, part of the SI joint, and intervertebral discs
   c. Diarthroses
      i. "Synovial joints"
         1. Most common and most mobile
         2. All have a synovial lining
      ii. Further classified into:
         1. Ball and socket – hip
         2. Hinge – interphalangeal
         3. Saddle – first carpometacarpal
         4. Plane – patellofemoral
2. Major tissues in a diarthroidal (synovial) joint
   a. Hyaline cartilage – covers the surfaces of opposing bones
   b. Capsule – varies in thickness from an inapparent membrane in some areas to strong ligamentous bands in others
   c. Synovium – lines the capsule
      i. The intima comprises the lining tissue (one to three cells deep) that surfaces all intracapsular structures, except the contact areas of articular cartilage
      ii. Normally the synovium is collapsed to minimize the volume, with no obvious pool of fluid

N.T. Colburn, *Review of Rheumatology*,
DOI 10.1007/978-1-84882-093-7_1, © Springer-Verlag London Limited 2012

     iii. The synovium does not have a limiting basement membrane

     iv. Contains

        1. Fat and lymphatic vessels

        2. Fenestrated microvessels which are terminal branches of an arterial plexus

        3. Nerve fibers derived from the capsule and periarticular tissues

  d. Synovial cells

     i. Reside in matrix-rich Type I collagen and proteoglycans

     ii. Two main types differentiated by the electron microscope

        1. Type A

           a. Macrophage-like with primarily a phagocytic function

           b. Monocyte derived with a high content of cytoplasmic organelles, including lysosomes, smooth-walled vacuoles, and micropinocytotic vesicles

        2. Type B

           a. Fibroblast-like with production of hyaluronate, which accounts for the increased viscosity of synovial fluid

           b. Have fewer organelles and a more extensive endoplasmic reticulum

        3. Other cells in the normal synovium include

           a. Antigen processing cells with a dendritic configuration

           b. Mast cells

           c. Occasional white blood cells

  e. Menisci

     i. Composed of fibrocartilage

3. Joint flexion and joint impact

  a. Eccentric contraction

     i. When the joint bends farther under an acute load as a response of the extensor muscle

     ii. A protective reflex mechanism

  b. Flexion distributes the stress

     i. In time by prolonging the deceleration of landing

     ii. In space by loading a large surface area of the convex member

  c. Loading energy at contact surfaces is transmitted mainly into bone, despite cartilages' viscoelastic properties (hydraulic shock)

  d. Stiff concave joint members can explode under overwhelming stress, whereas the more flexible convex mates are more protected

     i. Bone is thicker on the concave loading side

     ii. Articular cartilage is thicker on the convex side

        1. The concave articular cartilage tends to have more of a fibrous composition

  e. Synovial fluid contributes a significant stabilizing effect as an adhesive seal that permits sliding motion, but prevents distracting forces

     i. This stabilizing property is lost when the normally thin film enlarges, as with an effusion

  f. Synovial joints act as mechanical bearings with very low coefficients of friction

4. "Knuckle cracking"
    a. Reflects a fracture of the adhesive bond of synovial fluid
    b. Takes up to 30 min before the bond can be reestablished and the knuckle cracked again
    c. Secondary cavitation within the joint space causes a radiologically apparent bubble of gas
5. Intra-articular pressure
    a. Normal joint pressure is negative (-5.7 cm H_2O) compared with ambient atmospheric pressure
        i. About -4 mmHg in the resting knee
            1. This pressure falls further when the quadriceps muscle contracts
        ii. This pressure difference is a stabilizing force
    b. In an effusion, the resting pressure is above that of the atmosphere and rises further when surrounding muscles contract
        i. This reversal of pressure gradients is an additional destabilizing factor
6. Three major sources of lubrication in the synovial joint
    a. Hydrodynamic lubrication
        i. The dynamic motion of the bearing areas produces an aqueous layer that separates and protects the contact points
        ii. Articular cartilage is elastic, fluid-filled, and backed by an impervious layer of calcified cartilage and bone
        iii. Load induced compression of cartilage forces interstitial fluid to flow laterally within the tissue and to surface through adjacent cartilage
    b. Boundary layer lubrication
        i. Lubricin, a small glycoprotein produced by synovial lining cells, functions as a phospholipid carrier and binds to articular cartilage where it retains a protective layer of water molecules
        ii. A boundary lubrication based on phospholipids has been proposed as the common lubricating mechanism for many tissues
    c. Hyaluronic acid
        i. Lubricates the contact surface between synovium and cartilage
        ii. Produced by Type B synovial cells
        iii. Allows the synovium to sequentially contract and expand to cover non-loaded cartilage surfaces
        iv. Does not contribute to cartilage lubrication
        v. Through its viscosity augments hydrodynamic lubrication as it retards the outflow of load bearing fluid

Section B: Articular Cartilage

1. Extracellular matrix
    a. A load bearing connective tissue that can absorb impact and withstand shearing forces
    b. Composed of

      i. Collagen fibrils
        1. An extensive network confers tensile strength
     ii. Proteoglycans
        1. An interlocking mesh provides compressive stiffness through the ability to absorb and extrude water

2. Chondrocytes
   a. The sole cellular component of adult hyaline cartilage
   b. Comprise only 1–2% of the total cartilage volume
   c. Together with the surrounding dense extracellular matrix (ECM) form a functional unit termed the chondron
   d. Synthesize ECM macromolecules such as
      i. Fibrils of triple-helix Type II collagen
      ii. Aggrecan
      iii. Small proteoglycans
      iv. Matrix proteins both cartilage and non-cartilage specific
   e. Synthesize various enzymes, enzyme inhibitors, growth factors, and cytokines in response to biochemical, structural, and physical stimuli
   f. Have a limited capacity to replace lost collagen in mature cartilage
      i. May replace damaged or aging articular cartilage with type I collagen containing fibrotic tissue
   g. Receive nutrition through synovial fluid
      i. Nutrients are derived through diffusion, which is facilitated during joint loading
      ii. Chondrocytes are compromised when nutrient supply is minimal, in terms of the critical need for glucose (glycolysis for respiration), oxygen, or clearance of toxic waste
         1. Inflammatory tissue is low in glucose

3. Articular cartilage
   a. Composed of greater than 70% water
   b. The **dry** weight components are
      i. Type II collagen
         1. Makes up 50–60% of the **dry** weight of cartilage and 15–25% of the wet weight
         2. Forms a fiber network that provides shape and form to the cartilage tissue
      ii. Proteoglycan monomers (aggrecan)
         1. Makes up about 25% of the **dry** weight
         2. Large molecules (MW of 2 to 3 million) containing mostly keratan sulfate and chondroitin sulfate glycosaminoglycans (GAGs)
         3. Associated with large quantities of water bound to the hydrophilic GAG chains
         4. Contain a fixed negative charge to re-absorb water and small solutes into the matrix by osmosis, once compression is released
      iii. Minor collagens and small proteoglycans

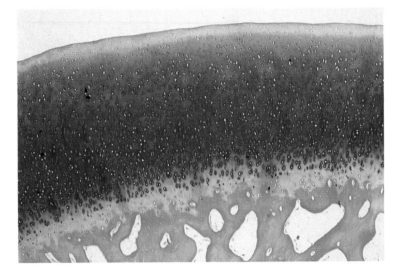

Fig. 1.1 Normal articular cartilage (Reproduced with permission from Osteoarthritis and crystal associated synovitis. *Atlas of Rheumatology*. ImagesMD; 2002-03-07)

   c. Avascular and aneural
      i. Patients with osteoarthritis (OA) have pain due to irritation of the subchondral bone, which is exposed as the cartilage degenerates
   d. Nourished by diffusion from the vasculature of the subchondral bone and, to a lesser degree from the synovial fluid
 4. Hyaline articular cartilage has four distinct regions
   a. Superficial tangential (gliding) zone (lamina splendens) (10% of the cartilage weight)
      i. Collagen fibers are thin and oriented horizontally to subchondral bone
      ii. A high concentration of the small proteoglycan decorin and a low concentration of aggrecan (low GAG content)
      iii. Chondrocytes are flattened
      iv. Collagen represents most of the dry weight of the superficial zone
   b. Middle (transitional) zone (40–60% of the cartilage weight)
      i. Largest zone
      ii. Collagen fibers are thicker and arranged in a radial bundle
      iii. High proteoglycan and water content
      iv. Rounded chondrocytes
   c. Deep (radial) zone
      i. Collagen bundles are the thickest and arranged in a radial fashion perpendicular to subchondral bone
      ii. The proportion of proteoglycan increases to 50% of the dry weight in the deep zone
      iii. Chondrocytes grouped in clusters and appear hypertrophic

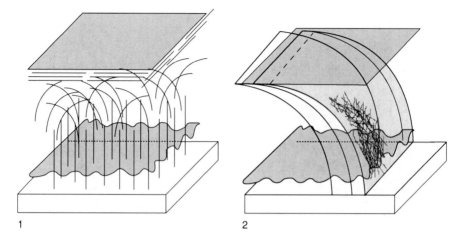

1   2

Fig. 1.2 Articular cartilage organized as a layered structure with four distinct regions (Reproduced with permission from Ultrastructural MR imaging techniques of the knee articular cartilage: problems for routine clinical application. *European Radiology.* DOI: 10.1007/s00330-003-2142-y. Springer; 2004-02-01)

    d. Calcified zone
       i. Separates cartilage from subchondral bone and provides an important mechanical buffer
      ii. Collagen fibers penetrate into this zone and anchor cartilage to the bone
5. Cell density progressively **decreases** from the superficial to the deep zone
   a. The deep zone is one-half to one-third of the density of the superficial zone
6. The concentration of collagen relative to proteoglycan progressively **decreases** from the superficial to the deep zone
7. The **wet** weight of cartilage is composed of the following
   a. Water content is 75–80% in the superficial zone and progressively **decreases** to 65–70% with zone depth
   b. Collagen accounts for 15–25%
   c. Proteoglycans, primarily aggrecan, account for up to 10%
8. Type II collagen
   a. Fibrils are composed of 300-nm tropocollagen molecules of three identical alpha chains, $[\alpha 1(II)]_3$, arranged in a triple helix and assembled in a quarter-stagger array
   b. A product of alternative splicing
      i. Lacks the 69 amino acid, cysteine-rich domain of the amino-terminal propeptide encoded by exon 2 in the type II collagen gene (COL2A1)
   c. Procollagen precursors
      i. Contains nonhelical amino- and carboxyl-terminal propeptides required for correct fibril assembly
     ii. Removed by specific proteinases

      iii. Speculated to play an inhibitory feedback role in collagen biosynthesis

      iv. Chondrocalcin is a carboxyl propeptide

         1. Remains transiently within the cartilage matrix after cleavage

         2. Proposed to play a role in mineralization as a calcium-binding protein

9. Minor collagen components of cartilage

  a. Type III

    i. Increased in OA cartilage

  b. Type VI

    i. Present as microfibrils in very small quantities localized around the chondrocytes

    ii. May play a role in cell attachment

    iii. Increased in OA cartilage

  c. Type IX

    i. Both a proteoglycan and a collagen

    ii. Contains a chondroitin-sulfate chain attachment site in one of the non-collagen domains

    iii. The helical domain forms covalent cross-links with type II collagen telopeptides and "decorates" the surface of the type II collagen fibril

    iv. Functions as a structural intermediate between type II collagen and proteoglycan aggregates

    v. Enhances the mechanical stability of the fibril network and resist swelling pressure of the entrapped proteoglycans

    vi. Regulates fibril size

       1. Destruction of this collagen may accelerate cartilage degradation

  d. Type X

    i. Not present in normal adult cartilage

    ii. Expressed in hypertrophic chondrocytes during calcification of the growth plate

  e. Type XI

    i. The $\alpha 3$ chain has the same primary sequence as the $\alpha 1(II)$ chain

    ii. A heterotrimeric molecule that is probably located in the same fibril as Type II

  f. Type XII and XIV

    i. Nonfibrillar collagens

    ii. Structurally related to type IX

    iii. Type XII associates with collagen fibrils in perichondrium and articular surface

    iv. Type XIV associates with collagen fibrils throughout

10. Proteoglycans

  a. Arranged into supramoleular aggregates

  b. Consist of a central hyaluronic acid (HA) filament to which multiple proteoglycan monomers are noncovalently attached

    i. May contain as many as 100 aggrecan monomers

  c. Stabilized by a small glycoprotein, link protein, an accessory protein

  d. Has the appearance of a large "bottle brush"

11. Aggrecan core protein
    a. 225–250 kDa encoded by 19 exons
    b. Covalently linked side chains of glycosaminoglycans (GAGS) which consti-
       tute 90% of the total mass
       i. GAGS include
          1. Approximately 100 chondroitin sulfate (CS) chains
          2. 30 keratan sulfate (KS) chains
          3. Shorter N- and O-linked oligosaccharides
    c. Separated into five functional units
       i. Three globular (G1, G2, and G3)
          1. G1 and G2 N-terminal (amino acid) and G3 C-terminal (carboxy)
             domains
             a. Have distinct structural properties
             b. Are cleavage products that accumulate with age or OA
          2. G1 domain
             a. Noncovalently linked by link protein to HA backbone
             b. A molecular mass of 38 kDa
             c. Composed of three subdomains that are encoded by exons 3, 4,
                and 5
             d. Together with link protein shares sequence homology with the
                immunoglobulin superfamily and a PTR double loop
                i. May function in cell adhesion and immune recognition
                ii. The PTR double loop interacts reversibly with five consecu-
                    tive HA disaccharide repeat units
          3. G2 domain
             a. Two proteoglycan tandem repeats and a PTR motif
             b. Does not bind to HA
             c. Separated from G1 by a linear interglobular domain
             d. No known function
          4. G3 domain
             a. Encoded by exons 13–18
             b. Contains three structural motifs
                i. An epidermal growth factor (EGF)-like domain
                ii. A lectin-like domain
                    1. Lecticans (versican, neurocan, and brevican) are HA bind-
                       ing proteoglycans that also contain a G3 domain
                iii. A complement regulatory protein (CRP)-like domain
             c. Participates in
                i. Growth regulation
                ii. Cell recognition
                iii. Intracellular trafficking
                iv. Extracellular matrix recognition, assembly, and stabilization
             d. One third of the aggrecan molecules in adult cartilage lack the G3
                domain
       ii. Two extended interglobular (E1 and E2)

1. E2 domain
   a. GAGs within are clustered primarily into two regions
      i. The chondroitin sulfate rich region
         1. Largest (260 nm)
            a. Over 100 chains and about 15–25 KS chains
         2. Located in the distal portion of E2
         3. Encoded by a single exon 12

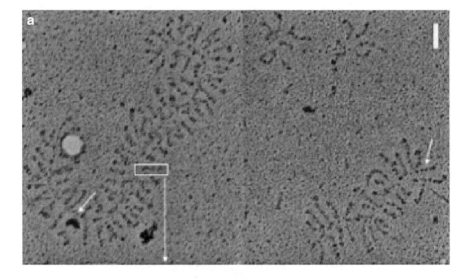

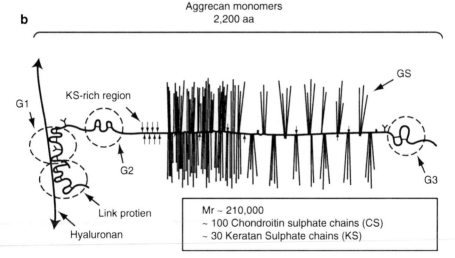

Fig. 1.3 The structure of aggrecan aggregate. (**a**) Aggrecan monomers (square) are attached on a hyaluronan backbone (arrow). (**b**) In the aggrecan monomer, three globular domains (G1, G2 and B3) are separated by two extended segments, which carry the glycosaminoglycans chrondroitin sulphage and keratan sulphate. (Reproduced with permission from Histology-ultrastructure-biology. *The Meniscus*. DOI: 10.1007/978-3-642-02450-4_3. Springer; 2010-01-01)

       ii. The KS rich region
          1. Located in the proximal portion of the E2 domain near the G2 domain
          2. Encoded by exon 11 and a small portion of the 5′ end of exon 12

12. Other large proteoglycans found in cartilage
   a. Versican
      i. Forms aggregates with HA
      ii. Core protein similar to aggrecan
         1. Except only two globular domains (analogous to G1 and G3) with one at each terminal
      iii. Low levels throughout life
      iv. Calcium-binding and selectin-like properties
         1. May have a space-filling role
      v. Derivatives may include
         1. Central nervous system (CNS) PTR proteoglycan
         2. Glial hyaluronan-binding protein
         3. Hyaluronectin
      vi. Common to most soft connective tissues, dermis, and mesentery
   b. Perlican
      i. Nonaggregating
      ii. Role in cell-adhesion

13. Small leucine-rich proteoglycan (SLRP) family
   a. Contains 10 or 11 hydrophobic leucine-rich repeat (LRR) sequences of 23 or 24 amino acids each flanked by cysteine residues
   b. Divided into several sub-families based on
      i. Gene organization
      ii. The number of leucine-rich repeats
      iii. The type of GAG chain substituent
   c. Nonaggregating subfamilies important in cartilage matrix include
      i. Biglycan
         1. GAG chains, CS, DS (dermatan sulfate), or both- attached near the N-terminus through two closely spaced serine-glycine dipeptides
         2. Binds transforming growth factor beta (TGF-β) and thereby may modulate growth, remodeling, and repair
         3. Displays affinity for Type IV collagen
         4. In mice knockout studies is a positive regulator of bone formation and bone mass
      ii. Decorin
         1. Only one CS or DS chain
         2. May also bind TGF-β
         3. Binds type II collagen fibers together
      iii. Fibromodulin
         1. Contains up to 4 KS chains linked to the central domain of the core protein and to several sulfated tyrosine residues in the N-terminus

      2. Stabilizes the collagen network with its negatively charged GAG side chains and the highly anionic tyrosine-sulfation sites with multiple-site linkage between collagen fibrils

      3. May help bind type II collagen to type IX

      4. Highly homologous with decorin

   iv. Lumican

      1. Similar to fibromodulin

   v. Proline arginine

      1. Rich end leucine-rich repeat protein (PRELP)

      2. N-terminal binding domain for heparin and heparin sulfate (HS)

      3. Mediates cell binding through HS in syndecan

   vi. Chondroadherin

      1. LRR core protein without N-terminal extension

      2. Binds to cells via $\alpha 2 \beta 1$ integrin

14. Noncollagenous matrix proteins important in cartilage matrix integrity include

  a. COMP (cartilage oligomeric matrix protein)

   i. A member of the thrombospondin family

   ii. Constitutes 10% of the noncollagenous, nonproteoglycan proteins in cartilage

   iii. A disulfide-bonded pentameric 550-kDa calcium-binding protein

   iv. Locations

      1. The interterritorial matrix of adult articular cartilage

      2. Pericellular in the proliferating region of the growth plate

         a. May have a role in cell–matrix interactions

   v. A possible marker of cartilage damage in arthritis

      1. Released in reactive arthritis

      2. High serum levels in early rheumatoid arthritis (RA) can distinguish an aggressive, destructive form of the disease

      3. May not be specific for cartilage because synovial cells also secrete COMP

  b. Cartilage matrix protein (matrilin 1 and 3)

   i. Expressed in cartilage at certain stages of development

      1. Tightly bound to aggrecan in immature cartilage

   ii. Located in tracheal cartilage

      1. Not found in adult articular cartilage or intervertebral disc

   iii. Three subunits with von Willebrand factor (vWF) and EGF domains

  c. CLIP (cartilage intermediate layer protein)

   i. Expressed in the middle to deep zones of articular cartilage as a precursor protein

      1. When cleaved at secretion forms the nucleotide pyrophosphohydrolase

   ii. Increased in early and late OA

  d. Glycoprotein 39 (gp39 or YKL-40)

   i. Found only in the superficial zone of normal cartilage

   ii. Synthesis or release often increased in cartilage that is undergoing repair or remodeling

      iii. Investigated as a marker of cartilage damage in arthritis

      iv. Chitinase homology

   e. Fibronectin

      i. Mediates cell–matrix interactions in cartilage by binding to cell-surface integrins and other membrane proteins

      ii. Alternate splicing of mRNA gives rise to different protein products at different stages of chondrocyte differentiation

      iii. Increased in OA cartilage

         1. May serve special functions in remodeling and repair

   f. Tenascin-c

      i. Similar to fibronectin

      ii. Six subunits form hexabrachion structure

      iii. Associated with chondrogenesis

      iv. Binds syndecan 3

15. Cell surface and integral membrane proteoglycans include

   a. CD44

      i. A lymphocyte homing receptor that binds HA, collagen, and fibronectin

      ii. Serves to anchor a substantial portion of aggrecan molecule within the pericellular matrix of chondrocytes

      iii. Participates in the receptor mediated catabolism of HA

      iv. Included in the PTR family, even though only half of the motif is present

      v. Extracellular HS/CS side chains with variable substitutions

   b. Syndecan 3

      i. Links to the cell surface via glycosyl phosphatidylinositol

      ii. Binds through the N-terminal heparan sulfate (HS) side chains on the extracellular domain to

         1. Tenascin-c during cartilage development

         2. Growth factors

         3. Proteases

         4. Inhibitors

         5. Other matrix molecules

      iii. Cytoplasmic tyrosine residues

   c. Anchorin CII (annexin V)

      i. 34 kDa integral membrane protein that binds Type II collagen

      ii. Shares extensive homology with the calcium binding proteins calpactin and lipocortin

   d. Integrins (α1, 2, 3, 5, 6, 10 and β1, 3, and 5)

      i. Two noncovalently linked transmembrane glycoproteins (α and β subunits)

      ii. Cell matrix interactions and intracellular signaling

16. Matrix turnover in articular cartilage

   a. Proteoglycans have a faster turnover rate (t1/2 of weeks) compared with collagen (t1/2 of months)

      i. The turnover rate for collagen is very slow, except in pericellular sites where there is evidence for ongoing type II collagen cleavage

      ii. The small, sulfated GAG components of proteoglycans are susceptible to enzymatic degradation and are resynthesized continuously

  b. Age related changes in articular cartilage include

      i. Increased damage to type II collagen

      ii. Major changes in the structure and content of the proteoglycan aggregate components

        1. Decreased size of aggregates

        2. Total content of sulfated GAGs does not change significantly

          a. Increased KS associated with decreased CS

        3. Increased amounts of free binding region

          a. G1 or G1 and G2 together with the KS-rich region

          b. Proteolytically cleaved link protein

        4. Increased content of HA of shorter chain length

17. Cartilage degradation

  a. Involves an imbalance between matrix metalloproteinases (MMPs) and their natural inhibitors (TIMP-1, 2, and 3)

  b. Collagenases

      i. MMP-1

      ii. MMP-8

        1. Can also degrade aggrecan

      iii. MMP-13

        1. Degrades Type II collagen more effectively than MMP-1

      iv. MMP-14 (membrane type I (MT1) MMP)

        1. Can also degrade aggrecan

  c. Aggrecan degradation

      i. An "aggrecanase" cleavage site in chondrocyte-mediated catabolism

      ii. Stromelysins

        1. MMP-3

        2. MMP-10

      iii. Proteinases

        1. ADAM-TS (a disintegrin and metalloprotease with thrombospondin motifs)

          a. ADAM-TS 4 and 11

            i. Aggrecanase 1 and 2

18. Matrix degradation

  a. Proteinases produced by chondrocytes that degrade matrix or participate in the proteinase activation cascade include

      i. Gelatinases

        1. MMP-2

        2. MMP-9

       ii. Cathepsins B, L, and D

      iii. Plasminogen activators

19. Cytokines and chondrocyte metabolism

  a. Degradation unregulated by interleukin-1 (IL-1) and tumor necrosis factor alpha (TNF-α)

  b. An anabolic effect with TGF-β and IGF-1

20. Measurements of proteoglycan and collagen degradation
    a. Monoclonal antibodies
        i. Recognize degradation (catabolic epitopes) or newly synthesized matrix components (anabolic neo-epitopes)
            1. Epitopes on denatured type II collagen at the collagenase cleavage site, the N-terminus of the three quarter fragment, are promising diagnostic reagents
        ii. Distinguish subtle biochemical differences in CS or KS chains
            1. In OA and RA the synovial fluid-to-serum ratio can be useful as a diagnostic indicator
        iii. Recognize specific aggrecanase or metalloproteinase cleavage sites in the aggrecan core protein
    b. Serum and synovial fluid levels of the carboxyl-terminal propeptide, CPII, or chondrocalcin can monitor the synthesis of type II collagen
    c. Urinary excretion of hydroxylysyl pyridinoline cross-links may indicate collagen degradation

Section C: Bone

1. Bone is a composite tissue consisting of mineral, matrix, cells, and water
    a. Mineral
        i. 62% of the weight
        ii. Hydroxyapatite $[Ca_5(PO_4)_3(OH)]$
            1. An analog of the naturally occurring crystalline calcium phosphate
                a. Fewer hydroxy groups
            2. Crystals
                a. Very small size
                b. Easy to dissolve
                c. Ideally suited for mineral ion homeostasis
            3. Imperfect compared to geologic apatites with many impurities such as
                a. Carbonate
                b. Fluoride
                c. Acid phosphate
                d. Magnesium
                e. Citrate
            4. Serves as a source of calcium (99% of total body), magnesium (80–85%), and phosphate (66%) ions
    b. Matrix
        i. Type I collagen predominantly (31% weight)
            1. Cross-links formed after fibrils are assembled in the ECM are specific for degradation
                a. Analyses of serum or urine cross-links are useful markers for diseases such as osteoporosis
        ii. Noncollagenous proteins (5% weight) composed of

      1. Osteocalcin (23%)
      2. BSP (21%)
      3. Osteopontin (12%)
      4. Decorin (10%)
      5. Osteonectin (9%)
      6. Biglycan (9%)
      7. Thrombospondin (8%)
      8. Other (7%)
c. Bone cells
   i. Osteoblasts
      1. Derived from mesenchymal cell lineage
      2. Synthesize matrix
   ii. Osteocytes
      1. Derived from mesenchymal cell lineage
      2. Enmeshed in bone matrix
      3. Convey nutrition throughout bone
      4. Sense mechanical signals
   iii. Osteoclasts
      1. Multinucleated giant cells of macrophage origin
      2. Remove bone
         a. Attach to the bone surface and seal off a microenvironment
         b. Release acid and degradative enzymes such as
            i. Acid phosphatase
            ii. Collagenase
            iii. Cathepsins
            iv. Specialized proteinases
   iv. Osteoprotegerin ligand (OPGL) (RANKL)
      1. A principal coupling factor between osteoblasts and osteoclasts
      2. A cell membrane-bound ligand on osteoblasts and activated T-cells
      3. Originally identified as a T-cell activator, RANKL (Receptor Activator for Nuclear Factor κ B Ligand)
         a. Also known as TNF-related activation-induced cytokine (TRANCE)
         b. A member of the TNF superfamily
      4. Binds to a receptor RANK on macrophages or immature osteoclasts
         a. Stimulates their maturation and activation
      5. Competitively bound by osteoprotegrin (OPG)
         a. A soluble secreted molecule that prevents binding to RANK
         b. Inhibits osteoclastogenesis
         c. May be useful as a therapy for osteoporosis
      6. Expression on osteoblasts is stimulated through
         a. Vitamin D receptor (1,25 OH vitamin D3)
         b. Protein kinase A (PGE2)
         c. Parathyroid hormone
         d. gp130 (IL-11)

      7. Upregulation on osteoblasts and T cells can lead to osteoclast activation and periarticular osteoporosis in inflammatory arthritis

         a. Influenced by local production of PGE2 and interleukins (TNF-alpha, IL-1)

    v. Three major hormone groups regulate the activities of bone cells

      1. Parathyroid hormone (PTH) and 1,25-dihydroxy-vitamin D

         a. Responsible for increasing Ca +2 levels through resorption and retention

         b. Stimulate osteoclasts to remodel bone via effects on osteoblastic synthesis of OPGL (RANKL)

      2. Calcitonin

         a. A PTH antagonist that suppresses osteoclast activity

      3. Estrogen and other sex steroids (corticosteroids)

         a. Directly affect osteoblast

2. Bone formation occurs through two distinct processes

    a. Endochondral ossification

      i. Bone replaces a cartilage model

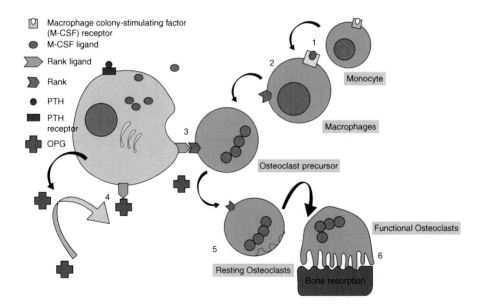

Fig. 1.4 Regulation of osteoclast differentiation *1*. Monocytes derived from vessels in the bone marrow express M-CSF receptor on their cell surface. *2*. M-CSF binds to M-CSF receptor and induces the expression of RANK. *3*. RANK ligand (RANKL) is produced by stromal cells/osteoblasts and binds to the receptor, RANK, on mononuclear osteoclast progenitors. *4*. OPG, a decoy receptor that binds to RANKL and inhibits osteoclast differentiation. *5*. Multiple factors including hormones and locally produced cytokines/growth factors and matrix proteins, mediate the activation (bone resorption) of osteoclasts (Reproduced with permission from Bone structure, development and bone biology. *Bone Pathology.* DOI: 10.1007/978-1-59745-347-9_1. Springer; 2009-01-01)

      ii. Seen in long bone formation and fracture healing

     iii. Begins when mesenchymal cells differentiate into chondrocytes

     iv. Process modulated by

       1. Indian hedgehog

       2. PTH-related peptide

       3. Bone morphogenic proteins (BMPs)

      v. Maturing chondrocytes hypertrophy and switch from Type II and IX collagen production to form type X collagen at the interface of cartilage and bone

       1. Type X collagen has a role in stabilizing the endochondral structure

         a. Defects in its production have been found in families with spondyloepiphyseal dysplasias

     vi. Proteoglycans' role in calcification and ossification

       1. Aggrecan associates with HA to form high-molecular weight space-filling aggregates that expand up to 50 times their volume

       2. Large proteoglycans (aggrecan and its aggregates and versican) keep the matrix hydrated and prevent unwanted calcification

         a. Effective inhibitors of mineral crystal growth and formation

           i. In severe OA calcification occurs around chondrocytes where proteoglycans have been degraded

       3. Smaller proteoglycans regulate collagen fibril formation

         a. Decorin and biglycan trim the surface of collagen fibrils

         b. Also bind growth factors (such as TGF-β) allowing them to persist in the matrix

     vii. Initial calcification in cartilage occurs in association with matrix vesicles

       1. Vesicles are enriched in enzymes that facilitate transport of calcium and phosphate ions and promote degradation of the matrix

       2. Mineral crystals break through the vesicles and fuse with collagen based mineral

    viii. Bone replaces calcified cartilage following vascular invasion

     ix. Remodeling

       1. Occurs according to Wolff's law

         a. A dynamic state that provides maximum strength with minimum mass

       2. Linked with interplay between osteoblast and osteoclasts

  b. Intramembranous ossification

      i. Bone forms directly

     ii. Seen in bones of the skull

3. Bone Mineralization

  a. For mineral crystals to form, their ion product within the crystal must exceed the solubility of the crystal (supersaturation)

      i. Alkaline phosphatase is an enzyme found on the outer membrane of osteoblasts and chondrocytes

       1. It can hydrolyze phosphate esters

      2. A deficiency of this enzyme can lead to hypophosphatasia and improper mineral deposition
- b. The smallest stable version of the crystal is called the nucleus
- c. Physiologic nucleation can be influenced in several ways
  - i. The synthesis or exposure of macromolecules that resemble the nucleus
    - 1. A phosphoprotein may resemble the phosphate-rich surface of the apatite crystal and bind Ca+
  - ii. Noncollagenous proteins provide nucleation sites
  - iii. Proteins that act as apatite nucleators at low concentrations can also inhibit crystal growth at high concentrations
  - iv. Collagen is not an effective nucleator
- d. Bone disorders linked to specific matrix proteins
  - i. Osteogenesis imperfecta
    - 1. Defects in Type I collagen
      - a. See impaired collagen fibrils and smaller abnormal mineral crystals
  - ii. Turner's syndrome
    - 1. Abnormal expression of biglycan
      - a. Excessive biglycan leads to Klinefelter's syndrome
  - iii. Osteopetrosis
    - 1. Multiple defects in expression and production of
      - a. Osteocalcin
      - b. Osteoprotegerin
      - c. Certain cytokines
        - i. Macrophage colony stimulating factor (M-CSF)
        - ii. Granulocyte colony-stimulating factor (CSF)
        - iii. IL-6
        - iv. TNF-alpha
  - iv. Odontogenesis imperfecta
    - 1. Abnormal dentin matrix protein I and dentin sialoprotein
  - v. Delayed osteogenesis
    - 1. Abnormal fetuin
      - a. α2-HS-glycoprotein

Section D: Synovium and Synovial Fluid

1. Synovium originates from the skeletal blastema
   - a. Synovium and bone marrow develop from a common perichondrial envelope
   - b. Within an embryonic skeletal blastemal element, precartilaginous foci form a perichondrium
   - c. Invasion of cartilage forms bone marrow stroma with maturation to periosteum
   - d. An interzone detaches from cartilage to form synovium
2. Synovium is a plane of cleavage rather than a cavity
   - a. The fluid-filled gap within normal synovial structures rarely is more than 50 μm thick

    b. If removed, this disconnective surface is replaced by adherent connection tissue, resulting in loss of motion

3. Synovial functions include

    a. The control of synovial fluid (SF) volume and composition

        i. The synovial surface has an absence of interstitial pores >1 μm in diameter that allows for fluid retention

    b. The provision of nutrition to chondrocytes

4. Synovium includes multiple layers held in place by atmospheric pressure without a limiting basement membrane

    a. Subintima

        i. Confers mobility and packing properties

        ii. Forms 95% of what can be felt clinically

        iii. Composed of different areas

            1. A superficial membrane that moves freely over deep structures

            2. Areolar areas may stretch, crimp, roll, or slide

            3. Fatty areas may provide elastically deformable packing

            4. Areas with folds or finger-like villi

            5. Fibrous, often avascular, areas form with villi; more common with aging

        iv. Stromal cells are seen with similar potential as intimal fibroblasts

        v. A capillary network lies within the subintima

            1. Derived from a plexus of arterioles and venules, together with lymphatics and associated nerve fibers

    b. Intima

        i. Contains synovial fluid

        ii. Contains two types of specialized cells surrounded by matrix rich in microfibrils consisting of fibrillins 1 and 2 and collagen VI

            1. (Type A) Intimal macrophages

                a. Monocyte derived with a primary phagocytic function

                b. A high content of cytoplasmic organelles, including lysosomes, smooth walled vacuoles, and micropinocytotic vesicles

                c. Express typical macrophage markers

                    i. CD14, CD68, CD163

                    ii. IgG Fc receptor FcγRIIIa (CD16a)

                        1. This receptor combined with complement decay-accelerating factor (DAF) may act as an "early warning system" for response to pathogens

                        2. Activation leads to the production of TNF and IL-1, important in the pathogenesis of RA

                        3. Expression is controlled by mechanical stress and seen in exposed sites where RA nodules occur

            2. (Type B) Intimal fibroblast

                a. Produces hyaluronate

                    i. Accounts for the increased viscosity of SF

                    ii. Uridine diphosphoglucose dehydrogenase (UDPGD) is the enzyme involved in hyaluronan synthesis

Fig. 1.5 Phase contrast microscopy of cultured synovial cells. (a) Typical fibroblast cultures with predominately bipolar morphology (b) Morphologically-distinct phenotypes such as type A cells with bipolar structure and type B cells with multiple cytoplasmic extensions are present. Vesicles surround the cell membrane (V) (Reproduced with permission from Macrophage-like synoviocytes display phenotypic polymorphisms in a serum-free tissue culture medium. *Rheumatology International*. DOI: 10.1007/ s00296-004-0545-y. Springer; 2006-01-01)

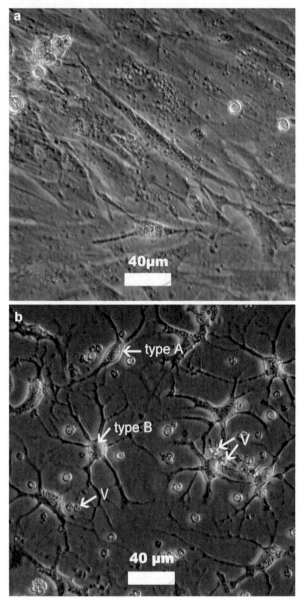

b. Expresses vascular cell adhesion molecule 1 (VCAM-1) and DAF
   i. VCAM-1 prevents mononuclear leukocytes from migrating into SF
   ii. Granulocytes that carry the coligand for VCAM-1, known as α4β1 and lymphocytes without VCAM-1 are allowed to pass
iii. Other cells in the synovium include
   1. Synovial stroma cells
      a. Express VCAM-1

         b. Capable of forming lymphoid follicles with the appearance of RA synovium

         c. Fewer organelles and a more extensive endoplasmic reticulum

     2. Antigen processing cells with a dendritic configuration and mast cells

     3. In normal tissue the majority are fibroblasts and the minority are macrophages

5. Synovial fluid

     a. The water in synovial fluid is a dialysate of plasma

     b. Synovial-fluid volume is determined by the amount of hyaluronan present

         i. The intimal network of collagen VI microfibrillar mesh obstructs the passage of hyaluronan but is leaky to water, crystalloids, and proteins

     c. Hyaluronan has two roles in the maintenance of synovial fluid volume

         i. Prevents formation of a high vacuum in the joint and allows synovium to slide, stretch, and crimp without becoming torn

         ii. Maintains a fluid film between cartilage surfaces under load

            1. Allows fluid-based (hydrodynamic) lubrication to occur

6. The physical characteristics of normal synovial fluid

     a. Colorless and transparent

     b. A thin film covering surfaces of synovium and cartilage

     c. Cell counts <200/mm^3 with <25% neutrophils

     d. Protein concentration between 1.3 and 1.7 g/dL

         i. 20% of normal plasma protein

     e. Glucose within 20 mg/dL of the serum glucose level after 6 h of fasting

     f. Temperature at 32°C

         i. Peripheral joints are cooler than core body temperature

     g. String sign of 1–2 in.

         i. A measure of viscosity

     h. pH of 7.4

Section E: Skeletal Muscle

1. There are 640 muscles in the human which constitute up to 40% of adult body mass

2. Skeletal muscle cells are called fibers

     a. Fibers are grouped into fascicles

     b. The endomysium is between fibers

     c. The perimysium covers fascicles

3. Muscle fibers are grouped into motor units

     a. Consist of a lower motor neuron originating in the spinal cord anterior horn cell and the muscle fiber that it innervates

     b. All muscle fibers within a motor unit are of the same type

4. Different fibers within a single fascicle are innervated by different motor neurons

5. Muscle fibers are divided among three types
   a. Type 1 (slow twitch, oxidative fibers)
      i. Respond to electrical stimuli slowly
      ii. Fatigue resistant with repeated stimulation
      iii. Many mitochondria and higher lipid content
      iv. Endurance training (long-distance running) enhances their metabolism
   b. Type 2a (fast twitch, oxidative-glycolytic fibers)
      i. Properties intermediate between type 1 and type 2b
   c. Type 2b (fast twitch, glycolytic fibers)
      i. White fibers
      ii. Respond rapidly and with greater force of contraction but fatigue rapidly
      iii. Contain more glycogen and have higher myophosphorylase and myoad-
      enylate deaminase activity
      iv. Strength training (weight-lifting, sprinters, jumpers) leads to their hyper-
      trophy
      v. Referred to as "default fibers"
         1. More prominent during periods of deconditioning and contract
         inefficiently
   d. Muscle contains 40% type 1 and 60% type 2 fibers on average
6. Determinants of fiber type distribution
   a. Reinnervation with a different type of motor neuron
   b. Physical training
   c. Disease processes
   d. Heredity
      i. Most important
7. Sarcolemma
   a. A plasma membrane which surrounds each muscle fiber
8. Myofilaments
   a. Contractile proteins
      i. Actin
      ii. Troponin
      iii. Tropomyosin
      iv. Myosin
   b. Bathed in cytosol called sarcoplasm
   c. Organized within fibrils
      i. Fibrils are enveloped by the sarcoplasmic reticulum
9. Communication between the sarcolemma and sarcoplasmic reticulum is through
   the T-tubule system
10. Muscle band organization
   a. Dark band
      i. Composed of thick myosin
   b. Light band (I band)
      i. Occupied by thin filaments
         1. Actin, troponin, and tropomyosin
         2. Not overlapped by myosin

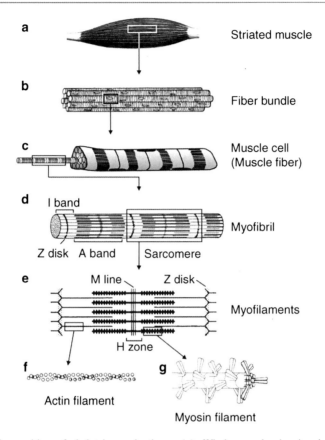

a Striated muscle

b Fiber bundle

c Muscle cell (Muscle fiber)

d I band · Myofibril

Z disk · A band · Sarcomere

e M line · Z disk · Myofilaments

H zone

f Actin filament

g Myosin filament

Fig. 1.6 Composition of skeletal muscle tissue. (**a**). Whole muscle showing longitudinally arranged muscle fiber bundles. (**b**) Muscle fiber bundle containing several muscle fibers (muscle cells). (**c**). Single muscle cell showing the typical striations and three nuclei close to the cell membrane. The box marks two sarcomeres that are shown in (**d**). at a higher magnification. Sarcomeres are the smallest functional units of a striated muscle; they extend from one Z line (or Z disk) to the next. (**e**). Components of a Sarcomere. Thick myosin molecules with spiny heads lie in the center. They interdigitate with thin actin molecules that are fixed to the Z disk. The isotropic (I) band on both sides of the Z line contains actin filaments, only (see **d**). The anisotropic (A) band contains both actin and myosin filaments with the exception of its middle portion (the lighter H zone) which is free from actin. The M-line (M-band) consists of proteins that are important for the stability of the sarcomere structure; they crosslink the myosin filaments. During contraction, the actin and myosin filaments slide against each other; thus, the I band and H zone become narrower whereas the A band maintains a constant width. (**f, g**) An actin filament consists of two chains of globular proteins, whereas the myosin filament is a bundle of many threadlike proteins from which the myosin heads protrude (Reproduced with permission from Functional anatomy of muscle: muscle, nociceptors and afferent fibers. *Muscle Pain: Understanding the Mechanisms.* DOI: 10.1007/978-3-540-85021-2_2. Springer; 2010-01-01)

    c. Z lines
       i. Middle of light band
      ii. Connect actin filament
    d. M line
       i. Middle of dark band
      ii. Middle of myosin filaments
    e. With contraction z lines move toward M line and I band becomes smaller
    f. Six actin filaments in a hexagonal pattern surround each myosin filament
11. Sarcomere
    a. The functional unit of the fiber
    b. Defined as the area between two Z lines
12. Energy for muscle function is generated in the mitochondria
    a. Located in the I bands on either side of the Z line
       i. Mitochondria contain their own DNA (mtDNA)
          1. mtDNA
             a. Circular
             b. Maternally derived
             c. Lacks a mechanism for repair
13. Muscle fibril contractions
    a. Action potentials transmitted along the sarcolemma, through the T-tubule to the sarcoplasmic reticulum, cause release of calcium into the sarcoplasm
    b. As calcium concentrations increase within the sarcoplasm, actin is released from an inhibited state, permitting actin–myosin cross-linking
    c. The muscle shortens until calcium is actively pumped back into the sarcoplasmic reticulum, which breaks the cross-links
14. Three ATPase proteins contribute to fiber contraction and relaxation
    a. Sodium potassium ATPase
       i. Maintains normal polarity of the sarcolemma
    b. A magnesium-dependent ATPase
       i. Controls actin–myosin cross-linking
    c. A calcium dependent ATPase
       i. Pumps calcium from the sarcoplasm into the sarcoplasmic reticulum permitting relaxation
15. Sources of ATP for muscle energy
    a. Free fatty acids
       i. Fasting intervals
      ii. At rest
     iii. Activities of low intensity and long duration
    b. Long chain fatty acids
       i. Combine with the carrier molecule carnitine to transfer across the mitochondrial membrane
          1. Process catalyzed by two enzymes found on the inner membrane
             a. Carnitine palmitoyltransferase (CPT) I
             b. CPT II
      ii. Once in the mitochondria, fatty acid and carnitine separate

      iii. Two carbon fragments of acetyl-CoA are split off by the process of beta-oxidation and metabolized by the tricarboxylic acid route and oxidative phosphorylation

         1. One molecule of palmitate results in the net gain of 131 molecules of ATP

  c. Glycogen

      i. Primarily when physical activity is intense or when anaerobic conditions exist

      ii. Mobilized to form glucose-6-phosphate by the process of glycogenolysis

         1. Initiated by myophosphorylase

         2. Glucose-6-phosphate is metabolized to lactate through the glycolytic pathway

            a. Under aerobic conditions, this pathway produces pyruvate which can enter the tricarboxylic acid cycle

            b. Aerobic metabolism of one molecule of glucose nets 38 molecules of ATP

            c. Anaerobic processing of one molecule of glucose results in only two molecules of ATP

16. Creatine phosphokinase (CK)

  a. Pivotal role in maintaining constant intracellular ATP concentrations

  b. Catalyzes the reversible transphosphorylation of creatine and adenine nucleotides

  c. At rest, the terminal phosphate of excess ATP is transferred to creatine, forming creatine phosphate and ADP

  d. During exercise, maintains ATP concentration at stable levels until creatine phosphate concentrations are depleted by 50%

      i. If activity continues and ATP concentrations continue to fall, then the purine nucleotide cycle begins

17. Purine nucleotide cycle

  a. The first step is conversion of AMP to inosine monophosphate (IMP) by myoadenylate deaminase activity with generation of ammonia

  b. Both IMP and ammonia stimulate glycolysis

      i. AMP is generated from IMP by a two-step process

         1. Fumarate is converted to malate

         2. Malate enters mitochondria and participates as an intermediate in the TCA cycle with efficient regeneration of ATP by oxidative phosphorylation

Section F: Vascular Endothelium

1. Endothelial dysfunction includes

  a. Enhanced permeability of the endothelium to plasma lipoproteins

  b. Oxidative modification of lipoproteins

    c. Increased adhesion of blood leukocytes

    d. Local functional imbalances between

        i. Pro- and anti-thrombotic factors

        ii. Growth stimulators and growth inhibitors

        iii. Vasoactive substances

2. Many factors alter endothelial gene expression during inflammation

    a. Altered hemodynamics

    b. Local cytokines or proteases

    c. Viral infection

    d. Free radicals

    e. Oxidized lipids

3. Dysfunctional endothelial cells produce

    a. Adhesive cofactors for platelets

        i. von Willebrand factor

        ii. Fibronectin

        iii. Thrombospondin

    b. Procoagulant components

        i. Factor V

    c. Plasminogen activator inhibitor-1

        i. Inhibitor of the fibrinolytic pathway

        ii. Reduces the rate of fibrin breakdown

4. Vasorelaxors include

    a. Nitric oxide

    b. Prostacyclin

5. Endothelial-derived vasoconstrictors include

    a. Angiotensin II

        i. Generated at the endothelial surface by angiotensin-converting enzyme

    b. Platelet-derived growth factor (PDGF)

        i. An agonist of smooth muscle contraction

        ii. Endothelial expression correlates with vascular dysfunction

        iii. The most effective natural inducer is α-thrombin, a protease component of the coagulation system

    c. Endothelin 1

6. The process of leukocyte attachment and diapedesis includes

    a. An initial rolling or tethering event (selectins)

    b. A signaling process (chemokines)

    c. A strong attachment step (the immunoglobulin family)

        i. Avid binding to the endothelial surface occurs in response to such activating agents as

            1. IL-1

            2. TNF alpha

            3. Lipopolysaccharide

            4. Oxidized lipids

    d. Transendothelial cell migration of the leukocyte

7. Vascular fibrosis occurs in a response to

    a. Insulin-like growth factor 1

    b. Basic fibroblast growth factor

    c. Transforming growth factor beta

8. Vascular endothelial growth factor (VEGF)

    a. Induces migration and proliferation of endothelium

    b. Increases the leakiness of new and pre-existing vessels

    c. Exacerbates the sequelae of inflammation

    d. A therapeutic target through its inhibition with

        i. Soluble receptors

        ii. Blocking antibodies

        iii. Gene therapy

Section G: Peripheral Nerves

1. Schwann cells

    a. Invest the length of each axon

    b. Gaps between these cells are called nodes of Ranvier

    c. Allow salutatory conduction of action potentials

2. Axons

    a. Large diameter

        i. 1–22 mm

        ii. Myelinated

        iii. Conduct nerve impulses rapidly

    b. Small diameter

        i. 0.2–2.4 mm

        ii. Unmyelinated

    c. Devoid of polyribosomes and rough ER

        i. Depend on the cell body for sustenance

3. Axonal transport

    a. Slow anterograde flow

        i. Transports proteins and microfilaments

    b. Axoplasmic flow of intermediate speed

        i. Transports mitochondria

    c. Fast axonal flow

        i. Transports substances contained within vesicles needed during neuro-transmission

    d. Retrograde flow

        i. Allows the periphery to provide feedback to the soma

        ii. Transports molecules and materials taken up by endocytosis

    e. Impaired axoplasmic flow

        i. Causes degeneration of distal axons

4. Epineurium

    a. A dense external fibrous coat which surrounds the nerve

    b. Disorders that lead to peripheral nerve damage, such as vasculitis, most frequently involve the epineurial arterioles

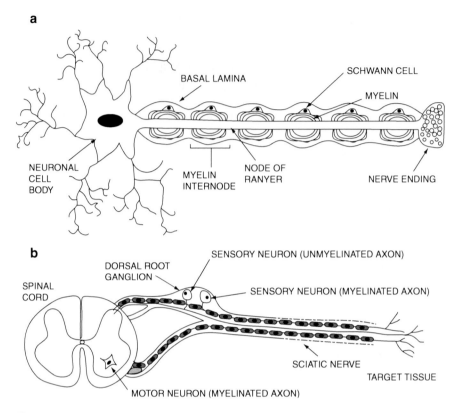

Fig. 1.7 (**a**) The neuron-Schwann cell functional unit of the peripheral nervous system. (**b**) Generalized diagram of the peripheral nervous system. The peripheral nervous system contains both myelinated and unmyelinated axons. Neuronal cell bodies from which PNS axons arise are located in either the dorsal root ganglia (sensory neurons) or in the ventral horn of the spinal cord (motor neurons). Sympathetic ganglia with their associated neurons, also part of the peripheral nervous system, are not shown (Reproduced with permission from Molecular probes for PNS neurotoxicity, degeneration, and regeneration. *Neurodegeneration Methods and Protocols.* DOI: 10.1385/0-89603-612-X: 67. Springer; 1999-01-01)

5. Perineurium
    a. Surrounds the neural fascicles
    b. A sleeve formed by layers of flattened epithelial-like cells
6. Endoneurium
    a. A thin layer of reticular fibers produced by Schwann cells
    b. Binds nerve fibers together
7. Motor nerves
    a. The axons of lower motor neurons
    b. Innervate extrafusal and intrafusal striated muscle fibers
    c. Spinal anterior horn cells
    d. Motor nerve cells of cranial nerves

8. Sensory nerves
   a. Axons of pseudo-unipolar sensory neurons
   b. Dorsal root or cranial nerve ganglia
9. Preganglionic sympathetic autonomic nerve cell bodies
   a. Reside in the intermediolateral gray columns of spinal cord segments T1–L2
   b. Fibers emerge with ventral roots and enter myelinated white rami
   c. Synapse with sympathetic ganglion cells
   d. Give rise to unmyelinated axons which emerge through gray rami
   e. Innervate such organs as smooth muscle and sweat glands
10. Preganglionic parasympathetic nerve bodies
    a. Located in the brainstem (cranial nerves III, VII, IX, and X) and in the S2–S4 segments of the spinal cord
    b. Cholinergic fibers include all the preganglionic autonomic fibers and post-ganglionic parasympathetic fibers
11. Sensory fibers are classified by their size and resultant conduction velocity
    a. 30–72 m/s
       i. A alpha
       ii. Myelinated
    b. 6–36 m/s
       i. A delta
       ii. Myelinated
    c. 0.5–2 m/s
       i. C fibers
       ii. Unmyelinated
12. Pain and temperature
    a. Transmitted by thinly myelinated (A delta) or small unmyelinated C fibers
13. Position and vibration
    a. Transmitted by large myelinated fibers
14. Touch
    a. Transmitted by medium-sized myelinated fibers
15. Neuronopathy
    a. The pathologic process resides in the cell body (neuron)
    b. The most well known motor neuronopathy is amyotropic lateral sclerosis (ALS)
16. Sensory neuronopathies
    a. Associated with pan-modality sensory losses (large- and small-fiber function)
    b. An example is Sjogren's
17. Axonopathy
    a. Pathology is in the axon
    b. Motor, sensory, and reflex changes are greatest in the distal extremities
    c. The most common neuropathy is seen in diabetes
18. Myelinopathy
    a. Pathology is in the Schwann cell or myelin
    b. Profound effects in conduction velocities

   c. Two classic forms
     i. Genetic
      1. Charcot-Marie-Tooth
     ii. Acquired
      1. Inflammatory demyelinating polyneuropathy

19. Wallerian degeneration
   a. Occurs in the nerve fiber and cell body as a result of anatomic axonal interruption
   b. Axon and myelin sheath distal to the injury degenerate and are removed by macrophages
   c. Axons just proximal to the sheath degenerate, but only for a short distance
   d. Schwann cells proliferate and give rise to solid cellular columns that serve as guides for sprouting axons
   e. The cell body undergoes a series of changes called chromatolysis
     i. Dissolution of Nissl substances leads to a decrease in cytoplasmic basophilia
     ii. Eccentric positioning of the nucleus
     iii. Swelling of the cell body

20. Mononeuropathy
   a. Pathology is in A single nerve
   b. Results from trauma or compression
     i. An example is carpal tunnel syndrome (CTS)

21. Multiple mononeuropathy
   a. Diagnosed when the clinical picture involves multiple individual nerves
   b. Examples include
     i. Vascular etiologies
      1. Highest on the differential
     ii. HIV
     iii. Acidosis
     iv. Lymphomatosis
     v. Meningeal carcinomatosis

22. Polyneuropathies
   a. Diffuse, symmetric, and involve distal nerves greater than proximal
   b. Acquired or hereditary
   c. Causes include
     i. Metabolic
     ii. Toxic
     iii. Infectious
     iv. Nutritional

23. Parameters assessed in a nerve conduction study (NCV)
   a. Distal latency
   b. Conduction velocity
     i. A function of axonal diameter and the degree of myelination

          1. Demyelination causes striking changes in conduction velocity

  c. Evoked response amplitude and duration

  d. Late responses

    i. F-wave

    ii. H-reflex

  e. Sensory studies

    i. Useful in localizing peripheral nerve lesions as either proximal or distal to the dorsal root ganglion

    ii. Standard sensory responses are unaffected by lesions proximal to the dorsal-root ganglia despite the presence of clinical sensory loss

24. Electromyogram (EMG)

  a. Differentiates neurogenic processes from myopathic disorders

  b. Separates active denervation from chronic

  c. Categorizes myopathies as irritable or non-irritable

  d. Detects the presence of abnormal discharges

25. Quantitative sensory testing

  a. Assesses small myelinated and unmyelinated nerve fibers

  b. A psychophysiologic test to evaluate heat and cooling thresholds and heat-pain sensation

  c. Quantitation of intraepidermal nerve fiber density by skin punch biopsy

26. Myelin has proteins and lipids that may become immunogenic

  a. Antibodies target specialized regions at the nodes of Ranvier and damage adjacent axons

  b. A complement-mediated humoral response against the myelin sheath

27. Demyelination

  a. Increases membrane capacitance

  b. Decreases membrane resistance

  c. Current leaks between the nodes of Ranvier

28. NCV features of demyelinating neuropathy

  a. Prolonged distal, F-wave, and H-reflex latencies

  b. Reduced conduction velocities

  c. Partial motor-conduction block

  d. Abnormal temporal dispersion

29. NCV features of axonopathies

  a. Result in loss of nerve fibers with little change to conduction

  b. Evoked response amplitudes are reduced

  c. Normal or near-normal distal, F-wave, and H-reflex latencies

  d. Little change in the shape and duration of evoked responses

30. Neuronal functional recovery varies

  a. Demyelinating neuropathies have rapid recovery with remyelination

  b. Distal axonal degeneration is slower

    i. Requires months to years

    ii. Axons regenerate at 1 mm/day

Section H: Collagen and Elastin

1. Collagen
   a. The major structural protein of the fibrillar component of the ECM
   b. The most abundant protein in the body
   c. Accounts for 20–30% of the total body mass
   d. Extracellular proteins with at least a portion of their structure as a triple-helix conformation
   e. Extensive posttranslational modifications
      i. Stabilizes the molecule
      ii. Maturation of fibrils via lysine-derived covalent cross-links
   f. 19 different types of collagen
      i. Divided into six subclasses
      ii. Based on the characteristics of the polymeric structures they form or their structural features
2. Fibril-forming collagens
   a. Types I, II, III, V, and XI
   b. Highly asymmetric flexible, rod-like structure
      i. Diameter of 1.5 nm
      ii. Length of 300 nm
      iii. Five charged regions 68 nm apart
   c. Composed of three polypeptide chains
      i. α chains
         1. About 95 kDa each
         2. Telopeptides at the NH2 and COOH termini
            a. Short nonhelical sequences of 15–20 residues
   d. Characterized by a repeating [Gly-X-Y]n structure
      i. X and Y residues can be any amino acid (AA)
         1. Most commonly proline and hydroxyproline (25%)
      ii. 338 triplets in type I chains and 341 triplets in type III chains
      iii. Type I and II triple helical region contains about 1,000 AA residues, $(Gly-X-Y)_{333}$
   e. Each alpha chain assumes a left-handed helical conformation (minor helix)
      i. The α carbon of the imino acid in the ring structure is not free to rotate
      ii. A residue repeat distance of 0.291 nm
      iii. A relative twist of 110°
      iv. 3.27 residues per turn of the helix
      v. 0.87 nm distance between glycine residues
   f. Glycine at every third residue occupies the center position along the common axis of the triple helix
      i. Lacks a bulky side chain
      ii. Because of this space restriction, any other AA would not be tolerated
   g. Fibril formation
      i. Collagen molecules are not soluble under physiologic ionic strength, pH, and temperature

      ii. Spontaneous parallel aggregation of collagen molecules into striated fibrils
          1. Each row of molecules is displaced along the long axis of the molecule by a distance of 68 nm
          2. Within the row, there is a gap of about 40 nm between the end of one molecule and the beginning of another
      iii. Charged regions align in a straight line
      iv. Individual molecules are staggered a quarter of their length in relation to each other

h. Type I collagen
    i. Commonly in heterotrimeric form [$\alpha 1(I)2\alpha 2(I)$]
    ii. Found in bone, tendon, skin (dermis), and joint capsule/synovium
    iii. Genes COL1A1 and COL1A2 located on chromosomes 17q21 and 7q21
    iv. Disease associations
       1. Osteogenesis imperfecta
         a. Brittle bones, thin blue sclerae, and abnormal tooth development
       2. Scleroderma
         a. T-cell sensitivity to type I collagen (and/or Type III)

i. Type II collagen
    i. Enriched in hydroxylysine and is highly glycosylated
    ii. Found in hyaline cartilage, disk, and vitreous humor
       1. The major fibrillar collagen of articular cartilage and the vitreous of the eye
    iii. Gene COL2A1 located on chromosome 12q13
    iv. Disease associations
       1. Chondrodysplasias
       2. Sticklers
       3. Premature OA
       4. Autoimmunity to Type II plays a role in
         a. RA
         b. Juvenile rheumatoid arthritis (JRA)
         c. Polychondritis

j. Type III collagen
    i. A homotrimer [$\alpha 1(III)$]3
    ii. Found in dermis, lung, blood vessels, and intestine, uterine wall
    iii. COL3A1 gene on chromosome 2q24
    iv. Disease associations
       1. Ehlers–Danlos syndrome Type IV
         a. Loose joints, rupture of bowel and major blood vessels
         b. Abnormal processing of the procollagen

k. Type V collagen
    i. Consist of two different α chains, $\alpha 1(V)$, and $\alpha 2(V)$
    ii. Found as either a heterotrimer of the two α chains or as homotrimers of either chain
    iii. Found in bone, tendon, skin (dermis), and joint capsule/synovium
       1. Same as Type I

      iv. Genes COL5A1 on chromosome 9q34 and COL5A2 and 3 on 2q34

      v. May play a role in influencing fibril size

      vi. Disease associations

         1. Ehlers–Danlos syndrome Types I and II

   l. Type XI collagen

      i. Consists of heterotrimers of three different chains, α1(XI), α2(XI), and α3(XI)

      ii. Found in articular cartilage and the ocular vitreous

         1. Same as Type II

      iii. Genes COL11A1 on chromosome 1p21, COL11A2 on 6p21, and COL2A1 on 12q13

      iv. Disease associations

         1. Spondyloepiphyseal dysplasia (SED)

3. FACIT collagens

   a. FACIT = Fibril associated collagens with interrupted triple-helix

   b. Type IX, XII, XIV, XVI, and XIX (9, 12, 14, 16, 19)

   c. Do not form fibrils independently

   d. Associate with the fibrillar collagens Types I, II, and III

   e. Contain triple-helical domains with disruptions in the Gly-X-Y sequence, producing interrupted triple helices

   f. Type IX, XII, and XIV all contain a single chondroitin sulfate polysaccharide chain

      i. Type XII and Type XIV have nearly identical amino-acid sequences and are both associated with type I collagen fibrils

      ii. Genes COL12A1 on chromosome 6 and COL14A1 on 8q23,24

   g. Type IX

      i. The most studied FACIT

      ii. Associates with Type II in articular cartilage

      iii. A heterodimer composed of three different chains, α1(IX), α2(IX), α3(IX)

         1. Contains a large noncollagenous (NC) domain at the NH2 terminus of α1(IX)

         2. A short NC3 segment creates a kink in the proteoglycan component region with the GAG chain (often a CS) extending from α2(IX) chain

         3. A large, positively charged NH2 terminal NC4 is exposed on the fibril surface and interacts with other matrix components

      iv. Genes COL9A1 on chromosome 6q12 and COL9A2 on 1p32

      v. Disease associations

         1. Type IX antibodies found in sera of patients with RA suggest a role in RA pathophysiology

         2. Multiple epiphyseal dysplasia (MED)

4. Network-forming collagens

   a. Tendency to form 3-D networks

   b. Types IV, VIII, and X (4,8,10)

   c. Type IV

      i. The best characterized

      ii. Found exclusively in basement membrane

    iii. Three molecular forms

       1. A heterotrimer $\alpha 1(IV)2$, $\alpha 2(IV)$ is the most abundant

    iv. Six genes for COL4A1 found on three different chromosomes 13q34, 2q35, and Xq22

    v. A long collagenous domain (400 nm) with multiple interruptions in the triple helix resulting in flexible regions

    vi. Assembled in a 3D, lattice-like network

       1. Head-to-head and tail-to-tail arrangement created by lysine- and cysteine-derived cross-links

       2. Dimerization with tail-to-tail interaction between 2 C-terminal non-collagenous domains (NC1) and tetramer-formation through N-terminal interactions

       3. Cross-link formation in the N-terminal region results in a proteinase-resistant region known as 7 s collagen

       4. Side-to-side interactions between different molecules and the network are important in the filtration function of basement membranes

    vii. Disease associations

       1. Goodpasture's syndrome

          a. Antibodies to the NC1 domain of the a3(IV) chain bind the glomerular and alveolar basement membranes causing immune complexes

       2. Alports syndrome

          a. Hereditary nephritis and deafness

          b. A mutation in the $\alpha 5(IV)$ gene

d. Type VIII collagen

    i. Found in sheet-like structures of Descemet's membrane

    ii. Separates the corneal epithelial cells from the corneal stoma and consists of stacks of collagen lattices

    iii. Contains a small triple-helical domain and two small lobular domains

    iv. Genes COL8A1 found on chromosome 3q12 and COL8A2 on 1p32

e. Type X collagen

    i. A short chain homotrimer

    ii. Gene COL 10A1 on chromosome 6q21

    iii. Role in endochondral ossification

       1. Found in calcifying hypertrophic cartilage

    iv. Disease associations

       1. OA

          a. Found at sites of osteophyte formation, surface fibrillation, and around clonal clusters of proliferative cells

       2. Metaphyseal dysplasia

5. Anchoring-Fibril-Forming collagen

a. Type VII

    i. Found in dermoepidermal, cornea, and oral mucosa

    ii. Forms anchoring fibrils that stabilize the attachment of basement membranes to the underlying connective tissues

      iii. Distinguished by its extraordinary length (nearly 467 nm)

         1. All but a small portion is triple helix

         2. Extends from the basement membrane to the papillary dermis

      iv. Contains a complex trident-like carboxy-terminal NC domain with fibrils formed by antiparallel dimerization

      v. Disease associations

         1. Mutations in the α1(VII) gene results in dystrophic forms of hereditary epidermolysis bullosa

         2. Type VII antibodies react with anchoring fibrils and produce epidermolysis bullosa acquisita in systemic lupus erythematosus (SLE)

  b. Beaded filament-forming collagen

    i. Type VI

      1. Found in most connective tissue

      2. A 336 residue triple helical region flanked by large globular domain

      3. Monomers contain three distinct α chains all with repeats similar to type A repeats in vWF

        a. α1(VI) (150 kDa)

        b. α2(VI) (140 kDa)

        c. α3(VI) (300 kDa and longer)

          i. 11 repeats and a 73 residue segment analogous to the platelet glycoprotein Ib

      4. A COOH terminus region flanked by a type III repeat of fibronectin

      5. A Kunitz-type proteinase inhibitor

        a. Suggest a role in cell adhesion and type I collagen binding

  c. Collagen with a transmembrane domain

    i. Prominent transmembrane domains

    ii. Types XIII and XVII (13, 17)

    iii. Type XIII

      1. Found in endomysium, placenta, and meninges

    iv. Type XVII

      1. Found in skin and cornea

      2. The protein of hemidesmosomes

      3. Disease association

        a. Previously referred to as the 180-kDa bullous pemphigoid antigen

6. Intracellular events in collagen biosynthesis

  a. 20 distinct genes encode the various collagen chains

  b. Prepro-α chains

    i. Processed mRNAs leave the nucleus and are transported to the polyribosomal apparatus in the rough ER for translation into polypeptide chains

    ii. A hydrophobic leader sequence is removed before secretion into the extracellular space

  c. Pro-α chains

    i. Longer (150,000 kDa) than the α chains (95,000 kDa)

    ii. Found in mature collagen fibrils

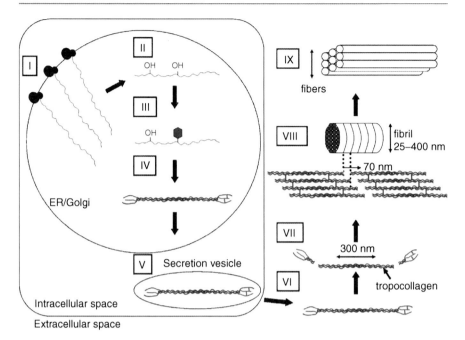

Fig. 1.8 Schematic of collagen biosynthesis. Prochains are synthesized in the ER (*I*) Selected prolines are hydroxylated (*II*). This is followed by glycosylation of selected hydroxylysines (*III*). The three pro-chains self assemble and form procollagen triple-helix (*IV*). The procollagen monomers travel via vesicles (*V*) from the Golgi apparatus to the extracellular space (*VI*), where they are cleaved to form tropocollagen monomers (*VII*). These monomers self-assemble into fibrils that can covalently crosslink to each other (*VIII*). Finally, the fibrils aggregate to form a collagen fiber (*IX*) (Reproduced with permission from Salsas-Escat, R. Stultz, C. M. The molecular mechanics of collagen degradation: implications for human disease. *Experimental Mechanics*. DOI: 10.1007/s11340-00. Springer; 2009-01-20)

    iii. Contain amino and carboxy-terminal propeptides that are largely nonhelical
    iv. Disulfide bonds at the carboxy terminals facilitate folding into a triple helix
  d. Polypeptide chains are hydroxylated by prolyl and lysine hydroxylases
    i. Require O_2, Fe, α-ketoglutarate, and ascorbic acid (vitamin C) as cofactors
    ii. Under-hydroxylated α chains form unstable helices that denature at body temperature (37°C)
    iii. Disease association
      1. Scurvy (ascorbic acid deficiency)
        a. A decrease in hydroxyproline content is seen
  e. Hydroxylysines are glycosylated
    i. Important for secretion of the procollagen monomer and later in stability of the cross-links
    ii. The enzyme UDP-**galactose**:hydroxylysine **galactosyl**transferase adds a galactose residue to the hydroxyl group of specific hydroxylysine residues

    iii. The UDP-**glucose**:galactose hydroxylysine **glucosyl**transferase then transfers a glucose to some of the hydroxylysine-linked **galactose** residues

    iv. Sequential glycosylation occurs during nascent chain formation

      1. Mature triple-helical collagen cannot act as a substrate for glycosylating enzymes

  f. Formation of C-terminal disulfide bridges and procollagen triple-helix

  g. Secretion of procollagen into the extracellular space

7. Extracellular events in collagen biosynthesis

  a. Conversion of procollagen to collagen by cleavage of N- and C-elopeptide termini by specific procollagen peptidases

    i. Proteolytic steps result in a reduction in the solubility of collagen

  b. Collagen molecules spontaneously assemble into fibrils by a near-quarter stagger shift

  c. Fibrils are stabilized by the formation of covalent intermolecular cross-links

    i. Lysyl and hydroxylysyl oxidase catalyze the oxidative deamination of specific lysine or hydroxylysine residues in the amino- or carboxy-terminal telopeptides

      1. Form aldehyde containing derivatives, allysine or hydroxyallysine

    ii. Aldehydes react with the ε-amino group of lysine or hydroxylysine residues on adjacent chains to form covalent cross-links

    iii. Disease association

      1. Failure to form intermolecular cross-links results in marked fragility of connective tissues

  d. End-to-end and lateral aggregation of fibrils form collagen fibers

8. Collagen Degradation

  a. Specific collagenases cleave the native molecule at a single position within the triple helix (between residues 775 and 776)

    i. Bisects each α chain into two fragments representing 75% and 25% of the intact molecule

    ii. Unfolded products are unstable and denature spontaneously at body temperature and pH

    iii. Increases susceptibility to gelatinases and stromelysins

  b. The most important collagenases for Type I collagen is the matrix metalloproteinase (MMP) group

    i. Consist of 28 distinct enzymes

    ii. Enzyme activation

      1. Many are secreted as enzymatically inactive proenzymes and activated by proteolytic cleavage of the proenzyme domain

      2. The membrane type of matrix metalloproteinases (MT-MMP) function as integral membrane proteins and are activated intracellularly

    iii. Synthesis is induced by proinflammatory cytokines

    iv. Constitutively secreted

    v. Regulated by a family of protein inhibitors known as tissue inhibitors of metalloproteinase (TIMP)

      1. Four family members (TIMP 1–4)

  c. α-macroglobulin is capable of inhibiting collagenase activity

    d. Measures of collagen turnover
       i. Serum procollagen peptides
      ii. Urinary hydroxyproline
     iii. Urinary pyridinoline/deoxypyridinoline cross-links
     iv. Serum and urinary N-telopeptides

9. Regulation of Collagen Gene Expression
    a. Transcriptional control
       i. Regulatory sequences on both sides of the transcription start site dictate the constitutive, tissue-specific, or inducible expression of collagen genes
      ii. Promoter function integrity is maintained in COL1A1 and COL1A2 genes by TATA and CCAAT boxes located at 25–30 and 75–80 bp upstream of the transcription start site
     iii. Important regulatory elements are found within the first intron of the human COL1A1 gene
        1. An Sp1-binding motif has been implicated in the enhanced activity of COL1A1 promoter in response to TGF-β1
          a. A polymorphic Sp1-binding site is seen in a subset of people with reduced bone density and osteoporosis
    b. Post-transcriptional control
       i. Collagen biosynthesis regulated by feedback mechanisms of amino- and carboxy-terminal propeptides
    c. Positive regulators
       i. TGF-β1
         1. Enhances type I gene expression by increasing the rate of transcription and stability of COL1A1 mRNA
    d. Negative regulators
       i. TNF-α
      ii. Interferon gamma (INF-γ)
        1. Reduces the stability and translation rate of COL1A1 mRNA

10. Elastin and Elastic Fibers
    a. Elastin fibers comprise a significant portion of the dry weight of ligaments
       i. Lungs (70–80%)
      ii. Large blood vessels such as aorta (30–60%)
     iii. Skin (2–5%)
    b. Disease associations
       i. Mutations in the elastin gene can cause cutis laxa and supravalvular aortic stenosis
    c. Two components of elastic fibers
       i. An amorphous element composed mainly of the protein tropoelastin
         1. Contains 850 amino acids
           a. Predominately hydrophobic domains of valine, proline, glycine, and alanine alternating with hydrophilic regions rich in lysine
         2. Lysine residues cross-link by forming desmosine and isodesmosine, unique to elastin
           a. Urine desmosine levels are used as a measure of elastin degradation.
           b. Oxidized enzymatically through the action of lysyl oxidase, a copper-dependent enzyme

      ii. A microfibrillar element composed of fibrillin and other proteins
         1. Fibrillin 1
           a. A 360 kDa glycoprotein
           b. Coded for by a gene located on chromosome 15
           c. Disease association
             i. Marfan's syndrome
               1. Loose-jointedness (ligaments)
               2. Aortic aneurysms (large blood vessels)
               3. Lens subluxation (Ocular zonule)
         2. Fibrillin 2
           a. Coded for by a gene located on chromosome 5
           b. Disease association
             i. Congenital contractual arachnodactyly
    d. Elastases
      i. Serine proteases
      ii. Capable of degrading elastase
      iii. Located in tissues, macrophages, leukocytes, and platelets
      iv. Contribute to the pathophysiology in the vasculitides
11. Adhesive cell-binding glycoproteins
    a. Bind cells by attaching to integrins
    b. Present in intracellular matrices and basement membranes
    c. Classical arginine-glycine-aspartic acid (RGD) cell binding sequence
    d. Examples include
      i. Fibronectin (connective tissue)
      ii. Laminin (basement membrane)
      iii. Chondroadherin (cartilage)
      iv. Osteoadherin (bone)

Section I: Proteoglycans

1. Proteoglycans
    a. Uniquely glycosylated proteins that often contain both N-linked and O-linked oligosaccharides
    b. The protein core
      i. One or more sulfated glycosaminoglycan side chains additions
      ii. Coded for by at least 20 distinct genes
    c. Nomenclature based on
      i. Named core protein plus glycosaminoglycan type
      ii. Tissue type of origin
    d. Provide a high-density source of fixed negative charges within the ECM
      i. The compression of a negative charge within a collagen network provides the osmotic pressure needed to withstand physiologic loads up to100–200 atm within milliseconds of standing

2. Glycosaminoglycans (GAG)
    a. Linear, anionic polysaccharides with repeating disaccharide units containing a hexosamine residue and usually a hexuronic acid residue
    b. Classified into three basic groups
        i. Chondroitin sulfate
            1. Contain a linear, repeating, N-acetylgalactosamine-glucuronic acid disaccharide structure commonly sulfated at the 4 or 6 position of the hexosamine residue
                a. Post-synthesis epimerization of glucuronic acid residues of chondroitin-4-sulfate to iduronic acid yields the GAG dermatan sulfate
        ii. Heparan sulfate
            1. A basic repeating glucuronic acid-N-acetylglucosamine disaccharide
                a. Linked via an O-glycosidic bond to a core protein via a common tetrasaccharide linkage unit
                    i. Xylosyl-galactose-galacotse-glucuronic acid
                b. Linkage region added co-translationally via interaction of the reducing end of the xylose with the hydroxyl of serine residue of the core protein
            2. Differentiated by the presence of alternating α- and β-glycosidic linkages
                a. All other GAGS typically are β-linkages
            3. Modifications to the basic heparin sequence include
                a. Unique sulfation patterns of the uronic acid and hexosamine hydroxyl group
                b. N-deacetylation followed by N-sulfation of the hexosamines
                c. Epimerization of particular glucuronic-acid residues to iduronic acid
                d. Lesser-modified heparin GAGs are called heparan sulfates
                e. More mature GAGs are called heparins
            4. Expressed on the surface of vasculature lining endothelial cells
                a. Binds
                    i. Antithrombin III
                    ii. Lipoprotein lipase
            5. Serglycin
                a. Heparin bearing
                b. Core protein with numerous serine/glycine repeats within the central portion of the molecule
                c. Exists as an intracellular proteoglycan localized within storage granules during resting states
                d. Mast cells substitute the core protein with CS rather than HS
        iii. Keratan sulfate
            1. Shorter GAGS (20–40 disaccharide units)
            2. Contain repeating galactose N-acetylglucosamine disaccharide units
            3. Contain sulfate residues at the 6 position of the galactose, the N-acetylglucosamine, or both

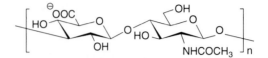

Fig. 1.9 Hyaluronic acid (Reproduced with permission from Novel approaches for glycodrug discovery. *Glycoscience.* DOI: 10.1007/978-3-540-30429-6_61. Springer; 2008-01-017-9105-1, 2008-01-01)

      4. Chain ends may be capped by sialic acid residues
      5. Two modes of attachment to the core protein
         a. Via a branched hexasaccharide linkage unit O-linked to serine residues (cartilage)
         b. Via a branched oligosaccharide linkage unit N-linked to asparagine residues (cornea)
   c. Hyaluronan (HA)
      i. A B-linked, repeating, glucuronic acid–N-acetyl glucosamine disaccharide structure
      ii. Not associated with a core protein
     iii. Not substituted with sulfate
     iv. A linear, non-branching polymer about 150 times longer than other GAGs
      v. Synthesized predominately within the Golgi via an HA synthase
3. Proteoglycans that interact with HA
   a. Possess a proteoglycan tandem repeat (PTR)
      i. A tandem repeat motif within the core protein at the amino-terminal region
      ii. Responsible for the specific, high-affinity binding to the HA filament
   b. Family includes
      i. Aggrecan
      ii. Versican
     iii. Brevican
     iv. Neurocan
      v. CD44
     vi. BEHAP
4. Proteoglycans that interact with collagen
   a. Horseshoe-shaped proteoglycans that interact with a single triple helix of collagen include
      i. Decorin
      ii. Biglycan
     iii. Fibromodulin
   b. Maintains proper spacing between fibrils
   c. Regulate hydration and movement of molecules
   d. Decorin deficient mice
      i. Reduced tensile strength of skin and tendons
      ii. Irregularities in fibril diameter

    e. Thin fibrils are decorated with Type IX collagen

    f. Fibrils of larger diameter are decorated with decorin

    g. Biglycan deficient mice

       i. Proteoglycan acts as a positive regulator of bone formation and bone mass

    h. The SLRP family

       i. Functions

          1. Regulate collagen fiber diameter

          2. Cross-link collagen lattices and other matrix components

          3. Serve as a repository for growth factors such as TGF-β

          4. Bind other macromolecules such as fibronectin

       ii. Members include

          1. Decorin

          2. Fibromodulin

          3. Lumican

          4. Epiphycan

          5. Keratocan

          6. Osteoadherin

5. Cell-surface proteoglycans

    a. Functions

       i. Local hydration and molecular movement

       ii. Bind basic growth factors and cytokines

       iii. Bind other matrix components

          1. Fibronectin

          2. Laminen

          3. Collagen

    b. Two groups ubiquitous to all cell types

       i. Transmembrane

          1. Represented by the syndecan family

          2. Articular chondrocytes express mRNA for syndecan-2 and 4, but little for syndecan-1

          3. Homologous core protein structures include

             a. A C-terminal cytoplasmic domain

             b. A hydrophobic transmembrane domain

             c. A large N-terminal extracellular domain that bears the GAG chain

          4. Contains a protease sensitive site within the proximal portion of the extracellular domain

             a. Allows for rapid regulation of functions via proteolytic shedding

          5. Syndecan core protein

             a. Two or more HS chains located on the distal end, alone or in combination with CS

             b. Typically located more centrally along the extracellular domain

       ii. Glypican

          1. Regulates expression of HS chains at the cell surface

          2. Does not exhibit hydrophobic transmembrane domains

        3. Glypiation
           a. Anchors to the plasma via covalent linkage to a glycosylphos-
              phatidylinositol attachment site
        4. Rapidly shed through the action of phospholipases
  6. Major roles of proteoglycan core proteins
    a. The type III TGF-β receptor
      i. Betaglycan
    b. Thrombomodulin
    c. Transferrin receptor
    d. HA receptor
      i. CD44
  7. Proteoglycan Metabolism
    a. Cartilage proteoglycans are regulated by resident chondrocytes
    b. Anabolism
      i. A cellular response to biomechanical stimuli and changes in the ECM
        composition
      ii. Mediated by
        1. Cell surface receptors
          a. Anchorin CII
          b. CD 44
          c. Integrins
        2. Peptide growth factors
          a. EGF
          b. FGF
          c. TGF-β
          d. PDGF
          e. TGF-α
          f. BMPs
    c. Catabolism
      i. Mediated by proinflammatory cytokines
        1. IL-1α and β
        2. IL-6
        3. TNF-α
        4. IFN-γ
  8. Distribution of proteoglycans
    a. Cell-associated proteoglycans
      i. Contain HS or CS as major GAG
      ii. Cell surface predominantly
        1. Syndecan
        2. Betaglycan
      iii. Intracellular
        1. Serglycin
      iv. Basement membrane
        1. Perlecan

   b. Proteoglycans secreted into the ECM
      i. Contain CS, DS, or KS as major GAG
      ii. Examples include
         1. Aggrecan
         2. Decorin
         3. Biglycan
         4. Fibromodulin
         5. Lumican
9. Proteoglycan Degradation
   a. Proteinases release GAGs
   b. GAGs are taken up by endocytosis
   c. Degraded in lysosomes by a series of glycosidase and sulfatase enzymes
   d. Average half life
      i. 25 days for newly synthesized aggrecan and HA in tissue
   e. Disease association
      i. Mucopolysaccharidoses
         1. Defects in degradation enzymes
   f. Aggrecan catabolism
      i. Primarily extracellularly
      ii. Involves proteolytic cleavage between the G1 and G2 domains of the core protein
      iii. MMPs are the proteolytic enzymes involved
         1. Characterized by a bound Zn at their active site and a requirement for calcium
   g. HA catabolism
      i. Primarily intracellularly
      ii. Follows endocytosis of HA receptors (CD44)
   h. Disease association
      i. Molecular fragments of collagen II and aggrecan are considered causal factors in joint disease

Mediators of Rheumatic Pathology

2

Section A: Cellular Constituents

1. The cardinal physical signs of inflammation were described by Celsius in the first century:
   a. Rubor (redness)
   b. Calor (heat)
   c. Dolor (pain)
   d. Tumor (swelling)
2. Neutrophils
   a. Highly condensed, segmented, multilobed nucleus
   b. Numerous cytoplasmic granules containing preformed mediators
      i. Phagocytize and digest foreign particles at sites of inflammation and antigens entry
      ii. Kill and dissolve microbes with release of enzymes and bactericidal products
      iii. Generate toxic oxygen radicals and hypohalous acids
   c. Cellular first line of defense
      i. Large numbers
      ii. Rapid mobilization
   d. Chemotaxis
      i. Directed migration to the inflammatory site
      ii. Occurs along a chemical gradient originating from the target
   e. Neutrophil chemoattractants
      i. Interact with specific guanosine triphosphate (GTP) binding protein linked (G-protein) surface receptors
      ii. Examples include
         1. Bacterial formylated peptides
         2. Activated complement components (C5a)
         3. Leukotrienes (LT B4)
         4. Chemokines (IL-8)

f. Neutrophil migration
  i. Rolling tethered interactions upon activation
    1. L-selectins (CD62L) on the neutrophil interact with carbohydrate gly-cosylated counterligands (sialyl-Lewis) on endothelial cells
    2. Glycoproteins on the neutrophil interact with endothelial cell E- and P-selectins (CD62E and CD62P)
  ii. At <2 h
    1. Neutrophils express L-selectin and P-selectin glycoprotein ligand-1 (PSGL-1) to activated endothelium's Sialomucin (CD34) and P-selectin (Weibel–Palade bodies)
g. Neutrophil adhesion
  i. Mediators
    1. Neutrophil β2 integrins adhesion molecules
      a. CD11b/CD18
      b. Leukocyte function–associated antigen-1 (LFA-1)
    2. Endothelial cell adhesion molecules
      a. Endothelial-leukocyte adhesion molecule-1 (ELAM-1)
      b. Intercellular adhesion molecule-1 (ICAM-1) (CD 54)
      c. Vascular cell adhesion molecule-1 (VCAM-1) (CD106)
  ii. Upon activation
    1. CD11b/CD18 binds ICAM-1 leading to neutrophil spreading and crawling
  iii. At <4 h
    1. Neutrophils express ESL-1 to activated endothelial cells' ELAM-1
  iv. At <12 h
    1. Neutrophils express LFA-1 to endothelial cells' ICAM-1
  v. At <24 h
    1. β2 integrin is expressed on monocytes to endothelial cells' ICAM-1
  vi. At <48 h
    1. β1 integrin is expressed on lymphocytes and monocytes to endothelial cells' VCAM-1
h. Neutrophil transmigration (diapedesis)
  i. Mediators
    1. Platelet-endothelial cell adhesion molecule-1 (PECAM-1/CD31) on neutrophils interact with PECAM-1 prominently expressed in the intercellular junctional areas of endothelial cells
  ii. Disease associations
    1. Abnormal activation of the endothelium seen in
      a. SLE
      b. Leukocytoclastic vasculitis (LCV)
      c. Giant cell arteritis
      d. Rheumatoid vasculitis
i. Phagocytosis
  i. Initiated by the binding of target particles to the cell surface

        1. Stimulus does not depend on **specific** recognition of an organism
- ii. Enclosure of the particle within a plasma membrane pouch
  1. Cytoplasmic vacuole called a phagosome
- iii. Enzymatic degradation of ingested materials
  1. Phagosome fuses with a lysosome to form phagolysosomes
- iv. Opsonization
  1. The coating of bacteria, cells, and debris with opsonins
     - a. Immunoglobulins (Igs)
     - b. Antibodies
     - c. Complement components
- v. Cell-surface receptors recognize coated particles
  1. Immunoglobulin
  2. Complement components
     - a. Complement receptor 1 (CR1) (CD35)
       - i. For fragments of the third component of complement (C3b)
     - b. Complement receptor 3 (CR3) (CD11b/CD18)
       - i. For inactivated cleavage product (iC3b)

j. Clearing immune complexes
- i. Receptors C3b and iC3 b are also important in the removal of immune complexes
- ii. 3 receptors that bind IgG-containing complexes via their Fc fragments
  1. FcγRI (CD64)
     - a. High-affinity receptor for monomeric IgG
     - b. Expressed on neutrophils only after INF-γ stimulation
       - i. Also expressed on unstimulated monocytes and macrophages
  2. FcγRIIa (CD32)
     - a. Low-affinity receptor that binds multimeric IgG
  3. FcγRIII (CD16)
     - a. Low-affinity receptor that binds multimeric IgG
- iii. Disease association
  1. FcγR polymorphisms affect phagocytic function and are susceptibility factors in the development of autoimmunity

k. Release of toxic proteolytic enzymes
- i. Three types of morphologically distinct granules involved in degranulation
  1. Primary azurophilic granules:
     - a. Contains microbicidal enzymes
       - i. Lysozyme
       - ii. Defensins
       - iii. Myeloperoxidase (MPO)
     - b. Contains proteases
       - i. Cathepsin G
       - ii. Proteinase 3
       - iii. Elastase

       2. Specific or secondary granules
         a. Degrade components of the ECM
           i. Lactoferrin
           ii. Gelatinase
           iii. Collagenase
       3. Tertiary granules
         a. Gelatinase
         b. Lysozyme
         c. Bacterial phospholipase A2
         d. Cathepsin
     ii. Degranulation is provoked by soluble stimuli
       1. C5a
       2. IL-8
       3. Immune complexes
 l. Disease associations
     i. Lysosomal enzymes contribute to tissue injury characterized by
       1. Immune complex deposition (RA)
       2. Uncontained neutrophil recruitment (gout)
     ii. Fc receptors engage immune complexes in articular cartilage
       1. Release proteinases and products of NAPDH oxidase protected from degradation by antiproteinases
     iii. Antineutrophil cytoplasmic antibodies (ANCA)
       1. Perinuclear ANCA (p-ANCA) detects neutrophil MPO
       2. Cytoplasmic ANCA (c-ANCA) detects proteinase 3
     iv. Superoxide anion radicals produced by the respiratory burst cause tissue injury
       1. MPO catalyzes the reaction of hydrogen peroxide with a halide (chloride) (hypochlorous acid) as neutrophils consume oxygen
3. Macrophages
  a. Monocyte/macrophage chemoattractants
     i. Formylated bacterial proteins
     ii. C5a
     iii. C-C chemokines
       1. RANTES
       2. Macrophage inflammatory protein (MIP-1 α and β)
       3. Monocyte chemoattractant protein (MCP-1)
     iv. TGF-β
     v. PDGF
  b. Monocyte/macrophage adhesion and transmigration facilitated by
     i. Monocyte β1 and β2 integrins
     ii. Endothelial cell ICAM-1
     iii. Vascular cell adhesion molecule (VCAM-1) (CD106)
  c. Monocyte differentiation and maturation influenced by
     i. Locally produced cytokines
       1. IL-1

      2. IL-3
      3. TNF-α
      4. IFN-γ
   ii. Growth factors
      1. M-CSF
      2. GM-CSF
  iii. Interactions with ECM proteins
      1. Fibronectin
      2. Collagen
      3. Laminin
d. Phagocytosis
   i. Macrophages possess three key properties that distinguish them from neutrophils
      1. Express major histocompatibility complex (MHC) class II on cell surface and function as antigen-presenting cells
      2. Produce proinflammatory and costimulatory cytokines that drive the acute phase response
        a. TNF-α
        b. IL-1
        c. IL-6
        d. IL-8
      3. Respond to certain cytokines (INF-γ from T cells) that increase their phagocytic capacity
        a. Causes aggregation into granulomas and multinucleated giant cells
   ii. Receptors that recognize opsonized particles
      1. FCγRI
      2. FCγRII
      3. FCγRIII
      4. CR1 and CR3
      5. Mannose receptor
        a. Recognizes glycoproteins on microbial cell surfaces
e. Activated macrophages produce a large number of substances
   i. Coagulation factors of both the intrinsic and extrinsic pathways
   ii. Procoagulant tissue factor
      1. Disease association
        a. Monocytes from RA patients have increased procoagulant activity
          i. Contributes to the deposition of fibrin at inflammatory sites
          ii. Formation of crescents in GN
  iii. Prothrombin activator
  iv. Plasmin inhibitors
   v. Proteases including collagenase and elastase
  vi. Bactericidal lysozyme
 vii. Proteins of the alternative and classical complement cascades
viii. Cytokines
      1. IL-1
        a. An endogenous pyrogen with proinflammatory effects

2. TNF-α
3. IL-6
   a. Activates lymphocytes and induces the synthesis of acute phase reactants by hepatocytes
4. IL-12
   a. Stimulates IFN-γ and the induction of Th1 lymphocyte response
5. IL-4
   a. A Th2 cytokine and a stimulus for antibody production
6. IL-10
   a. Predominantly anti-inflammatory

  ix. Neutrophil chemokine attractants
    1. IL-8

  x. Monocyte attractants
    1. MCP-1, -2, and -3
    2. RANTES
    3. MIP-1 α and β

  xi. Eicosanoid lipid mediators of inflammation derived from arachidonic acid (AA)
    1. Phospholipase (PLA2) liberates free AA and lyso-phospholipids from cell-membrane phospholipids
    2. AA is metabolized by 1 of 2 ways
      a. Via constitutive and inducible cyclooxygenases (COX, prostaglandin endoperoxide synthase)
        i. Generates prostaglandins and thromboxanes
        ii. Primary prostanoid product is prostaglandin E2 (PGE2)
          1. Vasodilates
          2. Increases vascular permeability
          3. Activates osteoclasts
        iii. Macrophages have both COX-1 and 2
      b. Via lipooxygenases
        i. Generates leukotrienes and lipoxin
          1. Leukotriene B4 (LTB4), LTC4 and platelet-activating factor (PAF)
          2. Important in regulation of platelet function

  xii. Nitric Oxide (NO)
    1. Increased by the macrophages' exposure to such cytokines as IL-1β and IFN-γ
    2. Vasodilates
    3. Reacts with superoxide anion to form toxic peroxynitrite compounds
    4. Disease associations
      a. Both RA and OA patients have increased NO by synovial macrophages and articular chondrocytes
      b. SLE patients have increased NO by endothelial cells

4. Platelets
  a. Chemotaxis

      i. PAF

      ii. Collagen fragments

  b. Adhesion

      i. Requires vWF which binds to platelet glycoprotein Ib/IX

  c. Activation

      i. Receptors for Ig and IgE

      ii. PAF

      iii. C-reactive protein (CRP)

      iv. Substance P

      v. Complement components

      vi. Leads to release of granular contents that promote clotting and further platelet aggregation

        1. Dense granules

          a. Contain adenosine diphosphate (ADP)

            i. An important platelet agonist

          b. Activates platelet fibrinogen-binding sites of the b3 integrin glycoprotein (GP) IIb/IIIa

          c. Activates serotonin

            i. A potent vasoconstrictor that activates neutrophils and endothelial cells

        2. Alpha granules

          a. Contains platelet factor 4 and beta thromboglobulin

          b. Activates peripheral mononuclear cells (PMNs) for sources of PDGF and TGF-β

        3. Other platelet granule products

          a. Thrombospondin

            i. Promotes neutrophil adhesion

          b. Coagulation factors V and VIII

          c. vWF

          d. Fibrinogen

          e. Fibronectin

5. Mast Cells

  a. Chemotaxis

      i. C-kit (or stem cell factor) is the major influential cytokine

  b. Activation

      i. A major stimulus is IgE through its high affinity receptor FcϵRI

      ii. Activated complement proteins C3a and C5a

      iii. Neuropeptides

      iv. Cytokines

  c. Degranulation

      i. Augmented by interactions with ECM proteins through integrins

      ii. Rapid exocytosis of secretory granules

      iii. Secretory granules contain two major products

        1. Proteoglycans

          a. Heparin

          b. Chondroitin sulfate

        2. Proteases
          a. Tryptase
          b. Chymase
          c. Carboxypeptidase
          d. May activate MMPs
     iv. Generation of eicosanoids
        1. LTC4
        2. PGD2
     v. Inhibits Th1 responses
        1. TNF-α
     vi. Promotes Th2 responses
        1. IL-4
        2. IL-5
        3. IL-6
   vii. Other molecules released
        1. Histamine
          a. Increased vasodilation and vasopermeability
        2. PAF
        3. PLA2
  d. Disease association
     i. Scleroderma
        1. Mast cells play an important role in fibrotic reactions through fibro-
          blast growth factor (FGF), TGF-β, and trypase
6. Eosinophils
  a. Bilobed nuclei
  b. Granules
     i. Contain cationic proteins, major basic protein, and eosinophil peroxidase
     ii. Stained with acidic dyes including eosin
     iii. Products are especially toxic to helminthes
  c. Major cytokine produced is IL-5
     i. Important growth, differentiation, and survival factor
  d. Chemotaxis
     i. LTB4
     ii. PAF
     iii. Chemokines
        1. Eotaxin
        2. RANTES
        3. MCP2, 3, and 4
     iv. Interaction between the very late antigens (VLA-4), $\alpha 4\beta 1$, or CD49b/
        CD29 integrins on eosinophils with VCAM-1 on endothelial cells
  e. Activation
     i. IgE
     ii. Low-affinity receptors for IgG
     iii. FcϵRI and II

        iv. FcγRII and III

        v. IgA receptor

        vi. Complement receptors CR1 and 3 and C5a

   f. Major source of

        i. Eosinophil peroxidase

          1. Generates hypobromous acid

            a. Toxic to parasites

        ii. Lipid-derived mediators

          1. LTC4

          2. Lipoxins

          3. PAF

   g. Disease associations

        i. Churg–Strauss syndrome and hypersensitivity vasculitides

          1. LTC4 in vascular injury

        ii. Eosinophilia myalgia syndrome and eosinophilic fasciitis

          1. TGF-β in fibrotic diseases

Section B: Growth Factors and Cytokines

1. Divided into categories based on function
   a. Colony-stimulating factors (CSF)
   b. Growth and differentiation factors
   c. Immunoregulatory cytokines
   d. Proinflammatory cytokines
2. Colony-stimulating factors
   a. Function primarily as hematopoietic growth factors
   b. Granulocyte-macrophage CSF (GM-CSF)
        i. Potentiates the growth of early bone marrow precursor cells together with IL-3
        ii. Production in monocytes, fibroblasts, and endothelial cells is enhanced by IL-1 and TNF-α
        iii. Influences the function of mature cells of the granulocytic and monocytic lineages
          1. Primes neutrophils, eosinophils, and basophils to respond to triggering agents with enhanced chemotaxis, oxygen radical production, and Phagocytosis
          2. Enhances eosinophil cytotoxicity
          3. Stimulates basophil release of histamine
          4. Enhances monocytes and macrophages to present antigen
            a. Increased expression of membrane-bound IL1-α
        iv. Disease association
          1. RA
            a. Both GM-CSF protein and mRNA are localized in damaged tissue and synovial fluid
            b. Enhances MHC II expression on synovium
            c. G-CSF
               i. Influences the growth and function of mature neutrophils

     d. M-CSF
        i. Influences the growth and function of mature monocytes and macrophages
3. Growth and differentiation factors
    a. PDGF
        i. Primarily a product of platelets
        ii. Also produced by macrophages and endothelial cells
        iii. Three different forms
        iv. Two different receptors
    b. Epidermal growth factor (EGF)
        i. Found throughout the body
        ii. A potent angiogenic factor
        iii. Induces the growth and proliferation of a variety of mesenchymal and epithelial cells
    c. Fibroblast growth factor (FGF)
        i. Two main forms
        ii. Induces the growth and proliferation of a variety of mesenchymal and epithelial cells
        iii. Disease association
            1. May stimulate osteoclast in RA synovium
    d. TGF-β
        i. Potent proinflammatory and anti-inflammatory effects
        ii. Macrophages and platelets are the main sources
        iii. Released in a latent form and must be activated in tissues by proteases
        iv. May enhance or inhibit growth and differentiation in fibroblast and is influenced by the presence of other cytokines
            1. TGF-β and EGF suppress the growth of particular types of fibroblasts
            2. TGF-β and PDGF stimulate fibroblast growth
        v. Induces production of collagen and fibronectin in fibroblasts
            1. TNF-α and INF-γ oppose this effect
        vi. Inhibits fibroblast production of collagenase and enhances production of inhibitor to these enzymes in the presence of PDGF, EGF, and FGF
        vii. Strongest known chemotactic agent for monocytes and enhances expression of Fc receptor III on these cells
        viii. Net effect on macrophage function is suppressive
            1. Decrease in HLA-DR expression
            2. Deactivation of H_2O_2
        ix. Exhibits immunosuppressive effects
            1. Inhibits IL-1-induced T-cell proliferation
            2. B-cell growth and Ig production after stimulation with IL-2 and 4
            3. Opposes IFN-γ-induced NK-cell function
        x. Disease associations
            1. Most important effects in rheumatic diseases include
               a. Recruitment of monocytes into tissues

    b. Dampening of lymphocyte and macrophage function

    c. Stimulation of tissue fibrosis

   2. Scleroderma

    a. Found in monocytes infiltrating skin and organ

     i. INF-γ inhibits TGF-β collagen production

      1. Not effective in clinical trials

   3. Pulmonary fibrosis

   4. Chronic glomerulonephritis (GN)

 e. Osteoclast differentiation factor (ODF)

   i. Synthesized by synovial fibroblasts and T cells

   ii. Acts with M-CSF to induce differentiation of synovial monocytes into osteoclasts

   iii. Inhibited by osteoprotegerin (OPG) which binds to both soluble and membrane ODF to prevent interaction with cell-surface receptors

   iv. Disease association

    1. Bone resorption in RA

 f. Growth factors' interactive role in disease processes

   i. Rheumatoid arthritis

    1. Proliferation of RA synovium

     a. PDGF, EGF, and FGF

    2. Enhanced growth of new capillaries in RA synovium

     a. FGF, IL-8, TNF-α, and VEGF

    3. Peripheral blood monocytes from patients produce enhanced amount of VEGF in response to TNF-α stimulation

    4. Synovial lining macrophages in RA contain large amounts of VEGF

     a. 50% reduction in release by IL-1R antagonist (IL-1Ra) and a monoclonal antibody to TNF-α

   ii. Scleroderma

    1. Tissue fibrosis

     a. PDGF, EGF, and FGF

4. Immunoregulatory cytokines

 a. T helper (Th) cells are divided into two subsets

   i. Th1 cells

    1. Produce IFN-γ, IL-2, TNF-α, and IL-1

    2. Differentiation is enhanced by IFN-γ and IL-12

     a. Produced by macrophages and NK cells

    3. Differentiation is suppressed by IL4 and 10

   ii. Th2 cells

    1. Produce IL-4, IL-5, and IL-10

    2. Differentiation is enhanced by IL-4

    3. Differentiation is suppressed by IFN-γ and IL-12

 b. IL-2

   i. Production stimulated by macrophage presentation of processed antigen in complex with a class II MHC molecule CD4+ helper

   ii. Binds to a specific two chain receptor on target cells

   iii. Functions
      1. Induces a clonal expansion of T cells
      2. Enhances B-cell growth
      3. Augments NK-cell function
      4. Activates macrophages
   iv. Disease associations
      1. SLE
         a. Soluble IL2 receptors are found in the circulation of patients
            i. Correlate with clinical activity
            ii. Reflect T-cell activation
            iii. Do not inhibit IL2
      2. Collagen-induced arthritis (CIA)
         a. Ameliorated by the administration of monoclonal antibodies to the IL2 receptor in mice

c. IL-4
   i. Produced by Th-2 and mast cells
   ii. A major influence on B cells
      1. Enhance IgG1 and IgE production
      2. Induce the expression of Fc receptors for IgE
      3. Stimulates the expression of class II MHC molecules
   iii. Exhibits suppressive effects
      1. Directly inhibits monocyte production of IL-1, 6, and TNF-α at the level of transcription (anti-inflammatory)
      2. Induces IL-1Ra production
      3. Inhibits the production of tissue-degrading neutral metalloproteinases by RA synovial cells in vitro
      4. Inhibits cartilage and bone destruction in CIA by recombinant protein or gene therapy

d. IL5
   i. Produced by T cells
   ii. Increases IL-2 receptor expression on T and B cells
   iii. Promotes antibody secretion by B cells
   iv. The most active known cytokine on eosinophils
      1. Induces chemotaxis
      2. Enhances growth
      3. Stimulates superoxide production

e. IL-10
   i. Overproduced in SLE, RA, and Sjogren
      1. May be involved in enhancing autoantibody production and in inhibiting T-cell function in SLE
      2. Anti IL-10 prevents and ameliorates murine models of SLE

f. Disease manifestations
   i. IL-4 and 5 may play a role in asthma
   ii. IL-4, IL-10, and IL-13 may dampen synovitis in RA

g. IL-14
  i. Potent growth factor for B cells
h. IL 7, 9, 11, 15, and 16
  i. Primarily growth factors for T lymphocytes
  ii. IL-7 and 11 are synthesized by bone marrow stromal cells
  iii. IL-7 is a requisite factor for IL-1-induced thymocyte proliferation
  iv. IL-9 induces proliferation of mast cells
  v. IL-11
    1. Synergizes with IL-3 stimulation of megakaryocytes
    2. Induces the hepatic synthesis of acute phase proteins like IL-1 and IL-6
    3. Enhances antigen-specific B-cell responses
  vi. IL-15
    1. Shares biologic properties with IL-2
    2. Present in high concentration in RA joints
      a. Responsible for attracting and activating T cells
  vii. IL-16 is a chemoattractant for CD4+ cells
i. IL-17
  i. Produced by activated memory CD4+ T cells
  ii. Stimulates IL-1 and TNF-α production in human monocytes and macrophages
  iii. Induces MMP 1and 9 production by synovial fibroblasts
  iv. Enhances nitric oxide production by chondrocytes
  v. Decreases chondrocyte proliferation and proteoglycan synthesis
  vi. Stimulates osteoclast differentiation into bone-resorbing cells
  vii. Disease association
    1. Protein and mRNA present in high levels in the rheumatoid synovium
    2. A potential therapeutic strategy in RA
      a. Single injection of IL-17 into normal rabbit knees led to proteoglycan degradation
j. IL-18
  i. Produced by macrophages, keratinocytes, chondrocytes, fibroblasts, and osteoblasts
  ii. Production stimulated by IL-1 and TNF-α
  iii. Stimulates IFN-γ production by Th1 and NK cells
    1. Promotes a Th1 phenotype in combination with IL-12 and IL-15
  iv. Induces GM-CSF, IL-1, and TNF-α production by synovial macrophages
  v. Stimulates nitric oxide production by synovial cells
  vi. Effects in vivo may be counteracted by IL-18-binding protein, a naturally occurring inhibitor
  vii. Disease association
    1. Protein and mRNA present in high levels in the rheumatoid synovium

k. IFN-γ
    i. Produced simultaneous with IL-2 by antigen-stimulated T cells
    ii. Enhances antigen presentation by stimulating the expression of MHC class I and II molecules on macrophages, endothelial cells, and fibroblasts
    iii. Potent activator of macrophages, cytotoxic T lymphocytes (CTLs), and NK cells
    iv. Stimulates antibody production by B cells
       1. Opposes the effects of IL-4
    v. Disease associations
       1. RA
          a. Antagonizes the stimulatory effects of TNF-α
       2. SLE
5. Proinflammatory cytokines
  a. TNF-α
    i. Structurally resembles a transmembrane molecule
    ii. Production
       1. 1–2% resides in the plasma membrane
       2. Product of monocytes, macrophages, and lymphocytes
       3. Stimulated by endotoxin, viruses, and other cytokines
    iii. Induces collagenase and PGE2 production in synovial fibroblasts together with IL-1
    iv. TNF-α receptors
       1. p55 and p75
       2. Present on a variety of target cells
       3. The extracellular portions are cleaved by proteases releasing soluble receptors
          a. Function as regulators of extracellular TNF-α
    v. Disease association
       1. RA
          a. Present in synovial tissues
          b. May induce muscle breakdown
  b. IL-1
    i. Family has three known members
       1. IL-1α
          a. Membrane-bound
       2. IL-1β
          a. The major extracellular product
       3. IL-1Ra
          a. A specific naturally occurring inhibitor
          b. Competitively inhibits receptor binding of IL-1
    ii. IL-1α and β are primarily products of monocytes and macrophages
    iii. Two different IL-1 receptors
       1. Type I
          a. Present on T cells, endothelial cells, and fibroblasts
          b. Functionally active

    2. Type II

       a. Predominate on B cells, monocytes, and neutrophils

       b. Not capable of inducing intracellular signal

  iv. Target cells are very sensitive to small concentrations of IL-1

    1. Occupancy of only 1–2% of receptors stimulates a complete response

  v. Expression is downregulated by TGF-β

  vi. Disease associations

    1. Systemic effects include fever, muscle breakdown, and induction of acute phase reactants

    2. May contribute to tissue destruction in the RA joint by inducing PGE2 and collagenase production by synovial fibroblasts and by chondrocytes

    3. Induces chemotaxis of neutrophils, monocytes, and lymphocytes into the synovium

    4. Enhances expression of adhesion molecules on endothelial cells

c. IL-6

  i. Produced by synovial cells stimulated by IL-1 and TNF-α

  ii. Major functions

    1. Induces hepatic synthesis of acute phase proteins

    2. Enhances Ig synthesis by B cells

  iii. Disease associations

    1. RA

       a. Enhances synthesis of a collagenase inhibitor

    2. Hypergammaglobulinemia of chronic disease

d. IL-8

  i. Member of a family of chemotactic peptides

  ii. TNF-α and IL-1 stimulates production by monocytes, macrophages, endothelial cells, and fibroblasts

  iii. Roles in neutrophil function

    1. An extremely potent chemotactic factor

    2. Expression of adhesion molecules

    3. Generation of oxygen radicals

    4. Release of lysosomal enzymes

  iv. Disease associations

    1. RA and gout

       a. Attracts neutrophils into the joints

6. Five different mechanisms regulate the actions of cytokines

a. Specific receptor antagonists

  i. IL-1Ra

    1. The first known naturally occurring molecule that functions as a specific receptor antagonist

    2. A secreted form is produced by monocytes, macrophages, and neutrophils

    3. An intracellular variant (icIL-1Ra) lacks the structural characteristics that lead to secretion

       a. Produced by keratinocytes and other epithelial cells

    4. A major product of tissue macrophages

a. Alveolar and synovial macrophages synthesize large amounts under the influence of GM-CSF
5. Does not effect normal T- or B-cell responses
6. Disease associations
   a. Therapeutic effects in RA, inflammatory bowel disease (IBD), diabetes mellitus (DM), and asthma
   b. Clinical trials in RA
      i. Safe and efficacious
      ii. 43% experiencing ACR 20 compared with 27% placebo
   b. Soluble cytokine receptors
      i. Etanercept
         1. Extracellular portion of the p75 TNF receptor coupled to the human IgG1
         2. Clinical trials in RA
            a. 20% ACR in 59% patients compared with 11% placebo
            b. Combined with methotrexate (MTX), 20% ACR in 71% patients compared with 27% MTX alone
   c. Antibodies to cytokines
      i. Serum of normal individuals have antibodies to IL-1α, TNF-α, and IL-6
         1. Relevance not established
      ii. Infliximab
         1. Chimeric murine/human monoclonal antibody to TNF-α
         2. Clinical trials in RA
            a. 20% ACR in 50% with infliximab and MTX and 20% MTX alone
            b. Radiologic regression after 6–12 months
         3. Other responsive diseases
            a. JRA
            b. Psoriatic arthritis
            c. Ankylosing spondylitis (AS)
      iii. Complications of anti-TNF therapy
         1. Should not be administered to patients with active or latent infections
         2. The long-term risk of developing malignancies is not known
         3. Up to 15% of patients have developed antinuclear antibodies
            a. A few exhibit a reversible clinical SLE syndrome
   d. Opposing actions of different cytokines
   e. Protein binding of cytokines

Section C: The Complement System

1. The complement system provides an innate defense against microbes and a "complement" to humoral immunity
2. Early reaction sequences behave as biologic cascades
   a. One component activates the next
   b. A rapid and robust amplification of the system
3. Critical roles

      a. Normal handling of immune complexes (ICs)

      b. Clearance of apoptotic cells and tissue injured by ischemia-reperfusion

4. Two major functions

      a. Modifies membranes with pathogen destruction (gram-negative bacteria and viruses)

          i. Alters the membrane of a pathogen by coating its surface with clusters of complement (opsonization)

          ii. Opsonic fragments are ligands for complement receptors

             1. Facilitates interactions known as immune adherence

          iii. Induces lysis

             1. Additionally, the membranes of some microorganisms can be disrupted by the terminal complement components

      b. Promotes the inflammatory response

          i. Complement fragments such as C3a and C5a can activate cells to release their contents

          ii. Facilitates migration to inflammation (chemotaxis)

5. Predates adaptive immunity

      a. An ancestral version emerged more than 600 million years ago as a host defense system

6. The complement system consists of plasma and membrane proteins

      a. Plasma proteins

          i. Synthesized primarily in the liver

          ii. Produced locally by monocytes, macrophages, fibroblasts, and many types of epithelial cells

      b. Membrane proteins

          i. Receptors with limited tissue distribution

          ii. Primarily on peripheral blood cells

          iii. Widely expressed regulatory proteins

7. Complement activation

      a. Anaphylatoxins

          i. C4a, C3a, and C5a fragments trigger release of mediators

             1. Histamine released from mast cells and basophils

             2. Cause smooth muscle contraction and vascular permeability

      b. Chemotactic factors

          i. C5a and C3a stimulate phagocytic cells and eosinophils to move

8. Three branches of the complement system lead to the C3 activation complex and proceed to a common lytic pathway called the membrane attack complex (MAC)

      a. Classical pathway (CP)

          i. Discovered first (1890)

          ii. Activated primarily by an interaction between C1 and immune complexes

             1. C1 is a large multicomponent protein

                 a. A single molecule of C1q with six globular heads

                 b. A serine protease tetramer C1s-C1r-C1s-C1r

                 c. An immunoglobulin-binding domain

       2. At least two of the globular regions of C1q attach to the Fc portion of an antibody

       3. Antibodies involved in activation include

         a. IgM

         b. IgG subclasses 1, 2, 3,

         c. **Not** activated by IgA, IgD, IgE, and IgG4

       4. Other proteins involved in activation

         a. C-reactive protein

         b. Serum amyloid P

         c. C4 nephritic factor

  iii. Enzyme Activation

       1. C1 binds to antibody

       2. The C1r subcomponent undergoes an autoactivation cleavage process and cleaves C1s

       3. C1s in turn cleaves C4 into C4b and C2 into C2a

       4. C4b and C2a assemble on the target surface and on antibody

         a. Forms C4b2a, the C3 convertase or C3-cleaving enzyme

       5. C4b covalently attaches via ester of amide linkages

       6. C3 binds substrate via an ester linkage

  iv. Amplification

       1. Each activated C1 generates many C4b and C2a fragments

         a. Most C4bs serve as opsonins

       2. C3 convertase rapidly generates many activated C3 molecules

       3. Concomitantly anaphylatoxins (C4a, C3a, and C5a) are generated

         a. Equal to the number of C4b, C3b, and C5b fragments

  v. Attack

       1. Most C3bs serve as opsonins

       2. C5 convertase, C4b2a3b, is generated when C3bs bind to C4b in the C4b2a, C3 convertase complex

       3. C5 is the substrate for the trimeric C5 convertase enzymatic complex

       4. Generation of C5b leads to the formation of the MAC

         a. MAC consists of C5b, C6, C7, and multiple C9s

         b. MAC assembly occurs through protein–protein interaction

           i. No proteolysis is involved after C5 cleavage

b. Alternative pathway (AP)

  i. The antibody-independent pathway

  ii. An important surveillance or sentry-like role

  iii. A small amount of auto-activated C3 continuously turns over ("C3 tickover")

  iv. C3 bound to a microbe serves as the nidus for engagement of the pathway

  v. Activation

       1. Activated by LPS on microbial cell surfaces in the absence of antibody

       2. Activated by IgA complexes and C3 nephritic factor

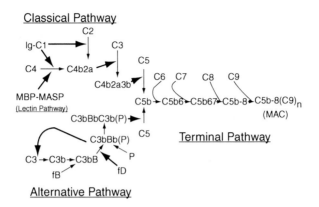

Fig. 2.1 The complement system and its control. Three constituent pathways and the component proteins are shown. Enzymatic cleavages are represented by thick arrows. The lectin pathway differs from the CP only in that the MBP–MASP complex replaces the C1 complex (Reproduced with permission from The complement system: an overview.*Complement Methods and Protocols.* DOI:10.1385/1-59259-056-X:1. Springer; 2000-01-01)

      3. Rapid amplification with foreign materials but blocked on host tissue by endogenous regulators

      4. Target-bound C3b binds factor B

      5. Factor B undergoes proteolytic cleavage mediated by the serine protease factor D and produces the fragments Bb and Ba

      6. Physiologic C3 convertase is formed (C3bBb) and stabilized by properdin

  vi. Amplification

      1. Auto-amplification with a feedback loop

        a. Stabilized C3 convertase cleaves more C3 into C3b

      2. Amplified C3b leads to large depositions on a target

      3. The MAC is also engaged

        a. C5 convertase (C3bBbC3bP) cleaves C5 to C5b and initiates assembly of the MAC

c. Lectin pathway

  i. Lectins are carbohydrate-binding proteins

  ii. Mannan-binding lectin (MBL)

      1. A serum protein secreted by the liver that preferentially binds to repeating mannoses on pathogens

      2. Resembles C1q (related to C1r and C1s)

      3. An oligomer with a terminal collagenous domain on one end and a globular domain on the other

      4. C-terminus possesses a carbohydrate-recognition domain

      5. Engagement leads to the activation of serine proteases called MASP-1 and MASP-2 (similar to C1r and C1s)

      6. MASP-1 and MASP-2 cleave C2 and C4

     7. Disease association

        a. Deficiency is associated with recurrent infections early in life

        b. A predisposing factor and a disease severity indicator for SLE and RA

9. Nomenclature

  a. CP proteins are identified by numbers

    i. C1, C2, C3, and C4

  b. AP proteins are identified by capital letters

    i. Factors B, D, and P

  c. MAC consists of C5, C6, C7, C8, and C9

  d. Smaller fragments are designated by a lowercase "a" (C3a)

  e. Larger fragments are noted with a "b" (C3b)

  f. Products further broken down are designated by lowercase letters

    i. C3b into iC3b

    ii. iC3b into C3c and C3dg

10. Complement Receptors

  a. Complement receptor 1 (CR1)

    i. An important role in IC clearance

    ii. Located on peripheral blood cells and follicular-dendritic cells

    iii. Functions

      1. Immune adherence

      2. Phagocytosis

      3. Antigen localization

    iv. On erythrocytes

      1. Primary ligand C3b/C4b

      2. Coated IC are processed and transported to the liver and spleen for transfer to tissue macrophages

    v. On granulocytes and monocytes

      1. Promote IC adherence

      2. Phagocytosis

    vi. On B lymphocytes, tissue macrophages, and follicular-dendritic cells

      1. Facilitates trapping and processing of ICs in lymphoid organs

  b. CR2

    i. Primary ligand C3dg/C3d

    ii. Expressed on B lymphocytes and follicular-dendritic cells

    iii. Facilitates antigen localization

    iv. A coreceptor for activation of the B-cell antigen receptor

  c. CR3/CR4

    i. Primary ligand iC3b

    ii. Located on the myeloid lineage

    iii. Functions in phagocytosis and adherence

11. Control of Complement

  a. Regulation of activation

    i. Excessive activation on one target

    ii. Fluid phase activation (no target)

         1. C1 inhibitor prevents excessive fluid phase C1 activation in the early phase of the CP

      iii. Activation on self (wrong target)

   b. Regulation of C3 and C5 convertases

      i. Membrane proteins decay-accelerating factor (CD55) and membrane cofactor protein (CD46)

         1. Disassemble the convertases (decay-accelerating activity)

      ii. Serum inhibitors C4b-binding protein and factor H

         1. Facilitate proteolytic inactivation of C4b or C3b

         2. Occurs in collaboration with serine protease factor I (cofactor activity)

   c. Regulation of MAC

      i. CD59 is a glycolipid-anchored protein that binds C8 and C9 to prevent proper MAC insertion

      ii. Vitronectin (S-protein) is a plasma protein that binds to and inactivates the fluid phase MAC

12. Inherited deficiencies of complement components predispose to bacterial infections (C3 deficiency) and autoimmunity (C1, 4, and 2 deficiency)

   a. C1q deficiency

      i. Inherited as autosomal codominant (recessive) trait

      ii. 90% present with lupus

      iii. Antibodies to C1q occur in 15–20% of SLE

         1. Pathogenesis unknown

      iv. Knockout mice develop a lupus syndrome with glomerulonephritis and ANA

      v. C1r or C1s deficiencies also present with SLE

   b. C1 inhibitor deficiency

      i. Inherited as autosomal dominant

      ii. Presents with hereditary angioedema

      iii. 40–50% present with lupus or a related rheumatic syndrome

   c. C2 deficiency

   d. C3 deficiency

      i. Presents with pyogenic infections

      ii. "C3 nephritic factor"

         1. An autoantibody against the AP C3 convertase

         2. Excessive C3 cleavage

         3. Clinical features

            a. Glomerulonephritis

            b. Partial lipodystrophy

            c. Frequent infections with capsulated bacteria

            d. Most are children

   e. Properdin deficiency

      i. Inherited as X-linked

      ii. Presents with *Neisseria meningitides*

 f. Factor D deficiency
  i. Inherited as X-linked
  ii. Presents with *Neisseria meningitides*
 g. Factor B deficiency
  i. Presents with *Neisseria meningitides*
 h. Factor H or I deficiency
  i. Presents with pyogenic infections
  ii. Secondary to deficiency of C3
 i. C4 deficiency
  i. 80% present with lupus
  ii. Partial deficiency also predisposes to lupus
  iii. C4 synthesized as two proteins
   1. C4A and C4B
    a. More than 99% homologous
  iv. C4 genes
   1. Two for C4A and two for C4B
    a. Tandemly arranged on chromosome 6 in the major histocompatibility locus
  v. C4A deficiency in SLE
   1. Part of a HLA haplotype containing B8 and DR3
   2. 10–15% of Caucasian SLE patients are homozygous for C4A deficiency
 j. MAC
  i. Deficiency of any one of the terminal complement components can result in recurrent infections with *Neisseria*
 k. Clinical features of lupus associated with complement deficiencies
  i. Early age of onset
  ii. Prominent cutaneous manifestations
  iii. Presence of anti-Ro antibodies
13. Complement Measurement
 a. Total hemolytic complement (THC) or CH50
  i. The most commonly used functional measurement
  ii. Based on the ability of the test serum to lyse sheep erythrocytes sensitized with rabbit antibody.
   1. A THC of 200 means that at a dilution of 1:200, the test serum lysed 50% of the antibody-coated sheep erythrocytes
  iii. All nine components of the CP (C1-C9) are required for a normal THC
  iv. A useful screening tool for detecting a homozygous deficiency of a complement component
   1. A total deficiency of any one of the C1-C8 components will produce a zero THC
   2. Deficiency of C9 will give a low but detectable THC
    b. C3, C4
     i. Widely available
     ii. Measured by nephelometric-based immunoassays

          iii. Various detection tests
             1. Activation fragments (C3a and C5a)
             2. Neoantigens
             3. Fragments of activation (C3d, C4d, and Bb)
       c. Complement inhibitors (used in trials)
          i. A monoclonal antibody to C5
          ii. A solubilized version of CR1

14. Interpretation of Complement Determinant Results
    a. Normal
       i. THC – 150–200 units/ml
      ii. C4 – 16–40 mg/dl
     iii. C3 – 100–180 mg/dl
    b. Acute Phase Response
       i. THC – 250 units/ml (INCREASED)
      ii. C4 – 40 mg/dl
     iii. C3 – 200 mg/dl (**INCREASED**)
    c. Classical Pathway Activation
       i. THC – 100 units/ml (DECREASED)
      ii. C4 – 10 mg/dl (DECREASED)
     iii. C3 – 80 mg/dl (**DECREASED**)
    d. Alternative Pathway Activation
       i. THC – 100 units/ml (**DECREASED**)
      ii. C4 – 30 mg/dl
     iii. C3 – 50 mg/dl (**DECREASED**)
    e. Inherited Deficiency or in vitro activation (more common)
       i. THC – <10 or 0 units/ml (**DECREASED**)
      ii. C4 – 30 mg/dl
     iii. C3 – 140 mg/dl
     iv. The lack of activity of THC in the setting of normal C4 and C3 suggests
          1. An improperly handled sample
          2. Cold activation (cryoglobulins) following collection
          3. Homozygous component deficiency
             a. C2 with a lupus presentation
             b. AP or MAC with a Neisserial infection
    f. Partial C4 deficiency or fluid phase activation
       i. THC – 50 units/ml (**DECREASED**)
      ii. C4 – <8 mg/dl (**DECREASED**)
     iii. C3 – 100 mg/dl (low normal)
     iv. Since THC is detectable, this is not a complete deficiency of C4 (partial C4A)
          1. A low value C2 suggests activation
          2. Normal C2 suggests an inherited partial C4 deficiency
      v. Types of ICs or a deficiency of the C1 inhibitor (hereditary angioedema) can also give this picture

Section D: Proteases and Their Inhibitors

1. There are three major degradative mechanisms for the turnover of ECM molecules
   a. Glycosidases
      i. Attack the carbohydrate components of proteoglycans and glycoproteins
      ii. Degraded by lysosomal enzymes only after endocytosis
      iii. Exception is heparanases
         1. Degrades GAGs of the HS proteoglycans extracellularly
   b. Free-radical attack and ROS
      i. Seen in inflammatory conditions
   c. Proteolytic enzymes (proteases, proteinases, or peptidases)
      i. Cleave peptide bonds with various degrees of selectivity
         1. Limited by the accessibility of the appropriate peptide bond
         2. Surface loops and unfolded areas are most susceptible to cleavage
      ii. Two modes of protein degradation
         1. Peptide chains trimmed from either end by exopeptidases
         2. Cleaved internally by endopeptidase action
            a. Immediate loss of function of most proteins
            b. Most important in joint destruction
2. Proteases classified into five major groups based on their catalytic centers provided by specific AA residues (serine, aspartic acid, or cysteine) or by a chelated metal ion (zinc)
   a. Serine Proteases
      i. The catalytic group is a hydroxyl moiety
      ii. The most abundant class
      iii. Active at neutral pH
      iv. Archetypical proteases of the digestive system
         1. Chymotrypsin
         2. Subtilisin
         3. Trypsin
      v. Proteases of PMNs
         1. Elastase
            a. Inhibited by alpha 1 proteinase inhibitor (antitrypsin)
         2. Cathepsin G
            a. Inhibited by alpha 1 antichymotrypsin and proteinase inhibitor
         3. Extremely destructive
      vi. Granzymes of mast cells and cytotoxic lymphocytes (A, B, M)
      vii. Plasmin
         1. The plasma protease in synovial fluid
         2. Cleaves fibrin and activates pro-MMPs
         3. Inhibited by protease nexins and alpha-1 antiplasmin
      viii. Plasminogen activators (tissue type and urokinase type)
         1. Generates plasmin
         2. Inhibited by protease nexins and plasminogen inhibitor 1 and 2

3. Kallikrein activates proplasminogen and factor XII
   a. Chemotaxic for neutrophils
   b. Inhibited by C1 inhibitor and alpha 2 macroglobulin
b. Threonine Proteases
   i. The catalytic group is a hydroxyl moiety provided by a threonine residue
   ii. Archetype – the proteasome
      1. Responsible for the turnover of such cytoplasmic proteins as NF-κB and its inhibitor IκB
      2. Participates in the processing of antigens for presentation through the class I pathway
c. Aspartic Proteases
   i. Catalytic group is COO-/COOH
   ii. Intracellular proteolysis
   iii. Requires low pH
   iv. Archetype – pepsin
   v. Major lysosomal protease cathepsin D
   vi. May play a role in the cleavage of amyloid precursor protein in Alzheimer's
d. Cysteine Proteases
   i. Catalytic group is S-
   ii. Divided into two structurally unrelated subclasses
      1. Caspase proteases- (**cysteine** protease, with specificity for**aspartic** acid, plus **"ase"** meaning enzyme)
         a. Mediators of the proteolytic events associated with programmed cell death (apoptosis)
         b. Caspase 1 (ICE), interleukin-converting enzyme, is responsible for activation of the precursor of IL-1
         c. All cleavage occurs following an aspartic acid residue
         d. Affected by the nature of other residues upstream and the sites overall accessibility
      2. Cathepsins – group of 11 human cysteine proteases
         a. Responsible for intracellular protein degradation in the lysosome
         b. Important role in antigen processing for presentation through the class II pathway
         c. Cathepsins B and L have extracellular roles
         d. Cathepsin K is the principal protease of the osteoclast
            i. Responsible for the degradation of the organic component of bone matrix
            ii. Can degrade native fibrillar collagen
e. Metalloproteases
   i. Most important mediators of extracellular degradation
   ii. Catalytic group is Zn2+ bound to the active site
   iii. Active at neutral pH
   iv. Either secreted in the ECM or anchored at the cell surface
   v. Divided into three families

1. Matrix metalloproteases (MMP)
   a. Responsible for degradation of collagen and matrix molecules
   b. 20 family members including four true collagenases (MMP1, 8, 13, and 14)
   c. Collagenases
      i. Hemopexin, a C-terminal domain, responsible for binding the enzyme to triple helical collagen
      ii. Cooperation between hemopexin and the catalytic domain allows individual chains to become accessible
   d. Gelatinases
      i. MMP-2 and 9
         1. MMP-9 involved in angiogenesis
      ii. Contain additional fibronectin type II repeats that aid in binding denatured collagen
   e. Stromelysins
      i. MMP-3 and 11
         1. MMP-11 has a furin activation cleavage site
      ii. Substrates are pro-MMP-3 and aggrecan
   f. MMP-7 (matrilysin)
      i. Substrates are proenzymes and fibronectin
      ii. Lacks hemopexin domain
      iii. Mainly in monocytes and epithelial cells
   g. MMP-12
      i. A macrophage elastase
      ii. Substrate elastin
      iii. Absence results in emphysema
   h. MT-MMPs
      i. Membrane type MMPs
      ii. Localized to the plasma membrane through a C-terminal trans-membrane domain
      iii. Restricted protease activity
      iv. MMP-14
         1. Substrate is pro-MMP-13
         2. Required for angiogenesis and bone development.
         3. A furin cleavage site
2. The ADAMs – a disintegrin and a metalloprotease
   a. Membrane localized
   b. Contain a disintegrin domain in addition to the catalytic unit
   c. Disintegrin domain binds to cell-surface integrins disrupting them from the ECM
   d. ADAM-17
      i. Tumor necrosis factor alpha converting enzyme (TACE)
      ii. Processes the cell surface form of TNF-α to the soluble cytokine
3. The ADAMTS – a disintegrin and a metalloprotease, with thrombos-pondin motif

   a. Lack a membrane-spanning domain
   b. Contain one or more thrombospondin motifs which assist with sub-
      strate binding to GAGs
   c. Aggrecanases, ADAMTS-4, and ADAMTS-5
      i. The principle mediators of aggrecan degradation
      ii. Cleave aggrecan core protein following glutamic acid residues
          at five unique sites
      iii. A furin activation/cleavage site
3. Protease Activation
   a. Proteases are synthesized as inactive proenzymes processed to their functional
      forms by two proteolytic mechanisms
      i. Autoprocessing
         1. Results in the removal of the inhibitory proregion of the cathepsin
            cysteine proteases
      ii. Propeptide cleavage by a processing protease
         1. Pro-hormone convertase furin, a Golgi-resident serine protease,
            cleaves at specific processing sites in MMP-11, 14, and aggrecanase
         2. The propiece of other MMPs is removed by the action of other active
            MMPs or serine proteases
            a. Pro-MMP-13 can be activated by MMP-2, 3 (in cartilage), or 14 (in
               bone and skin), or plasmin
            b. The proregion of the MMPs interacts with the active site zinc ion
               through a cysteine residue in the propeptide
               i. "Cysteine-switch" mechanism
                  1. Disrupted with organomercurial aminophenylmercuric acetate
                     (APMA)
4. Regulation of Metalloprotease Activity
   a. Synthesis or degradation modulated by the presence of extracellular signaling
      molecules and matrix molecule degradation products
      i. MMP upregulation
         1. IL-1 and/or TNF
         2. IL-1 with FGF-2 or oncostatin M
         3. FGF-2 upregulates IL-1 receptor expression
      ii. MMP suppression
         1. INF-γ, IGF-1, and TGF-β
            a. Negates the stimulatory effects of IL-1
            b. TGF-β suppresses IL-1 receptor expression
      iii. MMP activation and suppression
         1. Type I collagen and fibronectin fragments
         2. Mediated by different cell-surface integrin receptors
         3. Process determined by the sites of proteolysis
   b. Gene Expression for MMPs
      i. The first point of control for protease production is at the level of transcription
         1. Activated Protein-1 (AP-1) binding site

      a. Present within the promoter region of all MMPs except MMP-2

      b. Plays a dominant role in the suppression of MMP gene expression induced by TGF-β and glucocorticoids

        i. TGF-β inhibits MMP-3 through the TGF inhibitory element inducing Fos expression

    2. Fos and Jun transcription factors

      a. TNF-α induces a prolonged increase

    3. Cbfa1 (runt family member)

      a. Regulates MMP-13 expression in hypertrophic chondrocytes

5. Protease Inhibitors

  a. Inhibitors of cathepsin cysteine proteases

    i. The large cystatins family

  b. Inhibitors of serine proteases

    i. Alpha-1 antitrypsin and antichymotrypsin

      1. Present in synovial fluid

      2. Neutralizes soluble elastase and cathepsin G released from PMNs

  c. Tissue inhibitors of metalloproteases (TIMPs)

    i. Principal regulators of proteolysis in connective tissue

    ii. 2-domain proteins

      1. An inhibitory domain that binds to the active site of the MMP

      2. A second domain with alternate binding specificities

    iii. Activation of pro-MMP-2 requires a TIMP

      1. A trimolecular interaction with TIMP-2 links MMP-14 and pro-MMP-2 through its first and second domains allowing a second molecule of MMP-14 to cleave pro-MMP2

6. Mechanisms of Fibrillar Collagen Cleavage

  a. Collagen helix generally resistant to proteolysis

  b. Telopeptides susceptible to proteases

    i. Elastase

    ii. Cathepsin G

    iii. MMP-3

  c. Cleavage produces a characteristic ¾ and ¼ fragment (TCa and TCb)

  d. Collagenases cleave all three chains at a region three quarters distance along the molecule

  e. Primary cleavage sites of type I collagen

    i. Gly775-Ile in the a1i. chain

    ii. Gly775-Leu in the a2i. chain

  f. Cleavage of type II collagen

    i. Gly-Ile bond of the three a1(II) chains

  g. Cleavage of type III collagen

    i. Gly-Leu bond

  h. Once cleaved, chains unwind and are susceptible to stromelysin (MMP-3) and the gelatinases (MMP-2 and MMP-9)

7. Collagenases
    a. MMP-1
        i. Most effective collagenase for cleaving type III collagen
    b. MMP-8
        i. A PMN product
        ii. Digests both types I and II collagens
        iii. Does not cleave type II native fibrils
    c. MMP-13
        i. Most effective collagenase for cleaving type II collagen
    d. MMP-14
    e. Cathepsin K
        i. An osteoclast product
        ii. Functions optimally under acidic conditions
        iii. Cleaves the C-terminal telopeptide
        iv. Releases a telopeptide fragment and its accompanying intermolecular cross-links
        v. Able to cleave the triple helix at multiple sites
8. Sequence of Events During Extracellular Matrix Degradation
    a. Proteolysis is induced by inflammatory molecules such as TNF-α and IL-1
    b. Aggrecan is cleaved first
        i. Initially by aggrecanases of the ADAMTS family and later MMPs
    c. The NC4 (noncollagenous) domain of the a1(IX) chain is removed
    d. Followed by loss of COL2 (collagenous) domain of the a1(IX) chain
    e. Cleavage of type II collagen
        i. The delay after aggrecan cleavage may be up to 1 week in articular cartilage
    f. Type XI collagen degradation
        i. Occurs early together with cleavage of type II collagen
    g. Fibromodulin susceptible to early cleavage
    h. Leucine-rich fibrillar associated proteoglycans are very resistant to proteolysis
        i. Decorin
        ii. Biglycan
        iii. Lumican
    i. Disease Association
        i. Advanced OA fibril damage is accompanied by loss of biglycan and decorin
        ii. In established arthritis cleavage of aggrecan and type II collagen are seen at the same sites
        iii. Lost fibrils lead to permanent and irreparable damage to articular cartilage
            1. No effective way of retaining macromolecular aggregates of aggrecan
9. Articular Cartilage Resorption in Arthritis
    a. Hypertrophic chondrocytes produce MMP-13
        i. Capable of rapid cleavage of type II collagen fibrils in cartilage
    b. Principal intra-articular sources of MMPs and other proteases in arthritis
        i. Chondrocytes
        ii. PMNs

     iii. Synovial cells in RA

     iv. Chondrocytes in OA

  c. Neutrophils in RA

     i. Release elastase, cathepsin G, and MMP-1

     ii. Degrades aggrecan at the articular surface with adherence and activation of Fc receptors

     iii. No role in type II collagen degradation

  d. RA and OA have distinguishable sites in cartilage degradation

     i. RA

       1. Cleavage of aggrecan by MMPs occurs at the articular surface

         a. Accompanied by a loss of metachromatic staining toluidine blue

       2. Type II collagen denaturation is intense around chondrocytes adjacent to pannus and subchondral bone

       3. Chondrocytes generate or activate collagenases in response to inflammatory signals, such as IL-1 and TNF-α

     ii. OA

       1. Loss of aggrecan and type II collagen starts at and close to the articular surface around chondrocytes

       2. Loss extends progressively into the middle and deep zones

       3. Cleavage of collagen is accompanied by the loss of aggrecan and collagen fibril associated proteoglycans (decorin)

       4. Biglycan is lost from superficial sites

       5. Resorptive process driven by changes in the ECM and abnormal loading, not by inflammation

10. Proteases and Angiogenesis

  a. New vessels formation and capillary invasion is required for synovial hyperplasia

  b. MMP-9 is concentrated in sites of angiogenesis

  c. MMP-14 null mice exhibit a delay in the formation of the secondary center of ossification as a result of impaired vascular invasion

  d. Endothelial cells involved in angiogenesis need MMP-14 expressed on the cell surface to permit invasion

  e. MT1-MMP and MT2-MMP (MMP-15) expression permits invasion of type I collagen-rich tissues

  f. Disease Association

  i. Clinical trials for treatment of joint disease with MMP inhibitors

Section E: Arachidonic Acid Derivatives, Reactive Oxygen Species, and Others

1. Molecules linked by arachidonic acid (AA) derivation (prostaglandins, lipoxins, and leukotrienes) or signals necessary for their production (prostaglandins, reactive oxygen species, and nitric oxide)

2. Prostanoids are lipid mediators derived from arachidonic acid (arachidonyl-containing lipids)

    a. Prostaglandins (PGs)
       i. Short-lived active compounds
      ii. Act in an autocrine, paracrine, or endocrine manner
     iii. Derived predominantly from AA stored as phosphatidylinositol and phosphatidylcholine in the cellular membrane of all cells
    b. Thromboxanes
    c. Isoprostanes
3. Prostaglandin synthesis
    a. The first step is release of AA from membrane phospholipids
       i. The key rate-determining step
      ii. Occurs via the enzyme phospholipase A2 (or phospholipase C2)
         1. Lipomodulin is a natural inhibitor of phospholipase A2
         2. Lipomodulin expression is stimulated by glucocorticoids
    b. Fates for released AA
       i. Oxidized directly
      ii. Converted to prostaglandins, thromboxanes, or leukotrienes
4. Cyclooxygenase (COX) is the first enzyme from AA release to prostaglandin synthesis (also called prostaglandin H synthase (PGHS))
5. Two forms of COX
    a. COX1
       i. Expressed constitutively
      ii. Homeostatic roles
         1. Gastric mucosal protection
         2. Renal hemodynamics
         3. Platelet thrombogenesis
     iii. Message is long-lived and stable
    b. COX2
       i. Expressed in fibroblasts, endothelial cells, and macrophages
      ii. Induced by cytokines, mitogens, and tumor promoters
     iii. Induced in both physiologic and pathologic settings
         1. Human kidney during salt restriction
         2. Around atherosclerotic plaques
         3. Alzheimer's brain lesions
         4. Malignant neoplasms
            a. Can inhibit apoptosis and increase proliferation
6. Cyclooxygenases catalyze two sequential reactions that require heme as a cofactor
    a. First – oxygen is incorporated into AA, ring closure occurs, yielding the first unstable prostaglandin structure PGG2
    b. Second – PGG2 is reduced to PGH2
       i. Accelerated by the presence of lipid hydroperoxides or peroxynitrite
         1. Formed by inflammatory cells, such as PMNs and macrophages
      ii. PGH2 is converted by various isomerases to other biologically active PGs (or can be isomerized to thromboxane A2)
         1. PGD2
         2. PGI2

      3. PGE2
         a. A cytoplasmic, constitutively expressed isoform linked function-
            ally with COX1
         b. An inducible membrane-associated molecule linked functionally
            with COX-2 (role in inflammation)
      4. PGF2
7. Prostaglandin Receptors
   a. Members of the family of receptors characterized by seven membrane-span-
      ning domains
      i. Interact with G proteins for intracellular signal transduction
   b. There are eight surface receptors
      i. Four are PGE2 receptors
         1. EP1
         2. EP2
         3. EP3
         4. EP4
      ii. One is a PGD2 receptor
         1. DP
      iii. One is a PGI2 receptor
         1. IP
      iv. One is a PGF2a
         1. IF
      v. One is a TXA2 receptor
         1. TP
   c. All are expressed on smooth muscle
      i. EP1-4 and TP are expressed in the kidney
   d. Stimulation of EP2, EP4, IP, and DP
      i. Raises intracellular cAMP and leads to smooth muscle relaxation
      ii. IP inhibits platelet aggregation
      iii. EP2 and 4 are expressed in the glomerulus
         1. Role in reducing blood pressure
   e. Stimulation of EP1, FP, and TP
      i. Increase signaling via the inositol triphosphate/diacylglycerol pathway
        and leads to smooth muscle contraction
      ii. TP induces platelet aggregation
      iii. EP1 has a role in renal sodium transport
   f. Stimulation of EP3 reduces cAMP and leads to vasoconstrictive effects
8. PGE2 and PGI2 have proinflammatory effects leading to vasodilation and
  increased vascular permeability
   a. PGI2
      i. IP
         1. Knockout mice have impaired inflammation
   b. PGE2
      i. EP1 receptor
         1. Knockout fail to develop colon cancer

      ii. EP2 receptor
         1. Induced in macrophages by inflammatory stimuli
         2. Act in negative feedback
      iii. EP3 receptor
         1. Induces T-cell migration
         2. Influences production of metalloproteinases
         3. Plays a role in the febrile response
      iv. EP4 receptor
         1. Expressed constitutively by macrophages
         2. Act in negative feedback
           a. Knockout do not develop inflammatory osteoclast bone resorption

9. PGJ2 is formed by dehydration of PGD2
   a. Metabolites have anti-inflammatory properties
      i. The metabolite 15-deoxy D12, 14 PGJ2 is successful in treating adjuvant-induced arthritis in rats
   b. Acts in part through the nuclear receptor peroxisome proliferator activated receptor gamma (PPAR-γ)
      i. PPAR-γ agonist are diabetic drugs of the thiazolidinedione class (rosigitazone and pioglitazone)

10. Thromboxane A2 (TXA2)
   a. Derived from AA with the initial steps catalyzed by the COXs
   b. TX synthase converts PGH2 to TXA2
      i. Blocking TXA2 synthesis results in improvement in renal function
   c. TXA2 has a 6-carbon ring (5-member ring characterizes prostaglandins)
      i. Key mediator in inflammatory renal disease and asthma
      ii. High levels in murine lupus
      iii. High levels in the kidney lead to
         1. Vasoconstriction
         2. Platelet aggregation
         3. Mesangial cell contraction
         4. Increased production of ECM
         5. Decreased renal function
   d. TXA2 receptor TP
      i. Expressed in the kidney, on epithelial cells, platelets, smooth muscle of the arterial system, venous system, and pulmonary airways
      ii. Stimulation leads to
         1. Smooth muscle contraction
         2. Platelet aggregation
         3. Increased intestinal secretion
         4. Increased glomerular filtration
   e. Disease Associations
      i. Lupus
         1. Antagonism of the TP receptor in murine lupus nephritis reduces disease
      ii. Thymic development
         1. Induces cell death in developing thymocytes
         2. A role in negative selection

    iii. Asthma
1. Increased metabolites of TXA2
2. Agents that block production or the receptor are effective in treating bronchospasm
    iv. Systemic sclerosis
1. The role of TXA2 as a vasoconstrictor important in the development of Raynaud's phenomenon
2. Elevated levels of renally excreted systemic TXA2 metabolite
11. Leukotrienes (LTs)
   a. Produced primarily from AA released from phospholipase A2 in the cellular membrane
   b. Phospholipase–AA complex translocates to the nuclear membrane
   c. 5-lipooxygenase (5-LO) migrates from the cytoplasm to the nuclear membrane
   d. 5-lipooxygenase-activating protein (FLAP) is necessary for the series of reactions that convert AA to LTs
     i. Facilitates the transfer of AA from phospholipase A2 to 5-LO
   e. 5-LO converts AA to 5-hydroperoxyeicosa-tetranoic acid (5-HPETE) by a dioxygenase reaction
   f. 5-HPETE is transformed to LTA4 by a dehydrase activity
   g. LTA4 enters divergent pathways
     i. LTA4 hydrolase converts to LTB4 by the addition of H20
     ii. LTC4 is converted to LTD4 by the action of gamma-glutamyl transferase
     iii. LTD4 with removal of the terminal glycine by dipeptidase produces LTE4
   h. Cysteinyl or peptide leukotrienes
     i. The majority of biologic activity in the slow reacting substance of anaphylaxis (SRS-A)
     ii. Cause constriction of respiratory, gastrointestinal (GI), and vascular smooth muscle
     iii. Other actions include
1. Increase vascular permeability
2. Constrict mesangial cells
3. Stimulate bronchial mucus secretion
4. Inhibit ciliary function
5. Enhance mucosal edema
     iv. Examples include
1. LTE4
2. LTC4
3. LTD4
i. Noncysteinyl LT
     i. LTB4
     ii. Results in degranulation and release of reactive oxygen species and proteolytic enzymes
     iii. A potent chemoattractant for PMNs
     iv. Effects lymphocytes
1. Enhances the effect of gamma interferon on activation
2. Inhibits apoptosis of thymic T cells

      3. Induces differentiation of resting B cells

      4. Enhances proliferation and synthetic responses of B cells

  j. Receptors for LTs are the 7-domain transmembrane motif signaling through G proteins

    i. LTB4 receptors are found on PMN and lymphocytes

    ii. LTC4 receptors are found on respiratory, GI, and vascular epithelia

  k. Disease Associations

    i. Asthma

      1. Treatment includes pharmacologic agents, montelukast and zafirlukast, which targets the cysteinyl LT receptor

12. Lipoxins

  a. Derived from AA through lipooxygenase activity (like leukotrienes)

  b. Lipooxygenases 12-LO and 15-LO produce 12- or 15- HPETE

    i. Form LXA4 and LXB4

  c. Produced primarily by PMNs and platelets

  d. Vasodilatory and immunomodulatory

  e. Disease Associations

    i. Found in inflammatory lesions of arthritis and glomerulonephritis

13. Kinins

  a. A group of proteins activated in a sequence cascade

  b. Prekallikreins produce kallikrein when cleaved via trauma, immunologic signals or plasmin

  c. Plasma kallikrein acts on high molecular weight kininogen to produce bradykinin (a nonpeptide)

  d. Tissue kallikrein acts on low molecular weight kininogen to release kallidin (similar properties to bradykinin)

  e. Ubiquitous throughout all tissues with a wide spectrum of activities

    i. Stimulate smooth muscle contraction and bronchospasm

    ii. Increase vascular permeability and induce hypotension

    iii. Enhance the release of phospholipids,

      1. Frees AA for the production of PGs and LTs

  f. Dipeptidases are natural inhibitors of bradykinin

    i. Kininase II, a dipeptidase, is identical to angiotensin-converting enzyme (ACE)

    ii. ACE blocks the function of kinase II

      1. ACE inhibitors may block the metabolic breakdown of bradykinin

        a. Inhibits the inhibitor

        b. Bad in situations where bradykinin is overproduced

  g. Disease Association

    i. Proinflammatory in RA joints

14. Coagulation System

  a. Proinflammatory components of the coagulation and fibrinolytic systems

    i. Hageman factor activates the kinin system

    ii. Fibrin split products are potent chemoattractants for PMNs

    iii. Plasmin is capable of cleaving C3

    iv. Fibrin stimulates IL-1 and IL-8 and plays a key role in early scarring and fibrosis

15. Vasoactive Amines
   a. Histamine
       i. Stored in mast cell granules and released by IgE binding to antigen
      ii. Clinical effects
           1. Vasodilation
           2. Increased vascular permeability
           3. Bronchoconstriction
           4. Increased mucus
   b. Serotonin
       i. Stored primarily in dense body granules of platelets
      ii. Cause vasoconstriction and increased vascular permeability
     iii. Disease Association
           1. Blocking serotonin can cause fibrotic changes
           2. The drug methysergide maleate leads to retroperitoneal fibrosis
   c. Adenosine
       i. Anti-inflammatory effects at the site of its release
           1. Blocks AA release
           2. Limits PG and LT production
      ii. An agent used for blocking tachyarrhythmias
     iii. Methotrexate (MTX)
           1. Effects may be mediated by adenosine
           2. Promotes accumulation of the compound 5-aminoimidazole-4-car-
              boxamide ribonucleotide (AICAR)
              a. Enhances local release of adenosine
           3. Adding adenosine deaminase breaks down adenosine and decreases
              the anti-inflammatory action
      iv. Disease Associations
           1. Accumulation seen in adenosine deaminase deficiency leads to toxic
              effects on lymphocytes
16. Nitric Oxide (NO)
   a. The active moiety of nitroprusside and nitroglycerin
   b. Derived from the amino acid arginine through the enzyme NO synthase (NOS)
       i. Three forms of NOS derived from three genes
           1. Two forms, endothelial and neuronal, are expressed constitutively
              a. Depend on calcium and calmodulin
              b. Both produce NO that maintains vascular tone and neurotransmission
           2. Third form is inducible (iNOS)
              a. Primarily in immune cells, macrophages and macrophage-derived cells
                  i. Kills intracellular organisms and tumors
              b. Also on endothelial cells, some neuronal cells, PMNs, lymphocytes,
                 and NK cells
              c. Directly affects prostanoid synthesis
                  i. Peroxynitrite directly oxidizes arachidonyl-containing lipids to form
                     isoprostanes
                     1. 50% of increased PGF2 levels in iNOS knockout mice is iNOS
                        derived

    c. A potent vasodilator

    d. Causes direct tissue injury by interfering with the enzymes of the respiratory burst chain

    e. Interacts with superoxide to form peroxynitrite

      i. Peroxynitrite can nitrate tyrosine residues and oxidize cysteine, tryptophan, and tyrosine residues in protein altering their function

    f. Disease Associations

      i. Overproduction of NO is seen in patients with RA, SLE, and UC

      ii. Blocking the production of NO with arginine analogs, N-monomethyl arginine (NMMA), prevented or treated autoimmunity in animal models of arthritis, diabetes, MS, and SLE

17. Reactive Oxygen Species (ROS)

    a. Addition of one electron to oxygen forms the superoxide radical O_2^-

    b. Subtracting 2 electrons via superoxide dismutase (SOD) forms hydrogen peroxide

    c. When hydrogen peroxide reacts with iron (Fenton reaction), the hydroxyl radical is formed OH^-

    d. Oxygen radicals are important in PMN's ability to kill bacteria

    e. Disease Associations

      i. The pathogenesis of chronic granulomatous disease is the defect in the generation of superoxides by PMNs

      ii. PMNs from knockout mice with an inactivated subunit of cytochrome b oxidase could not produce superoxide

        1. Mice were susceptible to staph and fungal infections

Immunity

3

Section A: Molecular and Cellular Basis

1. Overview of the Immune System
   a. The innate immune response
      i. Skin and mucosa barriers
      ii. Phagocytic cells of the myelomonocytic lineage
      iii. Serum constituents such as complement
      iv. NK cells
         1. A lymphocyte subset that lack specific antigen receptors
         2. Recognize and kill virus-infected cells and tumors that lack or have low levels of MHC I molecules
         3. Not MHC restricted and not antigen specific
         4. Regulate adaptive immunity by the production of cytokines
         5. Activated by IL-15
         6. Large granular lymphocytes with numerous cytoplasmic granules
         7. Granules contain perforin (pore-forming protein) and granzymes
            a. Insert perforin into cells and secrete granzymes through the pore
            b. Granzymes attack the cell leading to apoptosis
         8. Classically express the CD16 and CD56 cell surface marker
         9. Also kill through antibody-dependent mechanism
            a. IgG bound to target cells interacts with Fc receptors (CD16) on NK cells causing release of lytic enzymes
         10. Disease Associations
            a. NK cells are numerous in skin biopsies of patients with graft-versus-host disease (GVHD)
            b. Expanded in LGL syndrome and in some patient with Felty's syndrome
   b. The adaptive response consists of
      i. T and B lymphocytes
      ii. Further divided into

---

    1. Humoral immunity
       a. B cell and immunoglobulins
    2. Cell-mediated immunity
       a. T cell and APC-dependent response
       b. Important in host defense against viruses, parasites, fungi, and mycobacteria
  c. Both systems include
    i. Antigen-presenting cells (APC)
      1. Direct host defense activity and promote T-cell responses
      2. Dendritic cells
      3. Macrophages
  d. Sites where B-cell differentiation occurs and T and B cells engage antigen
    i. Spleen
    ii. Lymph nodes
    iii. Peyer's patches in the intestine
  e. Chemokine receptors
    i. Varying levels of expression, responsiveness, and production affect migration patterns of immune cells
      1. HIV gains entry into permissive cells by CCR5 and CXCR4
2. Antigens and Antigen-Presenting Cells
  a. Lymphocytes recognize antigen by virtue of clonally specific antigen receptors
    i. B cells
      1. Recognize peptides, proteins, nucleic acids, polysaccharides, lipids, and small synthetic molecules
      2. Antigens bind directly to the B cell antigen receptor (BCR)
        a. A membrane associated form of immunoglobulin
      3. No need for APC
    ii. T-cells
      1. Need antigen to be presented
        a. T-cell receptor (TCR) recognizes peptide fragments of a processed larger protein antigen only when bound to the groove of MHC molecules
      2. Exception is the stimulation of T-cells by super antigen
        a. A superantigen is a molecule of bacterial or viral origin that directly interacts with MHC class II outside of the groove
         i. The V_β region in the TCR
        b. Results in direct T-cell activation and large amounts of T-cells
         i. An example is toxic shock syndrome caused by a staphylococcal exotoxin
3. MHC Molecules
  a. Two types of MHC molecules
    i. Class I
    ii. Class II
  b. The 3-D structure of both classes creates a cleft, or groove in which peptides are bound and recognized by T-cells

c. Each MHC molecule binds a single peptide, but the pool of MHC molecules produced can bind an array of peptides

d. Class I MHC molecules

   i. Primary function is to present **endogenous** peptides

   ii. Expressed on nearly all cells

   iii. Consist of two subunits

      1. An α chain encoded by genes within the HLA locus

         a. HLA-A

         b. HLA-B

         c. HLA-C

      2. A non-MHC-encoded protein

         a. β2-microglobulin

   iv. Bind degraded fragments of proteins, including peptides derived from pathogens (viruses), 9–11 AA in length

      1. Degraded cytosolic proteins in the proteasome are transported to the ER by peptide transporter molecules encoded within the MHC locus

      2. In the ER, class I molecules are synthesized and assembled

      3. Nascent MHC molecules associate with peptides and translocate to the plasma membrane

      4. MHC I/peptide complexes are recognized by T-cells

   v. CD-8

      1. A coreceptor

      2. T-cell accessory molecule that binds to class I molecules in a region distinct from the TCR

      3. Class I restricted

      4. Cytotoxic

         a. Destroys virally infected cells

e. Class II MHC molecules

   i. Primary function is to present **exogenous** peptides

   ii. Composed of two chains that are products of different MHC genes

      1. HLA-DR

      2. HLA-DQ

      3. HLA-DP

   iii. A limited array of cells express class II

      1. B-cells

      2. Macrophages

      3. DCs

      4. Activated T-cells

      5. Activated endothelial cells

   iv. Antigen processing occurs in three steps

      1. Ingested

      2. Internalized

      3. Proteolyzed

   v. The complex associates with a molecule called the invariant chain

      1. The invariant chain must be cleaved and removed by the action of proteases and HLA-DM

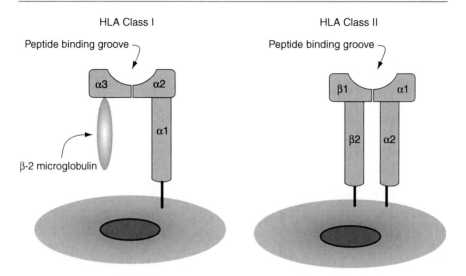

Fig. 3.1 Structure of class I and class II MHC proteins. HLA class I (Reproduced with permission from What is histocompatibility testing and how is it done?*Kidney Transplantation: A Guide to the Care of Kidney Transplant Recipients*. DOI:10.1007/978-1-4419-1690-7_4. Springer; 2010-01-01)

       2. Prevents endogenous peptide antigen binding
     vi. Binds peptides 10–30 AA in length
    vii. CD4
       1. A coreceptor
       2. Class II restricted
       3. 60% of all T-cells
  f. MHC-related CD1 family
     i. Lipid antigen presentation to T cells
    ii. γδ T-cells recognize nonpeptide antigen
      1. Prenyl pyrophosphate derivatives of mycobacteria
4. TCR Complex Antigen Recognition
  a. Subunits encoded by four TCR genes
     i. α
    ii. β
    iii. γ
    iv. δ
  b. Antigen-recognition unit combined as αβ and γδ heterodimeric receptors
  c. DNA rearrangement of variable (V), diversity (D), joining (J), and constant (C) region segments
     i. Recombination generated by
      1. Recombinase-activating genes
        a.RAG-1
        b.RAG-2

      2. Terminal deoxytransferase

        a. The insertion of random nucleotides at junctions

    ii. Allows for tremendous diversity

      1. Potentially 10^{16} $\alpha\beta$ receptors

    iii. V-regions are highly polymorphic

  d. Allelic exclusion by TCR genes

    i. If one chromosome undergoes rearrangement and produces a functional receptor chain, genes on the other chromosome are prevented from rearranging

    ii. Each T-cell clone expresses only one antigen receptor

    iii. Antigen-specific T cells develop in unimmunized or naïve individuals independent of exposure to antigen

    iv. Subsequent antigen exposure leads to clonal selection

      1. Improves the efficiency of the immune response

      2. Produces immunologic memory

  e. Antigen recognizing subunits associate with signaling subunits called invariant chains

    i. Not polymorphic

    ii. Include the CD3 family of molecules (γ, δ, ε, and ζ)

      1. The ζ chain can exist as a homodimer (ζ-ζ) or as a heterodimer (ζ-η)

        a. η is an alternative spliced form of ζ

      2. Usual TCR stoichiometry is TCR$\alpha\beta$/CD3$\gamma\delta\varepsilon_2\zeta_2$

5. TCR Complex Signal Transduction

  a. Invariant chains on tyrosine residues are phosphorylated by protein tyrosine kinases (PTK)

    i. Lck

      1. Binds CD4 and CD8

      2. Phosphorylates invariant chains

    ii. CD45

      1. A tyrosine phosphatase

    iii. Immune tyrosine-based activation motifs (ITAMs)

      1. Phosphorylated sites on the γ, δ, ε, and ζ subunits of CD3

      2. Consist of 17 AA with a duplicated sequence

        a. Tyrosine-X-X-leucine

        b. X denotes any AA

      3. Present on other receptors

        a. B-cell

        b. Fc receptors

      4. Docking sites for proteins with SH2 (Src homology 2) domains

    iv. Zeta-associated protein of 70 kDa (Zap 70) (PTK)

      1. Binds TCR ITAMs via SH2 domains

      2. Together with Itk leads to phosphorylation of the adapter protein LAT (linker of activated T-cells)

        a. Phosphorylated LAT binds other adaptor proteins that have SH2 domains

          i. Grb2

        ii. Gads

        iii. SLP-76

        iv. Affect other pathways

           1. The cascade of serine-threonine kinases activated by Ras

        v. Itk (PTK)

  b. Phospholipase C (PLC)γ catalyzes cleavage of phosphatidylinositol bisphosphate (PIP2)

     i. PIP2 produces

       1. Diacylglycerol

        a. Activates protein kinase C

       2. Inositol triphosphate

        a. Releases intracellular calcium

          i. Elevated calcium activates calcineurin

           1. Dephosphorylates nuclear factor of activated T cells (NFAT)

            a. NFAT translocates to the nucleus

           2. Blocked by the immunosuppressive drugs cyclosporine and FK506

  c. ITIMs (immunoreceptor tyrosine-based inhibitory motif)

     i. Inhibitory lymphocyte receptors motifs

     ii. Recruit phosphatases

     iii. NK inhibitory receptors

6. Costimulatory molecules (the second signal)

  a. CD28

     i. TCR stimulation in the absence of CD 28 leads to anergy (unresponsiveness)

     ii. Interference of CD28 signaling in murine lupus ameliorates autoimmune disease

     iii. Counter-receptors expressed on APC

       1. B7-1 (CD80)

       2. B7-2 (CD86)

  b. CTLA-4

     i. A molecule related to CD28

     ii. Also binds B7-1 and B7-2

     iii. Functions to downregulate the immune response

       1. CTLA-4 KO mice develop lethal lymphoproliferative disease

  c. CD11a/CD18

  d. CD2

     i. Interacts with CD58

  e. CD40 (on APCs and B-cells) and CD40 ligand (on activated T-cells)

     i. CD40

       1. Occupancy activates APCs to produce such cytokines as IL-12

     ii. CD40L (CD154)

       1. Mutations are the basis of the primary immunodeficiency X-linked hyper-IgM syndrome

        a. X-linked

       b. T cells cannot interact with CD40 on B-cells

         i. B cells fail to undergo isotype switching

     1. Produce only IgM

       c. Characterized by extremely low levels of IgG, IgA, and IgE

         i. Either a normal or markedly elevated concentration of polyclonal IgM

       d. Clinical characteristics

         i. Recurrent pyogenic infections

         ii. *P. carinii pneumonia*

         iii. Increased frequency of autoimmune disorders and malignancy

     iii. The CD40–CD40L interaction is a potential target for treating autoimmune disorders

7. T-cell Development

    a. Precursor T-cells originate in the bone marrow from stem cells and migrate to the thymus where they begin differentiation

    b. The vast majority of thymocytes entering the thymus die

    c. Most of the T-cell death that occurs in the thymus is due to programmed cell death (apoptosis)

    d. Immature cells

       i. Double negative

       ii. Lack CD4 and CD8

       iii. Express a pre-T receptor

    e. Mature Cells

       i. Double positive (DP) thymocytes

         1. Have both CD4 and CD8

         2. Express TCR

       ii. Single positive (SP) thymocytes

         1. DP thymocytes that mature to express either CD4 or CD8

         2. Mature TCR

    f. Positive selection

       i. TCRs recognize self-MHC molecules or undergo death by neglect

    g. Negative selection or clonal deletion

       i. TCRs recognize self-MHC molecules and self-peptides with high affinity and eliminate potentially autoreactive clones

    h. Central tolerance

       i. Both positive and negative selection occur at the DP and SP stages

       ii. Mechanism achieves tolerance to self

    i. Peripheral tolerance

       i. Tolerance achieved outside the thymus

8. Laboratory tests used to evaluate T-cell function

    a. Screen with an absolute lymphocyte count and perform a Candida skin test

       i. If both are normal, clinically significant T-cell dysfunction may be excluded

      ii. If Candida is negative, five other antigens are used to test cell-mediated function
        1. PPD
        2. Trichophyton
        3. Mumps
        4. Tetanus/diphtheria toxoid
        5. Keyhole-limpet hemocyanin
  b. If screening tests are abnormal, quantify
      i. Total T-cells
      ii. CD4 and CD8 cells
      iii. NK cells
      iv. Lymphocyte blastic transformation
        1. Radiolabeled thymidine uptake following stimulation with
          a. Lectins (PHA)
          b. Specific antigen (Candida)
          c. One-way mixed lymphocyte reaction
      v. Ability of T cells to synthesize IL-2 and IL-2 receptors
        1. Indicates successful T-cell activation
  c. HIV testing
      i. The prototypic acquired T-cell immunodeficiency state
      ii. Should be performed as part of the screening evaluation
9. Organisms responsible for infections in primary T-cell immunodeficiency (thymic hypoplasia (DiGeorge syndrome))
  a. Viruses (herpes viruses)
  b. Intracellular bacteria (mycobacteria)
  c. Fungi (*Candida*)
  d. Other (*Pneumocystis carinii*)
10. Immunoglobulin Molecules
  a. Responsible for the ability of B-cells to recognize antigen
  b. Assist in the clearance of pathogenic organisms
  c. Composed of two types of polypeptides
      i. Light chains
        1. Two isotypes
          a. κ
          b. λ
      ii. Heavy chains
        1. Nine distinct isotypes correspond to five different classes of Igs and the subclasses of IgG and IgA
          a. $\gamma = $IgG
            i. 4 subclasses
              1. $\gamma 1$
                a. IgG1 has two identical $\gamma 1$ chains and two identical L chains (either κ or λ)
              2. $\gamma 2$

                   3.γ3
                   4.γ4
         b. α = IgA
              i. Two subclasses
                 1.α1
                 2.a2
              ii. Functions at epithelial surfaces and associated with a secretory fragment
         c. μ = IgM
         d. δ = IgD
         e. ε = IgE
              iii. Each H and L chain has a variable and a constant region
                 1.Constant region
                   a. Binds to complement and Fc receptors
                 2.Variable
                   a. The antigen-binding capability of Ig resides in the variable regions of both the H and L chains

11. B-cell Development
   a. B-cell lymphopoiesis begins in the fetal liver and later switches to the bone marrow
   b. B2 B cells
      i. Conventional
      ii. Generated continuously in the adult bone marrow
   c. B1 B cells
      i. Produced early in ontogeny
   d. The rearrangement and expression of Ig genes are the two major events that occur in B cell development
   e. H chain genes
      i. All are on chromosome 14
      ii. Successful rearrangement requires joining of a Jh segment, a Dh segment, and a Vh segment
         1. DhJh rearrangements are first
         2. Vh is joined afterward
      iii. RAG-2
         1. Required for rearrangement of the Ig receptor
         2. Its lack results in the absence of mature lymphocytes
      iv. A mutation that impairs H chain rearrangement or expression will block B cell development
   f. Other factors important in B cell development
      i. Cytokine IL-7
      ii. Kinase Syk
      iii. Cell survival gene bcl-x
      iv. Transcription factors
         1. E2A

        2. EBF

        3. BSAP

     v. Bruton's tyrosine kinase (BTK) gene

        1. Mutations cause Bruton's X-linked agammaglobulinemia

          a. Characterized by impaired B cell development

  g. Pro-B cells (B-cell precursors)

     i. Have not initiated Ig rearrangement

     ii. Only DJ rearrangements

  h. Pre-B cells

     i. Precursors that have rearranged, transcribed, and translated an H chain

     ii. Translated μ chains are intracellular with small amount on the plasma membrane in conjunction with surrogate L chain

        1. Derived from the $\lambda 5$ and V pre-β gene products

        2. Compose the Pre-B cell receptor complex

     iii. The receptor complex signals the pre-B cells to proliferate and to rearrange one of its L chains

        1. κ and λ loci are on chromosomes 2 and 22, respectively

        2. Rearrangement requires a VJ joint

  i. Immature B-cell

     i. Express surface Ig with successful H and L gene rearrangement

     i. Cells die via apoptosis with unsuccessful rearrangements or expression of a functional pre-B cell receptor

  b. Fully mature B-cells

     i. Express surface IgD as well as IgM through alterative splicing of the pre-mRNA for IgM

12. B Cell Activation

  a. Once a B-cell precursor expresses surface Ig, it can respond to antigen

  b. Bound antigen to the BCR of an immature B-cell leads to self-tolerance

  c. Multivalent self-antigens (dsDNA) induce programmed cell death

  d. Oligovalent self-antigens render immature B-cells refractory to further stimulation

  e. Receptor editing (mechanisms to escape anergy)

     i. Rearrange another L-chain Ig gene

     ii. Change BCR specificity

     iii. Lose self-reactivity

  f. B-cell antigens are broadly divided into two types

     i. Thymus independent

        1. Do not require MHC class II T-cell help

        2. Multivalent and poorly degraded in vivo

          a. Bacterial polysaccharides

        3. Poor immunologic memory

        4. Induce minimal germinal center formation

        5. Trigger IgG2 secretion

        6. A distinct phenotype localized in the marginal zone of the spleen

          a. Marginal zone B-cells do not mature until about 2 years of age

   b. Poor response to polysaccharide antigen
      i. Seen in infants and splenectomized individuals
   ii. Thymus dependent
      1. Soluble protein antigens that require MHC class II–restricted T-cell help for antibody production
g. BCR
   i. Dual role
      1. Binds and internalizes antigen for processing into peptides that assemble with class II molecules for presentation to CD4 T-cells
      2. Activates the antigen-recognizing B cell
   ii. Signal transduction is mediated through two associated transmembrane proteins
      1. Ig-α
      2. Ig-β
   iii. Intracellular domains contain ITAM motifs
   iv. These heterodimers couple the BCR to the Src-related kinases
      1. Lyn
         a. Lyn-deficient mice
            i. Defective B-cell clonal expansion
            ii. Defective terminal differentiation
            iii. Fail to eliminate autoreactive B-cells
      2. Blk
      3. Fyn
      4. Zap-70-related tyrosine kinase Syk
         a. Syk- and Src-related kinases phosphorylate other downstream effectors and increase membrane levels of T-cell costimulatory ligands B7-1 and B7-2
13. B-cell Differentiation
   a. Exposure to a thymus-dependent antigen triggers two pathways
      i. Extrafollicular
         1. Leads to early antibody production
      ii. Germinal-center
         1. Leads to germinal center formation
         2. Immunologic memory
            a. Formation of memory B-cells
            b. CD40–CD40L interactions promote memory cell formation
         3. Generation of plasma-cell precursors
            a. IL-2, IL-10, and IL-6 promote differentiation into plasma cells
            b. Inhibited by CD40–CD40L interactions
         4. The light zone
            a. B-cells interact with helper T-cells and follicular dendritic cells
            b. B-cells possess high-affinity BCRs selected to survive
            c. Survival genes, bcl-x and bcl-2, result in the persistence of the selected cell

     5. Molecules with critical roles in germinal center formation
       a. B7-1
       b. CD19
       c. CD40 on B cells
       d. CD40L on activated T-cells
         i. Hyper-IgM Syndrome
           1. Absence of functional CD40L
           2. Do not form germinal centers
           3. Ig genes are unable to undergo class switching
  b. Isotype switching
     i. Successful B-cell–T-cell collaboration produces oligoclonal proliferative foci which secrete IgM
     ii. The H-chain constant regions exchange while the VDJ gene segments remain the same
     iii. IgM antibodies can then be converted to IgG, IgA, or IgE
     iv. Dependent on direct costimulatory signals
       1. CD40 and CD40L
     v. Dependent on cytokines
       1. TGF-β
         a. TGF-β enhances switching to IgA
       2. IL-2
       3. IL-4
         a. IL-4 enhances switching to IgE and IgG4
       4. IL-6
       5. IL-10
         a. IL-10 enhances switching to IgG1, IgG3, and IgA
  c. Somatic mutation
     i. Antibody affinity altered by the introduction of mutations in variable gene segments
     ii. Generate an autoreactive BCR that leads to B-cell death
  d. Plasma cells
     i. Lose their membrane Ig
     ii. Express high levels of CD38
     iii. Short lived
  e. Memory B cells
     i. Long lived
     ii. Contain somatically mutated V genes
     iii. Morphologically distinct from naïve B cells
     iv. Can be restimulated to rapidly generate a secondary antibody response
  f. B-cell migration into splenic and lymph node follicles
     i. Requires a chemokine B lymphocyte chemoattractant (BLC/BCA1) and its receptor CXCR5
14. Laboratory tests used to evaluate the integrity of B-cell function
  a. Screening tests

   i. Determine the serum IgA level

   ii. Perform in vivo functional tests

    1. Isohemagglutinin titers (anti-blood group A and B)

     a. Predominantly IgM

    2. Diphtheria and tetanus booster immunization

     a. Antibodies prior to and 2 weeks later

     b. Synthesize IgG against protein antigens

    3. Pneumococcal immunization

     a. Antibodies prior to and 3 weeks later

     b. Synthesize against polysaccharide antigens

   iii. If all of these tests are normal, then clinically significant B-cell dysfunction may be excluded

  b. If any of the screening tests are abnormal

   i. Quantify IgG and IgM levels

   ii. Perform in vitro testing

    1. Peripheral blood B-cell quantification

    2. Bone marrow pre-B-cell quantification

     a. Measures surface Ig negative, cytoplasmic u-chain-positive cells

    3. In vitro immunoglobulin synthesis

     a. Mononuclear cells stimulated with mitogen

15. Clinical presentation of patients with X-linked (Bruton's) agammaglobulinemia

  a. Acute and chronic infections of the upper and lower respiratory tracts, meningitis, and bacteremia

  b. Recurrent infections with the following organisms

   i. Extracellular, encapsulated, pyogenic bacteria (*Streptococcus pneumoniae*)

   ii. *Haemophilus influenzae*

16. Organisms responsible for septic arthritis in patients with hypogammaglobulinemia

  a. *Streptococcus pneumoniae*

  b. *Haemophilus influenzae*

  c. *Staphylococcus aureus*

  d. *Ureaplasma urealyticum*

  e. Other Mycoplasma organisms

17. Primary B-cell immunodeficiency syndromes commonly associated with autoimmune phenomena

  a. Selective IgA deficiency

  b. Common variable immunodeficiency

  c. X-linked agammaglobulinemia

  d. Hyper-IgM syndrome

18. Predominant T-cell immunodeficiencies do not manifest autoimmune phenomena

  a. Many do not survive infancy

19. X-linked agammaglobulinemia

  a. A rare disorder

  b. Absent or near absent levels of serum IgG, IgM, and IgA

  c. Abnormal in vivo B-cell functional tests

  d. Cell-mediated immunity is intact
  e. The molecular defect is mutation within the Bruton's tyrosine kinase gene
      i. Normally present within B cells at all stages of development
      ii. Leads to failure of B-cell maturation and absence of B cells
  f. Arthritis occurs in about 20%
      i. Half due to infection with typical pyogenic bacteria
      ii. Infections with enterovirus and Mycoplasma
      iii. Aseptic (possibly autoimmune arthritis)
          1. Mono- or oligoarticular large joints
          2. Rarely destructive
          3. RF and ANA are absent
  g. Associated dermatomyositis-like syndrome
      i. Progressive enterovirus CNS infection with rash and muscle weakness
  h. Therapy
      i. IVIG
          1. IVIG administered at a dose of 200–600 mg/kg every month
      ii. Aggressive treatment of bacterial infections
20. Selective IgA deficiency
  a. Most common primary immunodeficiency syndrome
      i. In the general population, a prevalence of 1/700
      ii. In patients with SLE, the prevalence ranges from 1% to 5%
          1. 10–20 times higher than the general population
  b. Characterized by absence or near absence of serum and secretory IgA
      i. Normal levels of IgG and IgM
  c. Cell-mediated immunity is intact
  d. Clinical presentations
      i. Asymptomatic
      ii. Recurrent respiratory and GI tract infections
      iii. Autoimmune phenomena
      iv. A genetic disorder present at birth
      v. Acquired later in life
          1. Associated with drug therapy (gold, penicillamine, sulfasalazine) or viral infections
          2. Often transient
  e. Rheumatologic manifestations
      i. Autoantibodies
          1. RF and ANA in the absence of clinically expressed autoimmune disease
          2. dsDNA and ssDNA
          3. Other antibodies against
              a. Cardiolipin
              b. Thyroglobulin
              c. Thyroid microsomes
              d. Smooth muscle
              e. Gastric parietal cell

        f. Striated muscle

        g. Acetylcholine receptor

        h. Bile canniculi

      4. Antibodies against IgA occur in up to 44%

    ii. Systemic autoimmune disorders occur in 7–36%

      1. SLE

      2. Aseptic arthritis

      3. JRA

      4. RA

      5. Sjogren's syndrome

      6. Dermatomyositis

      7. Vasculitic syndromes

   iii. Organ-specific autoimmune disorders

      1. Diabetes mellitus type I

      2. Myasthenia gravis

      3. IBD

      4. Autoimmune hepatitis

      5. Pernicious anemia

      6. Primary adrenal insufficiency

  f. Therapy

    i. Rigorous treatment of active bacterial infections with antibiotics

    ii. IVIG should not be administered

      1. Severe, occasionally fatal, anaphylaxis may occur since many patients have autoantibodies against IgA (including IgE anti-IgA)

   iii. Patients should ideally receive blood products obtained from other patients with IgA deficiency

21. Common variable immunodeficiency (CVID)

  a. A heterogeneous group of disorders characterized by IgG, IgM, and IgA hypogammaglobulinemia

  b. Features that distinguish CVID from X-linked agammaglobulinemia

    i. Equal sex distribution

    ii. Onset of symptoms later in life

   iii. Presence of circulating B-cells

  c. Most patients manifest a primary B-cell defect resulting in failure to mature into Ig-secreting plasma cells

  d. Clinical presentations

    i. A genetic disorder at birth

    ii. Acquired secondary to a viral infection or an adverse drug effect

   iii. Increased frequency of septic arthritis

      1. *Staphylococcus aureus*

      2. *Mycoplasma*

   iv. Associated cell-mediated immunodeficiency

      1. Fungi and mycobacterial pathogens

  e. Rheumatologic manifestations

    i. Autoantibodies

          1. Less often than in selective IgA deficiency

      ii. Polyarthritis

          1. No infectious organism detected

          2. Involvement of the large- and medium-sized joints with sparing of the small joints of the hands and feet

          3. Do not see rheumatoid nodules, erosions, or significant articular destruction

          4. Responds well to IVIG

      iii. Organ-specific autoimmune disorders in 20% patients

          1. Pernicious anemia

          2. Autoimmune hemolytic anemia

          3. Idiopathic thrombocytopenic purpura

   f. Therapy

      i. IVIG

          1. Recommended for patients who have low IgG levels and recurrent infections

          2. If there is a complete absence of IgA, along with anti-IgA antibodies, patients are at risk for anaphylaxis

22. Immunoregulation and Cytokines

   a. Factors that influence the immune response

      i. The nature of antigen

      ii. The route of exposure

      iii. The quantity of antigen

   b. Adjuvants activate antigen-presenting cells

   c. A major immunoregulatory mechanism is the production of a large number of cytokines that mediate innate immunity and inflammation

      i. IL-1 and TNF-α are major mediators of tissue injury

          1. Mutation in the TNF receptor in humans results in a periodic fever syndrome called TRAPS

23. T-Helper Cells (CD4+)

   a. Differentiate into one or two phenotypes

      i. Th1

          1. Produce IL-2, lymphotoxin α and IFN-γ

             a. Promotes a cell-mediated response

             b. INF-γ

                i. Activates macrophages

                ii. Upregulates class II

                iii. Suppresses Th2 response

             c. IL-2

                i. A key inducer of Th1 differentiation

                ii. Produced by B-cells and monocytes

                iii. Enhances T and NK cell cytolytic activity

                iv. Induces INF-γ secretion

             d. TNF is also secreted promoting inflammation

          2. Stimulate CD8+ cytotoxic T-cells to attack virally infected cells

     3. Therapies that inhibit Th1 cytokines (anti-TNFα) are used in Th1-mediated diseases (RA)

  ii. Th2

     1. Produces IL-4, IL-5, IL-6, IL-9, IL-10, and IL-13

     2. Promotes humoral or allergic responses

     3. IL-4, 10, and 13 inhibit macrophage activation and TNF-mediated inflammation

     4. IL-4

       a. A major regulator of allergic responses

       b. Inhibits macrophage activation

       c. Blocks the effects of IFN-γ

       d. A growth factor for mast cells

       e. Required for class switching of B-cells to produce IgE

       f. Influences Th2 differentiation

     5. IL-5

       a. Promotes the growth, differentiation, and activation of eosinophils

     6. IL-6

       a. Promotes B-cell maturation into a plasma cell

     7. IL-9

       a. Supports growth of T cells and bone mast cell precursors

     8. IL-10

       a. Opposite effects to INF-γ

       b. Inhibits macrophage antigen presentation

       c. Decreases expression of class II molecules

       d. An endogenous inhibitor of cell-mediated immunity

       e. Therapeutics

         i. Used to treat Th1 diseases (RA)

         ii. Antibodies against IL-10 have been used to treat Th2 diseases (SLE)

b. Transcription factors that can regulate Th differentiation

  i. GATA-3

  ii. c-Maf

  iii. NFAT

  iv. T-Bet

c. IL-2

  i. An autocrine T-cell growth factor

  ii. Determines the magnitude of T-cell and NK cell responses

  iii. Mice that lack IL-2

     1. Do not have immunodeficiency

     2. Display autoimmunity and lymphoproliferation

       a. Secondary to impaired apoptosis

d. IL-15

  i. Similar to IL-2

  ii. Binds the β and γ subunits of IL-2R

  iii. Produced by nonlymphoid cells

      iv. Important for NK and memory cell development
- e. Janus Kinases (JAKs)
  - i. A family of cytoplasmic protein tyrosine kinases (PTKs)
  - ii. Bind to cytokine receptors and phosphorylate the receptor after cytokine binding
  - iii. JAK3
    1. Binds to the cytokine subunit, γc
       a. A component of the receptors for IL-2, IL-4, IL-7, IL-9, and IL-15
    2. Deficiency of either γc or JAK3 leads to the same phenotype
       a. Severe combined immunodeficiency (SCID)
  - iv. Substrates for the JAKs are the signal transducers and activators of transcription (STATs)
- f. STATs
  - i. SH2 domains
  - ii. Bind phosphorylated cytokine receptors
  - iii. Phosphorylated by JAKs
  - iv. Translocate to the nucleus where they regulate gene expression
  - v. Mice deficient in STAT4
    1. Impaired Th1 differentiation (activated by IL-12)
  - vi. Mice deficient in STAT6
    1. Impaired Th2 responses (activated by IL-4)
  - vii. STAT1 and STAT2 knockouts have impaired IFN responses
24. Turning Off the Immune Response
    - a. ITIM-containing receptors inhibit signaling by recruiting protein tyrosine phosphatases
      - i. Counteract PTK
      - ii. CTLA-4 deficient mice
        1. Develop a fatal lymphoproliferative disorder
        2. CTLA-r recruits tyrosine phosphatases
    - b. TGF-β1 KO
      - i. Die of overwhelming immunologic disease
      - ii. Associated with autoantibodies characterized by lymphoid and mononuclear infiltration of the heart, lung, and other tissues
    - c. Suppressor of cytokine signaling (SOCS)
      - i. A family of cytokine-induced inhibitors that attenuate signaling
      - ii. KO mice have lethal immunologic disease
    - d. Fas
      - i. Induces T cells to undergo apoptosis
      - ii. Fas-dependent apoptosis is a mechanism of achieving peripheral tolerance
      - iii. Fas gene mutations, in humans, cause autoimmune lymphoproliferative syndrome (ALPS)
25. The Immune Response to Pathogenic Organisms
    - a. Tissue injury and disease can occur as a consequence of host response
    - b. Superantigens

       i. Foreign antigens capable of binding to the TCR and MHC Class II molecule outside the antigen-binding groove

         1. Particularly of bacterial or viral origin

       ii. Do not need to be processed and presented to stimulate T-cell activation

       iii. Do not appear to mediate the classic rheumatic diseases

       iv. Toxic shock syndrome

         1. Staphylococcal enterotoxins bind TCR variable regions ($V\beta$) and class II molecules activating T-cells

         2. Up to 10% of T-cells may share a common $V\beta$ region for which the superantigen is specific

         3. Clinical characteristics

           a. Fever

           b. Exfoliative skin disease

           c. Disseminated intravascular coagulation (DIC)

           d. Cardiovascular shock

c. Humor   al immune response to extracellular bacteria

       i. Toxins neutralized by antibody

       ii. Organisms lysed by complement

       iii. Organisms phagocytosed

       iv. Exaggerated response can lead to disease

         1. Post-streptococcal glomerulonephritis with immune complexes deposition

d. Cell-mediated response to pathogens

       i. The primary defense against intracellular pathogens like Mycobacteria

       ii. Recruitment of macrophages and multinucleated giant cells that participate in granuloma formation

       iii. Fibrin deposition and tissue induration is part of the delayed-type hypersensitivity (DHT)

       iv. Disease associations due to a cell-mediated response to an unknown organism

         1. Granulomatous disease

         2. Sarcoidosis

         3. Wegener's granulomatosis

e. Immune response to viruses

       i. Mediated by IFNα and β (innate immunity) and the production of specific antibodies (adaptive immunity)

       ii. Immune complex disease can occur (hepatitis B and arteritis)

f. Immune response to parasitic infections

       i. A Th-2 response

       ii. IL-4 and eosinophilia

26. Tolerance

a. Central tolerance

       i. A major function of the thymus

       ii. Deletion of potentially pathogenic T-cell clones with high avidity for self-antigens

b. Peripheral tolerance
    i. Achieved by anergy and Fas-mediated deletion of activated cells
27. Diseases Caused by Antibodies
    a. Type I (immediate) hypersensitivity
        i. IgE binds receptors on mast cells and basophils
        ii. Cross-linking of the receptor-bound IgE triggers the release of
            1. Histamine
            2. Proinflammatory lipid mediators
            3. Cytokines
        iii. Clinical presentations
            1. Allergic rhinits
            2. Anaphylaxis
    b. Type II hypersensitivity
        i. Antibody-mediated tissue injury with antibodies against circulating or fixed cells
        ii. Clinical presentations
            1. Autoimmune hemolytic anemia
            2. Autoimmune thrombocytopenia
            3. Goodpasture's syndrome
            4. Pemphigus pemphigoid
            5. Pernicious anemia
            6. Myasthenia gravis
            7. Grave's disease
    c. Type III hypersensitivity
        i. Immune complex disease
        ii. Deposited in organs and serosal surfaces
        iii. Clinical presentations
            1. SLE
            2. Polyarteritis nodusum (PAN)
            3. Post-streptococcal GN
            4. Serum sickness
    d. Type IV
        i. Delayed type hypersensitivity
        ii. Immune response to mycobacterial antigens
        iii. Positive PPD skin test
28. Diseases Caused by T–cells
    a. T-cell-mediated tissue injury include
        i. Delayed type hypersensitivity (DTH)
            1. Contact dermatitis is classic example
        ii. Direct lysis by cytolytic CD8 cells
29. The Acute Phase Response
    a. A complex cascade of primarily liver-synthesized proteins that increase in response to a variety of infectious or immunologic stimuli

b. Major acute phase proteins include
   i. Alpha-1 antitrypsin
   ii. C3
   iii. Ceruloplasmin
   iv. CRP
   v. Fibrinogen
   vi. Haptoglobin
   vii. SAA
c. The liver synthesizes acute phase proteins at the expense of albumin
   i. Albumin decreases during acute inflammation
d. Macrophages and monocytes are the principal cells involved in the initiation of the response
   i. Secrete IL-1, IL-6, and TNF
      1. IL-6 is a potent hepatocyte-stimulating factor resulting in the increased synthesis of acute phase proteins
      2. IL-1 enhances the effect of IL-6

Section B: Neuroendocrine Influences

1. The Hypothalamic-Pituitary-Adrenal Axis (HPA)
   a. Deficiencies in the neuroendocrine-immune (NEI) regulatory loop may result in increased autoimmune disease
   b. Cytokine stimulation increases HPA function by stimulating corticotropin-releasing hormone (CRH) production
      i. IL-1
         1. Stimulates CRH and arginine vasopressin (AVP)
      ii. IL-6
         1. Potent stimulator of HPA axis at the level of the hypothalamus
         2. Directly stimulates release of adrenocorticotropic hormone (ACTH) by the pituitary
         3. Synergizes with ACTH to increase production of cortisol by adrenocortical cells
         4. Produced by adrenal cells after stimulation with IL-1 or ACTH
      iii. HPA axis
         1. Acutely stimulated by TNF-α
         2. Delayed reaction with IL-2 and IFN-γ
2. Corticosteroids
   a. Inhibit immune and inflammatory responses at multiple steps
      i. Neutrophil and monocyte migration
      ii. Antigen presentation
      iii. Lymphocyte proliferation and differentiation
      iv. Cytokine production
      v. Synthesis of eicosanoids and other lipid mediators
      vi. Regulate thymocyte maturation and influence apoptosis

     vii. Production of nitric oxide
    viii. Production of metalloproteinases
      ix. Modulates activation, expansion, and clonal deletion of peripheral T-cells
       x. Shift response from Th1 to Th2
          1. Suppression of Th1 cytokines (IL-2 and IFN-γ)

3. The HPA Axis in Autoimmune Disease
  a. Premenopausal RA patients
       i. Subnormal serum cortisol responsiveness to adrenal stimulation by ACTH or insulin hypoglycemia
      ii. Adrenal hyporesponsiveness to elevated serum levels of IL-6
  b. Lewis rat (disease model for RA)
       i. Blunted CRH, ACTH, and cortisol secretion in response to many types of stressors (including IL-1)
  c. MLR lpr/lpr and NZB/NZW F1 (disease models for SLE)
       i. Blunted IL-1-stimulated corticosterone
  d. NOD (disease model for diabetes mellitus)
       i. Both T and B lymphocytes display extended survival
      ii. Thymocytes are resistant to corticosteroid-induced apoptosis
  e. OS chicken (disease model for Hashimoto's thyroiditis)
       i. Decreased free corticosterone
      ii. Blunted corticosterone response to IL-1
  f. UCD-200 chicken (disease model for scleroderma)
       i. Adrenal hyporesponsiveness to increased ACTH
      ii. Markedly increased ACTH production and normal levels of corticosterone in response to cytokines

4. Prolactin (PRL) and Growth Hormone (GH)
  a. Immunodeficiency from hypophysectomy can be reversed by PRL and GH
  b. PRL
       i. Promotes proliferation and differentiation of antigen-specific T-cells
      ii. Bromocriptine inhibits pituitary release of PRL and reduces lymphocyte reactivity
     iii. Stimulates the expression of IL-2 receptors and enhances the IL-2-induced proliferation of T-cells
     iv. Surface receptors homologous to cytokine receptors (such as IL-6)
      v. Cytokines have prolactin receptors
     vi. Levels modulate expression of autoimmune disease
  c. GH
       i. Promotes thymocyte proliferation
      ii. Surface receptors homologous to cytokine receptors (such as IL-6)
     iii. Cytokines have growth hormone receptors

5. The Hypothalamic-Pituitary-Gonadal Axis
  a. Estrogen is important in the pathogenesis of SLE
       i. Activates humoral immunity
      ii. SLE begins at menarche
     iii. Female preponderance

   iv. Exacerbation of symptoms during specific stages of the menstrual cycle or with pregnancy
   v. OCPs or estrogen replacement may exacerbate SLE
   vi. Disease remission at menopause
 b. Imbalances of sex steroid metabolism and modulation
   i. SLE
   ii. Klinefelter's syndrome associated with SLE
 c. Sex hormones and RA
   i. Risk increases in pubertal girls and premenopausal women
   ii. Pregnancy has an ameliorating effect on RA
   iii. Male RA
     1. Low serum total testosterone levels in active disease
     2. Combined low levels of cortisol and testosterone as disease predictors
6. Sex Steroid Influences on the Immune Response
 a. Estrogen
   i. An indirect influence through prolactin stimulation
   ii. Stimulates hyperreactivity in humoral immune responses
   iii. Favors a Th2 response
   iv. Estrogen receptors in lymphoid and thymic tissue
 b. Androgen
   i. Receptors present in thymic epithelial cells
   ii. Low levels a risk factor for an earlier onset age of RA
 c. Testosterone depresses humoral immunity
 d. Both estrogen and testosterone alter thymocyte development
 e. DHEA favor Th1 immune responsiveness
 f. Progesterone favors Th2 function
 g. During pregnancy, adrenal cortical function and hormonal production increases
   i. Placental CRH stimulates the HPA axis to increase cortisol and adrenal androgen production
   ii. Postpartum hypothalamic production of CRH is decreased
 h. Cell-mediated immune responses more active in women than in men
7. Sex Steroids in Animal Models of Autoimmune Disease
 a. NZB/NZW F1 mice
   i. Renal disease and autoantibody production progress more rapidly in females than in males
   ii. Castration or androgen therapy decreases disease activity in females
   iii. Castration or estrogen therapy increase disease activity in males
 b. MRL mice (SLE)
   i. Estrogens selectively enhance B-cell-mediated humoral immune responses
     1. Immunoglobulin levels
     2. Autoantibody production
     3. Immune complex glomerulonephritis
   ii. T-cell-mediated immune responses diminished by estrogens

8. Dehydroepiandrosterone (DHEA) and DHEA-sulfate (DHEAS)
   a. DHEAS is the predominant circulating adrenal androgen
   b. Levels lower in pubertal juvenile RA and premenopausal RA
   c. Levels inversely correlate with disease severity
   d. Therapeutic use in women with SLE resulted in modestly favorable clinical and immunological effects
      i. Not for patients with RA

Section C: Autoimmunity

1. Tolerance
   a. The phenomenon of antigen-specific unresponsiveness
   b. Innate Immune Response
      i. An evolutionary process
      ii. Best fit receptors link binding to foreign molecules with a proinflammatory response
      iii. Membrane complement regulatory proteins protect self-tissues from the alternative pathway
   c. Adaptive Immune Response
      i. A somatic process
      ii. Lymphocyte receptors and thresholds for activation selected during the lifetime of an individual
      iii. Tolerant of specific antigens (self) and intolerant of foreign antigens
      iv. Tolerance of autoantigens (self-nucleoproteins)
      v. Tolerance of exogenous antigens (dietary proteins)
2. Central Tolerance
   a. Determines the fate of lymphocytes in central lymphoid organs
   b. The affinity of antigen receptor binding
      i. Lymphocytes with no or very high affinity of binding die by apoptosis
      ii. Lymphocytes with intermediate affinity survive
      iii. Lymphocytes with the highest affinity are anergic in the periphery
   c. Sets the threshold for activation in the periphery
3. Peripheral Tolerance
   a. Lymphocytes require very low affinity binding to self-antigens to remain viable in the periphery
4. T-cell Fate
   a. Death by apoptosis
      i. No signal through the TCR
   b. Negative selection (deleted)
      i. Engage antigen with high affinity
   c. Positive selection
      i. Engages antigen with low affinity
      ii. Matures into either CD4 or CD8 T-cells
      iii. Occurs in the thymic medulla

      d. Clonal deletion

          i. Immature T-cells functionally deleted from the repertoire

          ii. An intrathymic process

      e. Anergy

          i. Interaction of the MHC–peptide complex with an autoreactive TCR

          ii. Costimulatory signals are not provided to the autoreactive cell

      f. Only about 5% survive the selection process

   5. B-cell Fate

      a. Death

          i. Faulty rearrangement of receptors in the pro- to pre-B-cell transition

          ii. High-affinity interaction with antigen

      b. Negative selection

          i. Antigens that cross-link sIgM (a transmembrane form of immunoglobulin M) most efficiently

      c. Receptor editing

          i. Self-reactive B-cells switch their light chain expression to avoid self-reactivity and death

      d. Anergy

          i. Functional inactivation so that re-exposure to an antigen in the periphery will result in failure to produce antibody

          ii. B-cells that bind to antigen with low affinity

          iii. B-cells that encounter oligovalent antigens unable to cross-link sIgM

      e. Clonal anergy

          i. Autoreactive cells are inactivated so that they cannot respond to antigen

      f. Tolerance

          i. Antigen encounter in the absence of specific T-cell help

             1. Particularly during early development

      g. Compared with T-cells, higher numbers of immature B cells seed the periphery

   6. Key Points on Lymphocyte Fate

      a. The avidity or relative affinity of the antigen receptor for antigen is key to determining the fate of immature lymphocytes

      b. Immature lymphoid cells in the central lymphoid organs cannot distinguish self from foreign antigens

          i. Renders them tolerant to foreign antigens by systemic immunization during the neonatal period

          ii. Autoreactive cells that bind antigen with moderate to high affinity are tolerized (deleted or inactivated)

      c. Signaling thresholds are established in the central lymphoid organs

          i. Emerging cells have higher thresholds for activation

   7. Clonal Encounter with Self and Induction of Anergy

      a. Brain

          i. Limited permeability of the blood–brain barrier

          ii. Minimal lymphoid drainage

          iii. Paucity of dendritic cells

          iv. Absent or low expression of MHC molecules on neurons

b. Eye
   i. Constitutive production of TGF-β in the anterior chamber suppresses immune responses
   ii. Constitutively expressed Fas ligand induces apoptosis of immune cells with rapid phagocytosis and suppression of inflammation
c. Testis
   i. Fas ligand is expressed constitutively
8. Immune Deviation and Suppression
   a. The largest exposure of the host to a diverse array of foreign antigens is by ingestion of food and microorganisms
   b. Ingestion of an antigen prior to immunization by a systemic route abrogates the immune response to that specific antigen by
      i. Immune deviation
      ii. Preferential production of TGF-β
      iii. Th2 cytokines
   c. Select subpopulations of CD4, CD8, or NK cells play a role in the maintenance of tolerance
   d. The immune system will respond to an individual antigen in different manners based on
      i. Chemical composition
      ii. The initial amount to which an individual is exposed
      iii. The initial route by which the antigen is introduced
      iv. The type of milieu within which the antigen encounters the immune system
   e. Characteristics of the antigen which favor the development of tolerance
      i. Intravenous or oral route
      ii. Monomeric antigen
      iii. Large dose
      iv. Immunologic immaturity
   f. Characteristics of the antigen which favor the development of an immune response (inflammation)
      i. Subcutaneous or intradermal route
      ii. Aggregated or polymeric antigen
      iii. Small dose
      iv. Surrounding inflammation
9. Discrimination Between Self and Foreign
   a. Response to a pathogen
      i. Phagocytes express pattern recognition receptors (PRR) with relative specificity for lipids or carbohydrates
      ii. Bacterial LPS interacts with macrophage receptors to initiate the release of reactive oxygen and nitrogen intermediates
      iii. Injury to the bacteria initiates release of proinflammatory cytokines (IL-1 and TNF)
      iv. These cytokines induce B7 on the macrophage which binds to CD28 on the T-cells providing the critical second signal

   v. INF-γ released by the macrophage enhances antigen presentation

  b. Response to dying host cells during normal cell turnover

   i. Dying cells undergo changes to their surface membranes

   ii. Phosphatidyl serine is translocated to the outer layer

   iii. Molecules that are recognized by different PRR trigger release of immunosuppressive TGF-β

   iv. An anti-inflammatory response is induced following phagocytosis of normal apoptotic cells

10. Termination of the Immune Response

  a. Cytokine withdrawal

   i. Destruction of microorganisms will reduce stimulation of inflammatory cytokines

  b. Inhibitory counter-receptors

   i. CTLA-4

    1. Expressed only on activated T-cells with a much higher affinity for binding to B7 than CD28

    2. Inhibits and down-modulates the immune response

  c. Active induction of death through death receptors

   i. Lymphocyte-mediated induction of activation-induced cell death (AICD)

    1. Occurs predominantly through the Fas and TNF receptors

     a. Fas receptor

      i. Expressed at low levels on resting T and B lymphocytes, as well as macrophages

      ii. Upregulated with cell activation

     b. FasL expressed predominantly on activated CD4+ Th1 and CD8+ T-cells

     c. See systemic autoimmunity (SLE) with mutations in Fas or FasL

     d. TNF-α receptor

      i. Expressed ubiquitously

      ii. Induces apoptosis of activated CD8+ T-cells

  d. Activated B-cells are subjected to a third round of selection in germinal centers

   i. Those triggered by antigen undergo somatic hypermutation and are positively selected (high-affinity clones)

   ii. Low affinity clones die by apoptosis

   iii. Mutations are generated randomly in the variable regions of the heavy and light chains

   iv. Autoreactive cells are eliminated by Fas

11. Apoptosis and Necrosis

  a. Necrosis

   i. Pathologic death due to inflammation

   ii. Results in rupture and fragmentation of the nucleus and cell

   iii. Cellular debris further contributes to the inflammatory reaction

  b. Apoptosis

   i. An orderly process of cell death with the activation of caspases

    ii. Seen during normal physiologic processes
      1. Embryogenesis
      2. Metamorphosis
    iii. Results in chromatin condensation, membrane blebbing, and fragmentation of cell and nucleus into smaller membrane-bound apoptotic bodies
    iv. Rapidly cleared by phagocytosis
      1. Apoptotic cells are rarely seen
      2. 95% of cells undergo apoptosis in thymus
    v. Does not trigger an inflammatory response
    vi. Seen in the induction and maintenance of tolerance
12. Autoimmune Models and Mechanisms
  a. Autoimmune disorders
    i. Broken self-tolerance and a loss of previously established tolerance
    ii. An antigen-driven processes characterized by
      1. Specificity
      2. High affinity
      3. Memory
  b. Autoimmunity develops with variations in an antigen's amino acid sequence
    i. Only a small peptide fits in the antigen-binding cleft of the MHC molecules
      1. 8–13 AA for MHC class I
      2. 13–25 AA for MHC class II
    ii. These positions are typically in polymorphic regions
  c. Molecular mimicry
    i. The peptide sequence of a foreign antigen may resemble a self-antigen
      1. Example: rheumatic heart disease
      2. Myocardial autoantigens, myosin and sarcolemmal membrane proteins resemble the streptococcal M protein
      3. Immune response directed against the strep M protein will also target myocardial tissue
      4. T- and B-cell clones continue to be stimulated by the cross-reactive autoantigens
    ii. Increased incidence in certain deficiency states (C1q)
    iii. Pathogen peptides have stretches of amino acids whose sequence is identical to the sequences in the antigen-binding cleft of MCH
      1. A string of 5 AA in a plasmid-derived peptide of *Shigella flexneri* with an identical sequence within HLA-B27
      2. Seen in dysentery and Reiter's syndrome
  d. Autoimmunity by Immunization
    i. Molecular mimicry
      1. The immunogen may share sequence similarity with self-antigens
    ii. Self-antigens in the presence of a powerful adjuvant
      1. Adjuvants activate innate immune system components such as TLR and complement
        a. Freund's complete adjuvant contains Mycobacteria

       2. Induces cytokines such as TNF and IFN-γ

         a. Enhanced antigen presentation in a proinflammatory context

         b. Upregulation of costimulatory molecules

       3. Loss of tolerance

       4. An autoantigen-driven specific immune response persists long after the trigger has been eliminated

e. Infection and Initiation of Autoimmunity

   i. Initiated by exposure to bacteria

       1. *Salmonella*

       2. *Shigella*

       3. *Yersinia*

   ii. Association between HLA-B27

       1. Bacterial peptide antigens presented by MHC class I induce immune responses that cross-react between host and bacterial products (molecular mimicry)

   iii. Ways that viruses manipulate the immune response

       1. Induce polyclonal B-cell activation

       2. Interfere with the complement cascade

       3. Modify cytokine expression and receptor function

       4. Inhibit MHC class I expression

       5. Subvert the regulation of cell survival and death leading to autoimmunity

         a. Bcl-2 homologue

         b. BHRF (Epstein–Barr virus (EBV))

         c. E1B 19-kDa protein (adenovirus)

f. Cryptic Epitopes

   i. Only a limited number of peptides derived from each protein are presented to T-cells (dominant peptide)

       1. Highly ordered degradation, transport, and binding of peptides to the MHC

       2. Tolerance induced to the dominant peptide

       3. Tolerance broken if a new "cryptic" peptide is presented

         a. Alters the processing or intracellular transport

         b. A vigorous immune response to self can occur if occurs in an inflammatory setting

g. Determinant (epitope) spreading

   i. The loss of tolerance

   ii. The generation of an active autoantigen-driven specific immune response to many epitopes of a single antigen or several physically associated antigens

       1. Linked autoantibody response to Sm and ribonuclear proteins (RNP) antigens

       2. Autoreactive T- and B-cell mediated response to a variety of autoantigens during the course of SLE

13. Autoantibodies
    a. The production of very low affinity autoantibodies (RF and ANA) increase transiently in the face of immune activation
        i. Mediated by CD5+ B-cells
    b. Increasing autoantibodies and increased prevalence of autoimmune diseases with advancing age
    c. Play a major pathologic role in the following diseases
        i. Hemolytic anemia and autoimmune thrombocytopenias
        ii. Diabetes mellitus (DM), myasthenia gravis (MG), and pernicious anemia
            1. Antibodies against cellular receptors
        iii. Goodpasture's syndrome and bullous pemphigoid
            1. Antibodies against basement membranes
            2. Immune complexes involving autoantibodies
        iv. SLE and Post-strep GN
14. Defined Mutations Predisposing to Autoimmunity
    a. Loss of function mutations of the early complement components predispose to SLE
        i. C1q
        ii. C2
        iii. C4
    b. Early complement deficiencies lead to defective clearance of apoptotic cells
    c. Mice with spontaneous mutations of the Fas receptor or its ligand develop massive lymphadenopathy and lupus like autoimmunity
    d. Background genes are important in the expression of a mutation with a great degree of variability
15. Strategies to avoid autoimmunity
    a. Minimize the opportunity for an immune response to self
    b. Active suppression of immune responses to self
    c. Mechanisms to terminate immune response

Genetics

4

1. Primary genes that determine immune response patterns
   a. Located within the MHC on chromosome 6
   b. Encode the HLA
2. An allele that confers increased risk
   a. When the conditional probability of disease (D) in a population (P) is greater in the presence of an allele (A) than it would be in the absence of the allele
      i. $P(D/A) > P(D/\text{not } A)$
3. Genetic Studies in Autoimmunity
   a. Aggregation in families is modest
   b. Monozygotic twins
      i. Genetically identical individuals
      ii. Concordance rates for autoimmune disease between 15% and 30%
      iii. Non-genetic factors play a role since <100% concordance
   c. Dizygotic twins and siblings
      i. Share approximately 50% of their genes in common
      ii. Concordance rates for autoimmune disease 2–5%
   d. Unrelated individuals
      i. Low overall degree of genetic similarity (at polymorphic loci)
         1. Approximately 0.1% difference over the entire genome
   e. Overall genetic risk
      i. Background population (genetically unrelated) prevalence in autoimmune disease range from 0.1% to 1%
      ii. Background prevalence used to calculate two ratios
         1. The relative risk to siblings (λs)
            a. Disease prevalence in siblings of affected individuals/Disease prevalence in general population
         2. The relative risk to MZ twins (λmz)
            a. Disease prevalence in co-twins of affected individuals/Disease prevalence in general population

N.T. Colburn, *Review of Rheumatology*,
DOI 10.1007/978-1-84882-093-7_4, © Springer-Verlag London Limited 2012

        iii. Compared with the general population

           1. An individual who has an identical twin or sibling with an autoimmune disease is at substantially increased risk

        iv. HLA linked genes account for 50% or less of this risk

    4. Genetic Terms

      a. Alleles

        i. Alternative forms of gene variants at a particular locus

      b. Haplotype

        i. A group of alleles located at adjacent or closely linked loci on the same chromosome

        ii. Usually inherited as a unit

        iii. Heterozygote

           1. An individual who inherits two different alleles at a given locus on two homologous chromosomes

        iv. Linkage disequilibrium

           1. In a population, the preferential association of two alleles or mutations more frequently than predicted by chance

        v. Linkage

           1. In a family, the coinheritance of two (nonallelic) genes or loci that lie close to one another

        vi. Polymorphism

           1. The degree of allelic variation at a locus

           2. The most frequent allele does not occur in more than 98% of the population

    5. The Human MHC

      a. Molecules that can bind specific antigen

        i. Innate Immune System

           1. CRP

           2. Mannose-binding protein

           3. High specificity binding to determinants such as repeating carbohydrates on foreign antigens

        ii. Adaptive immune system

           1. B-cell receptor (Igs)

           2. TCR

           3. MCH class I and II molecules

        iii. Transmembrane cell-surface molecules with two associated chains (dimers)

           1. Each chain based on a similar repeating structure derived from a common primordial gene

             a. The "immunoglobulin supergene"

           2. The amino terminus

             a. The furthest extracellular extension

             b. The site of antigen binding

             c. Three hypervariable regions

                i. Extraordinary diversity

                ii. The greatest diversity occurs in HRV3

       3. The carboxy terminus
         a. The intracellular end
       4. The remainder of the structure is conserved
  b. Located on chromosome 6
     i. A 3.4 million base-pair region
     ii. More than 200 loci
     iii. At least 128 functional genes
     iv. 40% of the genes are primarily involved in the immune response
     v. Divided into class I and class II regions with a "central" III MHC
  c. Genes of the central MHC
     i. Complement components
       1. C4A
       2. C4B
       3. C2
       4. Factor B
     ii. TNF-α and -β
     iii. Some of the heat shock proteins
  d. Class I region
     i. Expressed on all nucleated cells and platelets
     ii. Contains HLA-A, -B, -C
     iii. Approximately 2 million base pairs
     iv. Characteristics of the presented antigenic peptide fragment
       1. 8–13 amino acids in length
       2. Endogenous to the cytoplasm or nucleus of the cell expressing the MHC molecule
         a. "Self"-peptides
         b. Peptides of obligate intracellular pathogens (viruses and chlamydia)
         c. Tumor antigens
     v. Enables presentation of peptide antigens to T-cells
       1. CD8+ T-cells
         a. Cell-mediated killing
         b. Suppression of the MHC Class I presenting cell
     vi. Encodes only the MHC class I α-chain
       1. HLA-A α chain locus has 50 alleles
       2. HLA-B α chain locus has 200 alleles
       3. HLA-C α chain locus has 35 alleles
     vii. The total number of MHC class I molecules expressed in an individual is 6
       1. Given one heterozygous at each MHC class I β-chain allele
       2. Three maternal and three paternal
     viii. β2-microglobulin
       1. The β-chain
       2. Encoded by an invariant allele on chromosome 15

e. Class II region
  i. Molecules are expressed on certain immune cells
    1. APCs in particular
      a. B-cells
      b. Monocytes/macrophages
      c. Dendritic cells
      d. Thymic epithelial cells
    2. Activated T-cells
    3. Induced Class II expression during chronic inflammation
      a. Endothelial cells
      b. Synovial cells
  ii. Contains HLA-DR, -DQ, and -DP
  iii. Each class II molecule consists of two separate polypeptide chains designated α and β
    1. HLA-DRA
    2. HLA-DRB
  iv. Characteristics of the presented antigenic peptide fragment
    1. 13–25 AA in length
    2. Present in lysosomal compartments as a result of phagocytosis or receptor-mediated endocytosis
      a. Exogenous or foreign infectious material (bacterial)
  v. Enables presentation of peptide antigens to T-cells
    1. CD4+ T-cells
      a. T-cell coordinated phagocytosis
      b. Antibody response eradicates the antigen
  vi. Encodes both the α and β chains of Class II molecules
  vii. Each subregion contains its own cluster of genes
    1. HLA-DR subregion
      a. DR alpha chain
        i. Encoded by one gene (DRA)
        ii. DRA is generally not polymorphic
      b. DR beta chain
        i. Encoded by several genes
          1. Number varies according to haplotype
        ii. The HLA-DRB chain locus includes 200 alleles
        iii. Designated DRB1, DRB2, DRB3
          1. The DRB1 locus is the most variable
    2. HLA-DP and -DQ α-chain loci and HLA-DP, -DQ, and -DR β-chain loci
      a. All are polymorphic
      b. An individual with the greatest diversity will express two HLA-DR, 4 HLA-DP, and 4 HLA-DQ molecules
        i. A total of ten types of Class II molecules

6. HLA molecules
   a. Cell-surface proteins encoded by different MHC loci
   b. Highly polymorphic
   c. Defined as antigens (human leukocyte antigens)
       i. Specifically recognized as foreign by other individuals
   d. Major function is to present peptide antigen fragments for recognition by T-cells
   e. MHC restricted T-cell recognition
   f. Exhibit a high degree of structural (genetic) polymorphism
7. HLA and peptide antigen binding
   a. Each site has a similar configuration
       i. A groove
          1. α-helical walls
          2. Floor a series of anti-parallel strands (β-pleated sheet)
          3. Antigen binds at points on both the α-helical walls and the β-pleated floor
       ii. Three hypervariable regions of greatest genetic diversity
          1. Expressed in segments of each of the α-helices and the β-pleated sheet
          2. Selects which antigens can bind to specific molecules
          3. Selects which TCR can interact with specific combinations of MHC–antigen complex
             a. Referred to as trimolecular interaction
          4. A specific sequence of AA between position 67 and 74 of the HLA-DRB chain predisposes to RA
   b. MHC I configuration
       i. Formed between the two amino terminal domains of the same chain (α-chain)
   c. TCR and MHC II configuration
       i. Formed between the amino termini of both the α- and the β-chains
       ii. TCR binds the MHC–peptide complex
          1. Recognizes the unique conformation and charge of the antigen peptide and α-helices
          2. Cannot "see" the unique determinant of the β-pleated floor
   d. Immunoglobulin configuration
       i. Formed between the amino termini of the heavy and light chain
8. MHC allelic polymorphism
   a. Differences at multiple residues along the primary sequence
   b. Differences at multiple residues within the same functional domain in the three-dimensional structure
   c. MHC molecules may differ by 10% of their amino acids
   d. Differences occur primarily in hypervariable regions 1, 2, 3
       i. Responsible for specific binding
   e. Unusually high level of linkage disequilibrium

9. MHC codominant pattern of expression
   a. Both alleles are expressed
   b. Increased number of possible combinations
   c. Dominant effect
   d. Higher vulnerability to disease
      i. If two particular disease-associated HLA molecules are expressed
10. Association Studies and Relative Risk
    a. A cohort study
       i. Measures the probabilities that a particular allele confers risk for disease
       ii. A large number of subjects with or without an allele are followed over a lifetime and observed for disease
          1. Exposed with disease = a
          2. Exposed with no disease = b
          3. Not exposed with disease = c
          4. Not exposed with no disease = d
       iii. Relative risk
          1. A measure of how likely a person is to develop the disease if that person inherits allele A
             a. $RR = a/(a+b) \div c/(c+d)$
          2. If the disease is uncommon
             a. RR estimated from cross product $(a \times d) \div (c \times b)$
    b. A case control study
       i. Selected based on whether or not the test and control populations have disease
       ii. Frequency of the allele measured in each group
       iii. Design used in majority of data showing association between HLA alleles and autoimmune disease
       iv. Relative risk
          1. RR values in general less than 10
             a. Exception ankylosing spondylitis (AS) is 100
11. Linkage Disequilibrium
    a. Alleles located near one another (less than 200,000 base pairs apart) are found together in the same individual more often than would be expected by chance
       i. HLA-A3 is in linkage disequilibrium with common mutations in the HFE gene for hemochromatosis
       ii. HLA-A3 has no role in the pathogenesis of the disease
    b. RR > 1 between an allelic polymorphism and a disease
       i. Association statistically significant
       ii. Matched controls

12. Beyond the MHC
    a. Chromosome 1 has been an important candidate in SLE
    b. Major candidate genes outside the HLA
        i. IRF5
        ii. STAT4
        iii. ITGAM
    c. Linkage disequilibrium focuses on the association of particular alleles in populations of unrelated subjects
    d. Coinheritance of disease with a genetic marker within families
    e. Affected sibling pair (ASP) method
        i. The most widely utilized linkage analysis
        ii. Affected siblings are highly likely to be carriers of the same disease alleles
        iii. 50% probability that two siblings will share only one allele
        iv. 25% chance that siblings will share nothing in common
        v. Affected siblings would share more frequently than predicted by mendelian ratios a marker locus located near the disease gene
        vi. ASP develop statistical evidence for a given test marker locus using a x^2 analysis
            1. The null hypothesis being that there is no increased sharing at the marker locus

Rheumatoid Arthritis

5

Section A: Epidemiology, Pathology, and Pathogenesis

1. Epidemiology
   a. Peak incidence fourth and sixth decades (later in men)
   b. Classification criteria (1987 revised criteria from ACR)
      i. A sensitivity and specificity of about 90%
      ii. Must meet four of the following criteria
         1. Morning stiffness (joints) lasting 1 h, present 6 weeks
         2. Soft tissue swelling (arthritis) of three joint areas seen by physician, present 6 weeks
         3. Arthritis of the proximal interphalangeal (PIP), metacarpal phalangeal (MCP), or wrist joints, present 6 weeks
         4. Arthritis is symmetric, present 6 weeks
         5. Subcutaneous nodules
         6. Positive RF (85%)
         7. X-ray erosions or periarticular osteopenia in hand or wrist joints
            a. Most erosions within the first 2 years of disease
      iii. First five criteria are clinical
      iv. Defined as a symmetric polyarthritis involving the small joints of the hands, wrists, and feet (metatarsal phalangeals, MTPs)
   c. Prevalence 0.3–1.5% in North America
      i. 1% of adults in the USA
      ii. 5–6% in some Native American populations
      iii. Increases with age
   d. All races worldwide
   e. 2.5–3 times higher in women
   f. Familial aggregation
      i. Monozygotic twins have a concordance rate of 15–30% and a relative risk of 3.5%
      ii. The risk to unaffected sibling (if one sibling has RA) is 5–10 times that of the general population

N.T. Colburn, *Review of Rheumatology*,
DOI 10.1007/978-1-84882-093-7_5, © Springer-Verlag London Limited 2012

2. Pathology
   a. Earliest changes (electron microscopy)
      i. Injury to synovial microvasculature with occlusion of the lumen
      ii. Swelling of endothelial cells
      iii. Formation of gaps between endothelial cells
   b. The inflammatory stage
      i. Early cellular infiltration of lymphocytes and macrophages
      ii. Congestion
      iii. Edema
      iv. Fibrin exudation
      v. Mild hyperplasia of the superficial lining of both type A and B synoviocytes
      vi. Villous projections
      vii. Proliferative synovium (pannus)
   c. Aggregate formations
      i. One-third of patients acquire a topographical organization reminiscent of tertiary lymphoid tissues
      ii. T and B cells form aggregates with interspersed diffuse infiltrate
      iii. Enriched with CD4+ T cells
      iv. Characteristics of secondary lymphoid follicles
         1. Germinal center reactions with proliferating B cells grouped around a network of follicular dendritic cells
      v. Primary lymphoid follicles are absent
      vi. Diffuse zones consist of CD8+ T cells
      vii. 10–20% of cases form granulomas with histologic changes similar to rheumatoid nodules
   d. Synovial pannus
      i. Cell populations
         1. Plasma cells
            a. Some making RF in advanced cases
         2. Multinucleated giant cells
         3. Mast cells
         4. Few if any PMNs
            a. The predominant cell in inflammatory synovial fluid
      ii. Sublining characteristics
         1. Hyperplasia
         2. Lymphocytic infiltration
         3. Neoangiogenesis
         4. Correlates with disease activity rather than stages of disease
      iii. Extends and invades the cartilage and bone at the margin between the synovium and bone.
         1. Effector cells are synovial fibroblasts and macrophages
         2. Resorption lacunae
            a. Multinucleated cells with gene expression profiles identical to osteoclasts at focal bone erosions

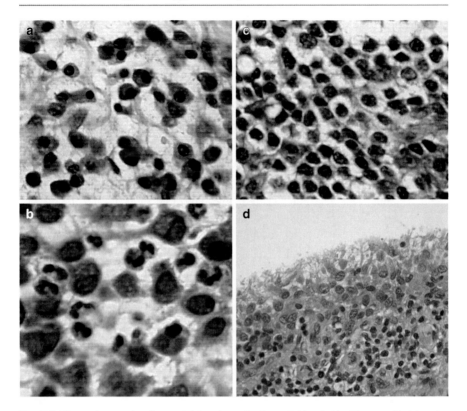

Fig. 5.1 Photomicrographs of synovial membrane in rheumatoid arthritis. Plasma cells (**a**), polymorphonuclear cells (**b**), lymphocytes (**c**), and hyperplasia of the lining layers (**d**). (Hematoxylin and eosin, ×400) (Reproduced with permission from Interleukin-6 levels in synovial fluids of patients with rheumatoid arthritis correlated with the infiltration of inflammatory cells in synovial membrane. *Rheumatology International.* DOI: 10.1007/s00296-006-0143-2. Springer; 2006-09-22)

    e. Histology of extra-articular manifestations
       i. Rheumatoid nodules
          1. Histologic appearance of a granulomatous reaction
             a. Multicentric fibrinoid necrosis surrounded by palisading elongated cells (modified macrophages) arranged radially (parallel to collagen fibers)
             b. Followed by a layer of granulation tissue with inflammatory cells
          2. Occur at pressure points
             a. Precipitated by minor trauma
       ii. Tenosynovitis
          1. Present in the majority
          2. A nonspecific inflammatory infiltrate
          3. Nodules with central necrosis (less frequent)
       iii. Pleurisy and pericarditis
          1. Diffuse mononuclear infiltration and fibrinoid necrosis

  iv. Vascular involvement

   1. Confined to small segments in terminal arteries

   2. Lack distinctive histologic characteristics

   3. Mononuclear infiltration in mid-sized and large arteries

  v. Interstitial pulmonary fibrosis

   1. Cannot be distinguished from the fibrosis of other connective tissue diseases

  vi. Sicca syndrome

   1. Histologically resembles Sjogren's

3. Genetic Basis

 a. Many different genes contribute to disease susceptibility

  i. Some genetic studies suggest that only 30% of increased risk can be ascribed to HLA, indicating a role for non-HLA genes

 b. Susceptibility regions for chromosomes 1, 3, 8, and 18

 c. Candidate gene associations

  i. PTPN22

  ii. PADI4

  iii. CTAL4

  iv. STAT4

 d. Genetic risk factors correlate with disease severity and phenotype

 e. Coefficient of familial clustering, λs

  i. A measure used to estimate the genetic component to disease

  ii. Defined as the ratio of the prevalence in affected siblings to the population prevalence

  iii. For RA, λs ranges from 2 to 12 for the entire genetic load

   1. Low compared to other autoimmune diseases or common genetic disorders

   2. Environmental or stochastic events pathogenesis

   3. The role of HLA accounted for a λs of 1.7

    a. Suggests the λs of other susceptibility genes would be small

 f. RA associated with HLA-DR4

  i. Disease conferring sequence encompasses amino acids 67–74 of the HLA-DRB1 gene

   1. A sequence motif in the third hypervariable region over-represented in RA

    a. Susceptibility gene or "shared epitope"

   2. Polymorphism characterized by a glutamine or arginine at position 70

    a. A lysine or arginine at position 71 and an alanine at position 74 (*positive charged AA*)

    b. Position 71 with the Lys/Arg dimorphism is associated with severe disease

   3. Alleles with a *negative charged AA* at any one of these positions are NOT associated with disease

    4. Disease associated alleles
      a. HLA-DRB1*0401
      b. HLA-DRB1*0404
      c. HLA-DRB1*0408
    5. Disease associated alleles in different populations
      a. Caucasians
        i. HLA-DRB1*0101/2
      b. Asians
        i. HLA-DRB1*0405
      c. Native Americans
        i. HLA-DRB1*1402
      d. Greeks
        i. HLA-DRB1*10
    6. HLA-DRB1*04 alleles
      a. Seen in severe joint disease and/or extra-articular manifestations
      b. Concordance rates in siblings who share both haplotypes are higher than in siblings who share only one
      c. Highest risk for seropositive RA with erosive and major organ disease in 0401/0401 and 0401/0404 (0401 > 0404)
ii. Crystallographic studies of HLA-DR peptide complexes
    1. The conserved sequence mapped to a helix that borders the antigen binding cleft of the HLA-DR molecule
    2. Side chains of the MHC molecules form pockets that interact with side chains of antigenic peptides
      a. Usually 9 AA in length
      b. Determines the peptide specificity of MHC binding
    3. The polymorphic AA of the shared epitope
      a. Forms the pocket that interacts with the side chains of the *fourth AA* in the bound peptide
      b. Preference for a *negatively charged* AA
    4. The positively charged AA at position 71 of the shared epitope favors the binding of peptides with a negatively charged AA
iii. Three functional models for disease associated polymorphisms
    1. Selective binding of autoantigenic peptides
      a. Antigenic peptides with a negatively charged AA at the fourth position trigger a disease inducing T cell response
        i. Peptides from pathogenic microorganisms cross-react with autoantigens
    2. Selective binding of TCR molecules
      a. The disease sequence directly interacts with contact AA of the TCR
      b. TCR-HLA-DR complex formation affected by the AA binding affinity
      c. The shared epitope selects for T cell repertoire in the thymus or T cell survival in the periphery

    3. The HLA molecule functions as a peptide donor
      a. The disease sequence functions as a peptide
         i. Influences the selection of T cells biased toward the recognition of cross-reactive peptides
        ii. Molecular mimicry between the disease sequence triggers proliferative synovial T cell responses
           1. AA sequence QKRAA and bacterial heat shock proteins *dnaJ*

4. Nongenomic Risk Factors
  a. Environmental factors
    i. All efforts to associate an infectious agent with RA have failed
      1. Isolation
      2. Electron microscopy
      3. Molecular biology
    ii. Several infectious agents induce chronic arthropathies in humans
      1. Lyme
      2. Parvovirus
      3. Rubella
      4. HTLV-1
        a. Arthropathy with incorporation of the *tax* gene into synoviocytes
  b. Stochastic events accumulated during the aging process
  c. Acquired genomic variability
    i. Gene arrangements that generate the antigen receptor repertoires of B and T cells

5. Antigen Specific Immune Responses in the Synovium
  a. Tissue infiltrating CD4+ T cells play a central role in the pathogenesis
  b. T cell proliferation in response to an antigen
    i. 30% of patients have tertiary lymphoid tissue with germinal centers
    ii. T cells are oligoclonally expanded
    iii. T cells expressing identical TCRs are found in distinct joints
  c. Synovial inflammation maintained by an antigen specific T cell response
    i. RA synovium engrafted into SCID mice
      1. T cell depleting antibodies reduced cytokines, metalloproteinases, and other inflammatory mediators
      2. Adoptive transfer of HLA-DR compatible T cell clones from the synovium boosted synovial inflammation
  d. T cell depletion in RA does not work
    i. Clonal expansion precluded suppression of the synovial response
    ii. Restorative capacity of the lymphoid system is exhausted
    iii. No change in the synovium despite profound lymphopenia
  e. Antigens recognized in RA have remained elusive
    i. Infectious agents
    ii. Rheumatoid factor in some germinal centers
    iii. Cartilage specific antigens (collagens and proteoglycans)
      1. GP39 is induced in cartilage after exposure to cytokines
    iv. MHC class II antigenic peptide tetramers failed to demonstrate a T cell response to antigens in synovium

     v. CD8 T cells respond to transcriptional transactivators encoded by EBV
       1. No evidence of EBV genes in RA synovium
    vi. Mouse model with erosions and joint specific inflammation to glucose-6-phosphate isomerase of the glycolytic pathway
6. The Cytokine Cascade in RA
  a. A highly complex network with cross-regulation of expression and function
  b. Two pathogenetic concepts of the significance of cytokines
    i. A cascade of events in which some cytokines are higher in the hierarchy than others
      1. IFN-γ
        a. A key mediator
        b. Controls synovial macrophage and fibroblast production of
          i. Monokines (TNF-α and IL-1β)
          ii. Metalloproteinases
      2. TNF-α and IL-1
        a. Two major proinflammatory cytokines
        b. Enhances synovial proliferation
        c. Stimulates secretion of
          i. Metalloproteinases
          ii. Other inflammatory cytokines
          iii. Adhesion molecules
          iv. PGE2
      3. Persistent inflammation correlates with tissue type
        a. Diffuse synovitis characterized by very low production of IFN-γ and IL-4
        b. Granuloma formation associated with the highest production of IFN- γ and IL-4
        c. Lymphoid aggregates produce IFN-γ and IL-10, but not IL-4
    ii. A balance between pro- and anti-inflammatory activities with less emphasis on single cytokines
      1. Feedback loops contribute to perpetuation of synovial inflammation
        a. IL-15
          i. Recruits, expands, and stimulates T cells that interact with synovial macrophages
          ii. Contact dependent (antigen independent)
          iii. Produce TNF-α and additional IL-15
        b. IL-18
          i. Antigen independent bystander T cell activation
        c. TNF-α
          i. Top of a cascade of proinflammatory cytokines
          ii. Blockade suppresses the production of other inflammatory mediators
            1. IL-1
            2. IL-6
            3. IL-8
          iii. TNF-α transgenic mice develop erosive arthritis
          iv. Anti-TNF agents control synovial inflammation

       d. The balance between other pro- and anti-inflammatory cytokines is shifted
          i. Blocking IL-1β or IL-6
         ii. Providing IL-4, IL-10, IL-11, or IL-13

7. Rheumatoid Factor (RF)
  a. A series of antibodies that recognize the FC portion of an IgG molecule as their antigen
  b. Any isotype (IgM, IgG, IgA, or IgE)
    i. IgM RFs (Most measured clinically)
  c. Mechanisms that initiate the production of RFs are unknown
    i. In RA
      1. A heterogeneous set of germline gene elements
      2. No identifiable genetic risk (Ig gene polymorphism)
    ii. Most are of the IgM isotype
      1. Polyclonal B cell activation as an early trigger
      2. Polyclonal stimulants (lectins and superantigens) induce RF production
    iii. Undergo T cell driven isotype switch and affinity maturation
    iv. Interact with the IgFc molecule and not with their antigen binding site (crystal structure)
  d. Effector functions
    i. RF expressing B cells capture antigens trapped in immune complexes
      1. Exist at high frequency in healthy individuals
      2. Unique localization in the lymph node mantle zone
    ii. RF producing B cells in RA
      1. Serve as antigen presenting cells for IgG complexed antigens
      2. Increase efficiency of immune responses to infrequent antigens
  e. Detected in healthy individuals
    i. Prevalence increases with age
  f. RF positivity associated with chronic inflammation and infection
    i. RA
      1. 70% are RF + at disease onset
      2. 10–15% become RF + over the first 2 years (overall 85%)
      3. A major laboratory hallmark
      4. Not a necessary requirement for disease development
      5. Associated with severe disease and extra-articular manifestations
        a. Almost exclusive RF + patients
        b. Subcutaneous nodules
        c. Increased mortality
    ii. Other diseases with positive RFs
      1. Hepatitis C (40%)
      2. SLE (20%)
      3. Sjogren's (70%)
      4. Subacute bacterial endocarditis

8. RA Synovial Membrane
   a. Synovial lining hyperplasia and extensive neoangiogenesis in the sublining
      i. Controlled by growth factors
   b. Activated endothelial cells
      i. Express adhesion molecules
      ii. Produce chemokines
      iii. Facilitate the influx of inflammatory cells
   c. High endothelial venules
      i. Usually seen in secondary lymphoid tissues
      ii. Specialize in lymphocyte recruitment
   d. p53 mutations found in synovial fibroblasts
      i. Evasiveness to apoptotic mechanisms
      ii. Increase proliferation and activation
   e. Immature mesenchymal cells
      i. Express embryonic growth factors of the *wingless* and *frizzled* families
      ii. Replace normal synovial fibroblasts
9. Mechanisms of Joint Destruction
   a. Inflammatory mediators and enzymes in synovial fluid have a direct effect on articular cartilage
   b. Pannus invasion
      i. Leads to focal bone erosions at the margin between bone and cartilage
      ii. Tissue destructive properties related to production of metalloproteinases and other proteinases
      iii. Controlled by IL-1, TNF-α, and TGF-β

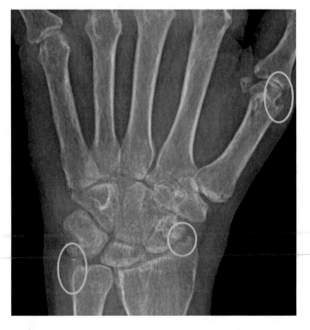

Fig. 5.2 Marginal joint erosions characteristic of rheumatoid arthritis (Reproduced with permission from Rheumatoid arthritis. *A Clinician's Pearls and Myths in Rheumatology.* DOI: 10.1007/978-1-84800-934-9_1. Springer; 2009-01-01)

    c. Subchondral osteolysis from adjacent bone marrow

    d. Chondrocytes and osteoclasts actively participate in the loss of ECM

        i. Chondrocytes decrease collagen and proteoglycan synthesis and increase synthesis of collagenase and stromolysin

       ii. Osteoclast differentiation is regulated by osteoclast differentiation factor

          1. Produced by T cells and fibroblast-like cells in the rheumatoid synovium

          2. Osteoprotegerin, a soluble receptor of osteoclast differentiation factor, can prevent bone erosions

    e. Neutrophils play a major mechanistic role

        i. Very few present in proliferating synovial tissue

       ii. The major cellular component of synovial fluid

      iii. Chemoattractants with neutrophil activating ability

          1. TGF-β and IL-8

            a. Important for adherence and transmigration

          2. Complement factor C5a

            a. Activated because of immune complex formation and LTB4

       iv. Phagocytosis of soluble immune complexes

          1. PG and LT production

          2. Degranulation

          3. Respiratory burst

       v. Targeted directly by immune complexes deposited in the upper cartilage layer

          1. Accumulate proteinases and oxygen metabolites

    f. Multinucleated giant cells

        i. Bony lesions produced by resorption lacunae

       ii. Express the entire repertoire of mature osteoclasts genes

          1. Acid phosphatase

          2. Cathepsin K

          3. Calcitonin receptor

10. The Systemic Component of RA

    a. Age-inappropriate reduction in thymic function

        i. Decreased production of new T cells that express T cell receptor excision circles

    b. Peripheral T cells show features of replicative senescence

        i. Shortened telomeres

       ii. Limited ability to clonally expand

    c. Contracted diversity of T and B cell compartments

    d. Clonal proliferation in the peripheral circulation

        i. CD28 (costimulatory molecule) is lost

       ii. T cells gain NK cell function

          1. Cytotoxic activity

          2. NK receptors

    e. The primary immunopathogenic defect lies in the failure of homeostatic control of the immune system

    f. Phenotypically and functionally identical CD4 T cells found both in patients with RA and acute coronary syndromes infiltrating the plaque

        i. Excess mortality in RA due to cardiovascular complications

Section B: Clinical and Laboratory Features

1. Early RA
   a. An insidious development of symptoms over a period of several weeks
      i. The most common mode of clinical development
   b. Acute monoarticular arthritis is rare
   c. Many findings not evident in the first month or two of disease
      i. Extra-articular features
      ii. Characteristic symmetry of inflammation
         1. Seen as the disease progresses to a more chronic state
      iii. Typical serological labs
   d. Diagnosis is one of exclusion
2. American College of Rheumatology (ACR) established criteria
   a. Diagnosis
   b. Classification of severity by radiographs
   c. Functional classes
   d. Definition of remission
3. Inflammatory synovitis (essential for diagnosis) documented by
   a. Synovial fluid leukocytosis
      i. Defined as WBC counts greater than 2,000/mm^3
   b. Histological evidence of synovitis
   c. Radiographic evidence of characteristic erosions

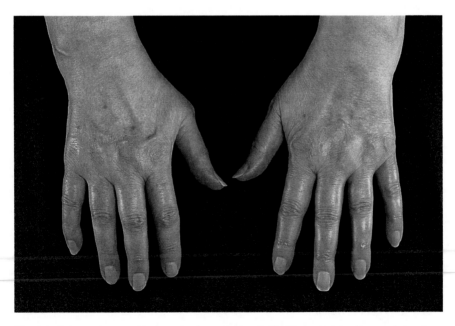

Fig. 5.3 Symmetric synovitis in early rheumatoid arthritis (Reproduced with permission from Rheumatoid arthritis, juvenile rheumatoid arthritis, and related conditions. *Atlas of Rheumatology.* ImagesMD; 2002-03-07)

Morning stiffness > 1 hr > 6 weeks
Arthritis of >3 joints simultaneously >6 weeks
Arthritis of wrist or finger joints >6 weeks
Symmetric arthritis >6 weeks
Rheumatoid factor
Subcutaneous rheumatoid nodules
X–ray signs of rheumatoid arthritis
In accordancce with the ARA criteria (1987), rheumatoid arthritis is diagonised when four of seven criteria are positive.

Fig. 5.4 ARA criteria (1987) for the diagnosis of rheumatoid arthritis (Reproduced with permission from Rheumatoid arthritis. *Encyclopedia of Diagnostic Imaging.* DOI: 10.1007/978-3-540-35280-8_2170. Springer; 2008-01-01)

4. Other causes of synovitis should be excluded
   a. SLE
   b. Psoriatic arthritis
   c. Arthritis associated with parvovirus or hepatitis B virus
   d. Crystalline disease
5. Joint deformities are not specific evidence for RA
   a. Occurs in SLE and non-inflammatory OA
6. Diagnosis established by a constellation of findings observed over a period of time
7. Clinical presentations inconsistent with a diagnosis of RA
   a. Asymmetric arthritis
   b. Migrating pattern
   c. Predominantly large joint arthritis
   d. Distal interphalangeal (DIP) joint involvement
      i. OA
      ii. Psoriatic arthritis
   e. Rash
   f. Back disease
      i. Seronegative spondyloarthropathy (SI joint)
   g. Back and DIP
      i. OA
   h. Renal disease
   i. RF negative status
   j. Leukopenia
   k. Hypocomplementemia
   l. Lack of erosions on radiographs after many months of disease
8. Laboratory Features
   a. Rheumatoid factor (RF)
      i. Found in the serum of about 85% of patients with RA
      ii. Titers correlate with
         1. Severe and unremitting disease
         2. Nodules
         3. Extraarticular lesions

    iii. Serial titers
      1. No value in following disease
      2. Do NOT correlate with disease activity
    iv. A small percentage of the patients who initially are RF negative become RF positive as the disease progresses
    v. Clinical features and prognosis parallel those of patients who were RF positive in early disease
    vi. RF negative disease
      1. Better prognosis
      2. Fewer extra-articular manifestations
      3. Better survival
      4. Sometimes found to have other diseases
        a. Psoriatic arthritis
        b. Lupus
        c. Calcium pyrophosphate crystal deposition disease
        d. Gout
        e. Hemochromatosis
      5. A positive anti-cyclic citrullinated peptide may be helpful

b. Anti-cyclic citrullinated peptide antibody
    i. Reacts with the common epitope identified in the past by other antibodies
      1. Anti-filaggrin
      2. Anti-perinuclear
      3. Anti-keratin
    ii. Highly specific for RA (98%)
    iii. Seen in up to 70% of patients with seropositive RA and 33% with seronegative RA
    iv. Can be present for years before articular manifestations
    v. Useful in differentiating RA from other disorders with articular symptoms plus RF + (hepatitis C)
    vi. Useful in the early diagnosis of RA in patients who are seronegative

c. ESR
    i. Correlates with the degree of synovial inflammation
    ii. Varies greatly

d. Both CRP and ESR
    i. Used to monitor the level and course of inflammation
    ii. The best correlation with disease activity

e. Anemia of chronic disease and elevated platelet counts are seen in patients with active RA
    i. Both correlate with disease activity

f. WBCs are generally normal
    i. May be low in Felty's

g. ANAs are positive in about 30% of patients
    i. Not directed against any of the typical antigens
      1. SS-A
      2. SS-B
      3. Sm

      4. RNP
      5. DNA
    ii. More severe disease and a poorer prognosis than ANA negative
  h. C3, C4, CH50 levels are usually normal or elevated
    i. Serum albumin is frequently low
  i. Acts as a negative acute phase reactant during active disease
  j. Lab abnormalities in patients with severe disease, high RF titer, rheumatoid nodules, and extra-articular manifestations include
    i. Hypergammaglobulinemia
    ii. Hypocomplementemia
      1. Severe vasculitis associated with RA
    iii. Thrombocytosis
    iv. Eosinophilia

9. Articular Manifestations
  a. Reversible signs and symptoms of inflammation
    i. A fluctuating pattern
  b. Irreversible and additive structural damage caused by synovitis
    i. Cartilage loss and erosion of periarticular bone are the characteristic features
    ii. Begins between the first and second year of disease
    iii. Progressive deterioration clinically
      1. Functionally and anatomically
      2. Loss of joint space on x-ray
      3. Crepitus on exam
    iv. Symptoms that fail to respond to aggressive anti-inflammatory treatment suggest structural damage
  c. Morning stiffness is a universal feature of synovial inflammation
    i. Prolonged in RA usually lasting >2 h
    ii. Related to immobilization
    iii. Duration correlates with the degree of synovial inflammation
    iv. Tends to disappear with remission
    v. Document presence and length of stiffness in the disease course

10. Synovial Inflammation
  a. Ankle and hip effusions are difficult to detect
  b. Chronic synovitis differs from synovitis of early disease
    i. Continuous inflammation with immobility
      1. Granulation tissue and fibrosis develop
      2. Vascularity of the synovium decreases
    ii. Obvious inflammation on exam is reduced significantly
      1. Phenomenon known as "burned-out" RA
    iii. Clinical manifestations
      1. Prolonged morning stiffness
      2. General malaise and chronic fatigue
      3. Anemia and elevated ESR
      4. Progressive joint destruction on x-rays
    iv. RA rarely remits spontaneously after the first year

11. Cervical Spine
    a. Common involvement
       i. 30–50% of patients
       ii. C1–2 the most frequently involved level
    b. Radiographs should be obtained prior to surgical procedures requiring intubation
    c. MRI or CT to document spinal cord compression
    d. Cervical spine disease parallels peripheral joint disease
    e. Clinical manifestations of early disease consist primarily of neck stiffness
       i. Perceived through the entire arc of motion
    f. Neck pain and neurological symptoms are not synchronous
    g. Cervical myelopathy
       i. Typically gradual in onset
       ii. Often unrelated to the development or accentuation in neck pain
       iii. Bilateral sensory paresthesia of the hands and motor weakness over weeks to months
       iv. Seen in patients with long-standing destructive disease
       v. Pathologic reflexes (Babinski's or Hoffmann's) and hyperactive DTRs
       vi. L'Hermitte's sign
           1. The sudden development of tingling paresthesia that descends the thoracolumbar spine as the cervical spine is flexed
    h. Patterns of cervical spine involvement
       i. Cervical subluxation
           1. Pain radiates to the occiput in the distribution of the C1–C3 nerve roots
              a. The earliest and most frequent symptom
       ii. C1–2 subluxation
           1. 50% of patients
           2. The most common is anterior subluxation
           3. Results in >3 mm between the arch of C1 and the odontoid of C2
              a. Caused by synovial proliferation around the articulation of the odontoid process with the anterior arch of C1
              b. Leads to stretching and rupture of the transverse and alar ligaments of C1
                 i. Stabilizes the odontoid process of C2
           4. Cervical myelopathy may occur with instability
           5. The risk of cord compression is greatest when
              a. The anterior atlanto-odontoid interval is ≥9 mm
              b. Posterior atlanto-odontoid interval is ≤14 mm
           6. Vertical atlantoaxial subluxation occurs as a result of collapse of the lateral articulations between C1 and C2
              a. The odontoid can impinge on the brainstem
              b. Occurs in <5% of RA patients
              c. The worst prognosis neurologically
                 i. When the odontoid is ≥5 mm above Ranawat's line
           7. Lateral (rotary) and posterior atlantoaxial subluxations can also occur

Fig. 5.5 Cervical spine involvement in rheumatoid arthritis (Reproduced with permission from Rheumatoid arthritis, juvenile rheumatoid arthritis, and related conditions. *Atlas of Rheumatology.* ImagesMD; 2005-01-18)

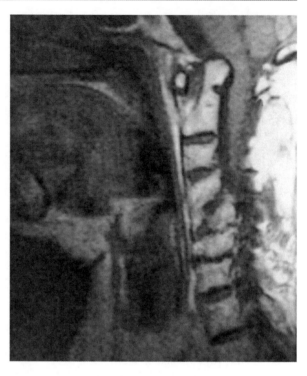

     iii. C1–2 Impaction
         1. 35% of patients
         2. Destruction between the occipitoatlantal and atlantoaxial joints
     iv. Subaxial involvement
         1. 10–20% of patients
         2. Typically C2–3 and C3–4 facets and intervertebral disks
         3. Subluxations related to apophyseal joint destruction
            a. "Stair-stepping" with vertebrae subluxation
            b. Most commonly at C4–5 or C5–6
            c. Lateral x-rays in flexion and extension confirm instability
12. Shoulders
    a. 50–60% involvement
    b. Effusions are difficult to detect
    c. The only objective finding is loss of motion
    d. Shoulder symptoms do not necessarily parallel cartilage destruction
    e. Frozen shoulder
       i. Restriction of shoulder motion in response to pain
      ii. Can develop rapidly
     iii. Treatment is aggressive range of motion (ROM) exercises
     iv. Symptoms are more severe at night

Fig. 5.6 AP radiograph of the left shoulder in a patient with rheumatoid arthritis (*RA*) showing marked destruction of the glenohumeral joint (Reproduced with permission from Arthropathies. *Bone Pathology*. DOI: 10.1007/978-1-59745-347-9_12. Springer; 2009-01-01)

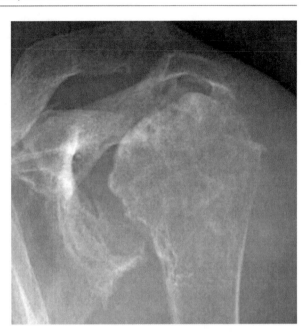

13. Elbow
    a. 40–50% of patients
    b. Easiest joint to detect inflammation
    c. Flexion deformities may develop in early RA
    d. Compression of the ulnar nerve by synovitis
       i. Paresthesia of the fourth and fifth digits
       ii. Weakness of the flexor digiti minimi
    e. Radiohumeral disease worse on pronation and supination
    f. Ulnohumeral disease worse on flexion and extension
14. Hand
    a. Wrists are affected virtually in all patients with RA (90%)
    b. PIP and MCPs are often involved (90–95%)
    c. Usual sparing of the DIP
    d. Ulna deviation at the MCP and radial deviation at the wrists
    e. Swan neck deformity
       i. Flexion contracture of the MCPs
       ii. Hyperextension of PIP
       iii. Flexion of the DIP
       iv. Caused by contraction of the flexors
    f. Boutonniére deformity
       i. Flexion of the PIP
       ii. Hyperextension of the DIP
       iii. Caused by weakening of the central slip of the extrinsic extensor tendon
          1. A palmar displacement of the lateral bands
       iv. Resembles a knuckle being pushed through a buttonhole

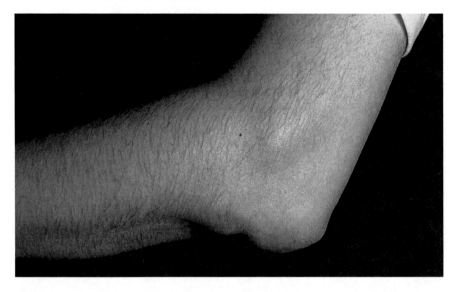

Fig. 5.7 Bursitis and nodulosis in rheumatoid arthritis (Reproduced with permission from Rheumatoid arthritis, juvenile rheumatoid arthritis, and related conditions. *Atlas of Rheumatology.* ImagesMD; 2002-03-07)

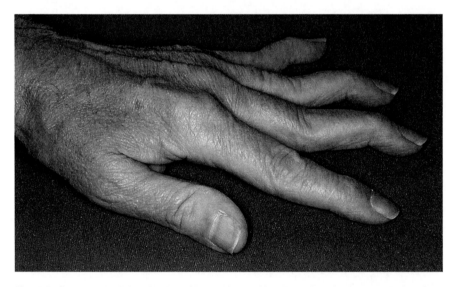

Fig. 5.8 Swan neck deformity in rheumatoid arthritis (Reproduced with permission from Rheumatoid arthritis, juvenile rheumatoid arthritis, and related conditions. *Atlas of Rheumatology.* ImagesMD; 2002-03-07)

    g. Fusiform swelling
       i. Synovitis of PIP joints appear spindle shaped
    h. "Piano key" ulna head
       i. Secondary to destruction of ulnar collateral ligament

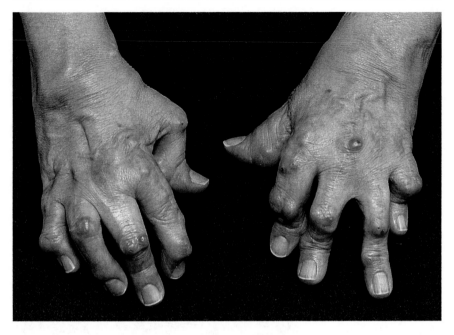

Fig. 5.9 Boutonniére deformity in rheumatoid arthritis (Reproduced with permission from Rheumatoid arthritis, juvenile rheumatoid arthritis, and related conditions. *Atlas of Rheumatology*. ImagesMD; 2002-03-07)

i. Compression neuropathies caused by synovitis
   i. Median nerve
      1. Carpal tunnel
      2. May improve as the retinaculum distends with disease progression
   ii. Ulnar nerve
      1. The nerve as it passes through Guyon's canal
      2. Distinguished from entrapment at the elbow by the absence of weakness of the fifth finger when flexed against resistance
j. Tenosynovitis and rheumatoid nodules can catch and lock as the nodule slides within the tendon sheath
k. Tendon rupture
   i. Inflammatory tenosynovitis erodes through the tendon
   ii. Most commonly in the extensor of the thumb DIP
   iii. Attrition rupture
      1. Extensors of the third, fourth, and fifth fingers abrade against an eroded ulna styloid
   iv. Clinical presentation
      1. History of an abrupt, usually painless, loss of function
      2. Detected by a discrepancy between active and passive motion

Fig. 5.10 Rupture of finger extensors in rheumatoid arthritis (Reproduced with permission from Rheumatoid arthritis, juvenile rheumatoid arthritis, and related conditions. *Atlas of Rheumatology.* ImagesMD; 2005-01-18)

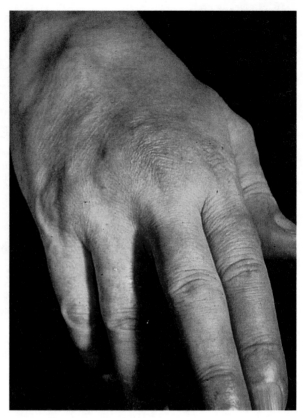

15. Hip
   a. 40–50%
   b. Early disease is often asymptomatic
   c. Subtle reduction in range of motion
      i. Difficulty putting on shoes and socks on the affected side
   d. Pain usually in the groin or thigh
      i. Also felt in the buttock, low back, or medial aspect of the knee
16. Knee
   a. 60–80%
   b. Popliteal (Baker's) cyst
      i. Posterior herniation of the capsule
      ii. May dissect or rupture into the calf muscles
      iii. Symptoms suggestive of thrombophlebitis distinguished by
         1. Characteristic history
         2. Absence of engorged collateral veins
         3. A distinct border of edema below the knee
      iv. Ultrasound
         1. Readily defines a Baker's cyst
         2. May not appear after rupture or dissection has occurred

Fig. 5.11 AP radiograph of the right hip showing axial joint space narrowing with irregular erosions along the femoral head and large lucencies consistent with geodes in a patient with rheumatoid arthritis (*RA*) (Reproduced with permission from Arthropathies. *Bone Pathology*. DOI: 10.1007/978-1-59745-347-9_12. Springer; 2009-01-01)

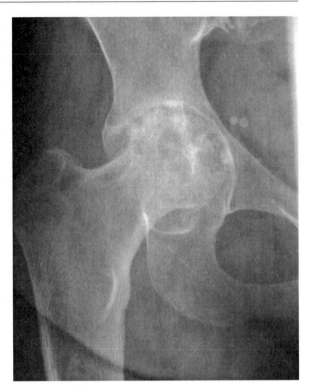

  v. Arthrography
    1. Contrast medium extends posteriorly into the distended gastrocnemio-semimembranous bursa
    2. Shows extension and/or rupture distally into the calf
 17. Foot and Ankle
  a. Joints that RA characteristically affects (in descending order of frequency)
   i. MTP (50–90%)
   ii. Talonavicular
   iii. Ankle (50–80%)
  b. MTP arthritis
   i. Cock-up deformities of the toes and subluxations of the MTP heads on the sole
   ii. Claw toe (hammertoe) is the most common deformity
   iii. Shoe wear leads to callous or ulcer formation
    1. Tops of the toes
    2. Inferior surface of the foot
   iv. Painful to walk
    1. "Walking on pebbles"
    2. Gait problems

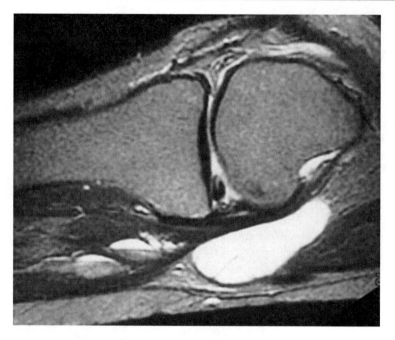

Fig. 5.12 Baker's cyst in rheumatoid arthritis (Reproduced with permission from Rheumatoid arthritis, juvenile rheumatoid arthritis, and related conditions. *Atlas of Rheumatology*. ImagesMD; 2005-01-18)

  c. Tarsal and subtalar joint arthritis
   i. Flattening of the arch and hindfoot valgus deformity
   ii. Ankle flexion and extension usually preserved in early RA
   iii. Tarsal tunnel syndrome
    1. Located posteroinferior to the medial malleolus
    2. Posterior tibial nerve is compressed by synovitis
    3. Paresthesias on the sole of the foot
    4. Worse with walking or standing
18. Joint Deformities
  a. Prolonged immobilization leads to tendon shortening and contraction of the articular capsule
   i. Maintaining motion may prevent the development of deformities
   ii. Shoulder, wrist, and elbows develop deformities early
    1. Patients still able to function with reduced range of motion
   iii. Pain is reduced when joints are positioned with maximum volume and decreased intra-articular pressure
  b. Muscles spasm and shorten in response to inflammation
   i. Intrinsic muscles of the hand
   ii. Anterior peroneal muscle of the foot
    1. Deformities of MCP flexion and tarsal pronation

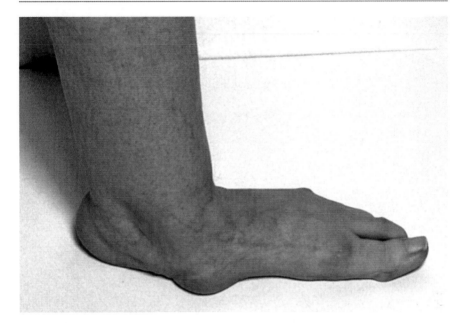

Fig. 5.13 Foot deformities in rheumatoid arthritis (Reproduced with permission from Rheumatoid arthritis, juvenile rheumatoid arthritis, and related conditions. *Atlas of Rheumatology*. ImagesMD; 2002-03-07)

    c. Fusion of incongruous articular surfaces secondary to
       i. Pannus destruction
      ii. Denuded cartilage surfaces
     iii. Eroded juxta-articular bone
19. Extra-articular Manifestations
    a. RA is a systemic disease
    b. General malaise or fatigue is common
       i. Rule out other causes
         1. Infections
         2. Malignancy
         3. Medications
    c. Risk factors for development of extra-articular manifestations
       i. RF+
      ii. Male
     iii. Rheumatoid nodules
     iv. Severe articular disease
      v. MHC class II HLA-DRB1*0401 allele
    d. Skin
       i. Rheumatoid Nodules
         1. Characteristic histology
           a. Central area of fibrinoid necrosis
           b. Surrounded by a zone of palisades of elongated histiocytes
           c. Peripheral layer of cellular connective tissue

      2. Develop in up to 50% of patients typically with
        a. RF+
        b. Severe disease
      3. Develop in crops during active phases
      4. May resolve when disease activity is controlled
      5. Locations
        a. Subcutaneous
        b. In bursae
        c. Along tendon sheaths
        d. Pressure points (typical)
          i. Predilection for the olecranon
            1. Distinguish from gout
          ii. Extensor surface of the forearm
          iii. Achilles tendon
          iv. Ischial area
          v. Sacrum
          vi. Occiput
          vii. MTP joint
          viii. Flexor surfaces of the fingers
      6. Methotrexate (MTX) may enhance or accelerate the development of nodules
        a. Even when the disease is well controlled
  ii. Granuloma annulare
      1. Lesions pathologically similar to rheumatoid nodules
      2. More common in childhood
      3. "Benign RA nodules"
      4. Not associated with arthritis
      5. RF negative
  iii. Vasculitis
      1. Occurs in patients with
        a. Long standing disease
        b. Significant joint involvement
        c. High titer RF
        d. Nodules
      2. Evaluate for evidence of other organ systems involvement
        a. Renal
        b. Neurological
      3. Leukocytoclastic vasculitis
        a. Most common
        b. Palpable purpura on exam
        c. Inflammation of postcapillary venules
      4. Small arteriolar vasculitis
        a. Small infarcts of digital pulp
        b. Associated with mild distal sensory neuropathy
        c. Vasculitis of the vasa nervorum

Fig. 5.14 Episcleritis in rheumatoid arthritis (Reproduced with permission from Rheumatoid arthritis, juvenile rheumatoid arthritis, and related conditions. *Atlas of Rheumatology.* ImagesMD; 2002-03-07)

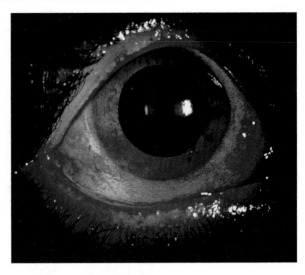

5. Medium vessel vasculitis
   a. Polyarteritis nodosa with visceral arteritis
   b. Mononeuritis multiplex
   c. Livedo reticularis
6. Pyoderma gangrenosum
iv. Skin abnormalities from drugs used to treat RA
   1. Ecchymoses
      a. Nonsteroidal anti-inflammatory drugs (NSAIDs) with platelet dysfunction
      b. Corticosteroids with capillary fragility
   2. Petechiae
      a. DMARDs cause thrombocytopenia
         i. Gold
         ii. Penicillamine
         iii. Sulfasalazine
   3. Cyanotic or grayish hue
      a. Chrysiasis (forehead cyanosis)
         i. Long-term gold use
      b. Grayish facial hue
         i. Chronic minocycline use
e. Ocular Manifestations
   i. Keratoconjunctivitis sicca
      1. Coexistent Sjogren syndrome is common
   ii. Episcleritis
      1. Commonly a benign, self-limited course

Fig. 5.15 Scleritis in
rheumatoid arthritis
(Reproduced with permission
from Rheumatoid arthritis,
juvenile rheumatoid arthritis,
and related conditions. *Atlas
of Rheumatology.*
ImagesMD; 2005-01-18)

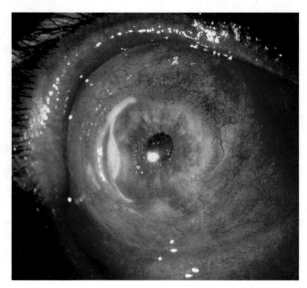

    iii. Scleritis
         1. Morbid prognosis
         2. Histologically resembles rheumatoid nodules
         3. Can erode through the sclera into the choroids
             a. Scleromalacia perforans
  f. Respiratory Manifestations
     i. Laryngeal manifestations
         1. Cricoarytenoid arthritis
             a. Pain
             b. Dysphagia
             c. Dysphonia
             d. Pain on swallowing
             e. Hoarseness
             f. Rarely stridor
             g. Usually episodic
             h. Accentuated in the morning
    ii. Pleural disease
         1. Pleurisy and pleural effusions may be the first manifestation of RA
         2. Usually self-limiting and episodic
         3. May be asymptomatic with small pleural effusions discovered
             incidentally
         4. Effusions characterized as cellular exudates
             a. WBC count < 5,000/mm^3
             b. High protein
             c. High lactate dehydrogenase levels
             d. Very low glucose
                  i. Due to a defect in the transport of glucose across the pleura
             e. Frequently a low pH

iii. Nodules
1. Solitary or multiple
2. Cavitate or resolve spontaneously
3. Caplan's syndrome
   a. Multiple rheumatoid nodules in patients who are coal miners
4. Bronchopleural fistula
   a. Rupture of a nodule
   b. May progress to pneumothorax or empyema
iv. Interstitial pulmonary fibrosis (IPF)
1. Fibrosing alveolitis occurs commonly in RA patients
   a. Symptomatic and progressive in <10%
2. Progressive dyspnea and velcro rales
3. Fibrosis primarily in the lower lobes on CXR
4. Hamman-Rich syndrome
   a. Rapidly progressive IPF

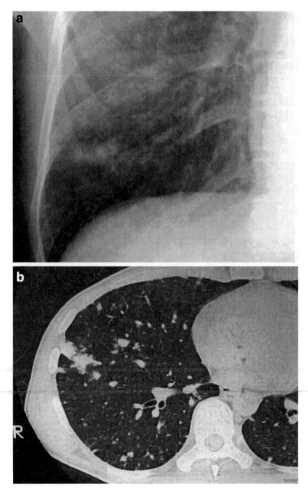

Fig. 5.16 Pulmonary nodules in a patient with RA on chronic steroid therapy. (**a**) Anteroposterior chest radiograph shows ill-defined nodular and linear opacities in the right lower lobe. (**b**) Corresponding CT shows multiple peripherally located well-marginated nodules of different sizes in association with subsegmental areas of air-space consolidation (Reproduced with permission from Respiratory infection in the AIDS and immuno-compromised patient. *European Radiology Supplements.* DOI: 10.1007/s00330-003-2044-z. Springer; 2004-03-01)

Fig. 5.17 Pulmonary fibrosis
in rheumatoid arthritis
(Reproduced with permission
from Rheumatoid arthritis,
juvenile rheumatoid arthritis,
and related conditions. *Atlas
of Rheumatology.* ImagesMD;
2002-03-07)

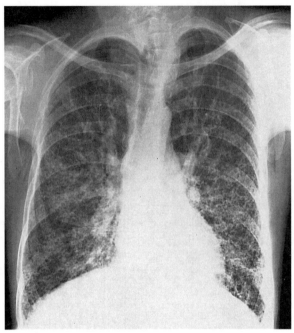

    v. Bronchiolitis obliterans (BO)
      1. Dyspnea
      2. Hyperinflated CXR
      3. Small airway obstruction on pulmonary function test
      4. Can be rapidly fatal
      5. Penicillamine therapy associated with causing this disease
   vi. Bronchiolitis obliterans with organizing pneumonia (BOOP) and nonspecific interstitial pneumonitis (NSIP)
      1. More responsive to corticosteroid therapy than IPF or BO
  vii. Drugs with pulmonary involvement identical to that seen in RA
      1. Penicillamine
        a. BO
      2. Gold
        a. IPF
      3. Methotrexate
        a. May improve if drug stopped
  g. Cardiac Manifestations
    i. Pericarditis
      1. The most common cardiac manifestation of RA
        a. Present in up to 50% at autopsy
      2. Presents with pain in 1% of RA patients
      3. Usually manifests as asymptomatic pericardial effusions
        a. Found by ECHO in about 30% of patients

     4. Episodes of pericarditis usually occur with disease flair

     5. Effusions are rarely large enough to cause tamponade

     6. Chronic constrictive pericarditis

        a. Late in the course

        b. Peripheral edema

        c. Signs of right sided heart failure

  ii. Nodules

     1. Form in and around the heart

     2. May cause conduction defects

     3. Occasional valvular insufficiency

     4. Embolic phenomena

     5. Possible myocardiopathy

  iii. Aortitis

     1. Involve segments or the entire aorta

     2. Aortic insufficiency related to dilation of the aortic root

     3. Aneurismal rupture

  iv. Coronary arteritis

     1. Presents as myocardial infarction

  v. Myocarditis

     1. Presents as heart failure

h. Gastrointestinal Manifestations (rare)

  i. Specific to RA

     1. Xerostomia with associated Sjogren's

     2. Ischemic bowel complication of rheumatoid vasculitis

  ii. Specific to RA therapy

     1. NSAIDs (major complications)

        a. Gastritis

        b. PUD

i. Renal Complications (rare)

  i. Glomerular disease (exceedingly rare)

  ii. Proteinuria

     1. Related to drug toxicity

        a. Gold and penicillamine can cause a membranous nephropathy

     2. Secondary to amyloidosis

  iii. Interstitial disease

     1. Occur with associated Sjogren's

     2. Related to drug toxicity

        a. Papillary necrosis

           i. NSAIDs

           ii. Acetaminophen

           iii. Other analgesics

j. Pathogenesis of Neurologic Disorders (1 of 3 mechanisms)

  i. Cervical spine instability (see above)

    ii. Peripheral nerve entrapment
- 1. Confirmed clinically by demonstrating a response to
  - a. Temporary splinting
  - b. Use of intra-articular corticosteroids
- 2. Compression sites
  - a. Median nerve
    - i. Carpal tunnel
  - b. Ulnar nerve
    - i. Guyon's canal
    - ii. Cubital tunnel
  - c. Posterior interosseous branch of the radial nerve
    - i. Antecubital fossa
  - d. Femoral nerve
    - i. Anterior to the hip joint
  - e. Peroneal nerve
    - i. At the MTP joint

   iii. Vasculitis (mononeuritis multiplex)
- 1. Marked by abrupt onset of a persistent peripheral neuropathy
  - a. Unaltered by change in the joint position or reduction in synovial inflammation
- 2. Concurrent evidence of rheumatoid vasculitis often seen
- 3. Neurophysiologic studies reveal an axonal lesion
  - a. May demonstrate several clinically inapparent mononeuropathies
- 4. A sural nerve biopsy confirms the diagnosis

k. Hematologic Manifestations

     i. Hypochromic microcytic anemia
- 1. Low serum ferritin
- 2. Low or normal iron binding capacity
- 3. An almost universal finding with active RA

    ii. Difficult to distinguish between an iron deficiency anemia
- 1. Fails to respond to iron therapy with a brisk reticulocytosis
- 2. Ferritin levels can be the same
- 3. Examine the bone marrow for iron stores (definitive answer)

   iii. Thrombocytopenia
- 1. Marrow suppression due to immunosuppressive or cytotoxic therapy
- 2. An autoimmune process in gold, penicillamine, or sulfasalazine therapy

   iv. Felty's Syndrome
- 1. Classic triad originally described as the combination of
  - a. *RA*
  - b. *Splenomegaly*
  - c. *Leukopenia*
  - d. (Leg ulcers)
- 2. Later descriptions added
  - a. Lymphadenopathy
  - b. Thrombocytopenia
  - c. The HLA-DR4 haplotype

3. Seen in 1% of RA patients
4. Most common in severe RA
    a. Nodule-forming
    b. Extra-articular manifestations
    c. RF+
        i. 95% are RF+ and HLA-DR4 positive
5. Leukopenia
    a. Pathogenesis poorly understood
    b. Selectively involves neutrophils ($<2,000/mm^3$)
6. Major complications
    a. Bacterial infections
        i. 20-fold increase compared with other RA patients
        ii. Severe infections correlate with neutrophil counts of $<1,000/mm^3$
    b. Chronic non-healing ulcers
7. Other complications
    a. A 13-fold increased risk of non-Hodgkin's lymphoma
    b. Nodular regenerative hyperplasia of the liver
        i. Portal hypertension
        ii. Bleeding varices
8. Treatment
    a. Same as for RA with joint disease
    b. Splenectomy and lithium are out of favor
        i. Previously used for severe recurring infections and non-healing ulcers
    c. Granulocyte colony stimulating factor (G-CSF)
        i. Effective at increasing WBC counts and decreasing infections in some patients
            1. Neutrophils $<1,000/mm^3$
        ii. Can cause arthritis and vasculitis in some patients when the WBC is raised
        iii. Filgrastim (Neupogen)
            1. Patients with recurrent infections
            2. Given at doses of 2–5 µg/kg/day until neutrophils $> 1,500/mm^3$
            3. Then weekly to maintain this level
v. Large granular lymphocyte (LGL) syndrome
    1. Shares some of the same features of Felty's
        a. Considered a subset of Felty's in RA
        b. 1/3 of Felty's patients
            i. Significant clonal expansion of LGLs on peripheral smear
            ii. HLA-DR4 positive
    2. Not exclusive to RA
    3. Syndrome characteristics
        a. Neutropenia
        b. Splenomegaly

      c. Susceptibility to infections

      d. Large granular lymphocytes

         i. Bear CD2, 3, 8, 16, and 57 surface phenotypes in the peripheral blood smear

         ii. Natural killer and antibody-dependent cell-mediated cytotoxic activity

20. Clinical problems frequently increased in RA

    a. Sjogren's

      i. Up to 30% develop secondary Sjogren's syndrome

        1. Dry eyes

        2. Dry mouth

      ii. Frequently ANA+

      iii. Typically do **NOT** have anti-SS-A or SS-B antibodies commonly seen in primary Sjogren's

    b. Amyloidosis

      i. Up to 5% develop secondary or AA associated amyloidosis

      ii. Occurs in long-standing, poorly controlled RA

      iii. Presents as nephritic syndrome

    c. Osteoporosis

      i. Seen in the majority of RA patients

      ii. Related to

        1. Disease activity

        2. Immobility

        3. Medications

      iii. Insufficiency fractures

        1. Spine and sacrum are common locations

        2. Long standing disease

    d. Ear ossicles

      i. Tinnitus

      ii. Decreased hearing

21. Course and Prognosis

    a. Factors that predict a severe persistent disease course

      i. The *best predictors* of disability and joint damage at presentation

        1. RF+

        2. Poor functional status

          a. High health assessment questionnaire (HAQ) score >1

      ii. Generalized polyarthritis involving both small and large joints

        1. >20 total joints

      iii. Extra-articular disease

        1. Rheumatoid nodules

        2. Vasculitis

      iv. Persistently elevated ESR or CRP

      v. Radiographic erosions within 2 years of disease onset

      vi. HLA-DR4 haplotype

      vii. Education level <11th grade

      viii. Manual labor jobs that contribute to joint damage

b. Disease remission
   i. Five or more of the following criteria must be fulfilled for at least 2 consecutive months
     1. Duration of morning stiffness not exceeding 15 min
     2. No fatigue
     3. No joint pain (by history)
     4. No joint tenderness or pain on motion
     5. No soft tissue swelling in joints or tendon sheaths
     6. ESR < 30 mm/h for a female or 20 mm/h for a male
   ii. The prevalence of remission is unknown
   iii. Two classic studies (1957 and 1959) found low rates of spontaneous remissions
     1. Only 10% of patients experienced clinical remission during more than a decade of follow-up
     2. Remission usually occurred within the first 2 years of disease onset
   iv. In patients who do not undergo spontaneous remission
     1. Joint destruction prognosis depends on the severity of synovial inflammation
c. Almost 90% of joints ultimately affected are involved during the first year of disease
d. Long-term prognosis
   i. About 50% of patients will be functional class III or IV within 10 years of disease onset
   ii. Over 33% who were working at the time of onset of disease will leave the workforce within 5 years
   iii. Standardized mortality ratio is 2–2.5:1 compared with people of same sex and age
   iv. RA shortens lifespan of patients by 5–10 (up to 15) years
   v. 5-year survival rate of 50% or less in patients with the poorest functional status and multiple joint involvement
   vi. Aggressive DMARD therapy can reduce disability by 30% over 10–20 years
e. Causes for increased mortality
   i. Cardiovascular (42%)
     1. Frequency not increased over the general population
   ii. Cancer and lymphoproliferative malignancies (14%)
     1. Increased 5–8 times over general population
     2. Associations not clear
       a. Chronic immunostimulation
       b. Immunosuppressive therapy
         i. MTX
         ii. Cyclosporine
         iii. Cyclophosphamide
     3. Consider infection and lymphoreticular malignancy with fever and lymphadenopathy
       a. Uncommon symptoms in RA

    iii. Infections (9%)
  1. Increased 5 times over general population
  2. Pneumonia is common
  3. Increased risk for joint infections
     a. Abnormal joint structure
     b. Immunosuppressive medications
     c. Suspect when one or two joints are swollen, red, and hot out of proportion to other joints
  4. Infections in total joint replacements (TJRs)
     a. A constant concern
     b. *Staph. aureus* is the most common infecting organism
    iv. Other causes of mortality
  1. Renal disease due to amyloidosis
  2. Gastrointestinal hemorrhage due to NSAIDs (4%)
  3. RA complications (5–10%) deaths due to RA itself
     a. Vasculitis
     b. Atlantoaxial dislocation
     c. RA involvement of the lungs and heart
     d. Medication induced
    v. Excess mortality has not changed in four decades
  1. Despite the general population's increased survival

Section C: Treatment

1. Major advances in the treatment of RA due to three trends
   a. Drug therapies used early in the disease can alter the outcome and reduce severity, disability, and mortality
   b. Improved understanding of pathogenetic mechanisms involved in immunologic and inflammatory responses
   c. Therapies specifically target the pathophysiologic processes and mediators
2. Gradual onset of disease occurs in more than 50% of patients
   a. About 20% have a monocyclic course that will abate within 2 years
   b. Long-term prognosis of abrupt onset disease is similar to that for gradual disease onset
   c. The median time between the onset of symptoms and diagnosis is 36 weeks
3. Successful management of RA
   a. An accurate diagnosis is the foundation for proper management
   b. Initiation of patient specific treatment early in the disease course
   c. Health care providers that work with health related beliefs to educate patients about their disease is fundamental
4. Clinical tools for monitoring disease activity
   a. Morning stiffness
   b. Severity of fatigue

    c. Health assessment questionnaire (HAQ) status
       i. Functional
      ii. Social
     iii. Emotional
     iv. Pain
    d. Visual analog scale
       i. A patient derived global assessment
    e. Number of tender and swollen joints
    f. Laboratory measures for the presence of
       i. Anemia
      ii. Thrombocytosis
     iii. Elevated ESR or CRP
    g. Serial radiographs of target joints (including hands) to assess disease progression
5. Major goals of therapy
    a. Relieve pain, swelling, and fatigue
    b. Improve joint function
    c. Stop joint damage
    d. Prevent disability and disease-related morbidity
6. ACR definition for improvement in RA treatment trials
    a. Required (both)
       i. ≥20% improvement in tender joint count
      ii. ≥20% improvement in swollen joint count
    b. Plus
       i. ≥ 20% improvement in three of the following five
         1. Patient pain assessment
         2. Patient global assessment
         3. Patient self-assessed disability (HAQ)
         4. Physician global assessment
         5. Acute-phase reactant
           a. ESR
           b. CRP
    c. ACR 20 criteria are met as defined above
    d. ACR 50 or ACR 70 criteria are met for patients improved by 50% or 70%
7. Occupational and physical therapy (PT) modalities
    a. Joint protection
    b. Functional enhancement
    c. Splints
    d. Orthotics and adaptive and adequate footwear
    e. Adaptive devices
    f. Exercises
       i. ROM
      ii. Stretching
     iii. Strengthening
     iv. Conditioning

8. Drug Therapy (two groups)
   a. Those used primarily for the control of pain and swelling
   b. Those intended to limit joint damage
9. NSAIDs
   a. Inhibits proinflammatory prostaglandins
   b. Effective treatments for pain, swelling, and stiffness
   c. No effect on disease course or risk of joint damage
   d. Inhibits one or both COX
      i. Results in decreased synthesis of PG
   e. Used primarily for symptom control
   f. Consider the patient's age, sex, and medical history
      i. Older females are at higher risk for GI complications
         1. Use of nonselective NSAIDS are contraindicated
      ii. Prescribe gastric protective agents
         1. Proton pump inhibitor (PPI)
         2. Misoprostol
         3. Selective COX
   g. NSAID gastropathy is common in RA
      i. Up to 30% chance of hospitalization or death from GI toxicity
10. Corticosteroids
   a. Inadequate as a sole therapy for RA
   b. Treatment for flairs or as a DMARD therapy bridge
      i. Brief course (15–20 mg a day) of prednisone tapering over 1–3 weeks
   c. Treatment for severe polyarticular disease
      i. 2–15 mg per day of prednisone in divided doses
      ii. Split dosing helps because of the short anti-inflammatory half-life
   d. Intra-articular injections
      i. Effective for reducing pain and inflammation in recalcitrant individual joints
11. DMARDs
   a. Prevent joint erosions and damage
   b. Control active synovitis and constitutional features
   c. No evidence to support that these drugs can
      i. Heal erosions
      ii. Reverse joint deformities
      iii. Cure disease
   d. 50% of patients remain on MTX therapy after 5–12 years
      i. Less than 20% remain on other DMARDs for 5 years
   e. Best time to initiate therapy
      i. When the diagnosis of RA is established
      ii. Before erosive changes appear on x-ray
   f. Two basic approaches in early treatment
      i. "Step-up" monotherapy
         1. Select a DMARD appropriate to disease severity
            a. Estimated by prognostic markers

      2. If monotherapy fails

        a. Switch to another DMARD

        b. Add one or two others

  ii. "Step-down"

      1. A combination of DMARDs and corticosteroids

        a. At the outset of disease

        b. Patients with a poor prognosis

      2. Eliminate each as disease control improves

g. Different treatment regimens for different stages of disease

  i. Newly diagnosed RA in a young woman with mild disease (few joints) RF+ and ESR < 30

      1. Hydroxychloroquine 400/day (OR sulfasalazine up to 3 g/day)

      2. +/− NSAID

      3. Prednisone 3–5 mg/day over 1–3 months

  ii. New onset RA with marked symptoms of fatigue, low-grade fever, weight loss, and polyarticular disease

      1. MTX

      2. NSAID

      3. Prednisone 5–15 mg/day

        a. Taper prednisone over 3–4 months

      4. Add hydroxychloroquine and/or sulfasalazine if unable to gain control in 6–8 weeks

  iii. Patient with established RA in whom MTX is partially effective

      1. Add NSAID or prednisone 5–15 mg/day

      2. Initiate combination therapy

        a. Hydroxychloroquine, sulfasalazine, or both

        b. TNF antagonist or leflunomide

  iv. Combination therapy with hydroxychloroquine, sulfasalazine, or both is ineffective

      1. Discontinue hydroxychloroquine and sulfasalazine

      2. Add leflunomide, azathioprine, cyclosporine, or anti-TNF

  v. Combination therapy with MTX and cyclosporine, leflunomide, or azathioprine is poorly tolerated or ineffective

      1. Continue MTX

      2. Discontinue the combination drug

      3. Add anti-TNF

  vi. Patient with established RA in whom MTX is ineffective, not tolerated, or contraindicated

      1. Mild disease

        a. Leflunomide

        b. Sulfasalazine

        c. Azathioprine

      2. Severe disease

        a. Cyclosporine

        b. Combinations of DMARDs

      c. Add anti-TNF

      d. Gold occasionally used

      e. Prednisone 5–15 mg/day may be needed

12. Hydroxychlroquine

    a. The first drug of choice for early, mild, and/or seronegative disease

    b. Favorable toxicity profile and ease of use

    c. Onset of activity within 3 or 4 months in about 50% of patients

      i. May take up to a year for full benefit

    d. Retinopathy is rare with appropriate dosages

13. Sulfasalazine

    a. Acceptable toxicity profile

    b. Used as initial treatment for early, mild, and/or seronegative disease

    c. Initial dose 500–1,000 mg/day

      i. Maximum 1,500 mg BID

    d. Side effects

      i. GI upset

      ii. Myelosuppression

    e. Frequently used in combination with hydroxychlroquine or MTX

14. Methotrexate

    a. Preferred choice for established disease or severe, newly diagnosed disease

      i. Patients who respond have significantly increased life expectancy

      ii. About 70% improvement as a single therapy

    b. Often used in combination

    c. Well-recognized, long-term efficacy and toxicity profile

    d. The lowest long-term drug discontinuation rate of any DMARD

    e. Dosing

      i. Initial dose is 7.5–10.0 mg/week

      ii. Titrated up to 17.5 mg/week average

      iii. Doses to 25 mg/week before considered failed

    f. Injectable MTX associated with less stomatitis and GI upset

    g. Side effects

      i. May occur in up to 70% of people

      ii. GI upset

      iii. Hepatotoxicity

        1. Rare

        2. Liver fibrosis

        3. Cirrhosis

        4. Avoid alcohol

      iv. Opportunistic infections

      v. B-cell non-Hodgkin's lymphoma

      vi. Accelerated nodulosis

        1. Especially on fingers

        2. No clear treatment

      vii. Avoid in certain patient populations

        1. Pregnant patients because of teratogenicity

       2. Patients with hepatic or renal insufficiency

       3. Patients with severe lung disease

  viii. Stomatits

    ix. Hair thinning

     x. Bone marrow suppression

    xi. Supplemental folate (1 mg/day) helps to reduce side effects

   xii. Avoid antifolate drugs (sulfamethoxazole)

       1. May precipitate pancytopenia

  h. Does not halt the progression of disease

    i. Long-term treatment with MTX compared to newer drugs

      i. Less expensive

     ii. Able to establish remission

    iii. Limits joint damage

15. Azathioprine

  a. Prescribed for moderate or severe RA

  b. Adequate toxicity and safety profile, but generally displaced by MTX

  c. No convincing evidence of true disease modifying capability

  d. May be used with refractory disease, or severe extra-articular disease manifestations such as vasculitis

16. Cyclosporine

  a. Effective in low doses (2.5–5.0 mg/kg/day)

    i. Solo

    ii. In combination with MTX

  b. Slows the progression of joint damage

    i. Even in severe, refractory RA

  c. Drawbacks

    i. High cost

    ii. Hypertension

    iii. Renal toxicity

    iv. Close monitoring

17. Cyclophosphamide

  a. Alkylating agent of limited benefit

  b. Poor toxicity profile

    i. Bone marrow toxicity

    ii. Infertility

    iii. Bladder toxicity

    iv. Oncogenicity

  c. Restricted to corticosteroid refractory systemic vasculitis

18. Leflunomide

  a. A pyrimidine synthesis inhibitor

  b. Clinical efficacy generally equivalent to that of MTX

  c. Slows the rate of radiographic progression of erosive disease

  d. Side effects

    i. Rash

    ii. Alopecia

   iii. Allergy
   iv. Weight loss
   v. Thrombocytopenia
   vi. Diarrhea
       1. Occurs early
       2. Usually abates
       3. Discontinue drug if unable to control
19. Anti-TNF
   a. Etanercept
      i. A fusion protein
      ii. Composed of two identical chains of recombinant human TNF-α fused
          with the Fc portion of human IgG1
      iii. Binds to soluble TNF-α in vitro
      iv. 70% of patients have substantial decreases in joint inflammation within
          1–2 weeks
          1. Enhanced by adding MTX
      v. Side effects
          1. Influenza-like symptoms
          2. Reactions at the injection site
             a. Usually abates
   b. Infliximab
      i. A chimeric monoclonal antibody to TNF-α
      ii. Maintenance dose 3 mg/kg every 8 weeks
      iii. Efficacy equivalent to etanercept
      iv. Associated with the development of autoantibodies
      v. Side effects
          1. Increased risk of active TB
          2. Demyelinating syndromes
   c. Improvement within 8–12 weeks
   d. Slows radiographic progression of disease
   e. High cost
   f. Avoid in certain patient populations
      i. Active serious infections
          1. Sepsis
          2. Osteomyelitis
      ii. History of TB
      iii. Myeloproliferative disease (lymphoma)
20. Abatacept and Rituximab
   a. Additional biologics for moderate-to-severe RA
   b. Approved for active RA with failed DMARD and anti-TNF therapy
   c. Abatacept
      i. Recombinant fusion protein
          1. Extracellular domain of human CTLA-4
          2. Fc domain of human IgG1
      ii. Binds to CD80/CD86 on APCs

      iii. Prevents second signal for T cell activation

      iv. An ACR20 response of 50% in active RA with failed anti-TNF response compared to placebo response of 19%

   d. Rituximab

      i. Chimeric anti-CD20 monoclonal antibody

      ii. Depletes B cells

      iii. Mechanism of action may involve

         1. Reduction of B cell cytokines

         2. Inhibition of T cell activation

      iv. Infused at a dose of 1,000 mg and repeated at 2 weeks

      v. Studied at 24 weeks with ACR 20 response for MTX alone (38%), rituximab alone (65%), MTX and rituximab (73%), and rituximab and cyclophosphamide (76%)

21. Therapies less used

   a. Minocycline

      i. Only antibiotic to be studied in RA

      ii. Improves mild to moderate symptoms

      iii. No documented DMARD properties

      iv. High rate of drug discontinuation secondary to side effects

         1. Skin discoloration

         2. Dizziness

         3. GI upset

         4. Autoimmune phenomena

            a. Hepatitis

   b. Chlorambucil

      i. Poor toxicity/efficacy profile

      ii. Used for severe extra-articular disease manifestations

         1. Systemic vasculitis

         2. Severe scleritis

   c. Immunosorbent column

      i. Weekly exchanges for 12 weeks

         1. Minority of patients

      ii. High risk

         1. Thrombophlebitis

         2. Syncope

         3. Thromboembolism

22. Combination therapies

   a. For patients with moderate to severe disease

      i. MTX used with other agents

         1. Most popular

         2. MTX, hydroxychloroquine, and sulfasalazine

   b. For acute and severe disease

      i. DMARD, corticosteroids, and NSAIDs

   c. 50% of patients receive combinations with two or three DMARDs

23. Extra-articular disease
    a. Vasculitis, scleritis, and recalcitrant serositis
    b. Require systemic corticosteroids
    c. May necessitate the use of immunosuppressive agents
        i. Cyclophosphamide
        ii. Cyclosporine
        iii. When controlled replace with MTX at 15–25 mg/week

Psoriatic Arthritis

6

1. Psoriasis
   a. Common in Caucasian
   b. Uncommon in Asians
   c. Overall prevalence is 2%
   d. Peak age 5–15 years
   e. Polygenetic
      i. Not a single gene Mendelian pattern
      ii. Multiple genetic or environmental influences affect phenotype
2. Arthritis occurs in about 5–7% of people with psoriasis
   a. Up to 40% in patients with extensive lesions that require hospitalization
   b. Overall prevalence is 0.1% in the US
   c. Male to female ratio is about equal
      i. Varies in subsets
   d. Peak age between 30 and 55 years
3. Genetic Factors for Psoriatic Arthritis (PA)
   a. Family studies
      i. Approximate 50-fold increased risk in first-degree relatives
      ii. Family members may develop psoriasis, arthritis, or both
      iii. Affected fathers are two times as likely to transmit the disease as affected mothers
   b. Animal studies
      i. HLA-B27 transgenic rat
         1. Psoriasiform skin and nail lesions
   c. HLA class I antigens
      i. Associated with and without arthritis
      ii. B13, B16, B17
         1. Linkage disequilibrium between these antigens and Cw6
      iii. Primary association is HLA-Cw*0602
   d. MICA-002 allele (class I MHC related gene) polymorphism
      i. Confers susceptibility to polyarticular PA independent of Cw*0602

N.T. Colburn, *Review of Rheumatology*,
DOI 10.1007/978-1-84882-093-7_6, © Springer-Verlag London Limited 2012

    e. HLA Class II antigen relationships
       i. HLA-DR7 and psoriasis
       ii. HLA-DR4 and PA
    f. A psoriasis-associated gene mapped to the long arm of chromosome 17
4. Environmental Factors
    a. Infectious agents
       i. Clinical similarities between reactive arthritis and PA
       ii. Precipitation of guttate psoriasis by strep infections in children
       iii. Reactive from psoriatic plaque flora (Strep and Staph)
    b. Trauma
       i. The deep Koebner effect
       ii. Release of putative autoantigens
       iii. Expression of heat-shock proteins resembling bacterial antigens
5. Immunologic Factors
    a. Similar histopathologic changes in the skin and synovium
       i. Activation and expansion of tissue-specific cells
          1. Keratinocytes
          2. Synoviocytes
       ii. Accumulation of inflammatory cells
          1. T-cells
          2. B-cells
          3. Macrophages
          4. Neutrophils
    b. T-cell activation
       i. Th1 phenotype and CD4 cells
       ii. Psoriasis improves with T-cell directed therapies
          1. Cyclosporine
          2. IL-2 fusion toxins
             a. Preferentially eliminates IL-2 receptor bearing cells
          3. CTLA4Ig
             a. Inhibits costimulatory signals for T-cell activation
    c. Skin and synovium dominated by monokines
       i. TNF-α, IL-1-α, IL-1β, IL-6, IL-15, and IL-10
       ii. Psoriatic arthritis compared to RA synovium
          1. TNF-α:IL-10 ratio is elevated
             a. A relative deficiency in IL-10
       iii. IL-15 in psoriatic skin
          1. Inhibits keratinocyte apoptosis
          2. Promote keratinocyte accumulation
6. Clinical Features
    a. Patients classified into three groups
       i. Mono- or oligoarthritis with enthesitis
          1. 30–50%
          2. Resembles reactive arthritis

   ii. Symmetric polyarthritis resembling RA
      1. 30–50%
   iii. Predominantly axial disease
      1. About 5%
      2. Spondylitis
      3. Sacroilitis
      4. Arthritis of hip and shoulder joints
      5. Resembles ankylosing spondylitis with or without peripheral disease
   b. With any of these subgroups
      i. DIPJ involvement (25%)
      ii. Arthritis mutilans (5%)
      iii. Sacroilitis (35%)
      iv. Spondylitis (30%)
   c. In about 70% of patients psoriasis is present many years before arthritis
      i. Psoriasis and arthritis appear concomitantly in about 15%
   d. Arthritis is usually insidious in onset
      i. 1/3 of patients have an acute onset
      ii. Constitutional symptoms are uncommon
   e. Arthritis sine psoriasis
      i. Arthritis appears before skin or nail changes
      ii. 15% of adults
      iii. More often in children
7. Joint Disease
   a. Mono- or oligoarticular
      i. The most common initial manifestation
         1. Observed in up to 2/3 of patients
         2. Usually a large joint (knee) with 1 or 2 IP joints and a dactylitic digit or toe

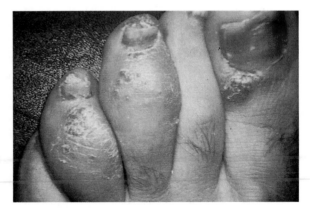

Fig. 6.1 Dactylitis in psoriatic arthritis (Reproduced with permission from Spondyloarthropathies. *Atlas of Rheumatology.* ImagesMD; 2005-01-18)

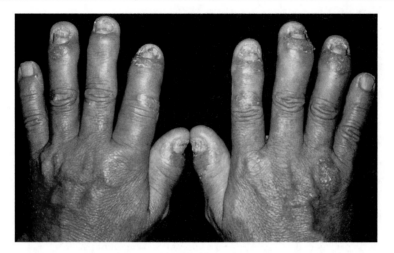

Fig. 6.2 Symmetrical hand deformities in psoriatic arthritis (Reproduced with permission from Spondyloarthropathies. *Atlas of Rheumatology*. ImagesMD; 2005-01-18)

    ii. Dactylitic
       1. A combination of tenosynovitis and arthritis of the DIP or PIP joint
    iii. Similar to the peripheral arthritis in spondyloarthropathies
    iv. 1/2 to 1/3 will evolve into a more symmetric polyarthritis
    v. Arthritis may follow an episode of trauma
       1. Family history of either psoriasis or guttate psoriasis in childhood
       2. Search hidden areas for psoriasis
         a. Scalp
         b. Umbilicus
         c. Perianal areas
    vi. DIP involvement
       1. Associated with psoriatic changes in the nails
  b. Polyarthritis
    i. The most common pattern is symmetric polyarthritis
       1. Small joints of the hands and feet, wrists, ankles, knees, and elbows
    ii. Distinguishable from RA by a higher frequency of
       1. DIP involvement
       2. Bony ankylosis of DIP and PIP
         a. "Claw" or "paddle" deformities of hands
  c. Arthritis Mutilans
    i. Rare
    ii. Highly characteristic of psoriatic arthritis
    iii. Osteolysis of the phalanges and metacarpals of the hands
       1. Or phalanges and metatarsals of the feet
    iv. Results in "telescoping" of the involved finger or toe
    v. Occurs in about 5% of patients with PA

Fig. 6.3 Arthritis mutilans (Reproduced with permission from Spondyloarthropathies. *Atlas of Rheumatology.* 2005-01-18)

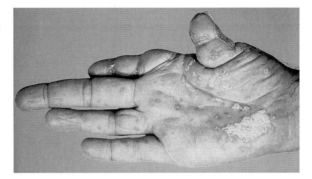

    d. Axial Disease
        i. Usually manifests after several years of peripheral arthritis
       ii. Spine symptoms rarely are a presenting feature
          1. Inflammatory back pain or chest wall pain may be absent or minimal
          2. Despite advanced radiographic changes
      iii. Sacroilitis
          1. Up to 1/3 of patients
          2. Occurs independent of spondylitis
          3. Frequently asymptomatic and asymmetric
      iv. Spondylitis
          1. Occurs independently
          2. Affects any portion of the spine randomly
          3. Results in fusions
       v. Cervical spine subluxations
          1. Rare
    e. Enthesitis
        i. Common
       ii. Achilles and plantar fascia
      iii. Frequently in the oligoarthritis form
    f. Ocular involvement
        i. Predominantly conjunctivitis
       ii. Up to 1/3
    g. Other complications (rare)
        i. Aortic insufficiency
       ii. Uveitis
      iii. Pulmonary fibrosis
          1. Involves the upper lobes
      iv. Amyloidosis
8. Dermatologic features
    a. Skin lesions
        i. Sharply demarcated erythematous plaque with a well marked silvery scale
       ii. Commonly involved areas
          1. Extensor surfaces of elbows and knees

Fig. 6.4 Nail pitting in psoriatic arthritis (Reproduced with permission from Spondyloarthropathies. *Atlas of Rheumatology.* 2005-01-18)

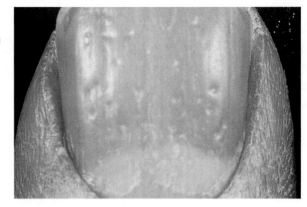

      2. Scalp

      3. Ears

      4. Presacral areas

   iii. Other sites of involvement

      1. Palms and soles

      2. Flexor areas

      3. Low back

      4. Hair line

      5. Perineum and genitalia

   iv. Variable size

    v. Gentle scraping usually produces pinpoint bleeding (Auspitz)

  b. Nail involvement

     i. The only clinical feature that identifies patients with psoriasis who are likely to develop arthritis

    ii. See pitting, onycholysis (separation of the nail from the underlying nail bed) transverse depression (ridging) and cracking, subungual keratosis, brown-yellow discoloration (oil-drop sign), and leukonychia

   iii. None of these nail findings are specific for psoriatic arthritis, even pitting can be seen in healthy individuals

   iv. However, multiple pits (>20) in a single nail in a digit affected by dactylitis or an inflamed DIP is characteristic of PA

9. Radiographic Features

  a. Bony changes

     i. A unique combination of erosion (differentiates from AS) and bone production in a specific distribution (distinguishes from RA)

  b. Distinguishing features

     i. Fusiform soft tissue swelling

      1. Bilateral asymmetric distribution

    ii. Maintenance of normal mineralization

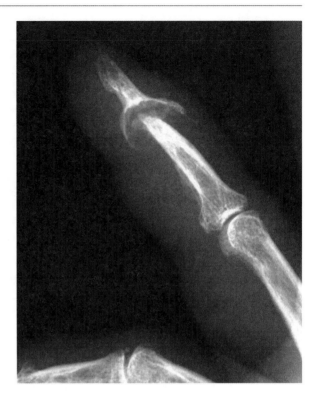

Fig. 6.5 Lateral radiograph showing pencil-in-cup deformity of the DIP of the third digit in psoriatic arthritis (Reproduced with permission from Systematic approach to arthropathies. *Diagnostic Imaging of Musculoskeletal Diseases.* DOI: 10.1007/978-1-59745-355-4_11; 2009-01-01)

      iii. Dramatic joint space loss
         1. With or without ankylosis
         2. IP joints of the hands and feet
         3. Widening of the joint spaces
      iv. Bone proliferation of the base of the distal phalanx
         1. Resorption of the tufts
      v. Joint erosions
         1. Pencil in cup deformities
      vi. Fluffy periostitis
   c. Sites of involvement (decreasing order of frequency)
      i. Hands
      ii. Feet
      iii. SI joints
      iv. Spine
   d. Syndesmophytes
      i. Isolated
      ii. Unusually bulky
      iii. Irregular marginal or nonmarginal
      iv. Appear at any portion of the spine

Fig. 6.6 Periosteal reaction in psoriatic arthritis (*arrows*) (Reproduced with permission from Systematic approach to arthropathies. *Diagnostic Imaging of Musculoskeletal Diseases.* DOI: 10.1007/978-1-59745-355-4_11)

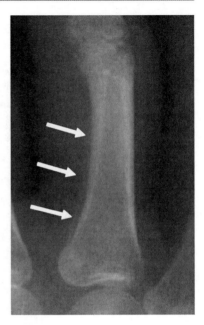

10. Differential Diagnosis
    a. Features that distinguish PA from RA
        i. Presence of dactylitis and enthesitis
        ii. Signs of psoriatic skin or nail lesion
        iii. Involvement of the DIPJ
        iv. Presence of spinal or SI disease
    b. Features that distinguish PA from other seronegative spondyloarthropathies
        i. Spine disease
            1. Less severe than AS
            2. Appears at a later age ≥30
        ii. Psoriatic skin or nail disease
        iii. FH of psoriasis
        iv. Less symmetric radiographic features
    c. Features that distinguish PA from reactive arthritis
        i. Lack of a preceding infectious episode
        ii. Predilection for joints of the upper extremities
        iii. Absence of balanitis and urethritis
        iv. Keratoderma blennorrhagica (reactive arthritis) and palmoplantar postural psoriasis are identical
        v. Hyperkeratotic changes in reactive arthritis involve only the soles and palms, not the nails
        vi. Rule out HIV in an unusually severe psoriasis and/or psoriatic arthritis
11. Treatment
    a. Skin disease
        i. Stable
            1. Initial treatment is topical

    2. Emollients
      a. Aqueous creams or petrolatum
      b. Cornerstone therapy
      c. Best BID
      d. Hydrates skin
      e. Soften scales
      f. Reduces itching
    3. Keratolytic agents
  ii. Extensive (>20%)
    1. Systemic therapy is indicated
    2. Topicals combined with
      a. Anthralin
      b. Corticosteroids
      c. Vitamin D derivatives
        i. Calcipotriene
      d. Topical retinoids
    3. Photochemotherapy PUVA therapy
      a. A psoralen (methoxsalen)
      b. 0.6 mg/kg
        i. Followed by 2 h with ultraviolet A radiation
      c. 3× weekly
        i. Then every 2–4 weeks for 2–3 months
 b. Joint Disease
   i. Splinting for persistent synovitis or enthesitis
   ii. NSAIDS initially
  iii. Local corticosteroids for 1 or 2 joints
  iv. DMARDs
    1. If unresponsive to NSAIDS and injections
    2. Start early as possible
    3. Progressive, erosive, polyarticular disease
    4. Oligoarticular disease of large joints
    5. MTX
      a. Effective for both skin and peripheral arthritis
      b. Same dosage as for RA
    6. Sulfasalazine
      a. 2–3 g/day
      b. Good for peripheral disease
      c. Not for axial or skin disease
    7. Other disease modifiers
      a. Antimalarials
      b. Gold
      c. Azathioprine
      d. Cyclosporine,
      e. Mycophenolate mofetil
      f. Leflunomide

     v. Retinoids and vitamin D may be effective

     vi. Avoid etretinate in axial disease

       1. Associated with spinal ligamentous calcification in long term use

     vii. Corticosteroids

     viii. Combination therapy

       1. For aggressive destructive disease with inadequate response to single therapy

       2. MTX with sulfasalazine, cyclosporine, or leflunomide

     ix. Enbrel

       1. Higher response rate than placebo (87% vs. 27%)

       2. Oligo- and polyarticular disease

       3. Both skin and join improvement at 12 weeks

12. Prognosis

    a. Overall more benign course than RA

    b. Worse (more aggressive treatment) with

      i. FH of psoriatic arthritis

      ii. Onset before 20

      iii. Presence of HLA-DR3 or DR4

      iv. Erosive or polyarticular disease

      v. Extensive skin involvement

Systemic Lupus Erythematosus (SLE)

7

Section A: Epidemiology, Immunopathology and Pathogenesis

1. Epidemiology
   a. Clinical manifestations
      i. Characterized by the production of antibodies to components of the cell nucleus
   b. A disease of young women of child bearing age
      i. Peak between the ages of 15 and 45
      ii. Sex hormones influence the probability of developing or expressing SLE
         1. Supported by animal models
   c. Female to male ratio
      i. 10:1
         1. Though less frequent male disease is **NOT** milder
      ii. 2:1
         1. Pediatric and older onset disease
   d. Disease risk
      i. Affects 1 in 2000
      ii. Varies with race, ethnicity, and socioeconomic status
      iii. White females
         1. Risk about 1 in 1000
      iv. Blacks and Hispanics
         1. 2–4 times greater than whites in the US
   e. Familial aggregation
      i. Increased frequency among first degree relatives
      ii. 25–50% concordant in monozygotic twins
      iii. 5% concordant in dizygotic twins
      iv. Occurs with other autoimmune diseases in extended families
         1. Hemolytic anemia
         2. Thyroiditis
         3. Idiopathic thrombocytopenia purpura

  f. Disease susceptibility
      i. Most cases are sporadic
     ii. Linked to particular class II genes of the MHC (HLA)
2. Renal Pathology
  a. Increases in mesangial cells and mesangial matrix
  b. Inflammation
  c. Cellular proliferation
  d. Basement membrane (BM) abnormalities
  e. Immune complex deposition
      i. In the mesangium, subendothelial and subepithelial sides of the glom-
         erular BM (electron microscope)
     ii. IgM
    iii. IgG
     iv. IgA
      v. Complement
  f. Classified according to two grading schemes
      i. World Health Organization (WHO) based on extent and location of pro-
         liferative changes within glomeruli and alterations in the BM
         1. Class I: Normal
         2. Class II: Mesangial Nephritis
         3. Class III: Focal proliferative glomerulonephritis (FPGN)
         4. Class IV: Diffuse proliferative glomerulonephritis (DPGN)
         5. Class V: Membranous nephropathy
         6. Class VI: Advance sclerosing GN
     ii. Classification based on signs of activity and chronicity
         1. Chronicity Index
            a. Each parameter graded 0–3 depending on severity
            b. Grades are added with a maximum score of 12
            c. Glomerulus sclerosis and fibrous crescents are graded as follows
                i. 0, absent
               ii. 1+, <25% of glomeruli involved
              iii. 2+, 25–50% of glomeruli involved
               iv. 3+, >75% of glomeruli involved
            d. Tubular atrophy and interstitial fibrosis are graded as follows
                i. 0, absent
               ii. 1+, mild
              iii. 2+, moderate
               iv. 3+, severe
         2. Activity Index
            a. Cellular proliferation
            b. Fibrinoid necrosis
            c. Cellular crescents
            d. Hyaline thrombi
            e. Leukocyte infiltration in the glomerulus
            f. Mononuclear cell infiltration in the interstitium

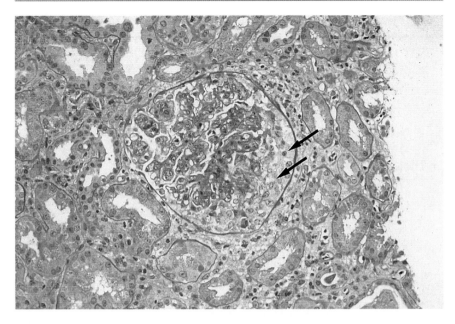

Fig. 7.1 Cellular crescent in lupus nephritis (Reproduced with permission from Systemic lupus erythematosus, scleroderma, and inflammatory myopathies. *Atlas of Rheumatology*. ImagesMD; 2005-01-18, 2009-01-01)

    g. Activity score
       i. Each graded 0–3 depending on severity
       ii. Grades are added with a maximum score of 24
       iii. Fibrinoid necrosis and cellular crescents have a weighting factor of 2
g. Histology predicts outcome
    i. Distinguishes reversible active inflammation from irreversible scarring
    ii. Correlates with clinical severity and prognosis
       1. Clinically adds little over lab studies
          a. Urinalysis (UA)
          b. Protein excretion
          c. Renal function studies
    iii. Biopsies reflect current status only
       1. Up to 40% change from one pathologic stage to another over time
    iv. Chronicity index
       1. Higher score associated with greater risk for renal failure
       2. Used as a guide to therapy aggressiveness
       3. Cyclophosphamide most beneficial for patients with intermediate scores
    v. Activity index
       1. Validity less clear
       2. Higher score correlates with increased risk of renal failure
       3. Identifies patients most likely to respond to aggressive therapy

3. Skin Pathology
   a. Inflammation and degeneration at the dermal-epidermal junction
   b. Basal or germinal layer is the primary site of injury
   c. Granular deposits of IgG and complement in a band like pattern
   d. Necrotizing vasculitis
4. CNS pathology (typical findings)
   a. Cortical microinfarcts
   b. Bland vasculopathy
   c. Degenerative or proliferative changes
5. Heart
   a. Nonspecific foci of inflammation even in the absence of clinical mani-
      festations
      i. Pericardium
      ii. Myocardium
      iii. Endocardium
   b. Verrucous endocarditis (Libman-Sacks)
      i. Classic
      ii. Manifested by vegetations
         1. Mostly at the mitral valve
         2. Immune complexes
         3. Inflammatory cells
         4. Fibrin
         5. Necrotic debris
6. Occlusive vasculopathy
   a. Venous and arterial thrombosis is common
   b. Thrombotic events may be triggered by inflammation or autoantibodies
   c. Autoantibodies include
      i. Antiphospholipid
      ii. Anticardiolipin
      iii. Lupus anticoagulants
      iv. Bound lipid antigens
      v. Bound serum protein B2-glycoprotein 1
         1. Form complexes with lipids
   d. See increases in endothelial cell adhesiveness
      i. Similar to Schwartzman reaction
7. Atherosclerosis
   a. Frequently in women with long standing disease
      i. Without the usual risk factors
   b. Postulated mechanisms
      i. Corticosteroid induced metabolic abnormalities
      ii. Hypertension
      iii. Vascular changes
         1. Immune complexes
         2. Pro-inflammatory mediators

8. Osteonecrosis
   a. Postulated mechanisms
      i. Vasculopathy
      ii. Drug side effects
      iii. Persistent immunologic insults
9. Neurodegeneration
   a. Postulated mechanisms
      i. Vasculopathy
      ii. Drug side effects
      iii. Persistent immunologic insults
10. Immunopathogenesis of Antinuclear Antibodies
    a. Autoantibody production directed to self molecules in the nucleus and cytoplasma
       i. The central immunologic disturbance
    b. Sera contains antibodies to
       i. IgG
       ii. Coagulation factor
       iii. ANA
    c. ANA
       i. Characteristic of SLE
       ii. Found in 95% of patients
       iii. Binds
          1. DNA
          2. RNA
          3. Nuclear proteins
          4. Protein nucleic acid complexes
       iv. Linkage
          1. Antibodies to certain nuclear antigens, DNA and histones frequently occur together
          2. The complex (not the individual components) are the driving antigen and the target of autoreactivity
    d. Two ANA are unique to SLE (included in the serological criteria for classification)
       i. dsDNA
          1. Frequently fluctuates over time
             a. May disappear with disease quiescence
          2. Reacts to a conserved nucleic acid determinant widely present on DNA
          3. The only ANA shown to correlate with the activity of GN
             a. Anti-dsDNA has been detected in the glomeruli of patients and animals with active disease
             b. Studies show enrichment of IgG anti-dsDNA in glomerular tissues relative to serum or other organs
             c. Longitudinal studies demonstrate high levels of circulating anti-dsDNA that frequently precede or coincide with active GN

      d. In animals injection of certain monoclonal IgG anti-dsDNA or expression of genes that encode pathogenic IgG anti-dsDNA can lead to GN

      e. GN can occur in the absence of elevated serum levels of anti-DNA

      f. Only some anti-DNA provoke GN (nephrogenic)

      g. Autoantibodies to non-DNA may participate in renal damage

    4. Features of anti-DNA that promote pathogenicity

      a. Isotype

      b. Charge

      c. Ability to fix complement

      d. Capacity to bind glomerular preparations

      e. Ability to bind to

        i. Nucleosomes

        ii. Immune deposits

        iii. Components of DNA and histones

    5. Anti-DNA antibodies not clearly associated with any other clinical event than nephritis

  ii. Sm

    1. A nuclear antigen

    2. Designated as small nuclear ribonucleoprotein (snRNP)

    3. A set of uridine rich RNA molecules complexed with a common group of core proteins

    4. Antibodies specifically target snRNP proteins and not RNA

    5. More constant over time

e. Associations of other autoantibodies with clinical events

  i. Antibodies to ribosomal P proteins (anti-P)

    1. Neuropsychiatric disease

    2. Hepatitis

  ii. Antibodies to Ro

    1. Neonatal Lupus

    2. Subacute cutaneous lupus

  iii. Antibodies to phospholipids

    1. Vascular thrombosis

    2. Thrombocytopenia

    3. Recurrent abortion

  iv. Antibodies to blood cells

    1. Cytopenias

f. Antigen location

  i. May translocate to the membrane and become accessible to antibody attack

  ii. ANA may enter cells and bind nuclear antigens to perturb cell function

g. Anti-DNA antibodies do **NOT** appear to mediate renal damage through deposition of circulating immune complexes

  i. DNA-anti-DNA complexes are difficult to detect in the circulation

    1. Even with increased amounts of anti-DNA in the glomerulus

Targeted Autoantigens	Prevalence in SLE (%)	Clinical Associations
DNA/DNA binding proteins		
dsDNA	50–60	Lupus nephritis and severe disease; can fluctuate with disease activity
Histone	50–70	Drug-induced lupus (>95%) and also in SLE
Nucleosome (can only be generated through apoptosis)	38–76	Lupus nephritis; IgG3 subclass is associated with disease activity
RNA/ribonucleo proteins		
Smith	Caucasians:10–20 African-Americans/ Asians: 30–40	Highly specific for SLE and more common in African-Americans and Asians
U1 RNP	30–40	Overlapping symptoms of SLE, myositis, and systemic sclerosis; seen in mixed connective tissue disease
Ro (SS-A)	25–35	Subacute cutaneous lupus, neonatal lupus; seen in Sjögren's syndrome
La (SS-B)	10–15	Neonatal lupus; seen in Sjögren's syndrome
Ribosomal-P	45–90 (general SLE:5–20)	Central nervous system (CNS) involvement (psychosis)
Cell membrane		

Fig. 7.2 Autoantibodies in SL(E) (Reproduced with permission from Autoantibodies, systemic lupus erythematosus. *Rheumatology and Immunology Therapy.* DOI: 10.1007/3-540-29662-X_359. Springer; 2004-01-01)

Blood cells and platelets	RBC: 44–65 Platelet: 62 (in one study)	Hemolytic anemia, leukopenia, thrombocytopenia; can have positive direct Coomb's test without clinical hemolytic anemia
Neuronal cells	30–92	Central nervous system (CNS) involvement (psychosis)
Phospholipids Lipoproteins (cardiolipin, β2- glycoprotein I, lupus anticoagulants)	17–87 (Varied greatly with different assays)	Vascular thrombosis, fetal loss, and CNS lupus

Fig. 7.2 (continued)

h. Two theories for the pathogenic mechanism of anti-DNA in GN
   i. DNA-anti-DNA complexes form in situ
      1. Assembled in the kidney on DNA or other nucleosomal components adherent to the glomerular BM
         a. Rather than being deposited from the blood
   ii. DNA or chromatin binds to the glomerulus and then recognized and bound by anti-DNA antibodies
      1. DNA of these complexes are likely nucleosomes
         a. Found circulating in increased amounts
      2. Charge structure and affinity for glomerular macromolecules
i. Autoantibodies not DNA in origin interact with glomerular antigens
   i. Anti-DNA antibodies contain other specificities and can bind to different glomerular structures
   ii. Activated complement incites inflammation and causes direct damage
      1. Complement fixing IgG anti-DNA antibodies are more pathogenic
   iii. Immune complexes can anchor to kidney sites
j. Vasculitis
   i. Immune complex mediated
   ii. Frequently seen with depressed complement
   iii. Cell mediated cytotoxicity
   iv. Direct antibody attack on tissue
11. Determinants of Disease Susceptibility
   a. Chromosomal regions associated with disease have been identified
   b. Gene polymorphisms occur in greater frequency with SLE than in controls
      i. Class II MHC polymorphisms
         1. HLA-DR2 and HLA-DR3
            a. Relative risk of 2–5

    2. MHC genes regulate in an antigen-specific manner

      a. More influence on the production of certain ANAs rather than disease susceptibility

      b. SLE is characterized by responses to self antigens of unrelated sequence

  c. Inherited complement deficiencies

    i. C4b

    ii. C4a

      1. Null alleles in 80% with SLE

        a. Irrespective of ethnicity

      2. Homozygous C4a deficiency confers a high risk for SLE

      3. Null alleles are a part of the extended HLA haplotype

        a. Markers HLA-B8 and HLA-DR3

        b. Class I and class II alleles reflect linkage disequilibrium with complement deficiency

    iii. C1q

    iv. C1r/s

    v. C2

  d. Pathogenesis of complement deficiency

    i. Impairs the neutralization and clearance of foreign antigen

      1. Leads to prolonged immune stimulation

    ii. Apoptotic cells persist and stimulate autoantibody responses

      1. C1q binds to apoptotic cells initiating complement's role in clearance

      2. C1q KO mice

        a. Elevated anti-DNA levels

        b. Glomerulonephritis

        c. Increased apoptotic cells in the tissue

12. Genetics of Murine SLE

  a. Inbred mice mimic human SLE

    i. ANA production

    ii. Immune complex GN

    iii. Lymphadenopathy

    iv. Abnormal B and T cell functions

  b. Full blown lupus syndrome requires multiple unlinked genes

  c. Lupus mice strains

    i. NZB

    ii. NZB/NZW

    iii. MRL-lpr/lpr

    iv. BXSB

    v. C3H-gld/gld

  d. Single mutation lpr and gld mice result in mutated proteins involved in

    i. Apoptosis

    ii. Maintenance of peripheral tolerance

    iii. Persistence of autoreactive cells

  e. lpr mutation

    i. Fas absence

      1. A cell surface molecule that triggers apoptosis in lymphocytes

      ii. Humans mutations in Fas
         1. Defects in apoptosis
         2. Autoimmune lymphoproliferative syndrome (ALPS)
            a. Lymphoproliferation of an unusual population of cells
               i. CD4-
               ii. CD8-
               iii. Thy.1+
               iv. B220+
            b. Not associated with autoantibody formation
            c. Not associated with clinical or serologic findings of SLE
   f. gld mutation
      i. Fas ligand Affects
   g. Clinical manifestations (nephritis) require other genes in the background
      i. MRL-lpr/lpr
         1. The only congenic strain with immune mediated GN
         2. High-level production of pathogenic anti-DNA
      ii. NSB/NZW (New Zealand)
         1. F1 mice develop an SLE-like illness from genes contributed by both
            NZB and NZW parents
         2. A series of genes promote autoimmunity and lead to expression of
            ANA
            a. *Sle2* and *sle3*
  h. Mice strains lack a common MHC class I or II marker susceptibility factor
      i. NZB mice with class II gene mutations
         1. Nephritis
         2. Enhanced anti-DNA production
      ii. NZB mice with MHC linked deficiency in TNF-α expression
         1. Administration of TNF-α ameliorates disease
13. Immune Cell Disturbances in SLE
   a. B cell hyperactivity
      i. Hyperglobulinemia
      ii. Increased numbers of antibody producing cells
      iii. Heightened responses to many antigens (both self and foreign)
   b. Abnormal tolerance
      i. Normally anti-DNA precursors are tolerized by anergy or deletion
      ii. SLE retains precursors that produce high affinity autoantibodies
   c. Pathogenic autoantibodies
      i. Hyperglobulinemia **not** a major mechanism in anti-DNA production
      ii. ANA antibody responses are antigen driven
         1. Antigen selection by a receptor driven mechanism
         2. Bind multiple independent determinants found in different regions of
            nuclear proteins
         3. Variable region somatic mutations increase DNA binding activity and
            specificity for dsDNA
         4. Preimmune repertoire composition affected
         5. Precursors mutated under self antigen drive

    iii. Molecular mimicry
       1. Autoantibody production stimulated by a foreign antigen bearing an AA sequence or antigenic structure resembling a self molecule
       2. Autoantibodies bind the entire molecule not only at sites of homology
       3. Self antigen sustains autoantibody production rather than a mimic
    iv. Cross reactivity
       1. Sequence similarity between certain nuclear antigens and viral and bacterial proteins
       2. Initiates an ANA response
       3. Induces a population of B cells
         a. Process self antigens
         b. Present determinants not subject to tolerance
         c. Stimulates autoreactive T cells
       4. Epstein Barr
         a. A possible infectious trigger
         b. SLE patients infected more commonly than controls
       5. Bacterial DNA has adjuvant properties
         a. Lack sequence motifs of mammalian DNA
    v. SLE patients autoantibody response
       1. May have a unique capacity to respond to DNA
       2. May be exposed to DNA with enhanced immunogenicity
         a. Surface blebs on apoptotic cells
         b. Nucleosomes
  d. T cells in disease pathogenesis
    i. T helper cell depletion abrogates autoantibody production and clinical disease in murine models of lupus
       1. Process not elucidated
    ii. T cell help by nonspecific activated T cells
       1. SLE antigen complexes contain multiple protein and nucleic acid species
       2. Complex antigens may trigger B cell activation by multivalent binding
    iii. T cell reactivity elicited to only one protein in a complex
14. Environmental or exogenous triggers for SLE
  a. Infectious agents
    i. Induce specific responses by molecular mimicry
    ii. Perturb overall immunoregulation
  b. Stress
    i. Neuroendocrine changes affecting immune cell function
  c. Diet
    i. Affects production of inflammatory mediators
  d. Toxins and drugs
    i. Modify cellular responsiveness
    ii. Modify the immunogenicity of self antigens
  e. Physical agents (sunlight)
    i. Cause inflammation and tissue damage

Section B: Clinical and Laboratory Features

1. ACR Diagnostic Criteria for SLE (11)
   a. Major clinical features
      i. Mucocutaneous
      ii. Articular
      iii. Serosal
      iv. Renal
      v. Neurologic
   b. Associated laboratory findings
      i. Hematologic
      ii. Immunologic
   c. Established for the purpose of clinical studies
   d. Not utilized strictly for diagnosis
   e. Greater than 90% sensitivity and specificity
2. Diagnosis made with 4 or more of the following 11 criteria (serially or simultaneously) during any observational interval
   a. Malar rash
      i. Tends to spare the nasolabial folds
   b. Discoid rash
   c. Photosensitivity
   d. Oral ulcers (or nasopharyngeal)
      i. Usually painless
      ii. Observed by a physician
   e. Arthritis
      i. Nonerosive
      ii. Two or more peripheral joints
   f. Serositis (either)
      i. Pleruitis
      ii. Pericarditis
   g. Renal disorder (either)
      i. Persistent proteinuria > 0.5 g/day
      ii. Cellular cast
   h. Neurologic disorder (either)
      i. Seizures
      ii. Psychosis
      iii. Both in the absence of offending drugs or metabolic derangements
   i. Hematologic disorder
      i. Hemolytic anemia
      ii. Leukopenia $< 4,000/mm^3$
      iii. Lymphopenia $< 1,500/mm^3$
      iv. Thrombocytopenia $< 100,000/mm^3$
   j. Immunologic disorder
      i. Positive LE prep
      ii. Anti-DNA
      iii. Anti-Sm

       iv. False + test for syphilis for 6 months
          1. Being replaced by positive test for antiphospholipid antibodies
   k. ANA
3. Nonspecific constitutional features of SLE
   a. Fatigue
   b. Fever
   c. Weight loss
4. Factors that precipitate the onset or exacerbation of disease
   a. Sun exposure
   b. Emotional stress
   c. Infection
   d. Certain drugs (sulfonamides)
5. Bimodal mortality curve
   a. Death within 5 years
      i. Active disease
      ii. High doses of corticosteroids and intense immunosuppression required
      iii. Develop concomitant infections
   b. 80–90% survival at 10 years
   c. Late deaths
      i. Often the result of cardiovascular disease
6. Mucocutaneous System
   a. One of the most commonly affected (80–90%)
   b. Four of the 11 formal criteria fulfilled with this system alone
   c. Three classifications of SLE specific skin lesions (based on clinical appearance and duration)
      i. Acute
      ii. Subacute
      iii. Chronic
7. Discoid lupus (DLE)
   a. Most common chronic form
   b. Two presentations
      i. Isolated in the absence of autoantibodies
         1. 2–10% will develop SLE
      ii. As part of the systemic disease
         1. 15–30% will have DLE
   c. Lesion characteristics
      i. Discrete papules or plaques
      ii. Evolve into larger coin-shaped (discoid) lesions
      iii. Often erythematous
      iv. Covered by scale
      v. Extend into dilated hair follicles
      vi. Erythematous inflammation at the periphery
      vii. Leave areas of scarring after healing
         1. Central atrophic scarring is characteristic
         2. Epithelial thinning and atrophy
         3. Follicular plugging and damage

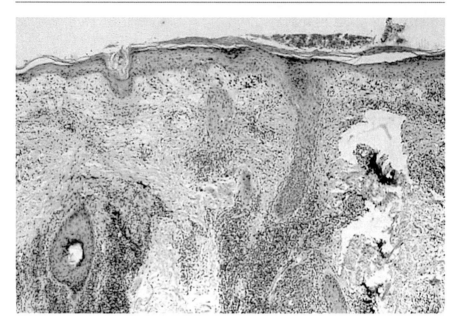

Fig. 7.3 Biopsy of discoid lupus erythematosus (Reproduced with permission from Systemic lupus erythematosus, scleroderma, and inflammatory myopathies. *Atlas of Rheumatology.* ImagesMD; 2005-01-18)

    viii. Depigmentation
     ix. Patches of alopecia
        1. Irreversible follicular destruction
   d. Typical sites of involvement
      i. Face (85%)
      ii. Scalp (50%)
     iii. Pinnae and behind the ears (50%)
      iv. Neck
       v. Extensor surface of the arms
      vi. Areas not exposed to sun
   e. Biopsy
       i. Inflammation around skin appendages (hair follicles)
      ii. Vacuolization at the dermal-epidermal junction
     iii. Characteristic positive lupus band test
        1. Immune reactants
           a. IgG
           b. IgM
           c. C3 > IgA
        2. Fibrin at the dermal-epidermal junction
   f. Treatment for resistant cases
       i. Chloroquine
      ii. Clofazimine (Lamprene)
     iii. Thalidomide

Fig. 7.4 Lupus profundus (Reproduced with permission from Systemic lupus erythematosus, scleroderma, and inflammatory myopathies. *Atlas of Rheumatology.* ImagesMD; 2005-01-18)

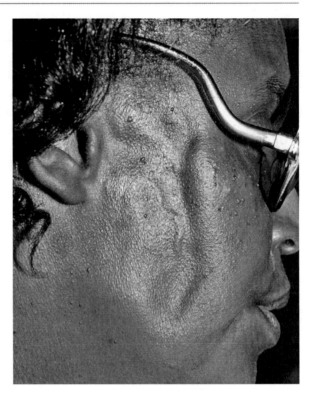

    iv. Cyclosporine
    v. Chronic lesions >50% of body
       1. Topical nitrogen mustard
       2. BCNU
       3. Tacrolimus
  g. Tumid lupus
    i. Seen early in DLE
    ii. Prominent dermal mucin
    iii. Edematous lesions
8. Lupus panniculitis (lupus profundus)
  a. Less common chronic form
  b. Spares the epidermis
  c. Involves the deep dermis and subcutaneous fat
  d. Firm nodules without surface change
  e. Attached to subcutaneous tissue with resultant deep depressions
  f. Treat resistant cases with dapsone
9. Subacute cutaneous lupus erythematosus (SCLE)
  a. The most common subacute form
  b. 7–27% of patients
  c. Primarily affects Caucasian women
  d. Lesion characteristics
    i. Symmetric

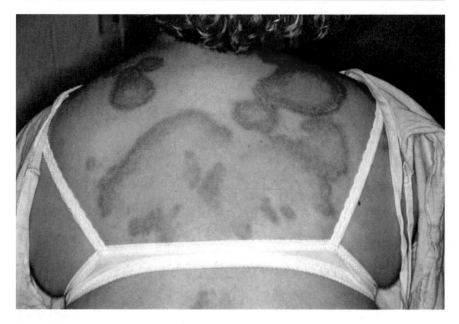

Fig. 7.5 Subacute cutaneous lupus (Reproduced with permission from Systemic lupus erythematosus, scleroderma, and inflammatory myopathies. *Atlas of Rheumatology*. ImagesMD; 2005-01-18)

    ii. Widespread
    iii. Superficial
    iv. Non-scarring
    v. Non-fixed
    vi. Begin as small, erythematous, scaly papules or plaques
    vii. Evolve into two forms
        1. Papulosquamous (psoriasiform)
        2. Annular or serpiginous polycyclic forms
            a. Coalesce to large confluent areas
            b. Central hypopigmentation and scaling
    viii. Both forms are nonscarring
    ix. Areas of depigmentation in dark skinned people
  e. Typical sites of involvement
    i. Most often in sun exposed areas
    ii. Shoulders
    iii. Extensor surfaces of arms
    iv. Upper chest and back
    v. Neck
    vi. Tends to spare midfacial areas
  f. Antibodies to SSA/Ro ribonucleoproteins are commonly found
  g. May have negative lupus band test on biopsy
  h. Treatment for resistant cases
    i. Mycophenylate mofetil
    ii. Retinoids
    iii. Cyclosporine

Fig. 7.6 Acute malar rash in SL(E) (Reproduced with permission from Systemic lupus erythematosus, scleroderma, and inflammatory myopathies. *Atlas of Rheumatology*. ImagesMD; 2005-01-18)

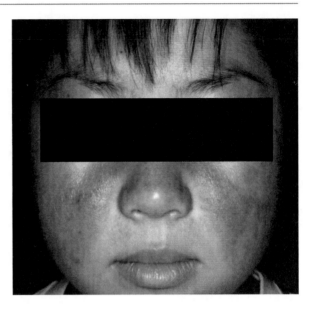

10. Malar (butterfly) rash
    a. The most classic of all acute rashes
    b. Lesion characteristics
        i. Erythematous and edematous eruption
        ii. Raised papules and /or plaques
        iii. Simulates the shape of a butterfly
        iv. Classically spares the nasolabial folds
        v. Heal without scarring
    c. Abrupt in onset and can last for days
        i. Indicates active systemic disease
    d. Initiated and/or exacerbated by exposure to sunlight
        i. Typifies acute photosensitive rashes
        ii. Criteria for photosensitivity and malar rash are independent
    e. Differential diagnosis
        i. Acne rosacea

            1. Pustules present
        ii. Seborrhea
        iii. Contact dermatitis
        iv. Atopic dermatitis
        v. Actinic dermatitis
11. Acute photosensitive rashes
    a. Sun exposed areas
    b. Heal without scarring
    c. Provide protection from UV light
        i. UV-B (290–320 nm)
            1. Greater problem for SLE than UV-A

        2. Blocked by sunscreen
           a. Shade Gel SPF 30 or equivalent
           b. No PABA
        3. Blocked by glass
        4. Avoid the hot part of day
           a. 10–4 pm
           b. Mostly UV-B light
    ii. UV-A (320–400 nm)
        1. Blocked only by clothing
        2. Some shorter waves can be blocked by sunscreens
        3. Cannot be blocked by glass
    iii. Avoid the sun
    iv. Use appropriate clothing
    v. Use camouflage cosmetics
12. Widespread morbilliform or exanthemous eruptions
  a. Less common acute form
13. Alopecia in SLE
  a. Diffuse or patchy
  b. Reversible or permanent scarring with discoid lesions
  c. Breakage of hair at the temples ("lupus fuzz")

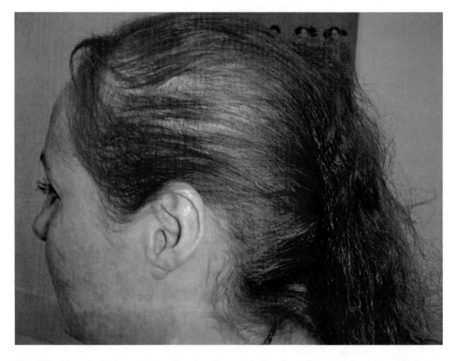

Fig. 7.7 Alopecia in lupus (Reproduced with permission from Systemic lupus erythematosus (Figure courtesy of Dr. Rachel Abuav). *A Clinician's Pearls and Myths in Rheumatology.* DOI: 10.1007/978-1-84800-934-9_13. Springer; 2009-01-01)

Fig. 7.8 Mucosal ulcers and erosions in SL(E) (Reproduced with permission from Rheumatology. *Atlas of Pediatrics.* ImagesMD; 2006-01-20)

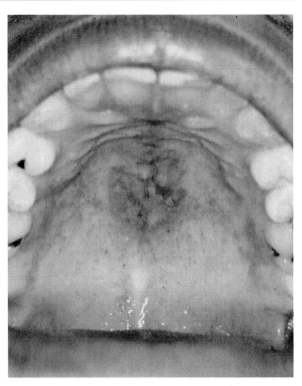

    d. Three causes of alopecia in SLE
        i. Active systemic disease
            1. Reversible once controlled
        ii. Discoid disease with patchy hair loss
            1. Permanent
            2. Hair follicles damaged by the inflammation
        iii. Drugs (cyclophosphamide)
            1. Diffuse hair loss
            2. Reversible after therapy stopped
14. Mucosal lesions
    a. Mouth
        i. Most commonly affected area
        ii. Buccal mucosa and tongue
        iii. Sores on the upper palate particularly characteristic
        iv. Typically painless
        v. Central depression often occurs with painful ulcerations
    b. Nose
    c. Anogenital area
15. Vasculitis
    a. Palpable purpura
    b. Urticaria

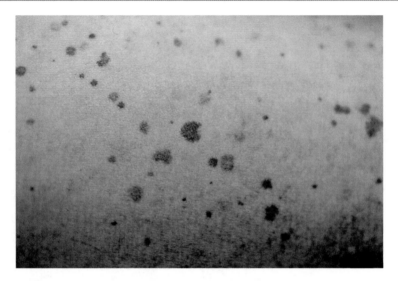

Fig. 7.9 Lesions of palpable purpura in SL(E) (Reproduced with permission from Systemic lupus erythematosus, scleroderma, and inflammatory myopathies. *Atlas of Rheumatology.* ImagesMD; 2005-01-18)

    c. Nailfold or digital ulceration
    d. Erythematous papules of the pulps of the fingers and palms
    e. Splinter hemorrhages
    f. Livedo reticularis
       i. Frequently associated with anti-phospholipid antibodies
16. Hand rash characteristic of lupus
    a. Erythematous lesions over the dorsum of the hands and fingers
    b. Affects the skin **BETWEEN** the joints
17. General and routine therapies for skin lesions in SLE
    a. Stop smoking so antimalarials work better
    b. Thiazides and sulfonylureals may exacerbate skin disease
    c. Topical and intralesional steroids
    d. Hydroxychloroquine
    e. Oral corticosteroids
    f. Dapsone for bullous lesions
18. Musculoskeletal System
    a. Arthralgia to arthritis
       i. The most common presenting symptom of SLE
       ii. Frequencies reported between 76% and 100%
    b. Complaints of pain may be out of proportion to the degree of synovitis
    c. Common presentations
       i. Symmetric
       ii. Involvement of the small joints of the hands
          1. PIP
          2. MCP

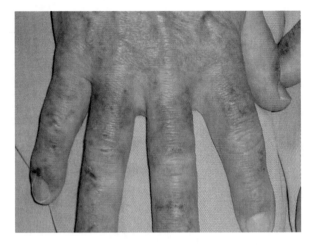

Fig. 7.10 Erythema over the phalanges in SL(E) The location of erythema in lupus contrasts with the Gottron's papules typical of dermatomyositis (Reproduced with permission from Systemic lupus erythematosus (Figure courtesy of Dr. John Stone). *A Clinician's Pearls and Myths in Rheumatology.* DOI: 10.1007/978-1-84800-934-9_13. Springer; 2009-01-01)

    iii. Wrists

    iv. Knees

    v. Spares the spine

    vi. Transient or persistent

    vii. Effusions

  viii. Non-erosive and non-deforming

 d. May be confused with early RA

    i. Deforming features can occur

      1. Ulnar deviation

      2. Hyperflexion

      3. Hyperextension

    ii. Secondary to involvement of para-articular tissues

      1. Joint capsule

      2. Ligament loosening

      3. Tendons

   iii. Reducible and hypermobile

   iv. Jaccoud's arthropathy

      1. Swan-neck deformities

      2. Ulna deviation

    v. If erosions are present

      1. Secondary to capsular and subluxation pressure

      2. Nonprogressive

 e. Treatment

    i. NSAIDs

      1. The first line of therapy in an SLE patient with arthritis and no evidence of internal organ involvement

      2. COX-2 may contribute to thrombotic risk in patients with antiphospholipid antibodies

    ii. Antimalarial drugs
       1. Hydroxychloroquine 200 mg BID
       2. Modest effects
  f. Synovial fluid
    i. Clear to slightly cloudy
    ii. Good viscosity and mucin clot
    iii. Absence of inflammation
    iv. ANAs can be present
    v. WBCs < 2,000/mm^3
       1. Predominance of mononuclear cells
    vi. Transudative or exudative
    vii. Serum/synovial fluid ratios
       1. Complement, total protein, and IgG can all be 1
       2. Only complement levels can be > 1
          a. Indicates local consumption
       3. Proportional escape of proteins into the joint space
    viii. Large effusion with warmth
       1. Consider septic arthritis
  g. Osteonecrosis
    i. Frequency 5–10%
    ii. Sites of involvement
       1. Femoral head
          a. Most common
       2. Femoral condyles
       3. Talus
       4. Humeral head
       5. Metatarsal heads
       6. Radial head
       7. Carpal bones
       8. Metacarpal bones
    iii. Bilaterality is frequent
    iv. Common symptoms
       1. Persistent painful motion
       2. Localized to one joint
       3. Often relieved with rest
    v. Causality
       1. Corticosteroids
          a. Most cases
       2. Raynaud's
       3. Small vessel vasculitis
       4. Fat emboli
       5. Anti-phospholipid antibodies
  h. Muscle
    i. Myalgia and muscle weakness of the deltoids and quadriceps
       1. Seen with disease flairs

      ii. Overt myositis
         1. Associated with elevations in CK
            a. Very high levels are rare
         2. Occurs in 15% of patients
         3. EMG and biopsy may be normal
            a. Compared to inflammatory myopathies
      iii. Myopathy with corticosteroid or antimalarial use
19. Renal Disease
   a. Present in 1/2 to 1/3rd of patients
   b. The most important predictor of poor outcome
   c. Based on the presence of proteinuria
      i. Dipstick 2+
      ii. Greater than 500 mg/24 h
   d. Clinical evaluation
      i. Urine dipstick and microscopic analysis
      ii. Baseline 24 h urine analysis for protein and creatinine
         1. Even with 1+ dipstick
         2. Especially important with dsDNA and low complement
   e. Sediment evaluation
      i. Bland
         1. Normal
         2. Mesangial disease
         3. Membranous disease
      ii. Active
         1. RBC casts
            a. Consistent with proliferative disease
         2. Both RBCs and WBCs
            a. Proliferative lesions
      iii. Persistent hematuria (> 5 RBCs/HPF) and/or pyuria (> 5 WBCs/HPF) **without** proteinuria is unusual unless
         1. Pathology is limited to mesangium in the case of RBCs
         2. Pathology is limited to interstitium in the case of WBCs
   f. Creatinine (Cr)
      i. Advanced renal insufficiency
         1. Elevated without concomitant proteinuria
      ii. Mesangial disease
         1. Normal
      iii. Focal proliferative
         1. Normal to mildly elevated
      iv. Diffuse proliferative
         1. Range from normal to dialysis dependent
      v. Membranous
         1. Range from normal to mild elevation
   g. Signs and symptoms
      i. Frequently insidious

    ii. Swollen ankles

    iii. Puffy eyes upon waking

    iv. Frequent urination

    v. A low serum albumin level

       1. An indicator of persistent proteinuria

    vi. Isolated hypertension

       1. Outside the norm for age, race, and gender

       2. Diffuse proliferative disease

       3. Focal proliferative disease

h. Biopsy

    i. Not required

    ii. Utilize

       1. When clinical parameters are not absolute

       2. When the result will make a clear difference in the therapeutic approach

i. Key histologic findings and their clinical implication

    i. Mesangial nephritis (WHO class II)

       1. Characterized by immune deposits in the mesangium

          a. Seen on immunofluorescence and electron microscope

       2. A and B additional classifications

          a. IIA

             i. Normal appearance on **light** microscope

          b. IIB

             i. Mesangial hypercellularity and/or increased matrix on **light** microscope

       3. **No** capillary loop deposits

       4. Demonstrates little clinical evidence of renal involvement

          a. Normal or near normal UA and renal function

       5. Rarely requires treatment

    ii. Focal proliferative glomerulonephritis (WHO class III)

       1. Characterized by hypercellularity

          a. Increases in mesangial, endocapillary, and/or infiltrating cells

       2. Encroachment of the glomerular capillary space

       3. Inflammatory lesions present in a segmental pattern

          a. Involving only one area of a glomerulus

          b. Involving <50% of the glomeruli

       4. Immune complexes present in the capillary loops

       5. Proteinuria and hematuria

          a. Severity less common than with diffuse disease

       6. A continuum with diffuse disease

          a. Lesions are qualitatively similar but less extensive

          b. Up to one-third will progress to diffuse disease

    iii. Diffuse proliferative glomerulonephritis (WHO class IV)

       1. Most patients who progress to renal failure

       2. Characterized by generalized hypercellularity of mesangial and endothelial cells

          a. Involvement of >50% of the glomeruli

3. Inflammatory cellular infiltrates and areas of necrosis
   a. Common
4. Obliteration of the capillary loops and sclerosis
5. Basement membrane thickening
6. Immunofluorescence
   a. Extensive deposition (full house pattern) of immunoglobulin (IgG, IgM, and IgA) and complement (C3, C1q)
   b. Mesangium and capillary loops
7. Electron microscope
   a. Immune complex deposits
   b. Both subendothelial and subepithelial distributions
8. Clinical
   a. Almost always have proteinuria (frequently nephrotic) and hematuria
   b. Decreases in renal function
   c. Hypertension is common

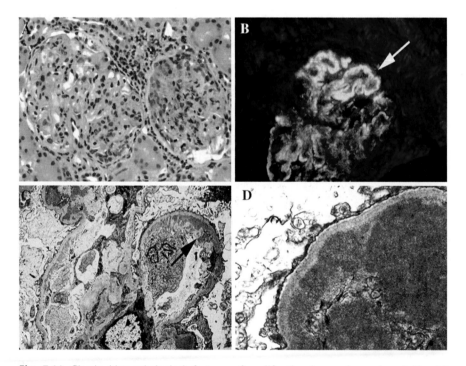

Fig. 7.11 Classic histopathological features of proliferative lupus glomerulonephritis. (**a**) Hypercellular glomeruli with increased mesangial and inflammatory cells, many of which are fragmented, a feature known as fibrinoid necrosis (×40). (**b**) Strong C3 deposits are focally linear and coalescing to produce "wire loops" (immunofluorescence microscopy ×40). (**c**) Electron microscopy demonstrates confluent predominantly subendothelial deposits (*arrow*) (×8K). (**d**) Fingerprint-like subendothelial deposits (electron microscopy ×20K) (Reproduced with permission from Pathology and immunology of lupus glomerulonephritis: can we bridge the two? *International Urology and Nephrology*. DOI: 10.1007/s11255-006-9170-x. Springer; 2007-04-12)

iv. Membranous nephropathy (WHO class V)
1. Characterized by diffuse thickening of the basement membrane
2. Glomeruli have normal cellularity
3. Immunoglobulin and complement deposits along the basement membrane
4. Clinical
   a. Extensive proteinuria
      i. Minimal hematuria
   b. Less renal function abnormalities
   c. A subset (10–30%) will slowly progress to chronic renal failure within a 10 year period
   d. A transition stage after treatment for proliferative GN
j. Prognosis
   i. Worst
      1. Diffuse proliferative GN
      2. Progressive forms of focal proliferative GN

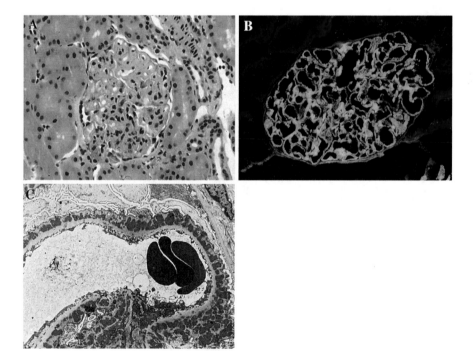

Fig. 7.12 Histopathological findings of membranous lupus glomerulonephritis. (**a**) Hematoxylin/ Eosin stain shows thick capillary loops and focal mesangial cell proliferation but no evidence of fibrinoid necrosis (×40). (**b**) IgG deposits are granular and present in the wall of the capillary loops. (**c**) Electron microscopy shows globular electron dense subepithelial deposits (×6K) and also the mesangium (immunofluorescence ×40) (Reproduced with permission from Pathology and immunology of lupus glomerulonephritis: can we bridge the two? *International Urology and Nephrology.* DOI: 10.1007/s11255-006-9170-x. Springer; 2007-04-12)

    ii. Best
       1. Membranous nephropathy
       2. Mesangial nephritis
  k. Urine protein
    i. A critical measurement of ongoing renal lupus activity
    ii. New proteinuria of 500 mg is significant
    iii. Membranous nephropathy can have continued proteinuria between 500 mg and 2 g
    iv. An exacerbation is best defined as at least a doubling of baseline proteinuria
  l. Serologic Tests
    i. dsDNA
       1. The only ANA shown to correlate with the activity of lupus nephritis
       2. Perform serial monitoring
       3. Present especially in focal and diffuse proliferative
    ii. Complement components (C3 and C4) and total hemolytic complement (CH50)
       1. Correlates with the activity of renal disease
       2. Many patients have partial C4 deficiency
         a. May always have a low C4
       3. Decreased especially in focal and diffuse proliferative
  m. Renal ultrasound
    i. A helpful guide to assess disease progression
    ii. Decreasing disease reversibility
       1. Decreased size and increased echogenicity of the kidneys
  n. Drug treatment
    i. Corticosteroids
       1. The first line of therapy in previously untreated patients with active disease
       2. Used in high doses to control disease quickly
       3. Prednisone at 1 mg/kg/day in three divided doses
    ii. Cytotoxic drug indications
       1. Corticosteroid failure
         a. A 6–8 week course of high dose prednisone has not restored serum creatinine to normal
         b. Proteinuria continues to be >1 g/day
         c. Perform a renal biopsy
       2. Poor prognostic indicators found on biopsy
         a. Glomerular sclerosis
         b. Fibrous crescents
         c. Irreversible tubulointerstitial changes
         d. Continued activity

    3. Patient subgroups
      a. Those with evidence of active and severe GN despite high dose prednisone
      b. Those who have responded to corticosteroids but required an unacceptable high dose
      c. Those with unacceptable side effects from corticosteroids
  iii. Cytoxic drugs most frequently used in lupus nephritis
    1. Oral azathioprine
      a. If nausea side effects use 6-mercaptopurine
    2. Oral cyclophosphamide
    3. Intermittent IV cyclophosphamide
    4. Oral chlorambucil
      a. An alternative to cyclophosphamide
    5. Mycophenylate mofetil or cyclosporine
      a. Especially with membranous GN
    6. Each of these drugs are given in association with prednisone (usually 0.5 mg/kg/day)
      a. Combination shown to prevent progression to renal failure more effectively than prednisone alone
    7. Severe drug toxicity
      a. Overall improvement in mortality difficult to show
o. End stage renal disease (ESRD)
  i. Over a 10-year follow-up 20–30% with severe lupus nephritis will progress
  ii. Lupus nephritis accounts for up to 3% requiring dialysis or transplantation
  iii. Dialysis
    1. With minimal disease the survival compares favorable with those of other patient groups
    2. SLE patients should wait 6 or 12 months on dialysis prior to transplantation
  iv. SLE may improve in progressive renal failure and on dialysis
    1. A decrease in nonrenal SLE
    2. A decrease in serologic markers of active disease
  v. Transplantation
    1. Lupus patients are excellent candidates
    2. The recurrence of active lupus nephritis in the transplant is unusual (<10%)
    3. Graft survival in SLE may be lower compared with other groups
    4. Recurrence in 10%
      a. Even in the absence of clinical or serologic evidence of active SLE
p. Prognostic indicators
  i. Good
    1. Baseline Cr < 1.4 mg/dl
    2. Activity index <12

        3. Chronicity index <4

        4. By 6 months of treatment

          a. Normalization of Cr

          b. Decrease in proteinuria to <1 g/day

        5. Stable Cr

        6. Decreased proteinuria to <2 g/day

        7. White race

    ii. Poor

        1. After 4 weeks of therapy

          a. Increase in Cr of 0.3 mg/dl

          b. Doubling of proteinuria over baseline

        2. Doubling of baseline Cr at any time

        3. Persistent nephrotic range proteinuria

        4. Crescents >50% of glomeruli

        5. High chronicity index

        6. Hypertension

        7. Black race

20. Nervous System

  a. About 2/3rd of SLE have neuropsychiatric manifestations

    i. Neurologic syndromes of the central, peripheral, and autonomic systems

    ii. Psychiatric disorders

  b. Formal ACR criteria include only seizures and psychosis

    i. Definitions for 19 neuropsychiatric syndromes have been developed

  c. Proposed mechanisms

    i. Vascular occlusion due to vasculopathy

    ii. Vasculitis

    iii. Leukoaggregation or thrombosis

    iv. Antibody mediated neuronal cell injury

  d. Present concomitantly with activity or exist in isolation

  e. Diffuse or focal

  f. Psychiatric disorders

    i. Mood disorders

    ii. Anxiety

    iii. Psychosis

    iv. Cognitive defects

        1. Attention deficit

        2. Poor concentration

        3. Impaired memory

        4. Difficulty in word finding

    v. Acute confusional state

        1. Disturbance of consciousness or level of arousal

        2. Reduced ability to focus, maintain, or shift attention

        3. Accompanied by cognitive disturbance and/or change in mood, behavior, or affect

    4. Develops over a brief time frame

    5. Fluctuates over the day

    6. Ranges from mild alterations of consciousness to coma

vi. Diagnosis

    1. Neuropsychological testing

    2. A decline from a higher formal level of function

vii. Differential diagnosis

    1. Difficult to attribute strictly to lupus

    2. Stress of chronic illness

    3. Drugs

    4. Infections

    5. Metabolic disorders

g. Neurologic manifestations

  i. Seizures

    1. Focal

    2. Generalized

  ii. Headache

    1. A common complaint

    2. "Lupus headache"

      a. Severe, disabling, and persistent

      b. Not responsive to narcotic analgesics

    3. Benign intracranial hypertension

  iii. "Lupoid sclerosis"

    1. A rare condition

    2. Patients exhibit complex neurologic deficits

    3. Similar to multiple sclerosis

  iv. Myelopathy and aseptic meningitis

    1. Rare

  v. Chorea

    1. Most common movement disorder

    2. Related to the presence of antiphospholipid antibodies

  vi. Cerebrovascular accidents

    1. Related to the presence of antiphospholipid antibodies

  vii. Cranial nerve disturbances

    1. Visual defects

    2. Blindness

    3. Papilledema

    4. Nystagmus or ptosis

    5. Tinnitus

    6. Vertigo

    7. Facial palsy

  viii. Peripheral neuropathy

    1. Motor

    2. Sensory

    3. Mixed motor-sensory

    4. Mononeuritis multiplex

        ix. Transverse myelitis
           1. Lower-extremity paralysis
           2. Sensory deficits
           3. Loss of sphincter control
        x. Acute inflammatory demyelinating polyradiculoneuropathy
           1. Guillain-Barre syndrome
  h. Cerebrospinal fluid
      i. Useful to rule out infection
      ii. Findings often nonspecific
          1. Elevated cell counts, protein levels, or both are found in only about one-third of patients
          2. May be normal in acute disease
  i. Imaging
      i. CT
          1. Mass lesions
          2. Hemorrhages
      ii. MRI
          1. Histopathologic findings of vascular injury
          2. White and grey matter lesions
          3. Abnormalities more likely with focal findings
          4. Clinical correlation is low
  j. Autoantibodies associated with CNS lupus (3)
      i. Serum anti-phospholipid antibodies
          1. Associated with focal neurologic manifestations
      ii. Cerebrospinal fluid anti-neuronal antibodies
          1. Associated with diffuse manifestations
      iii. Serum antibodies to ribosomal P proteins (anti-P antibodies)
          1. Associated with psychiatric problems
             a. Severe depression
             b. Psychosis
  k. Diffuse manifestations of CNS lupus
      i. Caused primarily by autoantibodies directed to neuronal cells or their products
          1. Affects neuronal function in a generalized manner
          2. Markers of abnormal autoantibody production
             a. Elevated levels of IgG
             b. Oligoclonal bands
      ii. Other causes
          1. Inflammatory cytokines
          2. Induction of nitric oxide production
          3. Oxidative stress
          4. Excitatory amino acid toxicity
      iii. Organic brain syndrome
          1. Elevated **anti-neuronal antibodies** in the CSF
      iv. Psychiatric disease
          1. **Serum anti-P antibodies** as a diagnostic marker

1. Clinical Presentations
   i. Patient with severe lupus treated 2 weeks with high dose prednisone becomes disoriented and demonstrates bizarre behavior with delusional thinking
      1. Differential diagnosis
         a. CNS lupus
         b. Prednisone induced psychosis
         c. A separate problem
            i. Infection
            ii. Metabolic disturbance
      2. Evaluation
         a. Examine for active lupus
         b. Rule out organic brain syndrome
            i. Decreased intellectual function
         c. Examine for focal neurological deficits
            i. Likely not the prednisone
      3. Labs
         a. Exclude a metabolic problem
         b. Determine lupus activity
         c. Evaluate for other organ involvement
      4. CNS directed studies
         a. MRI
         b. EEG
            i. Normal in steroid induced psychosis
         c. LP analysis of CSF
            i. Increased CNS IgG production
            ii. Oligoclonal bands
            iii. Anti-neuronal antibodies
      5. Serologies
         a. Anti-P antibody
            i. Associated with psychosis caused by lupus
         b. Studies for systemic disease activity
      6. Treatment
         a. If all studies are negative then likely steroid induced psychosis
            i. Decrease the dose
         b. Evidence for CNS lupus
            i. Increase the steroids and/or add cytotoxic drug
21. Cardiovascular System
   a. Pericarditis
      i. The most common occurrence
         1. 6–45%
         2. On average 25%
      ii. Presentation
         1. Complaints of substernal or pericardial pain

        2. Pain aggravated by motion
          a. Inspiration
          b. Coughing
          c. Swallowing
          d. Bending forward
        3. Hear a rub
        4. Typical T-wave abnormalities
        5. ECHO shows effusion
          a. Small to moderate
          b. Fluid straw colored to serosanguinous, exudative
          c. High WBC counts
            i. Up to 30,000 cells/mm^3
            ii. A predominance of neutrophils
          d. LE cells in the centrifuged cell sediment
      iii. Tamponade and constrictive pericarditis is rare
  b. Primary myocardial involvement
     i. Rare (<10%)
    ii. Fever
   iii. Dyspnea
   iv. Palpitations
    v. Heart murmurs
   vi. Sinus tachycardia
  vii. Ventricular arrhythmias
 viii. Conduction abnormalities
   ix. Congestive heart failure
    x. Percutaneous endomyocardial biopsy may be helpful
  c. Valvular disease
     i. Can be hemodynamically and clinically significant
    ii. More frequent in patients with antiphospholipid antibodies
   iii. Aortic insufficiency
      1. The most commonly reported lesion
      2. Multiple factors
        a. Fibrinoid degeneration
        b. Distortion of the valve by fibrosis
        c. Valvulitis
        d. Bacterial endocarditis
        e. Aortitis
        f. Libman-Sacks endocarditis
   iv. Libman-Sacks endocarditis
      1. The classic cardiac lesion of SLE
      2. "Atypical verrucous endocarditis"
      3. Verrucous vegetations ranging from 1 to 4 mm in diameter
      4. Initially reported on the tricuspid and mitral valve
    v. The presence or changes in valvular lesions
      1. Not related to the activity or the treatment of SLE

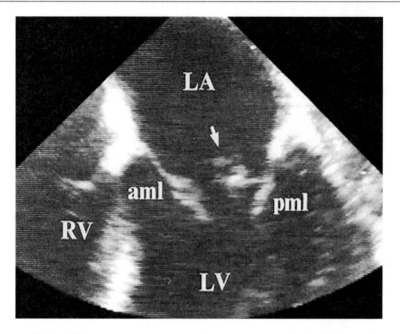

Fig. 7.13 Libman-Sacks vegetation and mitral valve thickening in systemic lupus erythematosus (Reproduced with permission from Rheumatic and connective tissue diseases and the heart. *Atlas of Heart Diseases.* ImagesMD; 2002-01-23)

     vi. Prophylactic antibiotics
        1. For surgical and dental procedures
        2. Recommended for all people with SLE
  d. Atherosclerosis
      i. An important cause of morbidity and mortality in SLE
     ii. 6–12% prevalence of angina and MI in some SLE cohorts
    iii. Myocardial infarct (MI) mortality about 10 times greater than the general age and sex-matched population
    iv. Severe coronary artery artherosclerosis in up to 40% with SLE
        1. 2% of controls
        2. Autopsy studies
     v. Risk factors
        1. Hypercholesterolemia
        2. Hypertension
        3. Lupus itself
     vi. Corticosteroids elevate plasma lipids
    vii. Antimalarials reduce cholesterol, LDL and VLDLs
   viii. Coronary arteritis may coexist with atherosclerotic heart disease
     ix. 40% of women (175) had focal plaque by B-mode ultrasound
        1. Measured carotid plaque and intima-media wall thickness
  e. Secondary hypertensive disease

22. Lungs and Pleura
   a. More than 30% have some form of pleural disease in their lifetime
      i. Pleuritis with chest pain
         1. A more common feature of serositis than pericarditis
      ii. Frank effusion
   b. Pleural effusions
      i. Often small and bilateral
      ii. Fluid character
         1. Usually clear and exudative
         2. Increased protein
         3. Normal glucose
         4. WBC count is elevated
            a. Less than 10,000
            b. A predominance of neutrophils or lymphocytes
         5. Decreased levels of complement
   c. Pulmonary involvement
      i. Pneumonitis
      ii. Pulmonary hemorrhage
      iii. Pulmonary embolism
         1. Especially with antiphospholipid antibodies
      iv. Pulmonary hypertension
   d. Shrinking-lung syndrome
      i. Decreased lung volumes without parenchymal disease
   e. Active lupus pneumonitis
      i. An abrupt febrile pneumonitic process
         1. Infection ruled out
      ii. Prominent features
         1. Pleuritic chest pain
         2. Cough with hemoptysis
         3. Dyspnea
      iii. Diffuse alveolar hemorrhage
         1. A manifestation of active disease
         2. Associated with a 50% mortality rate
         3. Occurs in the absence of hemoptysis
         4. Suggested by a falling hematocrit and pulmonary infiltrates
      iv. Occurs without pulmonary hemorrhage
      v. 10% develop a chronic syndrome
         1. Progressive dyspnea
         2. Nonproductive cough
         3. Basilar rales
         4. Diffuse interstitial lung infiltrates
   f. Pulmonary hypertension
      i. Progressive SOB
      ii. CXR is negative
      iii. Profound hypoxemia is absent

      iv. Pulmonary function tests (PFTs)
        1. Show a restrictive pattern
        2. A reduction in the diffusing capacity for carbon monoxide
      v. Diagnosis
        1. Doppler ultrasound studies
        2. Cardiac catheterization
      vi. Frequently associated with Raynaud's
     vii. Intrapulmonary clotting and/or multiple pulmonary emboli
        1. A causative factor
        2. Address and treat
        3. Especially in the setting of anti-phospholipid antibodies
        4. Gradually progressive over time
  g. Chronic interstitial lung disease and pulmonary fibrosis
  h. Secondary infections
23. Gastrointestinal Tract and Liver
  a. The peritoneum is the least likely of the serosal linings to be affected
  b. Abdominal pain
    i. Pancreatitis
    ii. Bowel vasculitis
      1. Rectal bleeding in mesenteric vasculitis
  c. Protein-losing enteropathy
    i. Uncommon
    ii. Low serum albumin
    iii. Pedal edema
    iv. Absence of proteinuria
  d. Parenchymal liver disease as a result of SLE is rare
  e. Elevated transaminases
    i. Seen during periods of active disease
    ii. With medications
      1. NSAIDs
      2. Azathioprine
      3. Methotrexate
    iii. With persistent signs of hepatitis in the absence of offending drugs
      1. Consider biopsy
  f. "Lupoid hepatitis"
    i. Originally coined in 1956 as a manifestation of SLE
    ii. Defined serologically and histologically as a subset of chronic active hepatitis
    iii. Need not have lupus
    iv. Seen in fewer than 10% with the ACR criteria for SLE
24. Ocular
  a. Retina cotton-wool spots
    i. The most common lesion in SLE
    ii. Results from focal ischemia
    iii. Not pathognomonic for lupus
    iv. Occurs preferentially in the posterior part of the retina

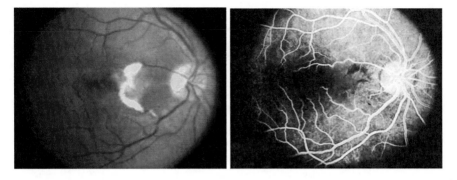

Fig. 7.14 Fundus photograph of cilioretinal artery occlusion in a patient with SLE with ischemic retinal whitening in the area of the papillomacular bundle, indicating more extensive ischemia than that producing cotton-wool spots, as well as periarterial sheathing (*left*). Fluorescein angiogram showing occlusion of the cilioretinal artery. The area of retinal ischemia appears hypofluorescent and obscures the background choroidal flush (*right*) (Reproduced with permission from A clinical approach to the diagnosis of retinal vasculitis. *International Ophthalmology.* DOI: 10.1007/s10792-009-9301-3. Springer; 2010-03-31)

     v. Often involves the optic nerve head
     vi. Grayish-white soft, fluffy exudates
     vii. About 1/3 of a disc diameter
     viii. "Cytoid bodies"
        1. Refers to the histologic features
  b. Other involvements by descending frequency
     i. Corneal
     ii. Conjunctival
     iii. Uveitis
     iv. Scleritis
  c. Retinal damage from antimalarials
     i. A greater cause of vision loss than the natural course of the disease
25. Hematologic Abnormalities
  a. The "Penias"
     i. Generally secondary to peripheral destruction
     ii. Not due to marrow suppression
     iii. Especially in the absence of offending medications
  b. Autoimmune hemolytic anemia
     i. Present in <10% of patients
     ii. Evaluate with a reticulocyte count
     iii. Active destruction of RBCs
     iv. Autoantibodies to RBCs
        1. Direct Coombs
  c. Coombs test
     i. Both direct and indirect can be positive in SLE
        1. Without active hemolysis
     ii. More patients will have a positive Coombs than hemolytic anemia

   d. Anemia of chronic disease
      i. Present in up to 80% of patients
      ii. Secondary to persistent inflammation
      iii. Careful patient follow-up
         1. More likely to demonstrate flairs of lupus activity
      iv. Mechanisms
         1. Decreased production of RBCs
         2. Slightly decreased RBC survival
         3. Abnormal iron processing by the reticuloendothelial system
            a. Serum iron usually low
            b. Low TIBC
            c. Ferritin normal or elevated
      v. Clinical Presentation
         1. HCT drops over several months to a steady level of 31%
         2. Normal RBC indices and CBC
         3. Medications include prednisone and prn low dose NSAIDs
         4. Anemia likely due to chronic disease
            a. Uncontrolled inflammation
   e. Leukopenia
      i. Seen in more than 50% of patients
      ii. Low counts with or without disease activity
      iii. Predisposition to infection
   f. Absolute lymphopenia
      i. Less than 1,500 cells/mm^3
      ii. More common than neutropenia
   g. Thrombocytopenia
      i. Degrees can vary
      ii. Sometimes the sole manifestation of disease activity
      iii. Rarely associated with qualitative defects in platelets
      iv. Life threatening bleeding is unusual
      v. Antiplatelet antibodies may be seen without thrombocytopenia
   h. Clinical Presentation
      i. SLE patient with low WBC
         1. 2,500 with 70 neutrophils, 20 lymphocytes, 8 monos, and 2 eosinophils
      ii. Prednisone tapered to 5 mg/day with no clinical manifestations of active disease
      iii. Review of systems (ROS) and physical exam (PE) are negative
         1. Except for a mild malar rash
      iv. Labs show no evidence for lupus nephritis or other internal organ involvement
      v. Evaluate and treat the leukopenia
         1. Leukopenia with neutropenia and lymphopenia is not uncommon
         2. Warrants no further evaluation or treatment
         3. Implies continued disease activity

i. Clinical Presentation
  i. Young SLE patient with severe thrombocytopenia
  ii. Bone marrow shows increased megakaryocytes
  iii. High dose prednisone increases platelets to normal
    1. Tapering prednisone results in a decline to <20,000
  iv. No other medications
  v. Normal PE
  vi. Diagnosis autoimmune thrombocytopenia
  vii. Therapeutic options
    1. Splenectomy
      a. Controversial in lupus
      b. For the young with no other problems of SLE
    2. Danazol
      a. An androgen
      b. Increases platelet count
      c. Doses up to 800 mg/day
    3. An immunosuppressive or cytotoxic drug
      a. Azathioprine
        i. Less toxic
      b. Cyclophosphamide
    4. IVIG
      a. For signs of bleeding
      b. Too costly for long term
j. Thrombocytopenic purpura (TTP)
  i. Five major manifestations
    1. Fever
    2. Altered mental status
    3. Worsening renal function
    4. Hemolytic anemia
    5. Thrombocytopenia
  ii. Can be misdiagnosed as a flare
    1. Examine the peripheral blood smear for schistocytes
      a. The quickest way to distinguish
    2. The presence of schistocytes will confirm a microangiopathic hemo-
      lytic anemia
      a. Coombs negative
      b. Seen in TTP
    3. Rules out autoimmune hemolytic anemia
      a. Coombs positive
      b. Seen in SLE
  iii. Etiology
    1. IgG autoantibody against a metalloprotease
      a. Cleaves the monomeric subunits of von Willebrand factor
    2. Large multimers of von Willebrand factors accumulates
      a. Endothelial cells secrete into the plasma

 3. Multimers bind to platelet glycoprotein receptors
  a. Cause adhesion and microthrombi
 iv. Treatment
  1. Plasmapheresis
   a. Removes the autoantibody and large multimers of von Willebrand factor
   b. Followed by FFP to replace the metalloprotease
  2. Corticosteroids and immunosuppressives
   a. Prevents recurrence
   b. Suppresses autoantibody formation
26. Hallmark Autoantibodies and Complement
 a. ANA
  i. The laboratory hallmark of SLE
  ii. Greater than 98% with SLE demonstrate elevated serum levels
  iii. Not specific for SLE
  iv. ANA in healthy individuals
   1. Frequency 32% at a 1:40 and 13% at 1:80
   2. Overall detected in about 2%
    a. Particularly in young women
  v. ANA in other rheumatic diseases
   1. Sjogren's
   2. MCTD
   3. Scleroderma
   4. RA
   5. Polymyositis
  vi. ANA in other inflammatory disorders
   1. Autoimmune hepatitis
   2. Hepatitis C
   3. Lymphoma
   4. IPF
  vii. False-positives increase with age
  viii. Serial measurements of ANA
   1. Not useful as a gauge of disease activity
  ix. Indirect immunofluorescence test
   1. The most common assay used to detect ANA
   2. Diluted serum is layered on a slide with fixed cells or tissue
   3. Unbound antibodies are washed off
   4. A secondary fluorescein-tagged antibody directed to immunoglobulin is added
   5. Patient antibody bound to the nucleus will be stained
    a. The nucleus will fluoresce
   6. Results are registered as positive or negative
   7. The strength of the positive reaction is recorded as a particular serum dilution
    a. Begins at 1:40

    x. Patterns of nuclear staining
       1. Rim (peripheral)
         a. The **most specific** pattern for SLE
         b. Autoantibodies to deoxynucleoproteins
       2. Diffuse
       3. Speckled
         a. The **most common** pattern in SLE
         b. The least specific for SLE
       4. Nucleolar
   xi. The best support for the diagnosis of SLE
       1. Positive test titers above 1:160
       2. Tests for specific types of ANA
       3. A negative ANA at 1:40 or 1:80
         a. Strongly suggest the diagnosis is **not** SLE
  b. Common autoantibodies in SLE and their major clinical associations
    i. dsDNA
      1. High diagnostic specificity for SLE
      2. A valuable means of predicting and assessing renal disease
    ii. SSA/Ro and SSA/La ribonucleoproteins
      1. Do not correlate with disease activity
      2. Seen in patients with dry eyes, dry mouth (secondary Sjogren) and neonatal lupus
      3. SSA/Ro
        a. Associated with subacute cutaneous lupus
        b. Photosensitivity
        c. Stains the cytoplasmic component of the cell
        d. Accounts for ANA-negative lupus
   iii. Histones
      1. H1, H2A, H2B, H3, H4
      2. SLE and drug induced lupus
    iv. Sm
      1. snRNP core proteins B, B', D, and E
      2. High diagnostic specificity for SLE
      3. No correlation with disease activity
    v. Antinucleosome antibodies
      1. A selective biologic marker of active lupus nephritis
    vi. Ku
      1. Diagnostic specificity for SLE
   vii. Proliferating cell nuclear antigen
      1. PCNA/cyclin
      2. High diagnostic specificity for SLE
  viii. Ribosomal P proteins
      1. High diagnostic specificity for SLE
      2. Cytoplasmic staining
      3. Psychiatric disease

ix. Phospholipids
    1. Anti-phospholipid antibodies (APAs)
    2. Detected by a test for anti-cardiolipin antibodies
    3. Mostly directed at B2-glycoprotein 1
       a. Usually with bound phospholipid
       b. The best characterized antigenic target
       c. Multiple inhibitory functions in coagulation pathways
    4. Inhibition of coagulation tests
       a. Lupus anticoagulant
       b. Picked up by an abnormal partial thromboplastin time (PTT)
       c. Further demonstrated by specific clotting studies
          i. The Russell viper venom test
       d. In vitro
          i. Prolonged clotting
          ii. Not corrected by mixing studies
       e. In vivo
          i. Thrombogenic
    5. Mechanism of APAs are unknown
    6. Clinical significance
       a. Primary anti-phospholipid antibody syndrome
       b. Thrombosis
          i. The major clinical association of APAs
             1. Not bleeding

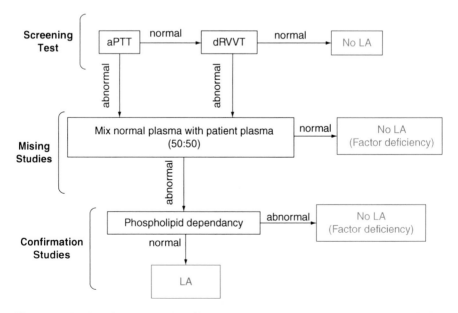

Fig. 7.15 Algorithm for the detection of lupus anticoagulant (*LA*) (Reproduced with permission from Antiphospholipid antibodies. *Antiphospholipid Syndrome Handbook.* DOI: 10.1007/978-1-84628-735-0_3. Springer; 2010-01-01)

ii. Arterial and venous
c. Recurrent abortions/fetal wasting
i. Intravascular thrombosis
ii. Placental insufficiency
d. Neurologic disease
i. Focal presentations
e. Thrombocytopenia
f. Livedo reticularis
g. Autoimmune hemolytic anemia
x. Cell surface antigens on RBC, platelets, lymphocytes lead to the respective penias
c. Complement
i. To discriminate between accelerated consumption and decreased synthesis of complement
1. Measure complement split products
ii. Complement split products provide an early diagnosis of lupus
1. C3a as a predictor of flair
27. SLE and Pregnancy
a. Sterility and fertility rates for SLE are comparable to controls
i. No increased rate of infertility as long as SLE is under control
b. Age-dependent premature ovarian failure
i. Occurs in those receiving cyclophosphamide
c. SLE compared to healthy women have higher rates of
i. Spontaneous abortion
ii. Intrauterine fetal death
iii. Premature birth
d. Clinical and serologic expression of SLE adversely altered by pregnancy
i. The placenta and fetus become targets of specific attack by maternal autoantibodies
e. Pregnancy outcome
i. Disease should be in clinical remission for 6–12 months prior to conception
1. Optimizes pregnancy outcome
2. Best when disease activity is quiet and medications are minimal
a. A patient on 5 mg/day of prednisone with quiescent disease
ii. Patients who conceive with **inactive** SLE are at increased risk
1. IUGR
2. Prematurity
3. Toxemia of pregnancy
iii. Stable SLE can relapse during pregnancy
1. 20–30% likelihood
iv. Poor fetal outcome
1. Development of SLE during pregnancy
a. Fetal death rate as high as 45%
2. Newly diagnosed lupus nephritis in the first trimester

   3. Active lupus nephritis
    a. Fetal mortality increased at least three fold
   4. Prematurity
    a. Occurs in most of the successful pregnancies
    b. Risk as high as 60% with active lupus
  v. Uncomplicated pregnancy
   1. Stable renal disease
   2. Creatinine <1.5 and 24 h <2 g
  vi. SLEDAI and SLAM
   1. Does not account for the physiologic adaptations of pregnancy
   2. Not validated for pregnant lupus patients
  vii. Close follow-up by a rheumatologist is advised
 f. Valid criteria attributable to a flare during pregnancy
  i. Characteristic dermatologic involvement
  ii. Arthritis
  iii. Fever not secondary to infection
  iv. Lymphadenopathy
  v. Leukopenia
  vi. Alternative pathway hypocomplementemia
  vii. Rising titers of DNA
 g. Invalid markers of disease activity
  i. Alopecia
  ii. Facial or palmer blush
  iii. Arthralgia
  iv. Musculoskeletal aching
  v. Mild anemia
  vi. Fatigue
 h. Active lupus nephritis versus preeclampsia
  i. Both have proteinuria
   1. Cellular casts and proteinuria more clearly represents an exacerbation of lupus nephritis
  ii. Both cause thrombocytopenia, hemolytic anemia, and convulsions
  iii. Preeclampsia (toxemia)
   1. Usually occurs in the 3rd trimester
   2. Hypertension
   3. Proteinuria
   4. Edema
   5. Consumptive coagulopathy
   6. Microangiopathic hemolytic anemia
   7. Convulsions
  iv. Making the diagnosis
   1. Normal pregnancy
    a. Proteinuria
     i. Associated rise in creatinine clearance
     ii. Corresponding fall in serum creatinine
    b. Complement values usually rise

    2. Preeclampsia
      a. SLE clinical manifestations are absent
      b. Lack of red cell casts
      c. Stable anti-DNA antibodies
      d. A high uric acid
      e. Remits upon delivery
        i. No further therapy
    3. Active lupus nephritis
      a. Complement values decrease
      b. CH50
        i. A decrease distinguishes lupus from preeclampsia or pregnancy induced hypertension
      c. Uric acid may be high or normal
      d. Continued therapy required
        i. High dose corticosteroids in combination with azathioprine during pregnancy
          1. Prednisone is the mainstay for serious lupus flares during pregnancy
        ii. Cyclophosphamide after pregnancy
    4. Useful labs
      a. Anti-dsDNA
      b. Complement
        i. CH50
i. Clinical Presentation
    i. A patient with active lupus nephritis and on 20 mg/day prednisone
      1. Counsel against pregnancy at this time
      2. Renal function can deteriorate with pregnancy
      3. Increased problems related to hypertension and pre-eclampsia
    ii. Patients with active lupus nephritis during pregnancy
      1. 50–60% chance of nephritis exacerbation
    iii. Patients with quiescent lupus
      1. The risk of nephritis exacerbation is<10%
    iv. Treatment
      1. Cyclophosphamide
        a. Contraindicated if renal disease worsens
      2. Azathioprine
        a Used successfully in pregnancy
        b. Metabolized by the placenta
        c. Little gets into the fetal circulation
j. SLE drugs used during pregnancy
    i. Corticosteroids
      1. Category B
      2. 90% metabolized by placental enzymes
      3. Low dose prednisone
        a. 5–10 mg/day

        b. Well tolerated

        c. May be protective from flare

    4. High dose steroids

        a. Cleft lip (< 1–4%)

        b. Premature birth may occur

  ii. NSAIDs

    1. Widely used for preterm labor without major adverse outcomes

    2. Side effects

        a. Premature ductus arteriosus closure

        b. Oligohydramnios

        c. Respiratory distress syndrome

        d. Pulmonary hypertension

        e. Fetal death

          i. With indomethacin

    3. Fetal abnormalities

        a. Associated with animal studies

        b. No evidence in human studies to involve

          i. Aspirin

          ii. Indomethacin

          iii. Diclofenac

          iv. Ibuprofen

          v. Sulindac

        c. Insufficient data on COX-2

    4. Low dose aspirin

        a. 80 mg/day

        b. Safe

        c. Effective prophylaxis

          i. Preeclampsia

          ii. IUGR

    5. Use in late term pregnancy

        a. Full dose aspirin at the time of delivery

          i. Prolonged labor

          ii. Anemia

          iii. Increased neonatal hemorrhage in premature infants

        b. Switch to low doses of prednisone (< 20 mg/day) at least 2 months before delivery

 iii. Hydroxychloroquine and chloroquine

    1. Category C

    2. Side effects

        a. Increased risk of miscarriages

        b. Retinal damage

        c. Ototoxicity

    3. Relative risk

        a. Low (4.5%) by recent studies

        b. Outweighed by potential benefits in certain circumstances

    iv. Sulfasalazine
      1. Category B
      2. For IBD
        a. Used safely throughout pregnancy and lactation
      3. For rheumatic diseases
        a. Probably safe
        b. Not extensively studied
      4. Folate supplementation recommended
      5. Can cause reversible oligospermia
    v. Etanercept, infliximab, anakinra
      1. All category B
      2. Used in pregnancy if clearly needed
      3. Secreted into breast milk
        a. Should not nurse while on these medications
   vi. Gold salts
      1. Category C
      2. Frequently associated with congenital malformations (10%)
        a. Cannot be routinely recommended
      3. Relatively safe in lactation
  vii. Cyclosporin
      1. Category C
      2. Crosses the placenta
        a. Associated with IUGR and prematurity (40%)
      3. Frequently used in pregnant transplant patients
        a. Teratogenesis not seen
      4. Secreted into breast milk
        a. Use during lactation not recommended
 viii. Azathioprine
      1. Category D
      2. Used in pregnancy for
        a. Renal transplants
        b. Hematologic malignancies
        c. IBD
        d. Lupus nephritis
      3. Metabolized by the placenta
      4. Adverse effects
        a. Fetal growth retardation
        b. Cytopenias
        c. Opportunistic infections
      5. For severe and life threatening rheumatic disease
        a. Lupus nephritis
      6. Close prenatal monitoring
      7. Long-term evaluation of the offspring
      8. Detected in breast milk
        a. Not considered safe in lactation
      9. Safe for men to conceive

   k. Drugs to avoid during pregnancy
      i. Penicillamine
        1. Category D
        2. Used in Wilson's disease and cysteinuria
        3. Severe adverse effects on the fetus
          a. Serious connective tissue disorders
          b. Neonatal sepsis
      ii. Methotrexate
        1. Category X
        2. Associated with spontaneous abortions and birth anomalies
        3. Both men and women should discontinue the drug at least 3 months before conception
          a. Prolonged retention of methotrexate in tissues
        4. Not recommended in lactation
     iii. Leflunomide
        1. Category X
        2. Increased fetal death and teratogenesis
        3. Elimination protocol for men and women desiring pregnancy
          a. Cholestyramine 8 g TID for 11 days
          b. Followed by two separate tests to verify negligible plasma levels
          c. Without elimination unsafe levels remain for up to 2 years
     iv. Cyclophosphamide and chlorambucil
        1. Both category D
        2. Contraindicated during pregnancy
          a. High risks of congenital malformations if used during the 1st trimester
          b. 22% and 33%, respectively
        3. Adverse effects if used later in pregnancy
          a. Neonatal bone marrow suppression
          b. Infection
          c. Hemorrhage
        4. Cyclophosphamide is secreted in breast milk
          a. Associated with leukopenia in the offspring
          b. Not recommended during lactation
        5. Chlorambucil during lactation
          a. Data is insufficient to recommend
28. Neonatal Lupus (NLE)
   a. Passively acquired autoimmunity to the fetus and neonate
      i. Immune abnormalities in the mother cross the placenta
   b. Anti-Ro/SSA antibodies
      i. Inhibit inward L-type calcium currents of cardiocytes
        1. Damage to the AV node leads to complete heart block
        2. Sinoatrial node can also be involved
      ii. Bind to fetal heart conducting cells
        1. Elicits an inflammatory injury

   c. Congenital heart block (CHB)
      i. The major morbidity and mortality of NLE (40%)
         1. Frequently the only manifestation
      ii. Most often 3rd degree
         1. Complete heart block is irreversible
      iii. Identified between 16 and 24 weeks of gestation
      iv. Mortality rate 20%
         1. A result of myocarditis
      v. Majority of children require pacing (50%)
   d. Cutaneous involvement
      i. Erythematous
      ii. Annular lesions
      iii. Predilection for the periorbital region (40%)
         1. Face
         2. Scalp
      iv. Similar to that of subacute cutaneous lupus erythematous
      v. Rash and CHB (10–20%)
   e. Hepatic and hematologic involvement (lesser extent)
      i. Hemolytic anemia
      ii. Thrombocytopenia
         1. Anti-platelet antibodies
         2. Associated hemorrhage
            a. Especially at the time of delivery
   f. Noncardiac manifestations are transient
      i. Resolve at about 6 months
      ii. Coincident with the disappearance of maternal autoantibodies
   g. Risk factors for mothers
      i. Anti-SSA/Ro
         1. High titers (4–5% overall)
         2. Incidence (1–2%)
         3. Frequently anti-52-kDa
         4. More common in those with associated Sjogren's
      ii. Anti-SSB/La
         1. 25–70%
      iii. Less than one-third of mothers of affected children actually have SLE
   h. Fetal risk factors
      i. Discordant dizygotic and monozygotic twins
      ii. 20–25% overall risk of CHB
         1. Once a SLE mother has had one child with CHB
   i. Surveillance for at risk mothers
      i. Weekly fetal echos from the 18th to 24th weeks of gestation
         1. Measure the mechanical PR interval
   j. Indications for treatment
      i. Heart block
      ii. Incomplete heart block

        iii. Signs of myocarditis

        iv. Congestive heart failure

        v. Hydrops

    k. Prenatal treatment

        i. Treat the mother with dexamethasone (4 mg/day)

        ii. Do not use prednisone

          1. Metabolized by placental 11-B hydroxygenase

        iii. Plasmapheresis

        iv. Occasionally reverses heart block

    l. Postnatal treatment

        i. High dose corticosteroids

        ii. Immune globulin

        iii. May prevent progression to complete heart block

        iv. No therapy effective in reversing complete heart block once established

        v. All infants born to mothers with anti-Ro/SSA antibodies should have an EKG

          1. Evaluate for 1st degree AV block

          2. Postnatal progression to CHB has been reported

29. Antiphospholipid Antibody Syndrome

    a. Primary anti-phospholipid syndrome

        i. Anti-phospholipid antibodies with one of the clinical features of recurrent fetal loss or thrombocytopenia (surface of activated platelets display the anionic phospholipid target antigens) in the absence of any other manifestations of SLE

    b. Secondary anti-phospholipid syndrome

        i. Anti-phospholipid antibodies in the context of SLE

30. Drug Related Lupus (DRL)

    a. Development of a lupus-like syndrome following exposure to certain drugs (estimated risk)

        i. Chlorpromazine (low)

        ii. Hydralazine (**high**)

        iii. Isoniazid (low)

        iv. Methyldopa (low)

        v. Minocycline (low)

        vi. Procainamide (**high**)

        vii. Quinidine (**moderate**)

    b. Potentially offending agents

        i. Diphenylhydantoin

        ii. Mephenytoin

        iii. Phenytoin

        iv. Beta-adrenergic blocking agents

        v. Penicillamine

        vi. Gold salts

        vii. Carbamazepine

        viii. Sulfasalazine

   c. These drugs **do not** appear to aggravate idiopathic SLE

   d. Requires a temporal association (weeks or months) between ingestion of drug and the beginning of symptoms

   e. Rapid resolution of the clinical features following drug removal

   f. Demographic features

      i. Reflect those of the disease for which the drug was prescribed

      ii. More frequent in the elderly

         1. Usual age 50

      iii. Slightly more frequent in females than males

      iv. More common in Caucasians (six fold higher) than African Americans (AA)

      v. Fewer than 4 SLE criteria (in general)

   g. ANAs in DRL

      i. Developing a + ANA depends on the dose and duration of therapy

      ii. 10–30% of ANA + patients develop symptoms of lupus

      iii. ANAs without clinical features

         1. Insufficient for the diagnosis

         2. Not a reason to stop the drug

      iv. Anti-histone antibodies

         1. The most common autoantibody specificity in DRL

         2. A diffuse homogenous pattern

            a. Represents binding of autoantibody to chromatin

            b. DNA and histones

         3. Most have elevated levels of IgG anti-histone antibodies

         4. Also seen in idiopathic SLE (50–80%)

         5. Anti-histone antibody specificity

            a. Individual histones

               i. H1

               ii. H2A

               iii. H2B

               iv. H3

               v. H4

            b. Histone complexes

            c. Intra-histone epitopes

      v. Antibodies to antiphospholipid and ssDNA

         1. Common in both types of SLE

      vi. Autoantibodies may persist for 6 months to 1 year

   h. Uncharacteristic autoantibodies in DRL (rare)

      i. Anti-dsDNA

      ii. Anti-Sm

      iii. Ro/SSA

      iv. La/SSB

   i. Procainamide-induced lupus

      i. 75% develop a + ANA within the first year of treatment

         1. Over 90% by 2 years

    ii. IgG antibodies to the H2A-H2B-DNA complex
       1. Seen also in 15% of idiopathic SLE
  j. Hydralazine-induced lupus
    i. 30–50% develop a + ANA after a year
    ii. Major targets
       1. H3
       2. H4
       3. H3-H4 complex
    iii. Autoantibodies directed more to determinants hidden within chromatin
       1. Rather than those exposed on the surface
       2. Contrast to procainamide-induced lupus
  k. Hypocomplementemia is uncommon in DLR
  l. No therapy needed if asymptomatic after stopping the drug
    i. May remain ANA+
  m. Symptoms
    i. Constitutional complaints
       1. Malaise
       2. Low-grade fever
       3. Myalgia
    ii. Articular complaints
       1. Present in >80%
       2. Arthralgia > arthritis
  n. Rare clinical features
    i. Dermatologic
    ii. Renal
    iii. Neurologic
  o. Procainamide-induced lupus
    i. Presents often with pleuropulmonary disease and pericarditis
    ii. Pleuritis
       1. 30–40% have acute pulmonary infiltrates
    iii. Most symptoms controlled with NSAIDs
       1. After discontinuing the drug
    iv. Severe symptoms require a short course of prednisone
       1. Especially with pleuritis or pericarditis
    v. Toxic immunosuppressants
       1. Almost never required
  p. Hydralazine-induced lupus
    i. Differs from procainamide induced disease
    ii. Serositis and pulmonary parenchymal involvement less common
    iii. Rashes more likely
       1. The classic malar rash and discoid lesion are unusual
  q. Minocycline-induced lupus
    i. Minocycline
       1. A semisynthetic tetracycline
       2. Used to treat acne

    ii. Affects ages 14–31

    iii. Female > male

    iv. Occurs after an average of 30 months

       1. Doses of 50–200 mg/day

    v. All patients have a positive ANA

    vi. pANCA

       1. 75–80%

    vii. Antihistone antibodies

       1. Only 10–15%

    viii. Symptoms

       1. Arthritis/arthralgia (all)

       2. Fever (33%)

       3. Rash (20%)

       4. Pleuritis (10%)

       5. Hepatitis and anticardiolipin antibodies (33%)

    ix. Treatment

       1. Discontinue the drug

r. Predisposing genetic factors

    i. Metabolism of these drugs involves the hepatic enzyme N-acetyltrans-ferase

       1. Catalyzes the acetylation of amine or hydrazine groups

       2. The rate of reaction is under genetic control

    ii. Acetylator phenotype

       1. The major risk for procainamide or hydralazine induced lupus

       2. Not involved in idiopathic SLE

    iii. 50% of the US white population are fast acetylators

    iv. Slow acetylators

       1. Develop + ANA earlier and at higher titers when treated with procain-amide or hydralazine

       2. More likely to develop symptomatic disease than fast acetylators

    v. N-acetylprocainamide

       1. Similar chemically to procainamide

       2. Not associated with DRL

s. Pathophysiology

    i. Activated neutrophils

       1. Enzymatic action of myeloperoxidase

       2. Converts lupus-inducing drugs to cytotoxic metabolites for lymphocytes

       3. Generates the release of autoantigens

    ii. The injection of an active metabolite of procainamide into the thymus (animal study)

       1. Induced anti-chromatin autoantibodies

       2. Disrupted central T-cell tolerance

       3. Inhibits DNA methylation

       4. T-cells alter their gene expression

Arthritis Associated with Calcium-Containing Crystals

8

1. Calcium Pyrophosphate Dihydrate (CPPD) Crystal Deposition Disease
   a. CPPD crystals may cause symptoms similar to
      i. Septic arthritis
      ii. Polyarticular inflammatory arthritis
      iii. Osteoarthritis
   b. Distinguishing CPPD deposition disease from other arthritides
      i. **Specific identification** of CPPD crystals
         1. $Ca_2P_2O_2\text{-}2H_2O$
      ii. Found in synovial fluid or articular tissue
   c. Chrondrocalcinosis
      i. Calcium containing crystals detected as radiodensities in articular cartilage
      ii. Characteristic radiographic patterns
         1. Wrist
            a. Triangular fibrocartilage complex
         2. Knees
            a. Hyaline cartilage
            b. Menisci
         3. Calcifications should be bilateral
   d. Other calcium containing crystals that can appear as chondrocalcinosis
      i. Calcium hydroxyapatite
         1. Calcium salts
      ii. Ochronosis
         1. Calcification of intervertebral disc cartilage
            a. Largely calcium hydroxyapatite
   e. Less frequent areas for CPPD crystal deposition
      i. Synovial lining
      ii. Ligaments
      iii. Tendons
      iv. Periarticular soft tissue
         1. Much like gouty tophi

N.T. Colburn, *Review of Rheumatology*,
DOI 10.1007/978-1-84882-093-7_8, © Springer-Verlag London Limited 2012

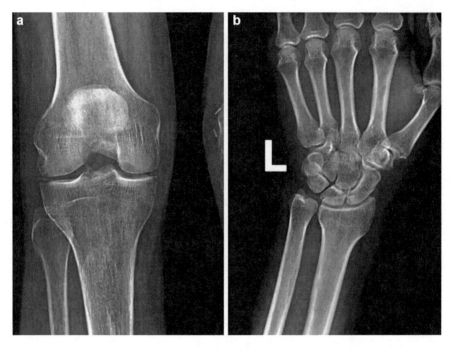

Fig. 8.1 Calcium pyrophosphate dehydrate (CPPD) deposition within the meniscal cartilage of the knee (**a**) and the triangular fibrocartilage of the wrist (**b**) (Reproduced with permission from Calcium pyrophosphate dihydrate (CPPD) crystal deposition disease (Courtesy of Dr. Richard Chou, Dartmouth-Hitchcock Medical Center). *A Clinician's Pearls and Myths in Rheumatology*. DOI: 10.1007/978-1-84800-934-9_37. Springer; 2009-01-01)

   f. Arthritis and CPPD deposition with normal X-rays
     i. Aspirate to distinguish gout from pseudogout
   g. Pseudogout
     i. Acute, gout-like attacks of inflammation
     ii. Occurs when CPPD is released as a crystal into a joint
   h. Pyrophosphate arthropathy
     i. Structural damage to a joint associated with CPPD deposition
       1. With or without chondrocalcinosis
   i. Calcium pyrophosphate dihydrate deposition disease
     i. Term used for all problems associated with CPPD deposition
       1. Chondrocalcinosis
       2. Pseudogout
       3. Pyrophosphate arthropathy
     ii. Clinical presentations
       1. Pseudogout
       2. Pseudo RA
       3. Pseudo OA
         a. With or without superimposed acute attacks of pseudogout

    4. Asymptomatic "lanthanic" radiographic form
    5. Pseudo Charcot or Pseudo-neuropathic arthritis
    6. Overlapping features of the above
 j. Prevalence of chondrocalcinosis
   i. Pathologic survey
    1. 4% of the adult population have CPPD at the time of death
   ii. Increases with age
    1. 30–50% by their ninth decade have chondrocalcinosis
   iii. Asymptomatic ("lanthanic") form of CPPD
    1. The most common clinical presentation of CPPD
   iv. Characteristic radiographs
    1. The knees and triangular fibrocartilage of the wrists (90%)
 k. Classification
   i. Hereditary
    1. Susceptibility to familial CPPD has been localized to the short arm of chromosome 5
   ii. Sporadic (idiopathic)
   iii. Associated with various metabolic diseases (none proven)
    1. Hyperparathyroidism
    2. Hypothyroidism
    3. Hypomagnesemia
    4. Hypophosphatasia
    5. Hemochromatosis
    6. Amyloidosis
   iv. Trauma
 l. Routine studies in newly diagnosed cases of CPPD deposition disease
   i. Serum calcium
   ii. Alkaline phosphatase
   iii. TSH
   iv. Magnesium
   v. Phosphorous
   vi. Ferritin
   vii. Iron
   viii. TIBC
 m. Clinical presentations for CPPD with an underlying metabolic cause
   i. Deposition is severe
   ii. Affects many joints
   iii. Patient younger than 55 years
   iv. Patients older than 55
    1. Hyperparathyroidism is a primary consideration
 n. Pathogenesis of cartilage degeneration and inflammation
   i. Acute pseudogout
    1. A dose related inflammatory host response to CPPD
    2. Crystals shed from cartilaginous tissues contiguous to the synovial cavity

    ii. Neutrophils
       1. Phagocytose crystals
       2. Release lysosomal enzymes and chemotactic factors
   iii. Synovial cells
       1. Phagocytose crystals
       2. Proliferate
       3. Release destructive mediators
         a. Prostaglandins
         b. Cytokines
         c. Proteases
           i. Collagenases and stromelysin
           ii. Able to degrade cartilage matrix
   iv. Colchicine
       1. Blocks release of chemotactic factors for neutrophils and mononu-
         clear cells
       2. Inhibits neutrophil-endothelial cell binding
       3. Stops inflammatory cell ingress
    v. CPPD and degenerative joint disease (DJD)
       1. Fibroblasts or synovial cell ingest crystals
       2. Crystal dissolve intracellularly and raise intracellular free-calcium
         levels
       3. A mitogenic response follows
         a. Tissue hypertrophy
         b. Lining cells secrete proteolytic enzymes (MMPs)
       4. Cytokine release leads to further protease release by lining cells or
         chondrocytes
       5. Compared to all forms of arthritis synovial fluid containing CPPD
         crystals have (on the average)
         a. The highest concentration of proteoglycan breakdown products
         b. The highest ratio of protease-to-protease inhibitor
  o. Pathogenesis of crystal deposition
    i. Inorganic pyrophosphate (PPi)
       1. Plasma levels and urinary excretion are not elevated
       2. Synovial fluid concentrations are elevated
       3. Articular chondrocytes liberate PPi into media
         a. Nonarticular tissues do not
       4. Liberation stimulated by
         a. Ascorbate
         b. TGF-β
         c. Retinoic acid
         d. Thyroid hormones
       5. Liberation inhibited by
         a. Probenecid
         b. Insulin-like growth factor 1
         c. Inhibitors of protein synthesis

        d. Isoforms of PTH related peptide

        e. IL-1

   6. Signaling pathways involved in PPi generation include

        a. Protein kinase C (up regulates)

        b. Adenylyl cyclase (down regulates)

   7. NTPPase

        a. An ectoenzyme which generates extracellular PPi

        b. Found in elevated amounts in CPPD disease

        c. Generates PPi from nucleoside triphosphate substrates

           i. ATP present in elevated amounts in fluid containing CPPD crystals

           ii. ATP added to cartilage explants induces formation of perichondral CPPD-like crystals

        d. Enriched in chondrocyte vesicles

           i. Grow monoclinic CPPD crystals in vitro

              1. With ATP

           ii. The vesicle associated NTPPase form is distinct

              1. Similar to intermediate layer cartilage protein

   8. Extracellular PPi formation

        a. Physiologic role in preventing excess articular structure apatite mineralization

        b. Decreased in mutations of ANK protein

  ii. Optimal environment CPPD crystal deposition

        1. Excess articular anion production

        2. Pericellular increase of anion with increased PPi generation

        3. Synthesis of molecules capable of heterologous CPPD crystal nucleation

        4. Absence of physiologic crystal inhibitors

p. Pseudogout pattern of CPPD crystal deposition disease

  i. Affects 25% of patients with CPPD

  ii. Marked by inflammation in one or more joints

  iii. Abrupt in onset

  iv. Last several days to 2 weeks

  v. Can be as severe as gout

        1. Usually less painful

        2. Takes longer to reach peak intensity

  vi. Anatomical distribution

        1. Documented in all joints

           a. Including the 1st MTP

        2. Large joints > small joints

           a. One half of all attacks involve the knees

        3. Usually only a single joint

           a. Oligoarticular and polyarticular described

  vii. Occurs spontaneously or provoked by trauma, surgery, or severe illness

  viii. Usually self-limited

        1. Untreated resolves within a month

    ix. Usually asymptomatic between episodes
     x. Simulates infection
         1. Overlying erythema (cellulitis)
         2. Systemic features
             a. Malaise
             b. Fever
    xi. Diagnosis
         1. Aspiration of the joint
         2. Synovial fluid
             a. Yellow and cloudy
             b. Opaque and chalky white from crystals
             c. Leukocytosis
                 i. Predominance of PMNs
         3. Synovial fluid analysis
             a. Cell count and differential
             b. Gram stain
             c. Bacterial culture
         4. CPPD crystals by light microscopy
             a. Rhomboid shaped or rectangular
             b. Ends blunt or square
             c. Compared to monosodium urate crystals
                 i. Needle shaped or pointed
         5. CPPD crystals by polarized light microscopy
             a. Intracellular CPPD crystals confirms the diagnosis
             b. Microscope must have a first order red compensator
             c. Weakly positively birefringent
                 i. Appears blue when viewed with the long axis of the crystal
                    parallel to the direction of slow vibration light
                    1. Aligned in the plane
                 ii. Mnemonic **ABC** (**A**ligned **B**lue **C**alcium)
                    1. Aligned crystal with the red compensator
                    2. Blue appearance
                    3. Calcium crystal
                 iii. Long axis of the crystal at a right angle to the direction of the
                    slow vibration
                    1. Appears yellow (rather than blue)
                    2. Rotate the microscope stage
         6. X-ray diffraction
             a. Rarely required for crystal identification
    xii. Systemic findings in an acute attack
         1. Fever
             a. Up to 103°
         2. Leukocytosis
             a. 12,000–15,000

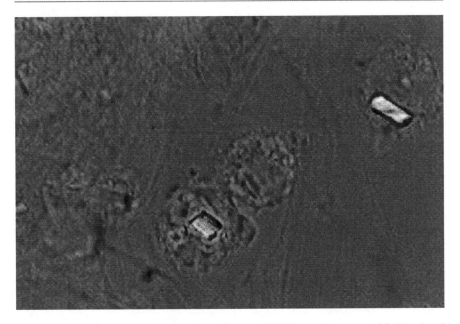

Fig. 8.2 Rod-shaped calcium pyrophosphate dihydrate (CPPD) crystals in synovial fluid analyzed by compensated polarized light microscopy (Reproduced with permission from Calcium pyrophosphate dihydrate, hydroxyapatite, and miscellaneous crystals. *Pocket Primer on the Rheumatic Diseases.* DOI: 10.1007/978-1-84882-856-8_15. Springer; 2010-01-01)

      3. Elevated ESR and serum acute phase reactants
         a. IL-6 may mediate some of these effects
  xiii. Pitfalls in diagnosis
      1. Simultaneous septic arthritis and CPPD
         a. Enzymes from infecting bacteria can degrade cartilage and release crystals
         b. Send fluid for gram stain (GS) and culture
      2. Simultaneous gout and pseudogout
         a. Diagnose with polarized light microscopy
      3. Acute pseudogout in wrist of elderly may cause carpal tunnel syndrome (CTS)
      4. Precipitate by an urgent medical illness (MI or surgery)
         a. Fluid shifts in calcium
      5. New joint pain in elderly hospitalized patient
         a. Evaluate for pseudogout
         b. Most idiopathic cases are older than 55–60 years
      6. Reported after intra-articular hyaluronate
         a. High concentrations of phosphate
      7. IV pamidronate rapidly normalizes attacks of hypercalcemia
         a. Precipitates pseudogout
      8. 20% of attack may not have chondrocalcinosis on X-rays

q. Pseudorheumatoid pattern of CPPD crystal deposition disease
   i. Seen in up to 5% of patients
   ii. Clinical presentation
      1. Multiple joint involvement
         a. Knees
         b. Wrists
         c. Elbows
      2. Symmetric distribution
      3. Low grade inflammation
      4. Can persist for weeks
      5. Morning stiffness
      6. Fatigue
      7. Synovial thickening
      8. Flexion contractures
      9. Elevated ESR
     10. Low titer RF + (10%)
   iii. Presentations that favor the diagnosis of RA
      1. High titer RF+
      2. Widespread synovitis involving the hands and feet
      3. Erosions
   iv. Rule out CPPD before diagnosing seronegative RA
      1. Review X-rays
      2. Aspirate a joint for crystals
   v. Seropositive RA and CPPD can coexist
   vi. Hemochromatosis with arthralgia
      1. One third of patients may be CPPD associated
r. Pseudo-OA pattern of CPPD crystal deposition disease
   i. One half of CPPD patients will have progressive degeneration of numerous joints
   ii. Knees are the most commonly affected
      1. Valgus knee deformities
         a. Pseudo-OA more likely to affect the lateral compartment
         b. Primary OA affects the medial compartment (varus deformities)
      2. Isolated patellofemoral OA
         a. Also a common presentation
   iii. Joints less commonly affected
      1. Wrists
      2. MCPs
      3. Hips
      4. Shoulders
      5. Elbows
      6. Ankles
   iv. Joints not involved (as in primary OA)
      1. DIP
      2. PIP

      3. 1st CMC
- v. Symmetric involvement is the rule
  - 1. Degeneration may be more advanced on one side
- vi. Flexion contractures of the involved joints are common
  - 1. Characteristic of CPPD pseudo-OA
- vii. Recurrent episodes of acute pseudogout
  - 1. Up to 50% of pseudo-OA patients
- viii. Radiographs
  - 1. Chondrocalcinosis
  - 2. Exuberant osteophyte formation
- s. Pseudo-neuropathic pattern of CPPD crystal deposition disease
  - i. Crowned dens syndrome
    - 1. Acute neck pain ascribed to CPPD
    - 2. Tomographic appearance of calcification surrounding the odontoid process
    - 3. May mimic meningitis
      - a. Neck pain with stiffness and fever
    - 4. After parathyroidectomy
      - a. Occurs in the postoperative period
  - ii. Cervical or lumbar spine
    - 1. Long tract signs and symptoms
    - 2. Deposits of CPPD and adjacent tissue hypertrophy
    - 3. Anatomical sites (lead to cord encroachment)
      - a. Ligamentum flavum
        - i. Most reported site in the cervical spine
      - b. Chondroid metaplastic growths
      - c. Facet joint osteophytes
      - d. Bulging disc
  - iii. Pseudo-Charcot joint
    - 1. True neuropathic joint
      - a. Pain is less than expected by severity of X-ray and clinical findings
      - b. Abnormal vibration and proprioception
      - c. Not a candidate for total joint arthroplasty (TJA)
    - 2. In pseudo-Charcot
      - a. Normal pain perception
      - b. A candidate for TJA
    - 3. Tabes dorsalis with CPPD
      - a. Develop true neuropathic joints
- t. Radiologic Features
  - i. Punctate and linear densities in articular hyaline or fibrocartilaginous tissues
    - 1. Typical appearance
  - ii. Typical sites
    - 1. Articular cartilage of the knee and hip

       2. Lateral and medial meniscus
       3. Acetabular labrum
       4. Fibrocartilaginous symphysis pubis
       5. Articular disc of the wrist
       6. Anulus fibrosus of intervertebral discs
   iii. Earliest deposits occur in normal cartilage
   iv. Radiographic screens for CPPD
       1. AP of both knees
          a. Preferably **NOT** standing
       2. AP of the pelvis
          a. Visualization of the symphysis pubis and hips
       3. PA of each hand with wrist
       4. If these views are negative
          a. Further study usually not needed
    v. Hemochromatosis associated radiographic changes
       1. Frequently seen together with CPPD
       2. MCP joint squaring of the metacarpal end
       3. Subchondral cysts
       4. Hook-like osteophytes
 u. Diagnostic Criteria for CPPD crystal deposition disease
    i. Demonstration of CPPD crystals in tissue

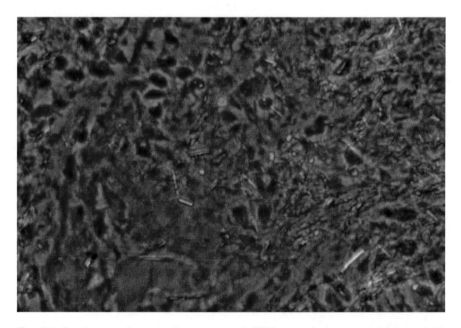

Fig. 8.3 Coexistence of monosodium urate and CPPD crystals in a synovial joint fluid. (Reproduced with permission from Systematic approach to arthropathies. *Diagnostic Imaging of Musculoskeletal Diseases.* DOI: 10.1007/978-1-59745-355-4_11. Springer; 2009-01-01)

        1. Monoclinic or triclinic crystals
          a. Weakly positive or no birefringence
        2. Typical radiographic calcifications
    ii. Acute arthritis
        1. Knees or large joint
   iii. Chronic arthritis (especially if accompanied by acute exacerbations)
        1. Knee
        2. Hip
        3. Wrist
        4. Carpus
        5. Elbow
        6. Shoulder
        7. MCP
   iv. Features that help differentiate chronic arthritis from OA
        1. Uncommon sites
        2. Radiographic joint space narrowing
          a. Radiocarpal
          b. Patellofemoral
            i. Patella wrapped around femur
        3. Subchondral cyst
        4. Severity of degeneration
          a. Progressive
          b. Collapse and fragmentation
          c. Loose bodies
        5. Osteophytes that are variable and inconstant

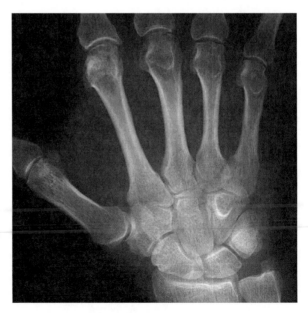

Fig. 8.4 Arthritis of hemochromatosis involving the second through the fourth MCP joints. Note the large hook-like osteophyte from the radial aspect of the second metacarpal head (Reproduced with permission from Arthropathies. *Essentials in Bone and Soft-Tissue Pathology.* DOI: 10.1007/978-0-387-89845-2_3. Springer; 2010-01-01)

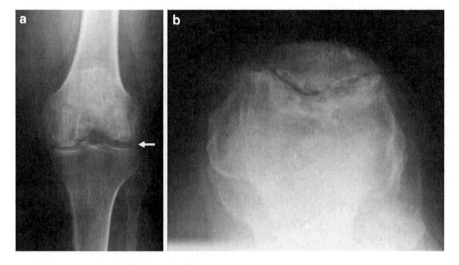

Fig. 8.5 AP (a) and skyline (b) radiographs of the knee of a patient with CPPD arthritis. The arthropathy is similar to osteoarthritis, but the patellofemoral joint is disproportionately affected. Note the chondrocalcinosis in the lateral joint space outlining the lateral meniscus (arrow, a)

      6. Tendon calcifications
        a. Triceps
        b. Achilles
        c. Obturators
  v. Treatment
     i. No practical way to remove CPPD crystals from the joint or prevent their deposition
       1. Phosphocitrate may inhibit crystal formation and cellular responses
       2. Unknown whether removal impacts degenerative changes
    ii. Treat the underlying associated disease
       1. Does not result in resorption of crystal deposits
   iii. Acute attacks in a large joint
       1. Aspiration alone
         a. Can halt an attack with crystal removal
       2. Aspiration plus injection
         a. Microcrystalline corticosteroid esters
    iv. Local injections
       1. Little risk for systemic effects
         a. Especially beneficial in the elderly
       2. Long acting corticosteroid (triamcinolone hexacetonide)
         a. 20–40 mg for large joints
         b. 10–20 mg for smaller joints
    v. Colchicine
       1. IV
         a. Effective in pseudogout

     2. Oral
       a. Less predictive
       b. Reduces number and duration of acute attacks
       c. Generally not favored
         i. Potential toxicity in the elderly
   vi. NSAIDs
     1. Recommended for most patients
     2. Indomethacin 50 mg tid or qid
       a. Classic for acute crystalline arthritis
     3. Others in full doses are as effective
     4. Check a creatinine before starting
   vii. Corticotropin or corticosteroids
     1. ACTH
       a. Intramuscular (IM) or IV at 40 U
       b. Relieves symptoms within 5 days
       c. Less effective if attack well established
     2. Triamcinolone acetonide
       a. IM 60 mg one to two times
       b. As effective as indomethacin
     3. Oral prednisone
       a. Consider if intra-articular or IM injection not desirable
         i. Patient with a bleeding diathesis
       b. Start 40 mg daily
       c. Taper to D/C in 10–14 days
  viii. Rest the affected joint
     1. Gradually resume activities as the attack subsides
   ix. Management of polyarticular attacks
     1. NSAIDs
     2. Systemic steroid regimens
     3. Colchicine
   x. Prophylaxis against pseudogout not required
     1. Most have few attacks widely separated in time
   xi. Frequent attacks
     1. Colchicine 0.6 mg BID
     2. Prevents recurrences
2. Basic Calcium Phosphates (BCP)
  a. BCP deposition
    i. Articular tissues
    ii. Skin
    iii. Arteries
    iv. Other tissues
  b. BCP types
    i. Carbonate-substituted hydroxyapatite
      1. $Ca_5(PO_4)3\text{-}2H_2O$

    ii. Octacalcium phosphate

    iii. Tricalcium phosphate

  c. Three groups of joint related problems

    i. Calcific tendonitis

    ii. Acute calcific periarthritis

    iii. BCP arthropathy

      1. Milwaukee shoulder syndrome

  d. Pathogenetic mechanisms

    i. Crystal directly cause arthritis

    ii. Crystals may accelerate or exacerbate preexisting arthritis

    iii. Crystals may exist as an epiphenomenon without a role

  e. Etiology and pathogenesis of BCP related conditions

    i. Calcification promoters

      1. Crystal nucleators

      2. Loss of inhibitors

    ii. Metastatic calcifications

      1. Occur in soft tissue

      2. High calcium x phosphate product (>70)

        a. Renal failure with high levels of phosphate

    iii. Dystrophic calcifications

      1. Occur in altered tissues

        a. Tissue damage

        b. Hypovascularity

        c. Tissue hypoxia

      2. Age-related changes

    iv. Genetic predispositions favoring calcification

    v. Calcinosis syndromes (soft tissue deposition)

      1. Systemic sclerosis

      2. Dermatomyositis

      3. Tumoral calcinosis

      4. SLE

    vi. Calcifications following severe neurological injury

    vii. Calcifications following triamcinolone hexactonide injection of joints

  f. Calcific tendonitis/periarthritis

    i. Chondrocytes or metaplastic synoviocytes produce calcifying matrix vesicles

      1. Similar to enchondral ossification

    ii. Acute calcific periarthritis

      1. BCP crystals cause pain and swelling

    iii. Calcific tendonitis

      1. Crystals may cause tendonitis

      2. BCP deposition in reaction to chronic strain in a poorly vascularized area

        a. Dystrophic calcification

g. The inflammatory response with BCP crystal
  i. Unusual
      1. Even with PMN engulfment of crystal
  ii. Synovial fluid
      1. Usually not inflammatory
      2. Leukocyte count low
          a. Predominantly mononuclear cells
  iii. Low grade inflammation
      1. Effusions
      2. Synovial lining cell hypertrophy
      3. Prostaglandin and protease release
      4. Chronic damage
h. BCP crystal identification
  i. X-ray
      1. Characteristic calcifications
  ii. Aspiration
      1. Yields material that looks like toothpaste
  iii. Light microscopy
      1. Crystals are so small they cannot be seen
          a. Length 50–500 nm
      2. Aggregates appear as refractile "shiny coins"
          a. Up to 5 mm in diameter
  iv. Polarized light microscopy
      1. Crystals are not birefringent
  v. Special stains
      1. Alizarin red will confirm calcium
          a. Not specific for BCP
  vi. Techniques for precise crystal identification
      1. Transmission electron microscopy
      2. Electron microprobe
      3. Fourier transform infrared spectroscopy
      4. Raman spectroscopy
      5. Atomic force microscopy
      6. Binding assay
          a. Utilizes carbon 14
              i. [^{14}C]ethane-1-hyroxy-1,1-diphosphonate
i. Clinical Features
  i. Shoulder joint destructive arthritis
      1. Milwaukee shoulder/cuff tear arthropathy
      2. Severe degenerative arthritis of the glenohumeral joint
      3. Loss of the rotator cuff
      4. Associated with the presence of BCP crystals
      5. Typically elderly women in their 70s
      6. Large, cool synovial effusions

7. Bilateral involvement is common
    a. The dominant side more severely affected
8. Severe radiographic changes
    a. Severe OA of the glenohumeral joint
    b. Periarticular soft tissue calcifications
    c. Upward subluxation of the humeral head
        i. With deformity
9. Large rotator cuff tears
10. Variable pain
    a. Frequent night pain
11. Limited ROM
12. Synovial fluid
    a. Often with streaks of blood
    b. Noninflammatory
        i. Low leukocyte counts
    c. Most contain BCP crystals
    d. Some contain CPPD crystals
13. Treatment
    a. Daily low dose NSAIDs
    b. Local heat
        i. Frequently beneficial
    c. Repeated arthrocenteses
        i. For large effusions
    d. Physical therapy
        i. Maintain ROM
        ii. Strengthen surrounding muscles
    e. Surgery
        i. For advanced DJD

ii. BCP arthropathy of other joints
    1. Knees
        a. Lateral compartment joint space loss
            i. Similar to CPPD
            ii. Distinguished from primary OA
    2. Finger (Philadelphia finger)
        a. Rapidly destructive arthritis

iii. Calcific Tendonitis
    1. Tendons affected
        a. Shoulder
            i. BCP deposition is common
            ii. Up to 5% of X-rays of adults have calcium deposits
            iii. Usually in the supraspinatus tendon
        b. Hand
        c. Wrist
        d. Hip
        e. Knee

   f. Foot

   g. Neck

    i. Longissimus colli insertion on anterior tubercle of the atlas

  2. Frequently found as incidental findings

   a. Shoulder X-rays for symptoms of bursitis or impingement

  3. Calcifications may be a result of chronic tendonitis rather than the cause

  4. Treatment

   a. NSAIDs

   b. PT

   c. Local injection of short acting corticosteroids

    i. Use sparingly

    ii. Steroids may promote calcifications

   d. Needle disruption of calcifications

    i. More rapid dissolution of the deposit

    ii. Stimulates phagocytosis of the BCP

   e. Surgical or arthroscopic debridement

    i. For very large or severely symptomatic calcific deposits

   f. Pulsed ultrasound

    i. May dissolve BCP crystals

iv. Calcific Periarthritis

  1. The most common site of calcification is the rotator cuff

  2. Symptoms

   a. Most are asymptomatic

   b. May subside over several weeks

    i. Spontaneous

    ii. With treatment

   c. Chronic shoulder pain

    i. Tendons of the rotator cuff

     1. Supraspinatus frequently

   d. Severe attacks

    i. Large deposits

    ii. Precipitated by crystal dispersal

     1. Surrounding tissues

     2. Subdeltoid bursa

     3. Shoulder joint

    iii. Intense local inflammatory reaction

     1. Swelling

     2. Warmth

     3. Erythema

    iv. Diagnosis

     1. X-rays

     2. Other imaging

     3. Needle aspiration

      a. Yields chalky material

      b. May shorten the course of the attack

     v. Differential diagnosis
        1. Sepsis
        2. Trauma
        3. Fracture
        4. Gout
        5. Pseudogout
  3. Treatment
    a. NSAIDS
      i. Given in full doses
      ii. The mainstay of therapy
    b. Colchicine,
      i. Either oral or IV
      ii. Successful for acute calcific periarthritis
    c. Aspiration with injection of corticosteroid
      i. Triamcinolone hexactonide for intra-articular injections
      ii. Betamethasone for soft tissue injections
v. Hydroxyapatite pseudopodagra
  1. Involves small joints
    a. 1st MTP
  2. Symptoms
    a. Identical to gout
  3. Diagnosis
    a. Younger **premenopausal** women
    b. Synovial fluid
      i. Absence of monosodium urate crystals
    c. X-ray
      i. Characteristic calcifications around the joint
vi. BCP crystals and osteoarthritis
  1. Present in 30–60% of OA joints
  2. May arise from exposed bone or metaplastic synovial tissue
  3. Observed in hyaline articular cartilage
    a. Not to the extent of CPPD
  4. OA severity correlates with the presence and amount of BCP crystal
  5. Whether BCP crystal contributes to the pathogenesis of OA is undetermined
  6. Subgroup of inflammatory OA
    a. DIP and PIP joints
    b. Erythema
    c. Synovial thickening
    d. Severe radiographic erosive damage

Gout

9

Section A: Epidemiology, Pathology and Pathogenesis

1. Gout
   a. A heterogeneous group of diseases
   b. Monosodium urate (MSU) crystals deposit in tissues
   c. Uric acid supersaturates in extracellular fluids
2. Clinical manifestations
   a. Gouty arthritis
      i. Recurrent attacks of inflammation
         1. Articular
         2. Periarticular
   b. Tophi
      i. Accumulation of crystalline deposits
         1. Articular
         2. Osseous
         3. Soft tissue
         4. Cartilaginous
   c. Uric acid nephrolithiasis
      i. Uric acid calculi in the urinary tract
   d. Gouty nephropathy
      i. Interstitial nephropathy
      ii. Renal function impairment
3. Hyperuricemia
   a. The metabolic disorder underlying gout
   b. Defined as urate concentration more than 2 standard deviations (SD) above the mean
      i. Greater than 7.0 mg/dl for men
      ii. Greater than 6.0 mg/dl for women
   c. Serum uric acid concentrations
      i. Both age and sex dependent
      ii. Associated with the onset of puberty in males and menopause in females

4. Age distribution
   a. Gout is rare in males <30 and in premenopausal females
   b. Peak age of onset
      i. Males 40–50 years old
      ii. Females after 60
5. Asymptomatic hyperuricemia in the absence of gout
   a. Not a disease
   b. Present in at least 5% of people
   c. Fewer than 1 in 4 will develop urate crystal deposits
6. Epidemiology
   a. Gout is predominantly a disease of adult men
      i. Peak incidence in the fifth decade
   b. Rarely occurs in men before adolescence or in women before menopause
   c. Prevalence
      i. 5–28 per 1,000 for males and 1–6 per 1,000 for females
      ii. Increases with age and increasing serum urate concentrations
      iii. Increasing in elderly women
         1. Increased longevity
         2. Use of thiazide diuretics
         3. Chronic renal insufficiency
      iv. Higher among AA men than Caucasian men
         1. Reflects the prevalence of hypertension
   d. Male to female ratio 2–7:1
   e. 15% of all patients with hyperuricemia develop gout
      i. Risk increases to 30–50% if serum uric acid concentration is >10 mg/dl
   f. Gout is the most common cause of inflammatory arthritis in men over 40
   g. Serum urate concentrations in males
      i. Childhood mean values of 3.5 mg/dl rise in puberty
      ii. Reach adult levels of 4.0 mg/dl
   h. Serum urate concentrations in women
      i. Remain constant until menopause
      ii. Estrogen promotes renal excretion of uric acid
      iii. Begin to rise post-menopausal
   i. Severe hyperuricemia
      i. 13 mg/dl men and 10 mg/dl women
      ii. Tolerated with little apparent jeopardy to renal function
7. Pathogenesis of Hyperuricemia
   a. Uric acid is the end product of purine degradation
   b. Uricase
      i. Oxidizes uric acid to the highly soluble compound allantoin
      ii. Humans lack the enzyme
         1. Subjects humans to the risk of tissue deposition
      iii. Humans possess the uricase gene
         1. Inactive gene but a hyperuricemic propensity
            a. Uric acid has powerful antioxidant and free radical scavenger properties

        2. Uricase gene KO mouse

          a. Develops severe uric acid nephrolithiasis

          b. Renal dysfunction during the first month of life

   c. Environmental factors that modify urate concentrations

      i. Body weight

      ii. Diet

      iii. Lifestyle

      iv. Social class

      v. Hemoglobin level

   d. Genetics

      i. The tendency toward hyperuricemia is inherited

        1. Manifested when a diet high in purine content is ingested

        2. Seen in Filipinos living in the US versus those living in the Philippines

      ii. Familial occurrence in about 20% of affected patients

      iii. One-fourth of first degree relatives of people with gout had hyperuricemia

8. Purine Metabolism and Biochemistry

   a. Uric acid is derived from

      i. The ingestion of foods containing purines

      ii. The endogenous synthesis of purine nucleotides

   b. Purine synthesis de novo

      i. A purine ring is synthesized from small molecule precursors

      ii. Precursors are added sequentially to a ribose-phosphate backbone donated by PRPP (5-phosphoribosyl-1-pyrophosphate)

      iii. The first reaction in the pathway is catalyzed by amidophosphoribosyltransferase

        1. A main site of pathway regulation

        2. Antagonistic interaction

          a. Inhibition by purine nucleotide products

          b. Activation by PRPP

      iv. Other sites of purine nucleotide production control

        1. At the level of PRPP synthesis

        2. At the distal branch point

          a. Distribution of newly formed nucleotides into adenylate and guanylate derivatives

   c. Other purine nucleotide synthesis pathways

      i. Through the activities of adenine phosphoribosyltransferase and hypoxanthine-guanine phosphoribosyltransferase (HGRPT)

      ii. Occurs in a single step

      iii. Catalyzes the reaction between PRPP and the respective purine base substrate

      iv. Governing factors

        1. The availability of PRPP

        2. Concentrations of the nucleotide products

   d. Catabolic steps that generate uric acid from nucleic acids and free purine nucleotides
      i. Degradation to hypoxanthine and xanthine through purine nucleoside intermediates
      ii. Intermediates oxidized to uric acid in sequential reactions
         1. Catalyzed by the enzyme xanthine oxidase
   e. Urate circulates in unbound form
      i. Miscible pool averages 1200 mg in men and 600 in women
      ii. Synthesis averages about 750 mg/day in men
         1. Two-thirds of the pool is turned over daily
   f. Major route of uric acid disposal
      i. Renal excretion accounts for about two-thirds of urate loss
      ii. Purine free diet
         1. About 425 mg/day excreted in the urine
      iii. Increased filtered urate load
         1. Normally excreted
   g. Minor route of uric acid disposal
      i. Bacterial oxidation of urate secreted into the gut
      ii. Limited ability to compensate for changes in urate-pool size and serum urate values >14.0 mg/dl
9. Causes and Classifications of Hyperuricemia
   a. Causes of hyperuricemia
      i. Increased uric acid production
      ii. Diminished uric acid excretion by the kidney
   b. Pathogenic processes of inherent disordered uric acid metabolism
      i. Overproduction of urate
         1. Endogenous purine precursors
         2. Exogenous (dietary) purine precursors
      ii. Underexcretion of urate
         1. Abnormal renal handling
         2. 90% with hyperuricemia and gout
      iii. A combination of both
   c. Urate overproduction
      i. A urate value >800 mg/24 h (on a regular purine diet)
         1. Suggests overproduction of uric acid
         2. 10% of individuals with hyperuricemia by isotopic labeling
      ii. Occurs in a variety of acquired disorders characterized by excessive rates of cell and nucleic-acid turnover
         1. Myeloproliferative and lymphoproliferative diseases
         2. Hemolytic anemias
         3. Anemias associated with ineffective erythpoiesis
         4. Paget's
         5. Psoriasis
         6. Excessive dietary purine consumption
         7. Alcohol abuse
            a. Accelerated ATP degradation

  iii. Inherited derangements of purine nucleotide synthesis
    1. Two enzyme abnormalities
      a. Superactivity of PRPP synthetase
      b. Partial deficiency of HGPRT
        i. Kelley-Seegmiller syndrome
    2. Partial deficiency of HGPRT and mild superactivity of PRPP synthetase
      a. Early adult onset gout (<30)
      b. High incidence of uric acid urinary tract stones
    3. Severe HGPRT deficiency
      a. Spasticity
      b. Choreoathetosis
      c. Mental retardation
      d. Compulsive self-mutilation
        i. Lesch-Nyhan syndrome
    4. Regulatory defects in PRPP synthetase
      a. Sensorineural deafness
      b. Neurodevelopmental defects
    5. Intracellular accumulation of PRPP in HGPRT deficiency
      a. Drives purine synthesis at an increased rate
    6. Variant forms of PRPP synthetase with excessive activity
      a. Increases uric acid synthesis by increasing PRPP availability
    7. Aberrations of each of these enzymes result in increased uric acid synthesis
      a. Increase PRPP availability
      b. Alter the balance of control of purine synthesis toward increased production
    8. Both enzymes produced from X-linked genes
      a. Homozygous males are affected
      b. Carrier females
        i. Postmenopausal gout and urinary stones
      c. Hyperuricemia in prepubertal boys
        i. Always suggest one of these enzymatic defects
  d. Uric acid underexcretion
    i. A urate value <800 mg/24 h (on a regular purine diet)
    1. Suggest underexcretion
    ii. More than 90% of primary hyperuricemia have a relative deficit in the renal excretion of uric acid
    iii. Drugs that cause hyperuricemia due to decreased renal excretion of urate (**CAN'T LEAP**)
    1. Cyclosporine
    2. Alcohol
      a. Associated with lactic acid production
        i. Reduces renal excretion of urate
      b. Increases synthesis of urate by accelerating the degradation of ATP
      c. Beer contains a lot of purine guanosine

  3. Nicotinic acid
  4. Thiazides
     a. Interferes with urate excretion at the proximal convoluted tubule
  5. Lasix
  6. Ethambutol
  7. Aspirin
     a. Low dose <2 g/day
  8. Pyrazinamide
iv. Other drugs that cause hyperuricemia by unknown mechanisms
  1. Levodopa
  2. Theophylline
  3. Didanosine (ddI)
v. Drugs that have a **hypo**uricemic effect
  1. Angiotensin receptor blockers (ARBs)
vi. 95% of filtered urate undergoes proximal tubular (presecretory) reabsorption
  1. 50% of the filtered urate load undergoes proximal tubular secretion
  2. Contributes the major share of excreted uric acid
vii. 40% of the filtered urate load undergoes postsecretory tubular reabsorption
viii. Hyperuricemia at the renal level
  1. Diminished tubular secretory rate
  2. Diminished uric acid filtration
ix. Renal urate excretion can be influenced by heredity
  1. Kindred with early onset gout and reduced fractional excretion
  2. A renal urate transporter gene identified
x. Chronic lead intoxication manifest with gouty arthritis
  1. Lead tainted moonshine results in chronic renal tubular damage
  2. Secondary hyperuricemia (saturnine gout)
xi. Decreased excretion of uric acid occurs in conditions where organic acids accumulate and compete with urate tubular secretion
  1. Diabetic ketoacidosis
  2. Starvation
  3. Ketosis
  4. Ethanol intoxication
  5. Lactic acidosis
xii. Diseases that predispose to renal insufficiency seen with gout
  1. Hypertension
     a. Increases tubular urate reabsorption
  2. Diabetes mellitus
     a. Insulin stimulates the renal tubular sodium hydrogen exchanger
        i. Promotes urate reabsorption
     b. Syndrome X
        i. NIDDM with elevated insulin levels
        ii. Abdominal obesity

          iii. Hypertension

          iv. Low LDL

           v. Hypertriglyceridemia

             1. Increases acetate

          vi. Increased risk for atherosclerosis

         vii. People with primary gout may have Syndrome X

      xiii. Miscellaneous causes of urate underexcretion

           1. Hyperparathyroidism

           2. Hypothyroidism

           3. Respiratory acidosis

   e. Combined overproduction and underexcretion

       i. Alcohol consumption

           1. High purine content in some alcoholic beverages

             a. Beer contains large quantities of guanosine

           2. Accelerated hepatic breakdown of ATP

           3. Hyperlactic acidemia

             a. Blocks uric acid secretion

      ii. Two inborn errors of metabolism produce hyperuricemia

           1. Glucose-6-phophatase deficiency (von Gierke's glycogen storage disease)

             a. Accelerated breakdown of ATP during hypoglycemia-induced glycogen degradation

             b. Resultant lactic acidosis

               i. Inhibition of renal tubular urate secretion as a result of competitive anions

           2. Fructose-1-phosphate aldolase deficiency

             a. Develop hyperuricemia in part because of accelerated ATP catabolism

             b. Resultant lactic acidosis

10. Pathogenesis of Tissue Manifestations

   a. Urate crystallizes as a monosodium salt in oversaturated joint tissues

   b. Only a minority with sustained hyperuricemia develop tophi and gouty arthropathy

   c. Deposition with decreased solubility of sodium urate at lower temperatures

       i. Peripheral acral structures

           1. Toes

           2. Ears

   d. Connective tissue structure plays a role in deposition

       i. The paretic side in hemiplegia is spared of tophi and acute gout

      ii. Urate tophi found in synovial membranes and in cartilage

   e. Declines in serum urate levels as effected by antihyperuricemic drugs

       i. Promote the release of urate crystals from tophi by decreasing the size of crystals

   f. Crystals may be found in joints that never had an attack

11. Histopathology of the Tophi

   a. A foreign-body granuloma surrounds a core of MSU crystal

b. An inflammatory reaction consisting mostly of mononuclear cells and giant cells surrounds the crystals

c. Erosion of cartilage and bone occur at sites of tophi

d. Needle shaped crystals are arranged radially in small clusters

e. DeGalantha stains urate black

f. Crystals identified by compensated polarized light microscopy

g. Other components of the tophi include

   i. Lipids

   ii. GAGs

   iii. Plasma proteins

12. Pathogenesis of Gouty Inflammation

a. Triggered by the precipitation of monosodium urate crystals

b. Inflammatory response determined by proteins that coat the crystal

   i. Crystals coated with IgG react with Fc receptors on corresponding cells and promote an inflammatory response

   ii. Crystal coated with apolipoprotein B inhibit phagocytosis and a cellular response

c. Crystals stimulate the production of chemotactic factors

   i. Cytokines

      1. IL-1, 6, and 8

      2. TNF

   ii. Prostaglandins

   iii. Leukotrienes

   iv. Oxygen radicals

d. Crystals activate complement and induce lysosomal enzyme release

e. Crystals generate soluble mediators via proteolysis of serum proteins

   i. C5a

   ii. Bradykinin

   iii. Kallikrein

f. Nonspecific activation of certain signal transduction pathways

   i. Membrane G protein

   ii. Cytosolic calcium mobilization

   iii. Various protein kinases

      1. Src-family tyrosine kinases

      2. Mitogen activated protein kinases

         a. ERK1/ERK2

         b. JNK

         c. p38

g. Neutrophil influx into the joint

   i. Promoted by endothelial-neutrophil adhesion

   ii. Triggered by IL-1 and TNF-α

   iii. Major mediators promoting ingress and activation

      1. IL-8

      2. Closely related chemokines that bind the IL-8 receptor

         a. CXCR2

        3. PAF

        4. C5a

        5. Leukotriene B4

    iv. Neutrophil-endothelial interaction

        1. The major therapeutic focus for colchicine

h. Systemic manifestations

    i. Fever

    ii. Leukocytosis

    iii. Hepatic acute phase protein response

    iv. Occurs with the release of

        1. IL-1

        2. TNF-α

        a. Accelerated neutrophil apoptosis

        3. IL-6

        4. IL-8

i. Attack self limited by

    i. Intraarticular neutrophil apoptosis

    ii. Cessation of neutrophil influx into the joint

    iii. Response modulated by different proteins coating the crystal

    iv. Phagocytosis and degradation of crystals by neutrophils

        1. Decrease crystal concentration

    v. Heat associated with inflammation

        1. Increases crystal solubility

    vi. Enhanced ACTH secretion

        1. Suppresses the inflammatory response

    vii. Resolution with a shift in balance between

        1. Proinflammatory factors

        a. Il-1 and TNF

        2. Anti-inflammatory factors

        a. Generation of lipoxins

        b. Release of IL1-RA and TGF-β

Section B: Clinical and Laboratory Features

1. Stages of Classic Gout

  a. Asymptomatic hyperuricemia

    i. Elevated serum uric acid level without

        1. Gouty arthritis

        2. Tophi

        3. Uric acid nephrolithiasis

    ii. 98% of uric acid at pH 7.4 is in the form of MSU

        1. Hyperuricemia occurs when the soluble concentration of MSU is exceeded

        2. Any level above 6.8 mg/dl

iii. Urate levels between 7.0 and 8.0 mg/dl
   1. 3% of subjects had cumulative incidence of gouty arthritis
iv. Urate levels of 9.0 mg/dl or more
   1. 22% of subjects had a 5 year cumulative incidence of gouty arthritis
b. Acute intermittent gout
  i. Initial episode usually follows decades of asymptomatic hyperuricemia
  ii. Acute gouty attack
    1. Rapid development of
      a. Warmth
      b. Swelling
      c. Erythema
      d. Pain
    2. Begins abruptly
      a. Often during the night or early morning
    3. Pain escalates over an 8–12 h period
    4. Monoarticular (85%)
    5. Involves the 1st MTP
      a. Half of patients
      b. "Podagra"
      c. Eventually affected in 90% with gout
    6. Other joints frequently involved in descending order
      a. Midfoot instep
      b. Ankles
      c. Heels
      d. Knees
      e. Wrists
      f. Fingers
      g. Elbows

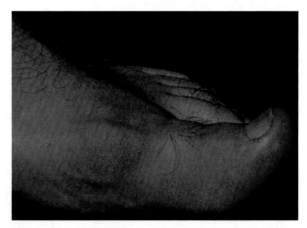

Fig. 9.1 Inflamed first metatarsophalangeal joint in a patient with gout (Reproduced with permission from Systematic approach to arthropathies. *Diagnostic Imaging of Musculoskeletal Diseases.* DOI: 10.1007/978-1-59745-355-4_11. Springer; 2009-01-01)

      7. Nonarticular sites
        a. Olecranon bursa
        b. Prepatellar bursa
        c. Achilles tendon
      8. Pain classically very severe
      9. Systemic symptoms
        a. Fever
        b. Chills
        c. Malaise
     10. Cutaneous erythema may be mistaken for cellulitis
       a. "Gouty cellulitis"
     11. Often spontaneously resolves over 3–10 days
     12. Skin desquamation overlying the affected joint
       a. With resolution of inflammation
  iii. The natural course of untreated acute gout varies
      1. Mild
        a. Resolving in several hours
      2. Severe
        a. Lasting 1–2 weeks
  iv. Early in the acute intermittent stage
      1. Infrequent episodes of acute arthritis
      2. Intervals between attacks sometimes last for years
   v. Attacks over time
      1. More frequent
      2. Longer in duration
      3. Involve more joints
  vi. Attacks precipitated by any rapid increase or reduction in serum urate level
      1. Allopurinol most responsible
      2. Microtophi destabilize and shed into the synovial fluid
c. Intercritical gout
   i. Asymptomatic intervals between acute attacks of gout
  ii. MSU crystals still identified in synovial fluid
  iii. Fluid containing crystals have higher mean cell counts
  iv. Reflects ongoing subclinical inflammation
d. Chronic tophaceous gout
   i. Develops after 10 or more years of acute intermittent gout
  ii. Intercritical period transition
      1. No longer free of pain
      2. Involved joint persistently swollen and uncomfortable
      3. Attacks continue to occur without therapy
        a. Often as every few weeks
  iii. Polyarticular involvement
      1. More common
      2. Sometimes symmetric
      3. Confused with RA

iv. Factors associated with deposition of tophaceous MSU
1. Function of the duration and severity of hyperuricemia
2. May or may not be detected on PE during the first years
3. Early age of gouty onset
4. Long periods of active but untreated gout
5. An average of four attacks per year
6. Tendency toward upper extremity involvement
7. Polyarticular episodes
v. Gouty tophi in subcutaneous sites
1. Digits of the hands and feet
2. Wrists
3. Ears (antihelix)
4. Knees
5. Olecranon bursa
6. Pressure points as the ulnar aspect of the forearm
7. Achilles tendon
8. Synovium
9. Subchondral bone
vi. Other sites of tophi occurrence
1. Heberden's nodes
2. Renal pyramids
3. Heart valves
4. Sclerae
vii. Development of the mature multilobulated gouty tophus
1. Crystal free macrophage acinus
a. A core of noncrystalline, amorphous material
b. Surrounded by a rosette of mononuclear phagocytes
c. Earliest organized phase
2. Radially arranged MSU crystals
a. Form in the amorphous core
b. A small, eccentric collection

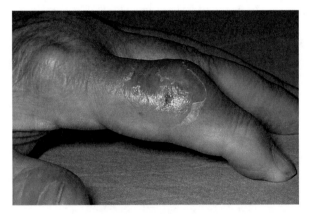

Fig. 9.2 Tophaceous gout
(Reproduced with permission
from Osteoarthritis and
crystal associated synovitis.
Atlas of Rheumatology.
ImagesMD; 2005-01-18)

        3. Corona
          a. A shell
          b. Cells proliferate to 8–10 cells thick
          c. Tightly packed
        4. Fibrous septae
          a. Replaces the corona as the tophus matures
        5. Multilobulated tophi
          a. Adjacent crystalline deposits coalesce
          b. Measures 1–10 cm in diameter
        6. Thick fibrous tissue encapsulates
     viii. Ulcerated tophi
        1. Extrude a white, chalky material
        2. Dense concentration of monosodium urate crystals

2. Early Onset Gout
  a. Symptom onset before age 25
     i. 3–6% of patients
     ii. A more accelerated clinical course
     iii. Requires more aggressive antihyperuricemic therapy
  b. A genetic component
     i. 80% incidence of family history
  c. Like classic gout caused by
     i. Overproduction of urate
     ii. Reduced renal clearance of uric acid
  d. Overproduction
     i. Enzymatic defects in purine pathway
        1. Complete deficiency of HGPRT
          a. X-linked inborn error of purine metabolism
            i. Lesch-Nyhan syndrome
          b. Treated with early allopurinol
        2. Partial deficiency of HGPRT
          a. X linked
            i. Kelley-Seegmiller syndrome
          b. Early onset gout or uric acid nephrolithiasis
          c. Minor or no neurologic problems
     ii. Glycogen storage diseases
        1. Type I, III, V, and VII
        2. Autosomal recessive
     iii. Hematologic disorders
        1. Hemoglobinopathies
        2. Leukemias
        3. Sickle cell
        4. B-thalassemia
        5. Non-lymphocytic leukemias

    e. Underexcretion
       i. Familial urate nephropathy
         1. Autosomal dominant
         2. Hyperuricemia at a young age
         a. Before evidence of renal insufficiency
         3. ESRD by age 40
       ii. Other nephropathies
         1. Polycystic kidney disease
         2. Chronic lead intoxication
         3. Medullary cystic disease
         4. Focal tubulointerstitial disease
3. Transplantation Gout
    a. Heart transplant recipients
       i. 75–80% on cyclosporine develop hyperuricemia
    b. Kidney and liver transplant recipients
       i. 50% on cyclosporine develops hyperuricemia
         1. Lower doses used
    c. Clinical stages in cyclosporin induced gout
       i. Asymptomatic hyperuricemia
         1. 1 of 6 progress to gout
         a. Compared with 1 of 30 in the general population
         2. Duration only 6 months to 4 years
         a. Compared with 20–30 years in classic gout
       ii. Acute intermittent stage
         1. Rapid appearance of tophi
         2. Duration only 1–4 years
         a. Compared with 8–15 years in classic gout
    d. Disease course
       i. Less dramatic in transplant patients
       ii. Use of other immunosuppressive drugs (steroids)
4. Gout in Women
    a. Approximately 5% of all patients with gout
    b. 90% are postmenopausal at the initial attack
    c. Polyarticular acute gouty attacks more common than men
    d. Tophi common in previously damaged joints
       i. Heberden's nodes
       ii. Finger pads
    e. Conditions associated with postmenopausal gout
       i. Diuretic use (95%)
       ii. Hypertension (73%)
      iii. Renal insufficiency (50%)
      iv. Pre-existing joint disease (OA)
       v. Strong hereditary component
    f. **Pre**menopausal gout and normal renal function evaluate for
       i. Autosomally inherited familial hyperuricemia nephropathy
       ii. Non-X linked inborn errors of purine metabolism

5. Normouricemic Gout
    a. Acute and chronic gout may have urate levels below 7.0 mg/dl
    b. Acute gout with normal serum urate
        i. Uricosuric effects of ACTH release and adrenal stimulation
            1. Caused by the stress of pain
        ii. Drugs that lower urate levels
            1. Allopurinol
            2. Probenecid
            3. Sulfinpyrazone
            4. High dose salicylates
            5. Corticosteroids
            6. Dicumarol
            7. Glycerol guaiacolate
            8. X-ray contrast agents
    c. Articular conditions that mimic gout
        i. CPPD
        ii. BCP
        iii. Liquid lipids
        iv. Infection
        v. Sarcoidosis
        vi. Trauma
6. Clinical Associations
    a. Renal Disease
        i. Hyperuricemia induced renal disease
            1. Chronic urate nephropathy
            2. Acute uric acid nephropathy
            3. Uric acid nephrolithiasis
        ii. Progressive renal failure
            1. 10% of deaths in gouty patients
            2. Associated with other comorbidities
                a. Hypertension
                b. Diabetes
                c. Obesity
                d. Ischemic heart disease
        iii. Chronic urate nephropathy
            1. A distinct entity
            2. Caused by deposition of MSU crystals in the renal medulla and interstitial tissue
            3. Mild and intermittent proteinuria
            4. Rarely causes renal dysfunction
                a. More often with associated hypertension
        iv. Acute uric acid nephropathy
            1. Acute tumor lysis syndrome
                a. Hyperuricemia with chemotherapy
                b. Especially lymphomas and leukemias

     2. Massive liberation of purines during cell lysis

     3. Acute renal failure with precipitation of uric acid crystals

        a. Distal tubules

        b. Collecting ducts

        c. Ureters

     4. Distinguished by uric acid to creatinine ratio

        a. Greater than 1.0 in a random 24 h collection

   v. Uric acid nephrolithiasis (renal stones)

     1. 10–25% of all gout

     2. Correlates

        a. Urate level

            i. 50% with a urate above 13 mg/dl

        b. Urine acidity

     3. 40% of patients have symptoms of stones before the development of gout

     4. Uric acid stones

        a. Radiolucent

        b. A nidus for **calcium** stone formation

            i. Increased incidence of calcium stones in patients with gout

           ii. Especially with hyperuricosuria

  vi. Other renal disease associated with hyperuricemia

     1. Polycystic kidney disease

        a. One third have gout

     2. Lead intoxication

     3. Familial urate nephropathy

  b. Hypertension

     i. Present in 25–50% of people with gout

     ii. 2–14% of people with hypertension have gout

     iii. Reduced blood flow may account for the association between hypertension and hyperuricemia

  c. Obesity

     i. Hyperuricemia and gout correlate highly with body weight

        1. Both men and women

     ii. Individuals with gout are commonly overweight

  d. Hyperlipidemia

     i. 80% of people with gout have elevated serum triglycerides

     ii. Decreased HDL in people with gout

7. Radiographic and Imaging Features

  a. Unremarkable early in the disease course

     i. The only finding may be soft tissue swelling around the joint in an acute attack

  b. Articular tophi

     i. Irregular soft tissue densities

        1. Occasionally calcified

     ii. Frequently asymmetric

       iii. Involved sites
          1. Feet
          2. Hands
          3. Wrists
          4. Elbows
          5. Knees
  c. Bony erosions of gout are radiographically distinct from the erosive changes of other inflammatory arthritides
     i. Gouty erosions are slightly removed from the joint
       1. RA erosions in the immediate proximity of the articular surface
     ii. Gouty erosions have both atrophic and hypertropic features
       1. Erosions with an "overhanging edge"
       2. Appear "punched out" with sclerotic margins
       3. Termed "rat bite erosions"
  d. Joint space preserved until very late in the disease
  e. Juxta-articular osteopenia absent or minimal
  f. Renal ultrasound
     i. Small and equally affected kidneys
     ii. Cortical area reduced in width

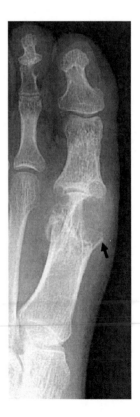

Fig. 9.3 PA radiograph of the foot showing para-articular erosions of the distal first metatarsal secondary to gout. Note the clasp shape appearance and overhanging edge (arrow) (Reproduced with permission from Systematic approach to arthropathies. *Diagnostic Imaging of Musculoskeletal Diseases.* DOI: 10.1007/978-1-59745-355-4_11. Springer; 2009-01-01)

        iii. Scars seen throughout the capsule

        iv. Primary locations for urate crystals

           1. Medullary interstitium

           2. Papillae

           3. Pyramids

8. Laboratory Features and Diagnosis

  a. Hyperuricemia

      i. Long considered a diagnostic cornerstone although

          1. The vast majority of hyperuricemic people will not develop gout

          2. Urate levels may be normal during gouty attacks

  b. Characteristic MSU crystals

      i. The definitive diagnosis of gout

      ii. Needle or rod shaped

      iii. Appear bright birefringent and yellow when parallel to the axis of slow vibration marked on the first order compensator

      iv. Crystals usually intracellular during acute attacks

  c. Synovial fluid

      i. Consistent with moderate to severe inflammation

      ii. Leukocyte count usually between 15,000 and 20,000

          1. Predominantly neutrophils

      iii. Bacterial infection can coexist with gouty crystals

  d. Laboratory evaluations

      i. CBC

      ii. SMA18

      iii. TSH

      iv. Lipid profile

      v. UA

      vi. 24 h urine

          1. Creatinine

          2. Uric acid

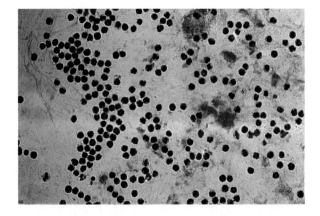

Fig. 9.4 Knee aspiration in gout

    e. Hematologic findings
       i. Elevated ESR
       ii. Mild neutrophil leukocytosis
       iii. Reactive thrombocytosis
    f. 24 h urine uric acid
       i. When considering uricosuric therapy
       ii. To investigate marked hyperuricemia (>11 mg/dl)
       iii. Avoid alcohol and contrast dyes before the study
    g. Urinary uric acid excretion of >800 mg in 24 h (on a regular diet) suggest a problem of urate overproduction
       i. In children and young adults
          1. Consider an enzymatic defect
       ii. Older patients
          1. Consider one of the diseases associated with rapid cellular turnover
             a. Myelo- or lymphoproliferative disorders

Section C: Treatment

1. Therapeutic goals
    a. Terminate acute attacks
    b. Provide rapid safe relief of pain and inflammation
       i. NSAIDs or colchicine
       ii. Corticosteroids
    c. Avert future attacks
    d. Prevent complications
       i. Tophi
       ii. Kidney stones
       iii. Destructive arthropathy
2. Tophaceous Gout
    a. Lower uric acid levels to permit urate resorption from tophi
    b. Requires long term treatment with allopurinol
       i. Keep levels at least 1.0 mg/dl below the supersaturation threshold of 7.0 mg/dl
    c. Probenecid may be added to allopurinol
       i. Helps the kidney excrete the uric acid load mobilized from resolving tophi
3. Acute Gout
    a. Eliminate pain and control symptoms
       i. NSAIDs
       ii. Colchicine
       iii. Systemic and intra-articular corticosteroids
    b. Urate-lowering drugs should not be instituted during an acute attack
       i. Patients already on allopurinol or a uricosuric drug should continue

c. NSAIDs
   i. The first choice in treating acute gout
   ii. Indomethacin is preferred
       1. Others may be as effective
   iii. Initiated at the maximum dosage at the first sign of an attack
       1. Dose is lowered as symptoms abate
   iv. Continue until pain and inflammation has been absent for at least 48 h
   v. Side effects are less common in treatment of acute gout
d. Colchicine
   i. An alkaloid derivative from the plant *Colchicum autumnale*
   ii. Used in the treatment of acute gout for nearly two centuries
       1. For joint pain since the sixth century
   iii. Treatment indications
       1. Acute gouty attacks
          a. Provides pain relief within 24 h in 90%
          b. Works best when instituted within minutes or hours of an attack
          c. Many will experience diarrhea with this regimen
       2. Prophylaxis against future attacks when hypouricemic therapy is initiated
   iv. Mechanism of Action
       1. **NO** effect on serum urate concentration or on urate metabolism
       2. Functions as an anti-inflammatory agent
       3. Inhibits microtubule polymerization
          a. Irreversible binding to tubulin dimers
          b. Prevents dimer assembly into protein subunits
       4. Disrupts neutrophil membrane dependent functions
          a. Chemotaxis
          b. Phagocytosis
       5. Inhibits phospholipase A2
          a. Leads to lower levels of inflammatory prostaglandins and leukotrienes
       6. Hinders crystal induced production of chemotactic factors and IL-6
       7. **NOT** bound to plasma proteins
          a. Highly lipid-soluble
          b. Readily passes into all tissues
   v. Pharmacology
       1. Half-life is 4 h following oral administration
          a. <1 h parenterally
       2. Concentrated intracellular
       3. Only 10% is excreted during the first 24 h
       4. Detected in granulocytes and urine for up to 10 days after a single dose
       5. Toxicity is a function of the cumulative dose
          a. Relative to renal function
       6. Hepatically metabolized

      7. Excreted principally in the bile
         a. 20% unchanged in urine
      8. Enters the enterohepatic circulation
         a. Toxic effects amplified in people with liver disease or extrahepatic biliary obstruction

vi. Dosing
      1. Oral
         a. 0.5- and 0.6-mg tablets
      2. Parenteral
         a. 0.5 mg/ml solution
      3. Administered in hourly doses of 0.5 or 0.6 mg
         a. Until symptoms are alleviated
      4. Small repeated doses minimize GI toxicity
         a. Occurs in up to 80% of patients
      5. Discontinue if GI symptoms lead to
         a. Hypovolemia
         b. Electrolyte disturbances
         c. Metabolic alkalosis
      6. Maximum cumulative dose
         a. 6.0 mg of oral colchicine
         b. Not to exceed 12 tablets
      7. Prophylaxis
         a. Average dose is 0.5 mg BID
         b. Minimal toxicity
         c. Can completely prevent attacks
         d. Lowers attack frequency in >90%

vii. IV colchicine
      1. Offers rapid onset of action
      2. Avoids GI toxicity
      3. Most hospitals have removed IV from their formularies
         a. Requires careful administration
         b. Narrow therapeutic window
         c. Serious adverse events
           i. Several deaths
           ii. Irreversible bone marrow suppression
         d. Alternative treatment options
           i. Corticosteroids
           ii. ACTH
      4. Dilute in 20 ml of 0.9% sodium chloride
         a. If not diluted properly thrombophlebitis can develop
      5. Administer over 20 min
      6. Skin sloughing at the site of an extravasation
      7. Single dose should not exceed 3 mg
      8. Cumulative dose should not exceed 4 mg in a 24 h period
      9. Additional colchicine should not be given for at least 7 days

10. Absolute contraindications
    a. Combined renal and hepatic disease
    b. Glomerular filtration rate (GFR) <10 ml/min
    c. Extrahepatic biliary obstruction
    d. Preexisting bone marrow suppression
    e. Sepsis
11. Relative contraindications
    a. Significant intercurrent infection
    b. Immediate prior use of colchicine within 7 days
    c. Hepatic or renal insufficiency
    d. Advanced age
12. Half the dose for patients with GFR < 50–60 ml/min
viii. Toxicity
    1. Gastrointestinal effects
       a. Usually following oral administration
       b. Nausea, vomiting, and diarrhea
       c. Malabsorption syndrome (rare)
       d. Hemorrhagic gastroenteritis (rare)
    2. Bone marrow suppression
       a. Thrombocytopenia
       b. Leukopenia
    3. Renal failure
    4. Shock and DIC
       a. Seen with parenteral use
    5. Hypocalcemia
    6. Cardiopulmonary failure
    7. Seizures
    8. Alopecia
    9. Neuromuscular syndrome
       a. Occurs almost exclusively in patients with chronic renal insuffi-
          ciency (serum creatinine >1.6 mg/dl) and prophylactic use
       b. Myopathy resembles polymyositis
          i. Proximal muscle weakness
          ii. Elevated CK
          iii. Abnormalities on EMG
          iv. Muscle biopsy characteristically reveals lysosomal vacuo-
              lated myopathy
          v. May resolve spontaneously within several weeks
       c. Peripheral neuropathy
          i. Takes longer to resolve
    10. CNS dysfunction
    11. Death
       a. Granulocytopenia is a major contributor to a fatal outcome

12. Most adverse effects are dose-related
    a. All reported cases of death, severe toxicity, or neuromuscular disease have involved
        i. Unusually high doses of colchicine
        ii. Renal insufficiency
        iii. Advanced age
        iv. The use of both oral and IV preparations
13. Overdose
    a. No antidotes
    b. Hemodialysis is ineffective
    c. Treat with colchicine specific Fab antibody fragments

e. Corticosteroids and ACTH
    i. For those in whom colchicine or NSAIDs are contraindicated or ineffective
    ii. Relapse or early recurrence has been reported
    iii. Prednisone
        1. 20–40 mg for 3–4 days
        2. Tapered over 3–4 days
    iv. ACTH
        1. IM injection of 40–80 IU every 6–12 h

f. Drug combinations
    i. Use if the attack is severe or therapy is delayed

g. Drugs that alter serum uric acid levels
    i. Allopurinol and probenecid
    ii. Never use in an acute attack
    iii. Do not stop if an acute attack occurs while the patient is on these medications

h. Joint drainage
    i. A non-toxic therapeutic option
        1. For recalcitrant gout
        2. For the elderly
    ii. Followed by an intra-articular injection
        1. Triamcinolone 10–40 mg
        2. Dexamethasone 2–10 mg
    iii. Culture first if suspected infection
    iv. Drain as much fluid as possible
    v. If on anticoagulants
        1. Use a small bore needle
            a. 22 gauge or smaller
        2. Apply direct pressure for 5 min

4. Prophylaxis
    a. Diet and lifestyle modifications
        i. Reduces the frequency of acute attacks
        ii. Decreases or negates the need for medication

      iii. Weight loss may reduce serum urate
      iv. Alcohol should be avoided
      v. In certain exercises or occupations
        1. Avoid dehydration and repetitive trauma
  b. Dietary specifics
      i. Purine content typically contributes only 1.0 mg/dl to the uric acid concentration
        1. Usually not used alone for disease prevention
      ii. Limit consumption of purine rich food
        1. Meats
          a. Particularly organ such as liver and kidney
        2. Seaford
        3. Shellfish
        4. Sardines
        5. Anchovies
        6. Vegetables and legumes
          a. Asparagus
          b. Cauliflower
          c. Spinach
          d. Beans
          e. Peas
          f. Mushrooms
  c. Eliminate medications known to contribute to hyperuricemia
      i. **CAN'T LEAP** as previously described
  d. Indications for chronic treatment of symptomatic hyperuricemia
      i. 2 or 3 acute attacks of gout within 1–2 years
      ii. Renal stones (urate or calcium)
      iii. Tophaceous gout
      iv. Chronic gouty arthritis with bony erosions
  e. Prophylactic colchicine
      i. Reduces the frequency of attacks by 75–90%
      ii. Mitigates the severity of attacks that do occur
      iii. Initiate only after an antihyperuricemic agent has been added
        1. Otherwise tophi can develop without the usual warning signs
      iv. May be used alone instead of a uricosuric agent or allopurinol
        1. If the patient does not meet the criteria for these drugs
        2. If the patient has a contraindication to these drugs
      v. May be used as urate lowering drugs are being initiated
        1. Often urate lowering drugs can precipitate an attack
      vi. Long term use of small daily doses (0.6 mg/day)
        1. Relatively safe
        2. Usually do not cause GI side effects
        3. Continue until no symptoms of gout for several months
        4. Prophylactic use and neuromuscular syndrome
          a. Almost exclusively in patients with chronic renal insufficiency (serum creatinine >1.6 mg/dl)

f. Urate-lowering drugs
   i. Agents used to maintain serum urate at <6.0 mg/dl
      1. Antihyperuricemic drugs
      2. Uricosuric drugs
      3. Xanthine oxidase inhibitors
   ii. Do not initiate during an acute attack
      1. Any change in serum urate may exacerbate or prolong the attack
   iii. Minimize changes in serum urate
      1. Gradual dose increases
      2. Prophylaxis with colchicine or NSAIDs
      3. Use at the lowest dosage necessary
   iv. Continue urate-lowering drugs **indefinitely** in individuals with chronic tophaceous gout
      1. Even if they have had no symptoms for years

g. Xanthine oxidase inhibitors
   i. Inhibit uric acid synthesis by inhibiting xanthine oxidase
      1. The final enzyme involved in the production of uric acid
   ii. Initiate only after an acute attack of gout has resolved entirely
   iii. Drugs include
      1. Allopurinol
      2. Oxipurinol

h. Allopurinol
   i. Recommended most often
   ii. Convenient single daily dose
   iii. Effective in both overproducers and underexcreters
      1. A 24 h urine collection is seldom performed in clinical practice
   iv. A hypoxanthine analogue
   v. Mechanism of Action
      1. Lowers blood and urine urate concentrations
         a. Inhibits the enzyme xanthine oxidase
         b. Leads to increases in the precursors xanthine and hypoxanthine
      2. Metabolized by xanthine oxidase to oxipurinol
         a. Oxipurinol is the active metabolite
         b. Oxipurinol can be measured to assess compliance
      3. Well absorbed from the GI tract
      4. Half-life of 40 min
      5. Maximum anti-hyperuricemic effect within 7–14 days
      6. Reduce by 50–75% other drugs that depend on xanthine oxidase for their metabolism if given concomitantly
         a. 6-mercaptopurine
         b. Azathioprine
   vi. Indications for use
      1. Urate overproduction
         a. Uric acid >700 mg in 24-h urine collection on a regular diet
      2. Tophus formation
         a. May take several months to resolve

      3. Nephrolithiasis

      4. Renal insufficiency

         a. Creatinine clearance < 50 ml/min

      5. Contraindications to uricosuric therapy

vii. Less common indications

      1. Hyperuricemia with nephrolithiasis of any type

      2. Prophylaxis against tumor lysis syndrome

      3. Lesch-Nyhan syndrome

         a. Hypoxanthine phosphoribosyltransferase (HPRT) deficiency

      4. Hyperuricemia due to myeloproliferative disorders

      5. Serum urate >12.0 mg/dl

         a. Or 24 h urine uric acid >1,100 mg

viii. Dosing

      1. Available orally in 100 and 300-mg tablets

      2. Usually given in once-daily doses

         a. To lower serum urate <6.0 mg/dl

      3. Initiated at 300 mg/day

      4. Maxed at 800 mg/day

      5. If >300 mg/day is required for adequate uric acid levels

         a. Investigate other correctable factors

         b. Non-compliance is the most common cause

      6. Lowest dose achievable

         a. Adjust to give 100 mg for each 30 ml/min of creatinine clearance

           i. Follow serum oxipurinol levels to titrate to therapeutic levels

         b. 200 mg/day

           i. GFR approaches 60 ml/min

         c. 100 mg or less appropriate for

           i. The elderly

           ii. Those with frequent attacks

           iii. GFR < 50 ml/min

ix. Combination use

      1. Allopurinol and a uricosuric agent

      2. Indicated in patients with extensive tophi and adequate renal function

      3. Urate diuretic enhances excretion of large quantities of solubilized urate

      4. Allopurinol reduces the formation of new urate

x. Common side effects

      1. Acute gouty arthritis

      2. Dyspepsia

      3. Headache

      4. Diarrhea

      5. Abnormal liver enzymes

      6. Cataracts

      7. Pruritic papular rash (3–10%)

    a. Particularly those with renal insufficiency

    b. Oral desensitization

       i. Stop drug and restart at a lower level

      ii. Start at 50 μg

     iii. Slowly increase to 100 mg by 1 month

     iv. Successful in 70–80% of patients

      v. Not done with serious reactions

    c. Stevens-Johnson syndrome

    d. Toxic epidermal necrolysis

    e. Vasculitis

    f. Hypersensitivity syndrome

    g. Risk three times higher if on ampicillin

xi. Less common side effects

1. Fever
2. Lymphadenopathy
3. Urticaria
4. Eosinophilia
5. Interstitial nephritis
6. Acute renal failure
7. Bone marrow suppression
8. Granulomatous hepatitis
9. Vasculitis
10. Toxic epidermal necrolysis
11. Peripheral neuropathy
12. Sarcoid-like reaction
13. Alopecia
14. Death

xii. Allopurinol hypersensitivity syndrome

1. Occurs in about 5–10% of patients who experience an allopurinol rash
2. Significant morbidity and mortality rate (20–30%)
3. Usually develops in patients who
    a. Have an associated renal insufficiency (75%)
    b. Are on diuretic therapy (50%)
4. Typically occurs 2–4 weeks after initiating therapy
5. Clinical manifestations
    a. Skin rash
    b. Fever
    c. Eosinophilia
    d. Hepatic necrosis
    e. Leukocytosis
    f. Worsening renal function
6. Treatment
    a. High-dose steroids
    b. Hemodialysis to remove oxipurinol

   i. Oxipurinol
       i. A xanthine analogue
       ii. The major metabolite of allopurinol
       iii. Patients intolerant of allopurinol may tolerate oxipurinol
       iv. Used in Europe
           1. Not widely available in the USA
       v. Poor GI absorption
       vi. Longer half-life (14–28 h) than allopurinol
       vii. Used in patients who have allergic reactions to allopurinol
           1. Up to 40% can have reaction to oxipurinol
           2. Avoid if serious toxicities are encountered with allopurinol
   j. Uricosuric Agents
       i. Mechanism of Action
           1. Weak organic acids
               a. Like uric acid
           2. Increases urinary excretion of uric acid
               a. Competitively inhibits tubular reabsorption of urate
           3. Lowers serum uric acid to <6.7 mg/dl in 75% of patients
           4. Minimizes uric acid nephropathy and nephrolithiasis
           5. Avoid low doses of aspirin or salicylates
               a. These inhibit urate secretion
           6. Most effective with
               a. Good urine alkalinization
               b. Urine flow >1,500 ml/day
       ii. Side effects
           1. Generally well tolerated by >90%
           2. Common
               a. Gastrointestinal symptoms (10%)
               b. Dermatitis (5%)
               c. Headache
               d. Drug fever
           3. Rare
               a. Hemolytic anemia
               b. Aplastic anemia
               c. Nephrotic syndrome
               d. Hepatic necrosis
               e. Anaphylaxis
           4. Preventable
               a. Acute gouty attacks
               b. Urate nephropathy and nephrolithiasis
       iii. Indications
           1. Hyperuricemia secondary to underexcretion of uric acid
               a. < 700 mg of uric acid in a 24 h urine collection
                   i. While on a regular diet
           2. GFR > 50–60 ml/min
           3. Willing to drink at least 2 l of fluids daily

      4. No history of nephrolithiasis or excessive urine acidity

      5. Avoid all salicylates

      6. Age < 60 years

        a. 65 years or older respond inadequately to most uricosuric drugs

  k. Probenecid

     i. The most commonly used uricosuric

     ii. Initial dose 0.5 g/day

     iii. Increase slowly to generally no more than 1 g BID

     iv. Compared with sulfinpyrazone

       1. Longer half-life (6–12 h)

       2. More extensively metabolized

     v. Common side effects

       1. Rash

       2. GI upset

       3. Urate nephrolithiasis

         a. Greatest concern

         b. Alkalinize the urine to pH 6.0–6.5 to increase urate solubility

         c. Use potassium citrate 30–80 mEq/day

         d. Use allopurinol instead

 l. Sulfinpyrazone

     i. An analogue of a phenylbutazone metabolite

     ii. **NO** anti-inflammatory properties

     iii. 98% bound to plasma proteins

     iv. Half-life 1–3 h

     v. 20–45% excreted unchanged in the urine

       1. Most as a uricosuric metabolite

     vi. Antiplatelet activity

       1. Through inhibition of thromboxane synthesis

     vii. Promotes urate nephrolithiasis

     viii. GI side effects in 5% of people

       1. Ulcerogenic

     ix. Bone marrow suppression may occur (rare)

     x. Dosing

       1. Available in 100 and 200 mg oral preparations

       2. Dosed initially at 50 mg twice daily

       3. Increased slowly from 100 to 800 mg daily in 3 or 4 divided doses

     xi. Compared with probenecid

       1. More effective in patients with renal insufficiency

       2. 3–6 times more potent

  m. Losartan

     i. An angiotensin II receptor antagonist

     ii. Promotes urate diuresis

     iii. May normalize serum urate levels

     iv. Can treat elderly for both gout and hypertension

5. Drug Interactions

  a. Concomitant use of allopurinol and ampicillin

       i. Associated with increased frequency of rash
- b. Probenecid prolongs the half-life and inhibits the excretion of
    - i. Penicillins
    - ii. Indomethacin
    - iii. Dapsone
    - iv. Acetazolamide
    - v. Sulfinpyrazone
- c. Probenecid affects the metabolism of
    - i. Rifampin
    - ii. Heparin
- d. Probenecid antagonizes the uricosuric effect of
    - i. Salicylates
    - ii. Pyrazinamide
- e. Allopurinol **increases** the half-life of probenecid and probenecid **accelerates the excretion** of allopurinol
- i. Prescribe higher doses of allopurinol and lower doses of probenecid
6. Asymptomatic Hyperuricemia
    - a. The finding of asymptomatic hyperuricemia is not an indication for treatment with urate-lowering drugs
    - b. The cause of hyperuricemia should be determined and associated problems addressed
        - i. Hypertension
        - ii. Alcoholism
        - iii. Hyperlipidemia
        - iv. Obesity
    - c. Indications for treatment
        - i. Situations where there may be an acute overproduction of uric acid
            1. Acute tumor lysis syndrome
        - ii. Where severe hyperuricemia exists
            1. > 12 mg/dl or 24 h uric acid >1,100 mg
            2. The prevalence of uric acid nephrolithiasis is 50%
7. Gout in the Transplant Patient
    - a. Therapeutic difficulties
        - i. NSAIDs and cyclosporin used together interfere with renal prostaglandin formation
            1. Decrease renal blood flow
        - ii. ACTH can not be used
            1. Lack of adrenal response on chronic corticosteroids
        - iii. Colchicine toxicity
            1. Hazardous in patients on azathioprine whose granulocytes count is decreased
            2. Associated with severe cases of myoneuropathy in patients on cyclosporin

        a. Even one tablet a day

     3. Cyclosporin is an inhibitor of the multidrug resistance MDR-mediated transport

        a. Colchicine depends on MDR-1 for hepatic and renal transport

        b. Toxic effects amplified as colchicine will not be excreted

  b. Best therapeutic choice

    i. Steroids

     1. Oral

     2. IM

     3. Intra-articular (IA)

        a. May be the safest alternative with marginal renal function and/or WBC count

    ii. Most are already on corticosteroid

    iii. Initial doses of up to 60 mg/day may be necessary

  c. Synovial fluid cultures should be performed routinely

  d. Managing hyperuricemia

    i. Poor response to uricosuric agents when GFR < 50 ml/min

    ii. Allopurinol causes potentiation of azathioprine

     1. Azathioprine is metabolized by xanthine oxidase

     2. Azathioprine should be reduced by 50–75% with the concomitant use of allopurinol

        a. Even with reduction a dangerous combination that can result in bone marrow failure

     3. Mycophenolate mofetil has supplanted azathioprine in many antirejection regimens

8. Other Therapies for Gout

  a. Benzbromarone

    i. A uricosuric agent

    ii. Effective even in patients with creatinine clearance as low as 25 mg/min

  b. Lisinopril

    i. ACE inhibitor

    ii. Mild uricosuric effect

  c. Urate oxidase

    i. An enzyme from *Asperillus flavus*

    ii. Catalyzes the conversion of uric acid to allantoin

    iii. 10 times more soluble and easier for the kidney to eliminate

    iv. Successful in the prevention and treatment of tumor lysis syndrome

  d. Febuxostat

    i. Inhibits xanthine oxidase

    ii. Blocks substrate access by occupying a channel

    iii. Potent inhibition of both oxidized and reduced forms

    iv. Minimal effects on other enzymes in the pathway

     v. Metabolized primarily by hepatic glucuronide formation
        and oxidation
    vi. Excreted in about equal amount in stool and urine
   vii. Given as 80 and 120 mg daily
  viii. Phase II study with comparison to allopuinol (300 mg) showed
       1. Superiority in patients with urate levels >8 mg/dl
       2. Primary endpoint <6 mg/dl
       3. After 1 year similar outcomes in incidence of flares and size of tophi

Vasculitides

10

Section A: Polyarteritis Nodosa, Microscopic Polyangiitis and Small-Vessel Vasculitides

1. Classification of the vasculitides based on
   a. The size of the blood vessel involved
   b. Current knowledge of disease pathophysiology
   c. The pattern of organ involvement
2. Subclassification of Vasculitides
   a. Based on certain pathophysiologic features
   b. Immune complex mediated
   c. Association with characteristic autoantibodies,
      i. Such as antineutrophil cytoplasmic antibodies (ANCA)
   d. The presence or absence of granulomatous inflammation
   e. Trophism of particular organs
      i. Microscopic polyangiitis (MPA) and cutaneous leukocytoclastic angiitis (CLA) both are similar clinically and pathologically
         1. Only CLA is confined to the skin
3. Characteristics of Small Vessel Vasculitides
   a. More numerous
   b. Affect blood vessels that are <50 µm in diameter
      i. Capillaries
      ii. Glomeruli
         1. Viewed as differentiated capillaries
      iii. Post-capillary venules
      iv. Nonmuscular arteries
4. Small Vessel Vasculitides
   a. Immune-complex mediated
      i. Cutaneous leukocytoclastic angiitis (hypersensitivity vasculitis)
      ii. Henoch-Schonlein purpura

N.T. Colburn, *Review of Rheumatology*,
DOI 10.1007/978-1-84882-093-7_10, © Springer-Verlag London Limited 2012

       iii. Urticarial vasculitis
       iv. Cryoglobulinemia
       v. Connective tissue disorders
   b. ANCA-associated disorders
       i. Wegener's granulomatosis
       ii. Microscopic polyangiitis
       iii. Churg-Strauss syndrome
       iv. Drug-induced ANCA-associated vasculitis
   c. Miscellaneous
       i. Behcet's
       ii. Erythema elevatum diutinum
       iii. Paraneoplastic
       iv. Bacterial, viral, or fungal infections
       v. Inflammatory bowel disease
5. Medium Vessel Vasculitides
   a. Polyarteritis Nodosa
   b. Kawasaki's disease
   c. Thromboangiitis obliterans (TO)
       i. "Buerger's disease"
   d. Primary angiitis of the CNS (PACNS)
6. Polyarteritis Nodosa
   a. The prime example of a medium-vessel vasculitis
   b. Involves arteries that contain muscular walls
       i. Corresponds to vessel diameter of about 50–150 μm
   c. First described in 1866 by Kussmaul and Maier in a journeyman tailor
       i. Had fever, weight loss, abdominal pain, and polyneuropathy
   d. The 1994 Chapel Hill Consensus Conference definition of classic PAN
       i. Necrotizing inflammation of medium sized or small arteries
       ii. Spares the smallest blood vessels
          1. Arterioles
          2. Venules
          3. Capillaries
       iii. **NOT** associated with glomerulonephritis
   e. An uncommon disease
       i. Reported annual incidence rates ranged from 2 to 9 cases per million people per year
       ii. 2:1 male to female ratio
       iii. All racial groups
       iv. Average age from mid 40s to mid 60s
   f. Pathological changes
       i. Pathologic lesion that defines PAN
          1. Focal segmental necrotizing vasculitis of medium-sized and small arteries
       ii. Limited to the **arterial circulation**
          1. Gross specimens show aneurysmal bulges of the arterial wall

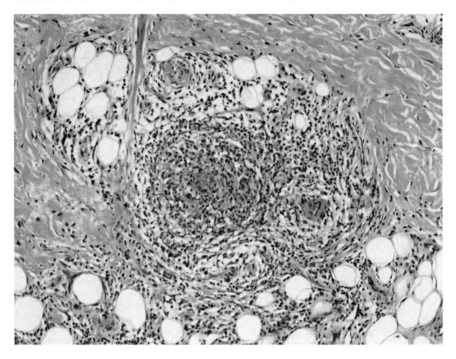

Fig. 10.1 Skin Biopsy shows a neutrophilic vasculitis affecting medium and small arteries in the deep dermis and subcutis consistent with PAN (Reproduced with permission from Medium-size-vessel vasculitis. *Pediatric Nephrology*. DOI: 10.1007/s00467-009-1336-1. Springer; 2010-07-21)

   iii. Histologic sections reveal
     1. Inflammatory cell infiltration of the blood vessel wall
     2. Accompanied by fibrinoid necrosis
   iv. Neutrophils are the principal component of the acute inflammatory infiltrate
     1. Mononuclear cells predominate in later stages
     2. May see variable numbers of lymphocytes and eosinophils
   v. Lesions are segmental
     1. Involve only parts of the arterial circumference
     2. Favor the branch points of arteries
   vi. The normal architecture of the vessel wall is disrupted
     1. Including the elastic laminae
   vii. Thrombosis or aneurysmal dilation occur at the site of the lesion
   viii. Healed areas of arteritis
     1. Proliferation of fibrous tissue and endothelial cells
     2. May lead to vessel occlusion
   ix. Infrequently seen in pulmonary and splenic arteries
   x. Histologically there must be the absence of granulomas or granulomatous inflammation

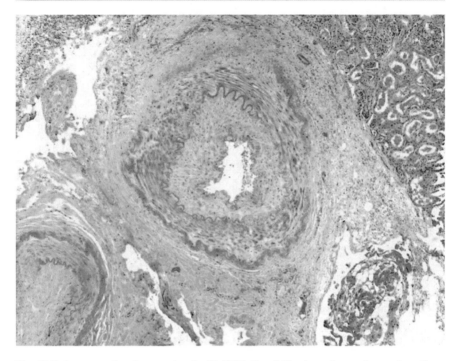

Fig. 10.2 Late vasculopathy associated with PAN. Renal histology shows abnormal medium-sized arteries with internal elastic lamina rupture, fibrosis and intimal thickening but no active vasculitis (Reproduced with permission from Medium-size-vessel vasculitis. *Pediatric Nephrology.* DOI: 10.1007/s00467-009-1336-1. Springer; 2010-07-21)

   g. PAN associations
      i. Hepatitis B virus
         1. A minority of cases (<10%)
         2. Usually occurs within 6 months of hepatitis B
         3. Accompanied by more
           a. Orchitis
           b. High blood pressure
           c. Renal infarcts
     ii. Other viral infections
         1. Cytomegalovirus virus (CMV)
         2. HTLV-1
         3. HIV
         4. Parvovirus
         5. EBV
         6. Hepatitis C
    iii. Autoimmune diseases
         1. RA
         2. SLE

    3. Dermatomyositis
    4. Cogan's
  iv. Medications
    1. Allopurinol
    2. Sulfa
  v. Hairy-cell leukemia
h. Etiology of PAN unknown
  i. No genetic susceptibility identified
  ii. Immune complexes seldom found
  iii. No trigger for inflammatory mediated damage defined
i. Clinical Features
  i. Usually begins with nonspecific symptoms
    1. Malaise
    2. Fatigue
    3. Fever
    4. Myalgias
    5. Weight loss
    6. Arthralgia
  ii. Overt signs of vasculitis may not occur until weeks or months after onset of first symptoms
  iii. Organ involvement
    1. Kidneys (70%)
      a. Medium sized renal and intrarenal arteries
      b. Causes a focal necrotizing glomerulonephritis
      c. Renin-mediated hypertension
        i. Caused by vasculitis of the interlobar renal vessels
        ii. Occasionally severe
    2. Skin (50%)
      a. Medium vessel vasculitis limited to the skin
      b. May occur in 10% of cases
      c. Mainly over the lower extremities
      d. Clinical presentation
        i. Multiple tender nodular skin lesions
        ii. 0.5–2 cm in diameter
        iii. Usually on the legs and feet
        iv. Can occur on arms and trunks
        v. Subcutaneous nodules
          1. Palpable purpura
        vi. Ulcers
        vii. Digital gangrene
        viii. Livedo reticularis found in 60%
        ix. Internal organ involvement is absent
          1. May have fever and arthralgia acutely
      e. Benign prognosis

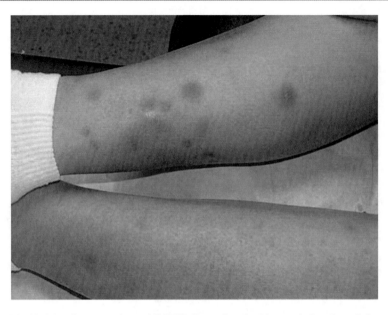

Fig. 10.3 Nodules from a patient with PAN (Reproduced with permission from Polyarteritis Nodosa. *A Clinician's Pearls and Myths in Rheumatology.* DOI: 10.1007/978-1-84800-934-9_26. Springer; 2009-01-01)

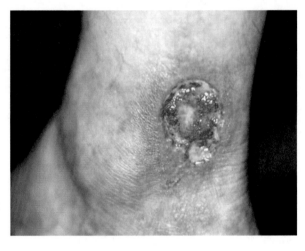

Fig. 10.4 Cutaneous ulcer in a patient with PAN (Reproduced with permission from Polyarteritis nodosa. *A Clinician's Pearls and Myths in Rheumatology.* DOI: 10.1007/978-1-84800-934-9_26. Springer; 2009-01-01)

    f. Treatment
        i. Prednisone 20–40 mg/day
       ii. Steroid sparing agents
          1. Low dose MTX
          2. Azathioprine
          3. Dapsone
          4. Colchicine
      iii. Cyclophosphamide is not needed

   3. Peripheral nerves
     a. A majority of people (>80%) have vasculitic neuropathy
     b. Mononeuritis multiplex (MM)
       i. Typical lesions
       ii. Most often affects
         1. Peroneal
         2. Tibial
         3. Ulnar
         4. Median
         5. Radial
       iii. Symptoms
         1. Foot or wrist drop
         2. Almost always causes sensory abnormalities
           a. Painful dysesthesias
         3. Motor involvement occurs in one-third
     c. EMG may show multiple axonal neuropathies
   4. GI tract (30%)
     a. Mesenteric arteritis
     b. Postprandial periumbilical pain
       i. The classic manifestation of "intestinal angina"
     c. Can be life threatening
       i. Perforation of an ischemic bowel
       ii. Rupture of a mesenteric aneurysm
     d. Other affected GI organs
       i. Gallbladder
       ii. Appendix
     e. Abnormal liver functions
   5. Muscle
     a. Myalgia (60%)
   6. Joint
     a. Arthralgias (50%)
     b. Arthritis (20%)
   7. Testicular pain
     a. Seen in 20%
     b. More common with associated hepatitis B
   8. Cardiac (low)
     a. Myocardial infarction
     b. Congestive heart failure (CHF)
     c. Usually remains subclinical
   9. CNS disease (low)
     a. Usually results from hypertension
       i. Rather than intracranial vasculitis
     b. Seizures
     c. Strokes
  10. Temporal artery (low)
     a. Jaw claudication

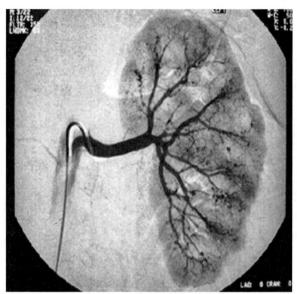

Fig. 10.5 Microaneurysms in a patient with PAN by renal angiography (Reproduced with permission from Polyarteritis nodosa. *Rheumatology and Immunology Therapy.* DOI: 10.1007/3-540-29662-X_2190. Springer; 2004-01-01)

   11. Eye (low)
       a. Retinal hemorrhage
   12. Typically **spares** the lungs
       a. Low incidence of intersitial pneumonitis
j. Laboratory features
   i. Often strikingly abnormal and nonspecific
   ii. Reflects systemic inflammation
       1. Normocytic normochromic anemia
       2. Thrombocytosis
       3. Elevated ESR/CRP
       4. Microscopic hematuria
          a. In the absence of GN
       5. Low levels of albumin
       6. Decreased levels of complement
          a. About 25% of cases during active disease
   iii. HBV associated PAN
       1. Hepatitis B surface antigen present in 10–50%
       2. HBeAg and HBV DNA positive
   iv. ANCA antibodies are **absent** (by definition)
k. Diagnosis
   i. A tissue biopsy or an angiogram demonstrating
       1. Microaneurysms
       2. Occlusion
       3. Stenoses of small and medium-sized vessels of the abdominal viscera
          a. Specifically kidney, liver, stomach, and small bowel

     ii. Other diseases with aneurysms on abdominal visceral angiography
        1. Segmental mediolytic arteriopathy
           a. A noninflammatory arterial disease that can mimic PAN
           b. Variant of fibromuscular dysplasia
           c. Affects hepatic, splenic, and celiac arteries
        2. Ehlers Danlos, type IV
           a. Vessel wall weakening
           b. Defect in production of type III collagen
        3. Fibromuscular dysplasia
   iii. Key clinical features
        1. Constitutional symptoms
        2. Multisystem involvement
        3. Palpable purpura
        4. Livedo
        5. Necrotic lesions
        6. Infarcts of the fingertips
        7. Peripheral neuropathy
           a. MM
        8. Renal sediment abnormalities
   iv. Simultaneous nerve and muscle biopsies of the sural nerve and gastroc-nemius muscle
        1. High yield if there is clinical MM
        2. Biopsy symptomatic and accessible sites
           a. Skin
           b. Sural nerve
           c. Skeletal muscle
           d. Liver
           e. Rectum
           f. Testicle
        3. Kidney biopsies are **NOT** diagnostic of PAN
           a. A renal biopsy will reveal a focal necrotizing GN with abnormalities in the urinary sediment or proteinuria
              i. Seen in almost all vasculitides
l. Treatment
   i. High-dose corticosteroids
        1. One half achieve remission
        2. Begin with 60 mg/day (1 mg/kg/day)
        3. May pulse with methylprednisolone (1 g/day for 3 days) at the start of therapy
   ii. Cyclophosphamide
        1. Indications
           a. Disease refractory to corticosteroids
           b. Serious major organ involvement
         2. 2 mg/kg/day oral or 500–1,000 mg/m^2 IV each month
        3. Monitor for neutropenia

4. Pneumocystis carinii prophylaxis is advised
   a. Bactrim
   iii. Combination therapy for HBV associated PAN
   1. Initial prednisone (30 mg/day) with rapid taper to suppress the inflammation
   2. Plasma exchange
      a. 6 week courses
      b. Simultaneously with the start of prednisone
      c. To remove circulating immune complexes
      d. About 3 exchanges per week
      e. 60 ml/kg exchanges
   3. Taper corticosteroids rapidly over 2 weeks total course
   4. Follow with antiviral therapy
      a. Lamivudine 100 mg/day or interferon α-2b
      b. To eliminate the virus
   5. Success accompanied by
      a. HBeAg to anti-Hbe
   6. Patients who do best are negative for
      a. HCV
      b. HIV
      c. Delta virus
m. Prognosis
   i. Depends on presence and extent of visceral and CNS involvement
   ii. Most deaths occur within the first year due to
   1. Uncontrolled vasculitis
   2. Delay in diagnosis
   3. Complication of treatment
   iii. Deaths after the first year due to
   1. Complications of treatment
   2. Vascular events
      a. MI
      b. Stroke
   iv. Overall 5 year survival
   1. Up to 75% with aggressive treatment
7. Microscopic Polyangiitis (MPA)
   a. Defined by the 1994 Chapel Hill Consensus Conference
      i. Necrotizing vasculitis with few or no immune deposits
      1. Pauci-immune
      ii. Affects the smallest blood vessels
      1. Capillaries
      2. Venules
      3. Arterioles
      iii. May affect medium-sized vessels
      iv. Tropism for the kidney (GN) and lungs (pulmonary capillaritis)

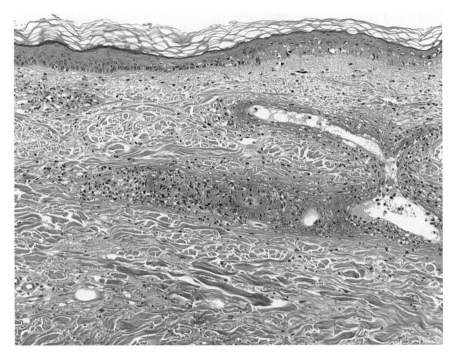

Fig. 10.6 Typical small-vessel leukocytoclastic vasculitis associated with microscopic polyangiitis with endothelial swelling, neutrophilic infiltrate with leukocytoclasia, extravasation of erythrocytes, and fibrinoid degeneration of the vessel wall of the upper dermis (Reproduced with permission from Dermatological manifestations associated with microscopic polyangiitis.*Rheumatology International.* DOI: 10.1007/s00296-007-0497-0. Springer; 2008-04-01)

    b. Characteristic histopathology
        i. Renal biopsy
            1. Focal, segmental necrotizing GN frequently with crescents
            2. Immunoflurorescence and electron microscopy show no immune deposits (pauci-immune GN)
       ii. Lung biopsy
            1. Pulmonary capillaritis with negative immunofluorescence
      iii. Skin biopsy
            1. Leukocytoclastic vasculitis
    c. Diagnosis
        i. Based on characteristic
            1. Clinical presentation
            2. Renal biopsy showing necrotizing GN without immune deposits
       ii. P-ANCA
            1. The most common staining pattern
            2. Supportive of the diagnosis

3. Found in up to 80% of patients
4. Corresponds to the presence antimyeloperoxidase antibodies

iii. C-ANCA
1. Found in a small minority of patients
2. Directed against serine proteinase 3
3. Does not present with upper respiratory tract involvement
a. Like Wegener's

iv. Differentiate from other pulmonary-renal syndromes which present with rapidly progressive renal dysfunction and pulmonary hemorrhage
1. SLE
a. Diffuse proliferative GN with immune complex deposits on kidney biopsy
b. Clinical and serologic manifestation of SLE
2. Goodpasture's
a. Linear pattern of immunofluorescence on kidney and lung biopsy
b. A positive anti-glomerular basement membrane antibody

d. Clinical Features
i. Affects males and females
ii. Peak age 30–50 years
1. Can occur at any age
iii. MPA (in contrast to PAN)
1. Does **NOT** cause microaneurysm formation of abdominal or renal vessels
2. Involves the lung (alveolar hemorrhage)
3. Rapidly progressive GN
4. Involves veins as well as arteries
5. Rarely causes severe hypertension
6. Commonly associated with p-ANCA (up to 80%)
7. Not associated with HBV
8. Nearly always requires cyclophosphamide
9. Relapses are common
10. Annual incidence of 2.4 cases per million
a. More common than classic PAN
iv. Pauci-immune, necrotizing GN is a dominant feature
1. Occurs in nearly four-fifths of all patients
2. Crescent formation and RBC casts
a. Found in renal tubules and urinary sediment
v. Pulmonary capillaritis
1. Leads to rapid life threatening alveolar hemorrhage and hemoptysis
2. About 12% develop this complication
vi. Common disease manifestation
1. GN (79%)
2. Weight loss (73%)
3. MM (58%)
4. Fever (55%)
5. Arthralgias (up to 65%)

Criteria	PAN	MPA
Histology		
• Type of vasculitis	Necrotizing with mixed cells, rarely granulomatous	Necrotizing with mixed cells, not granulomatous
• Type of vessels involved	Medium - and small - sized muscle arteries, sometimes arterioles	Small vessels (*ie*, capillaries, venules or arterioles)
		Small - and medium - sized arteries may be also affected
Distribution and localization		
Kidney		
• Renal vasculitis with renovascular hypertension, renal infarcts and microaneurysms	Yes	No
• Rapidly progressive glomerulonephiritis	No	Very common
Lung		
• Pulmonary hemorrhage	No	Yes
Peripheral neuropathy	50%–80%	10%–20%
Relapses	Rare	Frequent
Laboratory data		
pANCA	Rare (< 10%)	Yes (50%–80%)
HBV infection present	Yes (uncommon)	No
Abnormal angiography (microaneurysms, stenoses)	Yes (variable)	No

Fig. 10.7 Differential diagnosis of polyarteritis nodosa and microscopic polyangiitis (Reproduced with permission from Vasculitides. *Atlas of Rheumatology*. ImagesMD; 2002-03-07)

      6. Purpura (40%)

      7. Peripheral or CNS involvement (up to 30%)

    vii. Upper respiratory tract symptoms

      1. Milder than Wegener's

      2. **NOT** associated with

        a. Erosions of the sinuses

        b. Subglottic stenosis

        c. Saddle nose deformities

        d. Granulomatous inflammation

   viii. Typical clinical presentation

      1. Acute onset of rapidly progressive GN (100%)

      2. Pulmonary infiltrates and/or effusions (up to 50%)

      3. Diffuse alveolar hemorrhage with hemoptysis (up to 30%)

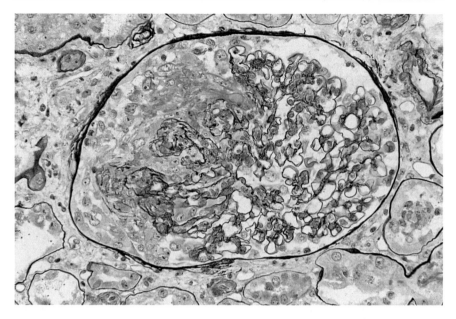

Fig. 10.8 Glomerulonephritis in microscopic polyangiitis (Reproduced with permission from Vasculitides. *Atlas of Rheumatology.* ImagesMD; 2002-03-07)

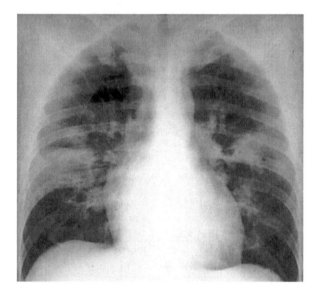

Fig. 10.9 Alveolar hemorrhage in microscopic polyangiitis (Reproduced with permission from Vasculitides. *Atlas of Rheumatology.* ImagesMD; 2002-03-07)

    e. Treatment
        i. Combination therapy with cyclophosphamide and corticosteroids
            1. Cyclophosphamide 750 mg/m^2 of body surface area
                a. Once a month for six treatments
            2. For patients with GN, alveolar hemorrhage, MM, or other severe manifestations

Fig. 10.10 Palpable purpura on lower leg of a man with microscopic polyangiitis (Reproduced with permission from Connective tissue diseases. *Therapy of Skin Diseases*. DOI: 10.1007/978-3-540-78814-0_37. Springer; 2010-01-01)

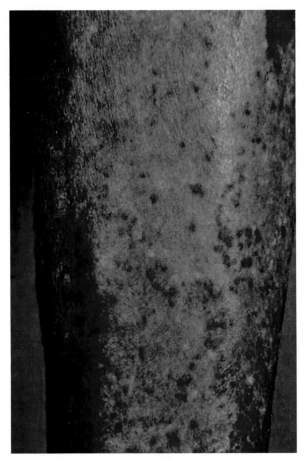

      ii. Plasmapharesis and IVIG
         1. Patients with progressive renal failure or pulmonary hemorrhage
   f. Prognosis
      i. Guarded
      ii. Relapses are common (33%)
      iii. Up to 45% end up on dialysis
      iv. Pulmonary hemorrhage can be life-threatening
      v. Overall 5 year survival is 65%
8. Cutaneous Leukocytoclastic Angiitis (CLA)
   a. Originally termed hypersensitivity vasculitis (HSV)
   b. Defined as a form of small vessel vasculitides confined to the skin
   c. Idiopathic or associated with a drug reaction
   d. Characteristic features
      i. Lesions typically occur in dependent regions
         1. Lower extremities
         2. Buttocks

    ii. Lesions occur in "crops"
        1. Groups of lesions similar in age
        2. Simultaneous exposure to the inciting antigen
    iii. Lesions usually accompanied by a burning or tingling sensation
        1. May be asymptomatic
  e. A wide array of skin lesions
     i. Palpable purpura
     ii. Papules
     iii. Urticaria
     iv. Erythema multiforme
     v. Vesicles
     vi. Pustules
     vii. Superficial ulcers
     viii. Necrosis
  f. Deep ulcers or livedo reticularis usually indicates involvement of medium-sized vessels
  g. Diagnosis
     i. Confirm by skin biopsy
        1. Leukocytoclastic vasculitis in the postcapillary venules
     ii. Both light and direct immunofluorescence (DIF)
        1. Variable patterns of Ig and complement deposition that is **NOT** distinctive
        2. Unlike HSP, urticarial vasculitis and Cryoglobulinemia
     iii. Should be active lesions (<48 h old)
  h. Two keys to the diagnosis and management of CLA
     i. Exclusion of systemic involvement by a careful history, PE, and selected laboratory tests
     ii. Identification and removal of the offending agent (medication)
        1. Removal usually leads to resolution within days to weeks
  i. Treatment
     i. Mild cases
        1. Leg elevation
        2. NSAIDs
        3. H1 antihistamine (fenofexadine)
     ii. For persistent disease (not associated with gangrene)
        1. Colchicine
        2. Hydroxychloroquine
        3. Dapsone
     iii. For refractory or more severe disease
        1. Immunosuppressive agents
        2. Begin with corticosteroids
        3. Azathioprine 2–2.5 mg/kg/day
           a. With excessive steroid use
9. Henoch-Schonlein Purpura (HSP)
  a. Characterized by the clinical tetrad (up to 80% of cases)
     i. Purpura
     ii. Arthritis

      iii. Abdominal pain

      iv. GN

  b. Defining histopathologic feature

      i. Deposition of immunoglobulin IgA around blood vessel walls

  c. The role of IgA in the pathogenesis of HSP

      i. The hinge region O-linked glycans of IgA1 are deficient in galactose and/or sialic acid content

      ii. Deficient IgA1 molecules form macromolecular complexes

        1. Activates the alternative complement pathway

        2. The kidney receptor on mesangial cells bind deficient IgA1 at its hinge region more readily

          a. Leads to proliferation and release of proinflammatory cytokines

      iii. Increased levels of IgA and IgA-containing immune complexes in the serum

      iv. HSP associated only with increases of IgA1 subclass

        1. Accounts for up to 90% of serum IgA but only 50% of secretory IgA

  d. Develops in any age

      i. Most frequent in children

        1. > 90% are less than 10 years of age

        2. Incidence in children is 135 cases/million/year

      ii. Incidence in adults is 1.2 cases/million/year

      iii. Two-thirds of people report antecedent upper respiratory illnesses

        1. Suggest an infectious trigger of the disease

  e. Clinical Features

      i. Typically presentations

        1. Acute onset of fever

        2. Palpable purpura on the lower extremities and buttocks

          a. May be extensive and confluent

          b. May involve the arms and trunk

          c. May begin as a macular erythema and urticarial lesion

            i. Progress rapidly or purpura

          d. Scrotal and scalp edema seen in children

        3. Abdominal pain

          a. Caused by either bowel edema or frank mesenteric ischemia

          b. Often colicky and may worsen after meals

          c. Nausea and vomiting

          d. Upper or lower GI bleeding

          e. Complications

            i. Intussusception

            ii. Hemorrhage

            iii. Ileal perforation (rare)

        4. Arthritis

          a. Arthralgias or arthritis in large joints

            i. Especially the knee and ankles

          b. Joints involved in up to 84% of patients

          c. Symmetrical involvement

    d. May also involve the wrists and elbows

    e. Often a migratory pattern

  5. Hematuria

    a. The clinical hallmark of GN is asymptomatic microscopic hematuria accompanied by proteinuria

    b. May see more marked findings such as nephrotic syndrome and acute renal failure

    c. GN almost always follows the appearance of cutaneous lesions

      i. Contrast to arthritis and GI disease which precedes the onset of purpura

  ii. Manifestations vary with age

    1. Primarily children between 2 and 10 years

    2. Infants have milder disease

    3. Less than 2 years of age less likely to develop GN or GI

    4. Children have more GI involvement

    5. Adults have more renal involvement

    6. Adults more likely to have renal insufficiency (13%)

  iii. Differential

    1. CLA

    2. Cryoglobulinemia

    3. ANCA-associated vasculitides

      a. If HSP is suspected, but no IgA on skin biopsy, evaluate for Wegener's

    4. Connective tissue disorders associated with vasculitis

    5. Infections (endocarditis)

  iv. Definitive diagnosis

    1. Skin biopsy demonstrates IgA deposits in blood vessel walls

    2. Leukocytoclastic vasculitis is the dominant finding on light microscopy

    3. Renal lesions range from minimal disease to focal or diffuse proliferative GN with crescents

      a. Immunofluorescence show mesangial IgA deposition

      b. Chronic renal failure is rare

        i. Except with adults who have >50% crescents on renal biopsy

f. Treatment

  i. Self-limited in 97% of cases

    1. Last an average of 4 weeks

  ii. NSAIDs alleviate arthralgia

    1. Avoid in GN

  iii. Corticosteroids help joint and GI symptoms

  iv. Progressive renal disease (severe GN)

    1. Does not respond to glucocorticoids

    2. Combination high-dose corticosteroid and a cytotoxic agent

  v. Poor prognostic factors

    1. Proteinuria >1 g/day

    2. Nephrotic syndrome

    3. Crescentic glomerulonephritis >50% crescents

10. Urticarial Vasculitis (UV)
   a. A small-vessel vasculitis
   b. Presents with urticarial lesions
      i. Not the typical palpable purpura
   c. Secondary UV (Most have an associated underlying disease)
      i. SLE
      ii. Sjogren's
      iii. Hepatitis B and C antigenemia
      iv. Drug reactions
      v. Sun exposure
   d. Primary or idiopathic UV
      i. A minority have a local process
      ii. Not associated with a specific disorder
   e. Clinical features
      i. Arthralgia and arthritis
      ii. Increased incidence of chronic obstructive pulmonary disease (COPD) (50%)
         1. Those who are also cigarette smokers
      iii. Uveitis (30%)
      iv. Episcleritis
      v. Fever
      vi. Angioedema (50%)
      vii. Peripheral neuropathy
      viii. Seizures
      ix. Increased ESR (66%)
   f. Three subtypes
      i. Normocomplementemic form
         1. Idiopathic
         2. Self-limited
         3. Benign
      ii. Hypocomplementemic form
         1. Often associated with a systemic inflammatory disease
         2. Most have this subtype
         3. Demonstrate low C3, C4, and CH50 during active disease
      iii. Hypocomplementemic urticarial vasculitis syndrome (HUVS)
         1. A potentially severe SLE-like condition
         2. Associated with autoantibodies
            a. To the collagen-like region of C1q
   g. UV compared to chronic idiopathic urticaria (CIU)
      i. 10% with CIU will have UV
      ii. UV lesions typically 0.5–5 cm in diameter
         1. True urticaria may coalesce into large lesions >10 cm
      iii. UV lesions last more than 48 h
         1. True urticaria last 2–8 h
      iv. CIU often have a purpuric (nonblanchable) component

     v. CIU associated with sensations of stinging and burning
        1. Rather than pruritus
     vi. CIU often leave postinflammatory hyperpigmentation
     vii. UV has systemic symptoms which are rare in allergic urticaria
        1. Fever
        2. Arthralgia
        3. Abdominal pain
        4. Lymphadenopathy
        5. Abnormal urine sediment
     viii. UV histology is LCV
        1. True urticaria involves edema of the upper dermis
     ix. Distinguish normocomplementemic UV from neutrophilic urticaria
  h. HUVS
     i. Disorder resembles SLE
     ii. Female predominance 8:1 ratio
     iii. SLE-specific autoantibodies do **NOT** occur in HUVS
        1. Anti-dsDNA
        2. Sm antigen
     iv. Clinical features that distinguish the two
        1. Symptoms associated with HUVS that are atypical for SLE
           a. Angioedema
           b. Uveitis
           c. COPD
        2. Renal biopsy may reveal mesangial inflammation or membranprolif-
          erative GN
           a. Progression to ESRD is unusual
     v. Most with HUVS have C1q precipitins
        1. IgG autoantibodies to the collagen-like region of C1q
        2. Also detected in up to one-third of SLE
 i. Treatment
     i. Conservative treatment (if no internal organ involvement)
        1. Antihistamines (both types)
           a. H1 (fexofenadine)
           b. H2 (ranitidine)
        2. NSAIDs
           a. Typically indomethacin
     ii. Normocomplementemic form usually requires little therapy
     iii. Hypocomplementemic form (limited to skin)
        1. Hydroxychloroquine
        2. Dapsone
        3. Low doses of corticosteroids
     iv. HUVS
        1. Intensive immunosuppression (life-threatening involvement of the
          lungs or other organs)
           a. Azathioprine and cyclophosphamide
              i. Reported in individual cases

        b. Cyclosporine

           i. Beneficial with progressive airway obstruction

11. Cryoglobulinemic Vasculitis

    a. Cryoglobulins (CG)

        i. Immunoglobulins or immunoglobulin-containing complexes (antibodies)

        ii. Spontaneously precipitate from serum under conditions of cold

        iii. Resolubilize upon warming

    b. Special requirements for the collection of CG specimens

        i. Collect at body temperature or significant quantities of CG may be lost

        ii. Drawn blood into a warmed syringe and immediately allow to clot for 1–2 h at 37°

        iii. After clotting, harvest serum at warm temperatures

        iv. Refrigerate serum at 4°C for 5–7 days before protein isolation

        v. Quantitation

           1. Direct measurement of packed volume of precipitate after centrifugation (cryocrit)

           2. Spectrophotometric determination of protein concentration

    c. Clinical complications

        i. Vasculitis

        ii. Hyperviscosity

    d. CGs classified into three types based on the presence or absence of monoclonality and rheumatoid factor (RF) activity

        i. Type I CGs (25%)

           1. A single homogeneous monoclonal immunoglobulin with only one class or subclass of heavy or light chain

           2. Lack RF activity

           3. Serum levels are usually high (5–30 mg/ml)

           4. Immunoglobulins readily precipitate in the cold

           5. Associated with certain hematopoietic malignancies

           6. Often lead to hyperviscosity (rather than vasculitis)

        ii. Type II CGs (25%)

           1. A "mixed" CG

             a. Consist of both IgG and IgM antibodies

           2. A monoclonal component that acts as an antibody against polyclonal IgG (possesses RF activity)

             a. Most are IgM-IgG

             b. Also IgG-IgG and IgA-IgG

           3. Serum levels usually high

             a. 40% at 1–5 mg/ml

             b. 40% with levels >5 mg/ml

           4. Associated with systemic vasculitis

             a. Involve small sized (and often medium-sized) blood vessels

             b. Deposition of CG-containing immune complexes in blood vessel walls

             c. Activation of complement

  iii. Type III (50%)
   1. Mixed polyclonal CGs consistently heterogeneous
   2. One or more classes of polyclonal immunoglobulins
   3. Sometimes non-immunoglobulin molecules
    a. Complement
    b. Lipoproteins
   4. Most are also immunoglobulin-antiimmunoglobulin CGs
   5. Difficult to detect
    a. Precipitate slowly
    b. Present in small quantities (0.1–1 mg/dl)
 e. Vasculitis secondary to mixed Cryoglobulinemia
  i. 90% are Hypocomplementemic
  ii. C4 levels characteristically more depressed than C3 levels
  iii. Often misdiagnosed
   1. Clinical symptoms similar to RA and SLE
   2. Presence of RF and hypocomplementemia
 f. Clinical Features
  i. Most common manifestations of CG vasculitis
   1. Recurrent crops of palpable purpura on the legs
  ii. May be associated with large painful ulcerations
  iii. Skin biopsies
   1. LCV
   2. Granular IgM and C3 deposits in and around small and medium sized blood vessels
  iv. Other common manifestations
   1. Vasculitic neuropathy
   2. GN
   3. Arthralgia
   4. Malaise
   5. Fatigue
   6. Mesenteric vasculitis
   7. Raynaud's
   8. Livedo reticularis
   9. Secondary Sjogren's
   10. CNS vasculitis (small minority)
  v. Clinical features of Type II and III are virtually indistinguishable
   1. GN almost always associated with Type II CGs
 g. CG vasculitis and HCV infection
  i. Accounts for 80% of cases
  ii. Possible causative role for hepatotrophic viruses in mixed cryoglobulinemia
  iii. Chronic hepatitis present in almost two-thirds of patients
  iv. Anti-HCV antibodies and HCV RNA in CG precipitates are concentrated 1,000-fold (compared to serum levels)

     v. Vasculitis occurs in only a minority of people with HCV
       1. 50% infected with HCV have demonstrable CGs
       2. Possibly related to host and infecting HCV genetic factors
     vi. Serum anti-HCV in mixed cryoglobulinemia ranges from 70% to 100% of cases
     vii. 36% prevalence of cryoglobulinemia with chronic hepatitis C
  h. Other infections reported in association with cryoglobulinemia
     i. Viruses
       1. HBV in <5% of people
       2. CMV
       3. Adenovirus
       4. HIV
     ii. Bacteria
       1. Subacute bacterial endocarditis
       2. Leprosy
       3. Post-strep
       4. Syphilis
       5. Q-fever
     iii. Fungi
       1. Coccidioidomycosis
     iv. Parasites
       1. Kala-azar
       2. Toxoplasmosis
       3. Echinococcosis
       4. Schistosomiasis
       5. Malaria
 i. Treatment
     i. Mild disease (frequent purpuric lesions, shallow cutaneous ulcers)
       1. Interferon α (3×10^6 units 3× per week)
       2. Alone or in combination with rebavirin (1,000–1,200 mg/day)
     ii. Antiviral therapy must be initiated after control of the inflammatory response with immunosuppression
       1. If not may see a temporary exacerbation of the vasculitic process
       2. Results from unfavorable alteration of the antigen:antibody ratio
     iii. Severe disease (MM)
       1. Corticosteroids and cyclophosphamide
       2. Plasmapheresis may be a useful adjunct
12. Thromboangiitis Obliterans (TO) (Buerger's disease)
  a. An inflammatory, obliterative, nonartheromatous vascular disease
  b. Most commonly affects small- and medium-sized arteries, veins, and nerves
  c. Acute phase characterized by
     i. Formation of a highly inflammatory thrombus
     ii. Mild inflammation in the blood vessels
       1. Not as prominent as other forms of vasculitis

d. Etiology
    i. Pathogenesis unknown
    ii. Tobacco plays a major role in the initiation and continuation of the disease process
    iii. Possible genetic predisposition and autoimmune mechanisms
e. Epidemiology
    i. More prevalent in the Middle East and Far East than in North America and Western Europe
    ii. Typically seen in young smokers aged 10–50 years
        1. Rarely beyond age 50
        2. Most are heavy smokers
            a. Using 3–6 cigarettes a day for a few years
    iii. Reported in pipe smokers and tobacco chewers
f. Clinical Features
    i. Initial manifestation usually ischemia or claudication of both legs (sometimes hands)
        1. Begins distally and progresses cephalad
        2. Two or more limbs are commonly involved
    ii. 40% of cases have superficial thrombophlebitis and Raynaud's phenomenon
    iii. Symptoms (require medical intervention)
        1. Claudication
        2. Pain at rest
        3. Digital ulceration
        4. Dysesthesias
        5. Sensitivity to cold
        6. Rubor
        7. Cyanosis
        8. Pedal (instep) claudication characteristic
        9. Gangrene and ulceration
            a. Seen in one-third of patients
            b. Usually in the toes and fingers
            c. Occurs spontaneously or follows trauma
                i. Nail trimming
                ii. Pressure from tight shoes
       10. Superficial migratory thrombophlebitis
g. Diagnosis
    i. Exclude conditions that mimic TO
        1. Atherosclerosis
        2. Emboli
        3. Autoimmune diseases
        4. Hypercoagulable states
        5. Diabetes
    ii. Differential diagnosis
        1. SLE, RA, scleroderma
        2. PAN, GCA or Takayasu's

    3. Small-vessel vasculitides

    4. APS

    5. Blood dyscrasias (hyperviscosity syndromes)

    6. Occupational hazards

    7. Hypothenar hammer syndrome and thoracic outlet syndrome

    8. Embolic disease

    9. Premature atherosclerosis

iii. **NO** specific tests

iv. Labs are usually normal

    1. CBC

    2. Liver function tests (LFTs)

    3. UA

    4. Fasting blood glucose

    5. Acute phase reactants

    6. Serologic tests (ANA, RF)

v. ECHO to rule out cardiac thrombi

vi. Arteriogram

    1. Rules out atherosclerosis

    2. Helps confirm the clinical diagnosis

       a. Certain findings are suggestive (though not pathognomonic)

       b. Involvement of small- and medium-sized blood vessels

       c. Most commonly the digital arteries of the fingers and toes

       d. Also involvement of the palmar, plantar, tibial, peroneal, radial, and ulnar arteries

       e. Bilateral focal segments of stenosis or occlusion with normal proximal or intervening vessels

          i. Proximal vessels should have no evidence of artherosclerosis or emboli

          ii. An increase in collateral vessels often occurs around the areas of occlusion

             1. Gives a tree root, spider web, or corkscrew appearance

vii. Pathology

    1. Acute Phase

       a. Biopsies not usually obtained during the acute phase

          i. Fear of ulceration in an ischemic area

       b. Panvasculitis is present

       c. A highly cellular thrombus with microabscesses

    2. Subacute phase

       a. Thrombus is less cellular

       b. Recanalization is apparent

       c. Perivascular fibrosis

    3. Late phase

       a. Organized and recanalized thrombus

       b. Perivascular fibrosis

       c. Internal elastic membrane is preserved

       d. Venulitis is frequently found

viii. Treatment
  1. Complete discontinuation of smoking or tobacco use in any form
    a. Including nicotine replacements
  2. Treatment of local ischemic ulceration
    a. Foot care
    b. Trial of calcium channel blockers and/or pentoxifylline
    c. Iloprost
    d. Sympathectomy
  3. Treat cellulitis with antibiotics
  4. Treat superficial phlebitis with NSAIDS
  5. Amputate when all else fails
  6. Surgical revascularization usually **NOT** an option
    a. Vascular involvement is distal
    b. Appropriate sites for bypass not generally present
    c. Long-term prognosis is poor if attempted

Section B: Wegener's Granulomatosis and Churg-Strauss Vasculitis

1. Distinguishing Pathologic Features
  a. Medium-sized and small vessels are affected
  b. The inflammatory infiltrate can be granulomatous and necrotizing
  c. Associated with the production of antibodies to neutrophil cytoplasmic antigens (ANCA)
    i. Churg-Strauss associated with
      1. Eosinophilia
      2. Atopy
      3. Asthma
2. Wegener's Granulomatosis
  a. A clinicopathologic syndrome of unknown etiology characterized by
    i. Inflammation
      1. Extravascular granulomatous inflammation
      2. Granulomatous vasculitis of predominantly small-sized vessels
      3. Necrosis of the upper and lower respiratory tracts
    ii. Glomerulonephritis
      1. Usually pauci-immune
      2. Focal and segmental
      3. Necrotizing
    iii. Variable involvement of other organ systems
      1. Granulomatous vasculitis of mostly small-sized vessels
      2. Extravascular granulomatous inflammation
      3. Necrosis
    iv. Strong association with C-ANCA and anti-proteinase three antibodies

b. Disease manifestations result from aseptic inflammation and tissue injury
   i. Nonspecific
      1. Pleomorphic infiltrates and necrosis
   ii. Characteristic
      1. Granuloma formation
      2. Vasculitis
   iii. Occur in parenchymal sites outside vessel walls
      1. May be the predominant lesion
c. Etiology remains unknown
   i. No infectious or noninfectious agent identified
   ii. An airborne agent suggested
      1. Disease usually begins with the upper respiratory tract
d. Sites most commonly affected
   i. The upper and lower respiratory tract
   ii. The kidneys (glomerulonephritis)
e. Limited disease
   i. Defined as absence of renal involvement
f. Generalized disease
   i. Implies involvement of all three major end organs
g. Epidemiology
   i. Affects about 1 in 20,000–30,000 people (rare)
   ii. All ages can be affected
      1. Range 5–78
      2. Majority are adults
      3. Mean age at diagnosis 41 years
      4. Only 16% of patients are <18 years
   iii. Male to female ratio 1:1
      1. No significant preferences in regard to gender
   iv. Recognized predominantly in Caucasians (97%)
      1. African Americans about 2–3%
      2. Can occur in all ethnic and racial backgrounds
h. ACR classification
   i. 88% sensitivity and 92% specificity if two or more of the following four criteria are met
      1. Nasal or oral inflammation characterized as oral ulcers or purulent or bloody nasal discharge
      2. Abnormal CXR showing nodules, fixed infiltrates, or cavities
      3. Abnormal urinary sediment showing microhematuria or RBC casts
      4. Characteristic granulomatous inflammation in the wall of an artery or in perivascular/extravascular areas
i. Pathophysiology
   i. Unknown
   ii. **NOT** due to immune complex disease or autoantibodies against structural components

       iii. The presence of granulomata and numerous CD4+ T cells suggests the possibility of cell-mediated immunopathology

       iv. Neutrophils and endothelial cells express proteinase 3 on their surface under certain conditions

          1. Viral or bacterial infections

       v. Anti-proteinase 3 antibodies

          1. Bind to surface proteinase 3 on endothelial cells

          2. Fix complement

          3. Initiate an inflammatory event within vessel walls

          4. Bind and activate neutrophils

j. Prognosis (Natural History)

       i. Highly variable

          1. Mild disease limited to the upper respiratory tract

          2. Fulminant life-threatening involvement of end-organs

       ii. A uniformly fatal disorder if left untreated

          1. Mean survival time of <1 year

       iii. Death from

          1. Respiratory or renal failure

          2. Infection

          3. A complication of treatment

       iv. Mortality prior to the 1970s

          1. Only 50% survived 5 months from the time of diagnosis

          2. 82% died within 1 year

       v. Mortality in 1991 with the NIH treatment protocol

          1. 13% from disease or treatment

k. Differential Diagnosis

       i. Churg-Strauss syndrome

          1. Distinguished by atopy and marked eosinophilia

       ii. Microscopic polyangiitis

          1. Unusual to have destructive airway disease or cavitary pulmonary nodules

          2. No granulomas

       iii. Angiocentric immuno-proliferative lesions (lymphomatoid granulomatosis)

          1. Unusual to see glomerulonephritis

       iv. Pulmonary renal syndromes (SLE or Goodpasture's)

          1. Immunofluorescence show granular deposition or linear deposition

       v. Granulomatous infections

       vi. Intranasal drug abuse

       vii. Pseudovasculitis syndromes (subacute bacterial endocarditis or cholesterol emboli syndrome)

l. Laboratory Features

       i. C-ANCA and anti-proteinase 3 antibodies (95%)

          1. The only specific abnormal lab tests

          2. Sensitivity and specificity 30–90% for C-ANCA

          3. Sensitivity and specificity 98% due to anti-proteinase-3

    ii. Sensitivity related to disease extent, severity, and activity
        1. Limited disease have lower C-ANCA titers and more false-negatives
        2. Titers correlate with disease activity in 60% of cases
        3. A rise in titers of clinically inactive disease can herald an exacerbation
           a. Not seen in an acute infection
           b. Allows distinction between an exacerbation and an infectious process
   iii. ANCA contribution to the development of disease is unknown
        1. IL-1 and TNF-α cause neutrophils to transport serine proteinase 3 (PR3) to their surfaces
        2. C-ANCA can react with PR-3 causing activation of neutrophils
        3. IL-1 and TNF-α upregulate adhesion molecules on endothelial cells, which bind activated neutrophils
        4. Activated neutrophils transmigrate into the vessel wall and cause vasculitis
    iv. Some patients have detectable P-ANCA (5–20%)
     v. Three categories of ANCA
        1. C-ANCA
           a. Characterized by diffuse, coarse, granular, centrally accentuated staining of the neutrophil cytoplasm
           b. Proteinase-3 is the protein nearly always recognized
              i. A neutral serine proteinase in primary azurophil granules
        2. P-ANCA
           a. Characterized by perinuclear cytoplasmic staining
           b. Due in part to an artifact of ethanol fixation of PMN
              i. Altered granule integrity with release of constituents
             ii. Positively charged granule proteins are displaced to the negatively charged nuclear membrane
            iii. Perinuclear rearrangement of charged antigens are prevented by cross-linking fixatives such as formalin
            iv. Allow true P-ANCA to be distinguished from ANA
           c. Myeloperoxidase is the protein recognized most often
              i. Especially in vasculitides
           d. Elastase, cathepsin G, lactoferrin, and B-glucuronidase are less common
        3. Atypical
           a. Those not clearly P- or C-ANCA
           b. Protein target unclear
           c. Common to P-ANCA
    vi. Evaluations for an ANCA-associated vasculitis
        1. Indirect immunofluorescence ANCA
        2. Specific ELISA for proteinase-3 antibodies
        3. Specific ELISA for myeloperoxidase antibodies
   vii. Other pauci-immune disorders associated with C-ANCA

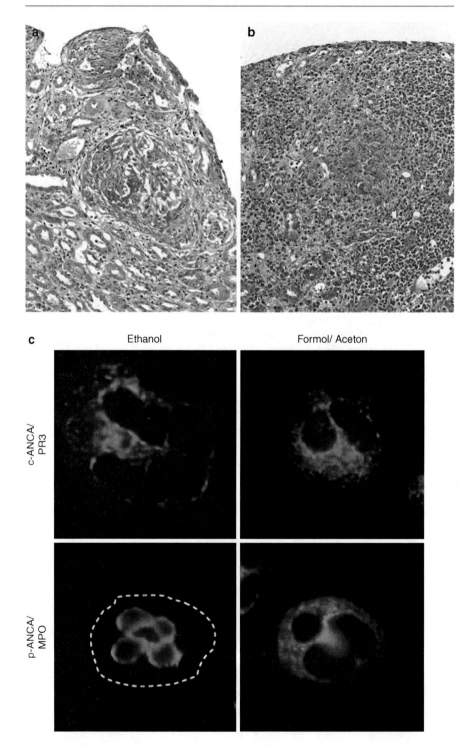

       1. Microscopic polyangiitis
         a. Anti-P3 (15–45%)
         b. Anti-MPO (45–80%)
       2. Idiopathic crescentic glomerulonephritis
         a. Anti-P3 (25%)
         b. Anti-MPO (65%)
   viii. Labs for systemic inflammation and end-organ involvement
       1. Anemia of chronic inflammation
       2. Leuko**cytosis**
       3. Thrombo**cytosis**
       4. Elevation of the ESR
       5. Low serum albumin
       6. Elevated globulin levels
       7. Cytokines
         a. IL-1
         b. IL-6
         c. TNF-α
   ix. Labs for evidence of glomerulonephritis
       1. Hematuria
       2. Pyuria
       3. Cellular casts
       4. Proteinuria
  m. Clinical Features
    i. Joint pain often disproportionate to signs of inflammation
       1. Joint destruction rare
    ii. 25% have peripheral or CNS disease
   iii. Constitutional symptoms
       1. Anorexia
       2. Weight loss
       3. Fatigue
       4. Malaise
       5. Fever
       6. Likely due to circulating cytokines
         a. IL-1
         b. IL-6
         c. TNF-α

Fig. 10.11 (a) Necrotizing glomerulonephritis in ANCA-associated vasculitis. (b) Renal granulomatosis in Wegener's disease. (c) Classical (c)-ANCA/PR3+ and perinuclear (p)-ANCA/MPO+ patterns by indirect immunofluorescence. Left, ethanol-fixed neutrophils and right, formaldehyde–acetone fixed neutrophils (Reproduced with permission from Renal involvement in Wegener's granulomatosis. *Clinical Reviews in Allergy & Immunology.* DOI: 10.1007/s12016-007-8066-6. Springer; 2008-09-02)

Fig. 10.12 Sinusitis in
Wegener's granulomatosis
(Reproduced with permission
from Vasculitides. *Atlas of
Rheumatology.* ImagesMD;
2002-03-07)

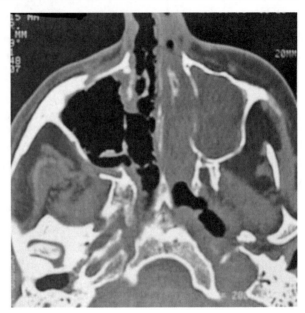

iv. 80–90% develop pulmonary and/or renal disease
v. Upper respiratory tract involvement
   1. Characteristic clinical manifestations secondary to chronic inflammation
     of the mucosa
     a. Granulomatous inflammation
     b. Vasculitis
     c. Necrosis
   2. Nasal, sinus, tracheal, and ear abnormalities are the presenting com-
     plaints in >70%
     a. Up to 90% eventually involved
   3. Chronic paranasal sinusitis (up to 80%)
     a. Most often due to Staph aureus
     b. Due to obstruction of the paranasal sinus ostia
   4. Chronic purulent nasal discharge
   5. Recurrent epistaxis
   6. Mucosal ulcerations
   7. Nasal septal perforation
   8. Nasal deformity (saddle-nose)
   9. Oral ulcers may or may not be painful
  10. Obstruction of the auditory canal
     a. Acute suppurative otitis media
     b. Chronic serous otitis media
     c. New onset otitis media in an adult = WG

Fig. 10.13 Saddle nose deformity in Wegener's granulomatosis (Reproduced with permission from Vasculitides. *Atlas of Rheumatology.* ImagesMD; 2002-03-07)

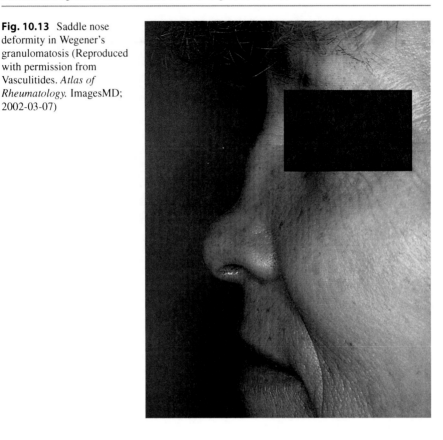

11. Subglottic stenosis
    a. Stridor
    b. Respiratory insufficiency
12. Check for ANCA and/or obtain a biopsy with otolaryngeal involvement and the following
    a. Active urine sediment
    b. Pulmonary abnormalities
    c. Elevated ESR
    d. Unexplained anemia
vi. Pulmonary involvement
    1. Characterized by variable degrees of
       a. Chronic (granulomatous) inflammation
       b. Acute (neutrophilic) inflammation
       c. Necrosis of the alveolar septa
       d. Small blood vessel necrosis
    2. Airways and larger blood vessels involved less commonly
    3. Up to 90% develop lung disease

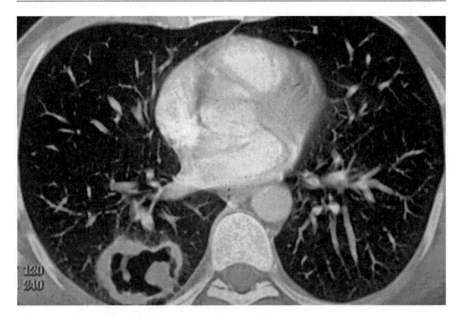

Fig. 10.14 Pulmonary nodules in Wegener's granulomatosis (Reproduced with permission from Vasculitides. *Atlas of Rheumatology.* ImagesMD; 2005-01-18)

4. Infiltrates or nodules present initially in about 50%
   a. Obstruction by nodules or intrabronchial lesions leads to postobstructive suppurative bacterial pneumonia
5. Granulomas typically occur in the extravascular interstitium of the alveolar septa
6. Neutrophil infiltration in
   a. Vessel walls
   b. Extravascular interstitium
   c. Alveolar spaces
7. Chronic fibrinous pleuritis
   a. Inflammation adjacent to the serosal surface of the lung
8. Symptoms
   a. Asymptomatic (one-third)
   b. Chronic cough
   c. Hemoptysis
   d. Alveolar hemorrhage (uncommon)
   e. Acute/subacute pneumonitis (uncommon)
   f. Chronic respiratory insufficiency (uncommon)
   g. Pleuritis (uncommon)
   h. Dyspnea

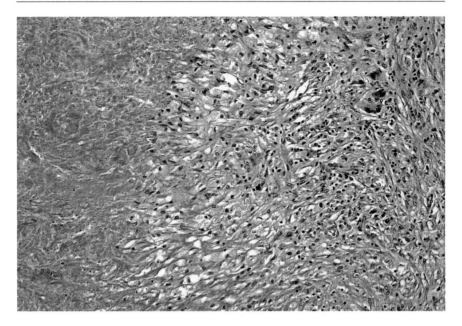

Fig. 10.15 Lung biopsy in Wegener's granulomatosis (Reproduced with permission from Vasculitides. *Atlas of Rheumatology*. ImagesMD; 2002-03-07)

    vii. Renal involvement
        1. Glomerulonephritis (75%)
           a. Typical renal lesion
           b. Pauci-immune
           c. Focal and segmental
           d. Necrotizing
           e. Crescentic in more severe cases
        2. Little or no deposition of
           a. Immunoglobulins
           b. Immune complexes
           c. Complement
        3. Asymptomatic until advanced uremia
        4. Manifests as an "active" urinary sediment with variable degrees of renal function compromise
           a. Hematuria
           b. Pyuria
           c. Proteinuria
           d. Cellular casts
        5. Renal vasculitis less common
           a. Characterized as necrotizing vasculitis
           b. With or without granulomatous infiltration

      6. For early detection of glomerulonephritis
        a. Biweekly dipstick analyses of urine
  viii. Pulmonary-renal syndrome
      1. Prototypic glomerulonephritis and alveolar hemorrhage
        a. Wegener's
        b. Goodpasture's
        c. SLE
      2. Wegener's
        a. Usually negative for Ig deposition
        b. Areas of necrosis may have scant Ig
      3. SLE
        a. Granular (lumpy) deposition of Ig
        b. Characteristic of immune complexes
      4. Goodpasture's
        a. Linear deposition of Ig in the glomerular BM
        b. Circulating anti-basement membrane antibodies bind to epitopes in the glomeruli and alveoli
        c. Antibody-antigen interaction leads to fixation of complement and initiation of inflammation
  ix. Eye
      1. Commonly involved (50%)
      2. Eye involvement may be the initial presentation
      3. Proptosis
        a. Due to infiltrations of the retro-orbital space
          i. Retro-orbital pseudotumor
        b. Affects 15%
        c. May result in loss of visual acuity
          i. Optic nerve impingement
        d. May result in loss of conjugate gaze
          i. Infiltration of the extra-ocular muscles
      4. Less common
        a. Scleritis
        b. Episcleritis
        c. Uveitis
        d. Conjunctivitis
        e. Optic neuritis
        f. Retinal artery thombosis
  x. Skin
      1. Involved in up to 50%
      2. Palpable purpura
        a. Children may be misdiagnosed as HSP
      3. Ulcers
      4. Subcutaneous nodules
      5. Vesicles

      6. Pathology
        a. Necrotizing vasculitis
        b. With or without granulomatous infiltration of vessel walls
        c. Extravascular infiltration
  xi. Musculoskeletal
      1. Arthralgia and myalgia up to 67%
      2. Synovitis less common
        a. Does **not** result in erosive joint disease
  xii. PNS and CNS
      1. Occurs in 15% and 8%, respectively
      2. Mononeuritis multiplex (most common)
      3. Less common
        a. Cranial neuropathy
        b. CVA
        c. Seizures
        d. Diffuse white matter disease due to vasculitis
  xiii. Pericarditis
      1. About 5% of patients
      2. Rarely results in interference with ventricular filling
n. Treatment
  i. Immunosuppressive therapy
      1. Effective at controlling disease progression
      2. May not produce sustained remissions
  ii. The NIH protocol for Wegener's
      1. The standard for critical organ involvement
      2. 1991 Wegener's NIH experience
        a. 158 patients with up to 8 year mean follow-up
        b. Treated with daily cyclophosphamide and corticosteroids
        c. 91% had marked improvement
        d. 75% achieved remission
        e. 44% had remissions of >5 years' duration
        f. 50% of remissions were associated with one or more relapses up
          to 16 years later
  iii. Daily oral cyclophosphamide and high-dose prednisone
      1. Best to induce remission in patients with severe disease
      2. Switch to less toxic medications to maintain remission
  iv. Initial therapy
      1. Cyclophosphamide (2 mg/kg/day, orally)
      2. In combination with prednisone (1 mg/kg/day, orally)
  v. Rapidly progressive disease
      1. Start cyclophosphamide at 3–5 mg/kg/day for 2–3 days
      2. Leukocyte count guides subsequent dosage adjustments
      3. Prednisone from 2 to 15 mg/kg/day for the first few days

    4. Prednisone at 1 mg/kg/day for about 4 weeks
      a. Alternate-day regimen over 1–2 months with a substantial clinical response
      b. Gradual taper over 3–6 months as tolerated
    5. Cyclophosphamide continued for about 1 year after complete clinical response
    6. Persistent C-ANCA positivity even in clinical remission should be maintained on weekly MTX to prevent relapses
    7. Before considering kidney transplant, disease should be under control and the C-ANCA titer low or absent
o. Side effects of long-term daily cyclophosphamide therapy
   i. Bladder cystitis (50%)
   ii. Bladder cancer
    1. 5% at 10-year follow-up and 16% at 15 years
    2. All with previous microscopic or gross hematuria
    3. Cytoscopic examination of the bladder is recommended
      a. Especially if hematuria not clearly due to GN
    4. Urine cytology relatively insensitive
   iii. Myelodysplasia (2%)
   iv. Cancer risk
    1. 2.4 fold increase in all malignancies
    2. 33-fold increase in bladder cancer
    3. 11-fold increase in lymphomas
   v. Severe infections
    1. 50% of patients in the NIH series
    2. 6% developed *Pneumocystis carinii* pneumonia
      a. All were in the earliest phase of treatment
      b. All were lymphopenic
        i. Mean lymphocyte count, 303 cells/mm^3
    3. *Pneumocystis* chemoprophylaxis
      a. Currently recommended during immunosuppression
      b. One double-strength tablet three times a week
      c. Limits recurrent sinus infections
        i. Cause exacerbations of Wegener's
   vi. Infertility
   vii. Mortality
p. Start therapy to prevent osteoporosis with prednisone use
q. Alternative therapeutic approaches
   i. High-dose intravenous (pulse) cyclophosphamide
    1. With daily corticosteroids
    2. May provide substantial initial improvement
    3. Not as effective as daily low-dose therapy in maintaining improvement
      a. Relapses more common
    4. Used in life-threatening disease
      a. Severe diffuse pulmonary infiltrates
      b. Potential or actual ventilator dependency

      c. Rapidly progressive glomerulonephritis
         i. Serum creatinine in excess of 2.5 mg/dl
   ii. Intermittent (weekly) low-dose (15–25 mg) methotrexate
     1. With corticosteroid
     2. Used in non-life-threatening disease with little renal compromise
     3. Reasonable alternative to cyclophosphamide
     4. Initiate MTX at 0.3 mg/kg/week
     5. Gradually increase dose
       a. Not to exceed 25 mg/week
     6. Lower dose for mild to moderate renal impairment
     7. 71% achieved remission within mean period of 4.2 months
     8. 36% subsequently relapsed over a mean period of 29 months
  iii. Induction therapy with daily cyclophosphamide
     1. Disease brought under control in 3–6 months
     2. Followed with maintenance MTX or azathioprine
     3. 80% maintenance of remission for up to 2 years
  iv. Cyclosporin
     1. Used alone or in combination with cyclophosphamide
     2. Not used if significant kidney disease
     3. Does not cause leukopenia
   v. Anti-tumor necrosis factor therapy
     1. High levels of TNF in Wegener's lesions
     2. Not effective alone
     3. Investigated in combination with cyclophosphamide or MTX
3. Principals for Monitoring Cytotoxic Therapy
  a. Leukocyte counts
    i. Guide adjustments of cyclophosphamide, MTX, and azathioprine
    ii. Should not be allowed to drop below 3,500 cells/mm^3
   iii. At early induction monitor about every 3 days
   iv. After counts stabilize, check at intervals no longer than every 2 weeks
    v. Monitor the elderly more frequently
  b. Neutrophil count
    i. Should not be allowed to drop below 1,000–1,500 cells/mm^3
    ii. Reduce dosages when approaching neutropenic levels
  c. Therapeutic benefits do **not** depend on the production of leukopenia or neutropenia
4. Churg-Strauss Syndrome (CSS)
  a. Allergic granulomatosis and angiitis
  b. A granulomatous inflammation of small- and medium-sized vessels
    i. Predilection for smaller arteries, arterioles, capillaries, and venules
    ii. Frequently involving the skin, peripheral nerves, and lungs
   iii. Associated with peripheral eosinophilia
  c. Epidemiology
    i. Analyses are scant
    ii. One UK study estimates annual incidence to be about 3 per million people

        iii. No clear sexual preference

        iv. Any age may be affected

    d. Pathophysiology

        i. Elements important in the pathogenesis

           1. Cytokines that affect the eosinophil (IL-5)

           2. Eosinophil granule proteins

              a. Major basic protein

              b. Cationic protein

        ii. Pathology

           1. Characteristic small necrotizing granulomas and vasculitis of small arteries and veins

           2. Intra- and/or extravascular granulomas

              a. Usually extravascular near small arteries and veins

              b. Highly specific with a central **eosinophilic** core surrounded radially by macrophages and giant cells

                  i. Contrast to a granuloma with **basophilic** core seen in other diseases

           3. Inflammatory lesions rich in eosinophils

        iii. Leukotriene antagonists associated with the precipitation of CSS

           1. Cysteinyl leukotriene type I receptor antagonists

              a. Zafirlukast (Accolate)

              b. Montelukast (Singulair)

              c. Pranlukast

           2. Whether there is a direct cause is controversial

              a. CSS occurs in uniquely susceptible people

              b. Subclinical CSS manifested with corticosteroid withdrawal facilitated by these antagonists

           3. Avoid their use in patients with established CSS

    e. Clinical Features

        i. Primarily in patients with a previous history of allergic manifestations

           1. Acute or chronic paranasal sinus pain or tenderness

           2. Rhinitis (often with nasal polyps) (70%)

           3. Adult-onset asthma (>95%)

        ii. Systemic vasculitis in association with

           1. Eosinophilia

           2. Patchy and shifting pulmonary infiltrates

           3. Allergic rhinitis

         iii. Asthma usually precedes vasculitis by months to many years

           1. In 20% both processes may occur simultaneously

        iv. Lungs

           1. Pleural effusions and diffuse interstitial lung disease

           2. Non-cavitating pulmonary nodules

           3. Pulmonary hemorrhage

        v. Nervous system (60%)

           1. Mononeuritis multiplex

           2. Symmetric polyneuropathy

           3. Rarely CNS

    vi. Skin (50%) (vasculitic phase)
      1. Subcutaneous nodules
      2. Petechiae
      3. Purpura
      4. Infarction
   vii. Joints
      1. Arthralgia
      2. Rarely arthritis
  viii. GI
      1. Abdominal pain
      2. Bloody diarrhea
      3. Abdominal masses
    ix. Distinguished from Wegener's
      1. CSS has a prominent eosinophilia
        a. 10% of peripheral leukocytes
      2. CSS is not a destructive process
      3. CSS more likely to have fleeting infiltrates than pulmonary nodules
      4. CSS pulmonary nodules do not cavitate
      5. CSS more likely to have coronary arteritis, myocarditis, and gut involvement
      6. Cardiac involvement is a major cause of death in CSS
        a. Pulmonary and renal in Wegener's
      7. CSS renal involvement is uncommon
      8. CSS has associated P-ANCA (67%)
        a. C-ANCA in Wegener's (90%)
      9. CSS histology shows eosinophilic necrotizing granuloma
        a. Necrotizing epithelioid granuloma in Wegener's
    x. Three clinical phases (may appear simultaneously)
      1. Prodromal phase
        a. Allergic manifestations of rhinitis, polyposis, and asthma
        b. May persist for years (3–7)
      2. Peripheral blood and tissue eosinophilia
        a. Resembles Loffler's syndrome
        b. Shifting pulmonary infiltrates and eosinophilia
        c. Chronic eosinophilic pneumonia
        d. Eosinophilic gastroenteritis
        e. May remit or recur over years
      3. Life-threatening systemic vasculitis
        a. Asthma may abruptly abate going into this stage
f. Laboratory abnormalities
    i. Eosinophilia
      1. Characteristic abnormality
      2. No direct correlation between degree of eosinophilia and disease activity
   ii. Anemia
  iii. Elevated ESR

      iv. Elevated IgE

      v. P-ANCA present in 67%

         1. Directed primarily against myeloperoxidase

  g. Diagnosis

      i. Previous history of allergy or asthma

      ii. Eosinophilia (> 1,500/mm^3)

      iii. Systemic vasculitis involving two or more organs

      iv. Corroborate with biopsy of involved tissue

  h. Treatment

      i. High-dose prednisone (1 mg/kg/day)

         1. Usually a prompt response

      ii. Cytotoxic agents

         1. Cyclophosphamide

         2. Reserved for severe, progressive disease

            a. Kidneys

            b. Gut

            c. Heart

            d. Lungs (diffuse pulmonary hemorrhage)

      iii. Interferon alpha

         1. 7.5–63 million units per week

         2. Beneficial in those who fail cytotoxic therapy

  i. Prognosis

      i. 5 year survival rate 78%

      ii. Cardiac involvement is the major cause of death (50%)

         1. MI

         2. CHF

Section C: Giant Cell Arteritis, Polymyalgia Rheumatica and Takayasu's Arteritis

1. Characteristics of giant cell arteritis (GCA) and Takayasu's arteritis (TA)
   a. Inflammatory attack on vessel walls
   b. Tissue tropism for defined vascular territories
      i. GCA
         1. Predominant in the aortic second- to fifth-order branches
         2. Often involve the extracranial arteries of the head
         3. Less often involves the aorta
      ii. TA
         1. The aorta and its major branches are prime targets
2. Giant Cell Arteritis
   a. Epidemiology
      i. Almost exclusively in individuals older than 50 years
         1. Incidence increases with age
         2. Almost ten times more common in the 80s

Giant cell arteritis: 5 criteria	Takayasu's arteritis: 6 criteria
Age at onset of disease ≥ 50 yr	Age at onset of disease ≤40 yr
New headache	Claudication of an extremity
Temporal artery abnormality	Decreased brachial artery pulse
Elevated erythrocyte sedimentation rate	Difference in systolic blood pressure between arms
Abnormal findings on biopsy of temporal artery	A bruit over the subclavian arteries or the aorta
	Arteriographic evidence of narrowing or occlusion of the entire aorta
Diagnosis: at least 3/5 criteria	Diagnosis: at least 3/6 criteria
Sensitivity =93.5%	Sensitivity =90.5%
Specificity =91.2%	Specificity =97.8%

Fig. 10.16 The American College of Rheumatology 1990 criteria for the classification of giant cell arteritis and Takayasu's arteritis (Reproduced with permission from Imaging of large vessel vasculitis with 18FDG PET: illusion or reality? A critical review of the literature data. *European Journal of Nuclear Medicine and Molecular Imaging.* DOI: 10.1007/s00259-003-1209-y. Springer; 2003-09-01)

    ii. Women affected twice more likely than men
   iii. Siblings of a patient with GCA at 10-fold increased risk
   iv. Highest prevalence in Scandinavian countries and of Northern European descent
      1. Incidence 15–25 cases per 100,000 aged ≥50 years
    v. Less frequent in Southern Europeans
      1. Incidence six cases per 100,000 individuals
   vi. Rare in blacks and Hispanics
      1. Incidence 1–2 cases per 100,000 individuals
 b. Etiology and pathogenesis
    i. Lesion characteristics
      1. Patchy or segmental arterial involvement
      2. **Fragmented internal elastic lamina**
   ii. Histologic hallmarks
      1. Mononuclear cell infiltrate
        a. Lack a complex organization
      2. Dominated by **T lymphocytes and macrophages**
      3. All layers of the arterial wall are penetrated
   iii. Two major histological patterns
      1. Granulomatous
        a. Mononuclear infiltrate
        b. Fragmentation of the internal elastic membrane
        c. Accumulation of histiocytes and multinucleated giant cells
        d. Multinucleated giant cells
          i. Occur in two thirds of the cases
          ii. Lie in close proximity to the fragmented internal elastic lamina
          iii. Active secretory cells

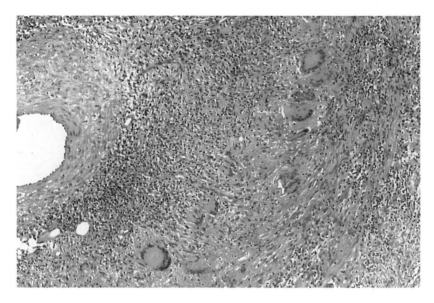

Fig. 10.17 Temporal artery biopsy in giant cell arteritis (Reproduced with permission from Vasculitides. *Atlas of Rheumatology.* ImagesMD; 2002-03-07)

        iv. Correlates with increased risk for ischemic complications

        v. Corresponds to high adventitial levels of IFN-γ

    2. Nonspecific panarteritis with mixed inflammatory infiltrate

      a. Composed largely of lymphocytes and macrophages

      b. Admixed with some neutrophils and eosinophils

      c. No giant cells

  iv. Other histological changes

    1. Perivascular cuffing of the vasa vasorum

    2. T-cell-macrophage infiltrates in the adventitia

      a. Along the external elastic lamina

      b. Studies suggest the adventitia is a critical site in the disease process

  v. Structural changes to the arterial wall

    1. Medial smooth muscle cell layer loses thickness

    2. Hyperplastic intima

      a. Compromises or occludes the lumen

    3. Luminal thrombosis is uncommon

    4. Fragmentation of the elastic laminae

  vi. Immune response in the arterial wall

    1. Experimental evidence supports a T cell mediated immunopathology

      a. Primarily **CD4+ T-lymphocytes of Th1 type**

        i. 25% activated

      b. Vasa vasorum is the site of entrance

2. Humoral immunity **not** important with absence of
   a. B-cells
   b. Pathognomonic antibodies
   c. Hypergammaglobulinemia
3. Animal model
   a. Human temporal arteries implanted into SCID mice
   b. Inflammatory response disrupted with depletion of T-cells
   c. IFN-γ from CD4+ cells of the adventitia critical to regulatory control
4. Macrophages also important in the pathogenesis
   a. In the adventitia produce
      i. IL-1
      ii. IL-6
      iii. TGF-β
   b. In the medial layer produce
      i. Metalloproteinases
         1. Oxidative injury by oxygen radicals
         2. Lipid peroxidation on medial smooth-muscle cells
   c. In the intimal layer produce
      i. Nitric oxide synthase 2
         1. Tissue injury
         2. Cellular activation
         3. Vascular remodeling

vii. Systemic immune response
   1. Highly activated monocytes produce IL-1 and IL-6
   2. IL-6
      a. A potent inducer of the acute phase response
      b. An independent disease manifestation apart from vessel involvement

c. Clinical disease related to nonthrombotic luminal occlusion
   i. Rapid and concentric growth of the intima
      1. Intimal hyperplasia generated by the mobilization of smooth-muscle cells
   ii. PDGF from macrophages support out-growth
      1. Patients with low PDGF have minimal or no lumen-occlusive intimal proliferation
      2. Patients with high PDGF are at risk for ischemic complications
   iii. Formation of new capillaries
      1. Intense neoangiogenesis induced in GCA
      2. VEGF from macrophages leads to profound structural arterial abnormalities
      3. Subsequent stenosis and tissue ischemia
   iv. Regulation of aldose reductase
      1. Protective response aimed at healing and tissue repair
      2. Metabolizes and detoxifies end products of oxidative damage

   d. Genetic risk factors
      i. High incidence rates in regions of Scandinavian ethnicity
      ii. HLA-DR4 haplotypes
         1. Associated with increased disease risk (60–70%)
         2. Several allelic variants are enriched among patients
      iii. HLA polymorphisms **not** correlated with disease severity (unlike RA)
      iv. HLA-DRB1 may confer increased susceptibility
   e. Clinical features
      i. Suspect in individuals with
         1. Age over 50
         2. A new type of headache
         3. Jaw claudication
         4. Unexplained fever
         5. Polymyalgia rheumatica
      ii. Two major symptomatic complexes
         1. Signs of vascular insufficiency resulting from impaired blood flow
         2. Signs of systemic inflammation
   f. Two major diagnostic variants
      i. Cranial GCA (20%)
         1. Extracranial branches of the carotid arteries
            a. Targeted preferentially (80–90%)
         2. Intracranial arteries
            a. Lack an internal elastic lamina
            b. Involvement is unusual
         3. Arteries most frequently involved
            a. Superficial temporal
            b. Vertebral
            c. Ophthalmic
            d. Posterior ciliary arteries
         4. Arteries less frequently involved
            a. Internal and external carotid
            b. Central retinal arteries
         5. Headaches
            a. Throbbing, sharp or dull
            b. Often severe enough to prompt evaluation
            c. The most common presenting clinical manifestation
            d. May or may not be associated with scalp tenderness
            e. In most cases the headache will cease promptly in response to corticosteroid therapy
         6. Temporal artery abnormalities
            a. A reduction in the pulse in conjunction with palpable tenderness
               i. The greatest sensitivity for diagnosis
            b. Vessels are thickened, tender and nodular
            c. Pulses are reduced or absent

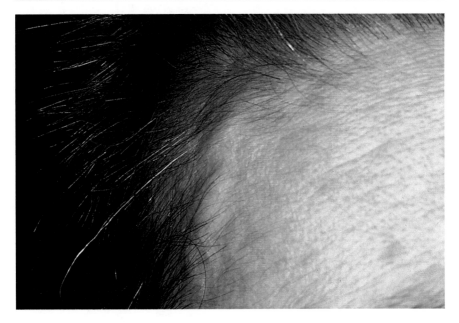

Fig. 10.18 Temporal artery in giant cell arteritis (Reproduced with permission from Vasculitides. *Atlas of Rheumatology*. ImagesMD; 2002 03-07)

    d. Most frequently in the temporal arterial branches

    e. In one third the temporal arteries appear normal

7. Vision abnormalities

    a. Focal arteritic lesions in the ophthalmic artery

    b. Without visual loss

       i. One of the five most common presenting clinical manifestations

    c. Lends additional support for the diagnosis

    d. Less sensitive than temporal artery involvement

    e. Prompt recognition and treatment prevents blindness

    f. Blindness occurs in less than 1% after corticosteroid therapy started

    g. Loss of vision

       i. Sudden, painless, and usually permanent

       ii. Occurs in 15% of patients

       iii. Can be an early symptom

       iv. Ischemic optic neuropathy the most common cause

       v. Posterior ciliary branches of the ophthalmic arteries

         1. Most common anatomic lesions

       vi. Retinal and ophthalmic artery thromboses

         1. Relatively less common

    h. Amaurosis fugax

       i. A warning sign that may precede blindness for months

       ii. A fleeting visual blurring with heat or exercise

       iii. Posture-related visual blurring and diplopia

    i. Ophthalmologic exam
      i. Optic-disc edema
      ii. Sectoral or generalized optic atrophy
      iii. Optic-disc cupping
    j. Spectrum of ophthalmic complications
      i. Pupillary defects
      ii. Orbital ischemia
      iii. Ocular motor ischemia with ophthalmoplegia
      iv. Anterior- and posterior-segment ischemia
      v. Iritis
      vi. Conjunctivitis
      vii. Scintillating scotomata
      viii. Photophobia
      ix. Glaucoma
8. Claudication of the masseter and temporalis muscles
  a. Relatively disease-specific manifestation
  b. Present in about one-half of patients
  c. Caused by compromised blood flow in the extracranial branches of the carotid
  d. Intermittent jaw claudication and even trismus with prolonged talking and chewing
  e. Claudication of the tongue and painful dysphagia (less frequent)
9. Vasoocclusive disease of the carotid and vertebrobasilar arteries
  a. TIAs
  b. Strokes
  c. Seizures
  d. Acute hearing loss
  e. Vertigo
  f. Cerebral dysfunction
  g. Depression

ii. GCA involving **both** large and medium-sized vessels
1. Neurological manifestations (20–30%)
2. Absent pulses with subclavian involvement
3. Hypertension with renal artery involvement
4. Angina pectoris with coronary involvement
5. Lower extremity claudication with iliac involvement
6. Abdominal pain with mesenteric involvement
7. Vasculitis of the pulmonary artery branches
  a. Respiratory symptoms
    i. Cough
    ii. Chronic, nonproductive cough can be an initial presentation
    iii. Hoarseness
    iv. Chest pain
  b. Frank pulmonary infiltrates (rare)

   8. Skin manifestations (rare)
      a. Small-artery involvement uncommon
   9. Clinical presentations in about 5% of patients
      a. Cough
      b. Claudication (upper > lower)
      c. Synovitis
iii. GCA as Fever of Unknown Origin (FUO) (15%)
   1. Fever and systemic symptoms without any localized symptoms
   2. Spiking temperatures and chills prompt a FUO work-up
   3. Symptoms
      a. Low-grade fever
      b. Malaise
      c. Anorexia
      d. Weight loss
      e. Fatigue
   4. Symptoms of vascular insufficiency can be absent
   5. Physical exam of the scalp arteries often negative
iv. Large-vessel variant GCA
   1. Large arteries targeted in 10–15%
   2. Arteries most frequently involved
      a. Carotid
      b. Subclavian
      c. Axillary arteries
   3. Arteries less frequently involved
      a. Femoral arteries
   4. Lack evidence of cranial involvement
      a. Do not complain of headaches
   5. Temporal arteries
      a. Appear normal on exam
      b. Almost 50% of biopsies are negative for vasculitis
   6. Angiography
      a. Diagnostic procedure of choice
   7. PET scan
      a. May suggest aortic involvement
      b. Even if not detected clinically
   8. Stenotic vascular lesions
      a. Typically located at the subclavian axillary junction
      b. Unilateral
   9. Aortic arch syndrome
      a. The major clinical presentation
      b. Claudication of the arms
      c. Absent or asymmetrical pulses
      d. Paresthesias
      e. Raynaud's phenomenon

            f. Peripheral gangrene

            g. Aortitis can coexist with cranial arteritis

        10. Thoracic aortic aneurysm

            a. A 17 fold increased risk

            b. Elastic membranes destroyed

                i. Replaced by fibrotic tissue

            c. Clinical spectrum

                i. Silent aneurysm

                ii. Aortic dissection

                iii. Fatal rupture

  g. Laboratory features

      i. A pathognomonic laboratory test does not exist

      ii. Acute phase reactants

        1. Typically highly elevated

      iii. ESR

        1. The most useful laboratory test

        2. A sensitive indicator of GCA

        3. Specificity <50%

        4. Tends to be higher in GCA than other vasculitides

            a. Almost always >50 mm/h

            b. Averages 80–100 mm/h (Westergren method)

        5. May be normal (rare)

            a. Associated with corticosteroid treatment for other conditions (polymyalgia rheumatica (PMR))

      iv. CRP

        1. Elevated levels may be more sensitive for the acute phase response

        2. Frequently at high levels (>10 mg/dl)

      v. IL-6 (serum)

        1. Marker with the highest sensitivity for detecting ongoing systemic inflammation

        2. Taken before and after corticosteroid therapy

        3. A strong inducer of acute phase reactants

      vi. Anemia

        1. Mild to moderate

        2. Normochromic or hypochromic

      vii. Platelet counts

        1. Commonly elevated

      viii. Liver function tests

        1. Abnormal alkaline phosphatase

  h. Diagnosis

      i. Suspect in individuals with

        1. Age 50 years or older

        2. Recent onset of unexplained headache

        3. Signs of tissue ischemia in extracranial vascular territory

        4. Loss of vision

    5. PMR
    6. Laboratory evidence for acute phase response
  ii. Biopsy
    1. Histological proof of arteritis
    2. Technique of choice
    3. Defines the need for therapy in 80–85%
    4. Sites
      a. Clinically abnormal arteries preferred
      b. Usually superficial temporal artery
      c. Patients with posterior headaches
        i. Positive superficial occipital artery biopsy
    5. Hampered by patchy or segmental arterial involvement
    6. Minimize the rate of false-negatives
      a. Take a sufficient length
        i. 3–6 cm
      b. Examine serial sections
        i. Slice like salami at 1–2 mm intervals
      c. Biopsy contralateral artery when first is negative
        i. Positive in 10–15% of cases
      d. Biopsy within 7 days of starting therapy
    7. Pitfalls in histological exams
      a. Up to 40% show diffuse lymphocytic infiltrate
        i. Without granulomas or giant cells
      b. An inflammatory infiltrate is needed to diagnose temporal arteritis
      c. Fragmentation of the internal elastic lamina is also a feature of aging arteries
      d. Diagnosis of healed temporal arteritis
        i. Intimal fibrosis
        ii. Medial scarring
        iii. Eccentric destruction of the internal elastic lamina
        iv. Corticosteroid therapy eliminates the inflammatory infiltrate
  iii. Angiography
    1. May support the diagnosis in the absence of a confirmatory biopsy
    2. Utilized in the presence of extracranial involvement
    3. Documents vasoocclusive disease
  iv. CT and MRI
    1. Sensitive enough to detect wall abnormalities
  v. Color duplex ultrasound and PET
    1. Utilized for diagnostic confirmation
i. Treatment
  i. Corticosteroids
    1. The cornerstone of therapy
    2. Initial doses of 60 mg/day
    3. Maintain high doses until reversible disease has responded

    4. Alternate-day regimens **not** effective

    5. Cannot reverse intimal hyperplasia

    6. Reduces ischemic insult by reducing tissue edema

  ii. Early therapy advocated

    1. Decreases the rate of GCA-related blindness

    2. Start before biopsy in cases of

      a. Visual loss

      b. Stroke

      c. Angina

    3. High dose corticosteroids started within 24 h

      a. Reversed sudden blindness and stroke-like events

      b. 1 g of IV methylprednisolone daily for 3 days

    4. Biopsies show arteritis after more than 14 days of therapy

 iii. Therapeutic response

    1. Complete relief within 12–48 h in almost all patients

    2. Localized manifestations of arteritis may take longer

      a. Headaches

      b. Scalp tenderness

      c. Jaw or tongue claudication

    3. An excellent response suggested as a diagnostic criterion

  iv. Medication taper

    1. When symptoms and laboratory evidence of inflammation have subsided

      a. Particularly the ESR has normalized

    2. Dose may be tapered by 10% every 1–2 weeks

    3. A typical taper

      a. By 5 mg every 1–2 weeks to 30 mg qd

      b. By 2.5 mg every 1–2 weeks to 15 mg qd

      c. By 2.5 mg every 4 weeks to 7.5 mg daily

      d. By 2.5 mg every 12 weeks until off

    4. Consider additional immunosuppressants

      a. If unable to tolerate tapering

      b. Remission not achieved

    5. Low-dose weekly pulse methotrexate

      a. Instituted with corticosteroids

      b. May allow more rapid tapers

  v. Discontinuing medications

    1. Continue for at least 6 months

    2. Often low-dose prednisone is needed for years

      a. Up to 40%

      b. Especially women

    3. Discontinuing too early associated with worsening of disease activity

  vi. Relapses are common

    1. Up to 60% of patients throughout the course of treatment

       2. Can occur several years after the completion of an appropriate therapeutic regimen

       3. Requires chronic monitoring and management

       4. Typically see symptoms of systemic inflammation

       a. No vascular complications

       5. IL-6

          a. The most sensitive in detecting inflammation prior to and during therapy

          b. Remains elevated after discontinuing therapy

          c. Indicates smoldering disease

   vii. No other rheumatic immunosuppressant useful in treating GCA

       1. Methotrexate's role as a steroid sparing agent is unclear

       2. Anti-TNF therapy being investigated

  viii. Limit corticosteroid side-effects

       1. Calcium and vitamin D therapy

       2. Bisphosphonates for osteoporosis

       3. Histologic or angiographic verification of vasculitis

  j. Prognosis

    i. Significant morbidity relates to reduced blood flow

       1. Eye

       2. Optic nerve

       3. Brain

    ii. Within the first 4 months of starting therapy

       1. Risk of death increased (3×)

   iii. After 4 months or therapy

       1. Mortality similar to age-matched general population

   iv. Typically die of vascular complications (MI)

    v. Increased prevalence (17×) of thoracic aortic aneurysm and aortic dissection

       1. Follow closely for new aortic insufficiency murmurs

       2. Surgery indications

          a. When the aneurysm enlarges to greater than 5 cm

          b. Dissection

3. Polymyalgia Rheumatica (PMR)

  a. A clinical diagnosis in patients with the following presentation

    i. Age > 50 years

    ii. Bilateral pain and stiffness in muscles of the (2 of 3 areas)

       1. Neck

       2. Shoulder girdle

       3. Pelvic girdle

   iii. Symptoms present for at least 4 weeks

   iv. Signs of systemic inflammation

       1. Malaise

       2. Weight loss

        3. Sweats
        4. Low-grade fever
     v. Laboratory abnormalities of an acute phase response
        1. Elevated ESR (>40 mm/h)
        2. Elevated CRP
        3. Anemia
        4. Pathognomonic test not available
     vi. Prompt response to corticosteroid therapy
        1. Prednisone 10–15 mg/daily
        2. Considered a diagnostic criterion
     vii. Exclusion of other diagnoses in the differential
        1. Except temporal arteritis
b. **"SECRET"** clinical features
     i. **S**=Stiffness and pain
     ii. **E**=Elderly individuals
     iii. **C**=Constitutional symptoms, Caucasians
     iv. **R**=Arthritis (rheumatism)
     v. **E**=Elevated erythrocyte sedimentation rate (ESR)
     vi. **T**=Temporal arteritis
c. Pathomechanisms closely related to GCA
     i. Considered a form of GCA that lacks fully developed vasculitis
d. Epidemiology
     i. Mean age of onset about 70 years
        1. Rarely affects those under age 50
        2. More common with increasing age
        3. Most are >60 years
     ii. Women affected twice as often as men
     iii. Largely affects white populations
        1. High risk include those of Scandinavian and Northern European descent
        2. Whites in the southern USA less frequently affected than those of the northern states
        3. Uncommon in black, Hispanic, Asian, and Native Americans
     iv. Two fold to threefold more frequent than GCA
     v. Annual incidence rates
        1. In high risk populations estimated at 20–53 per 100,000
           a. Persons older than 50 years
        2. In low risk populations (Italians) about 10 cases per 100,000
e. Etiology and pathogenesis
     i. No causative agent has been identified
        1. Despite the sudden onset of intense inflammation
     ii. Association with aging is unclear
     iii. PMR considered a GCA variant
        1. PMR noted in 40–60% of temporal arteritis (TA) patients
           a. May be the initial symptom in 20%

     2. TA may occur in patients with PMR
       a. Histologic evidence of TA seen in patients with no clinical evidence of arteritis
       b. PET scans show increased uptake in the aorta of PMR patients with subclinical arteritis
       c. Scandinavia studies show TA to occur in 50% of PMR patients
         i. 20% in North America with coexistent TA
     3. Genetic risk factors same as GCA
       a. HLA polymorphisms (HLA-DR4)
   iv. Temporal artery biopsies from patients with PMR
     1. In situ transcription of proinflammatory cytokines
     2. Typical infiltrates **not** identified on histomorphology
     3. Lack tissue production of IFN-γ
       a. Could be the critical event that would transform subclinical vasculitis into arteritis
   v. Immune system's role in the pathogenesis
     1. No immune defect or characteristic antibody identified
     2. Highly activated monocytes spontaneously produce IL-1 and IL-6
 f. Clinical features
   i. Typical pain and stiffness
     1. Usually involve more than one area
       a. Neck
       b. Shoulders
       c. Pelvic girdle
     2. Onset can be both abrupt and insidious
     3. Myalgia are symmetrical
     4. Initially affect the shoulders
     5. Magnitude of the pain limits mobility
     6. Dramatic stiffness and gelling phenomena
     7. Night pain common
     8. Complain of muscle weakness due to the pain and stiffness
   ii. Weight loss
   iii. Anorexia
   iv. Malaise
   v. Depression
   vi. Synovitis
     1. 31% in one series followed over 16 years
     2. Frequently involved joints
       a. Hips and shoulders
         i. Difficult to detect
         ii. Possible cause of proximal pain and stiffness
       b. Knee effusions
         i. Can be large (30–150 ml)
         ii. Inflammatory
         iii. Poor mucin clot

           iv. Leukocyte count varies
              1. 1,000–20,000 cell/mm^3
           v. Culture and crystals negative
        c. Wrist synovitis
          i. Often associated with CTS
        d. Sternoclavicular synovitis
     3. Demonstrated by
        a. Scintigraphic evidence of axial synovitis
        b. Clinical observation
        c. Synovial fluid analysis
        d. Synovial biopsy
  vii. Peripheral arthritis
     1. Presents with pitting edema (38%)
     2. Initial presentation or occur later
     3. Often polyarticular
 viii. Tenosynovitis and bursitis
     1. Demonstrated by MRI as a source of symptoms
   ix. Diffuse edema of the hands and feet
     1. Seen in men
    x. Physical exam
     1. Findings less striking than history would suggest
     2. May appear chronically ill
     3. Neck and shoulders often tender
     4. Shoulder ROM
        a. Active ROM (AROM) limited by pain
        b. Passive ROM (PROM) limited by capsular contracture and muscle atrophy
     5. Manual motor testing confounded by pain
   xi. A heterogeneous syndrome
     1. Disease that is mild and responds promptly to therapy
        a. Monophasic
     2. Disease that remits within a few months
        a. Remittive
     3. Disease that requires higher than typical initial doses of steroids
  xii. Symptoms mimicked by
     1. Other arthropathies
     2. Shoulder disorders
     3. Inflammatory myopathies
        a. Elevated CK
        b. Abnormal EMG
        c. Weakness predominates
     4. Hypothyroidism
        a. Elevated TSH
        b. Normal ESR
     5. Parkinson's

     6. Malignancies
       a. Clinical evidence of neoplasm
       b. No association of cancer with PMR
     7. Infections
       a. Clinical suspicion of infection
       b. Positive cultures
     8. Fibromyalgia syndrome
       a. Tender points
       b. Normal ESR
     9. Depression
       a. Normal ESR
    10. Rheumatoid arthritis
       a. Often difficult to distinguish from PMR
       b. Response to corticosteroids is **NOT** a reliable distinguishing feature
       c. Features that support PMR
         i. Negative RF
         ii. Lack of involvement of small joints of hands and feet
         iii. Lack of joint damage
         iv. Absence of erosive disease
    11. GCA
       a. Consider a temporal artery biopsy with features that support GCA
         i. Pyrexia and chills
         ii. Arteries on exam
           1. Enlarged
           2. Tender
         iii. Signs of vascular insufficiency
           1. Claudication in the extremities
           2. Bruits over arteries
           3. Discrepant blood pressure readings
         iv. Failure of prednisone (15–20 mg/day) to
           1. Significantly improve symptoms
           2. Normalize the ESR/CRP within 1 month
       b. A negative temporal artery biopsy doses **not** exclude the possibility of large-vessel vasculitis
         i. Subclavian
         ii. Axillary
         iii. Aorta
   g. Laboratory
     i. Elevated ESR
       1. Often >100 mm/h
       2. The characteristic finding
       3. May be normal or mildly elevated
     ii. Abnormalities reflecting the systemic response
       1. Normochromic normocytic anemia
       2. Thrombocytosis

       3. Increased gamma globulins
       4. Elevated acute phase reactants
  iii. Abnormal LFT's
       1. Seen in up to a one-third of patients
       2. Increased alkaline phosphatase level (most common)
  iv. Normal
       1. Renal function
       2. UA
       3. CK
   v. Negative ANA and RF
h. Treatment
   i. Corticosteroids
       1. Doses for long-term treatment are low
       2. Single daily doses more effective than alternate-day dosing
       3. Steroid requirements vary among patients
       4. Prednisone 20 mg/day
         a. Two thirds of patients respond
         b. Usually evokes a dramatic and rapid response
           i. Most improve within 1–2 days
       5. Taper dose with resolution of symptoms
         a. 2.5 mg every 10–15 days
         b. Patient's response is the most reliable parameter
           i. Symptoms
           ii. ESR
           iii. CRP
         c. Taper by 1 mg increments
           i. When daily doses reach 7–8 mg
       6. Dosages up to 40 mg/day
         a. Persistently elevated inflammatory markers on 20 mg/day
         b. For those at higher risk to develop GCA
       7. Discontinuing prednisone
         a. Observe the patient for about 1 year after a dose of about 5 mg/day
           is attained
         b. Taper prednisone by 1 mg every 1–2 months
           i. If no evidence of disease recurrence
         c. Relapses
           i. Unusual
           ii. Small increases in dose
           iii. Further tapering again after a period of 6 months to 1 year
       8. Some require low doses for extended periods
       9. Steroid-sparing medications
         a. No data
         b. May use MTX
  ii. NSAIDs
       1. Effective in only 10–20% of patients

       2. Best for those with mild symptoms

       3. Selection based on tolerability and safety

          a. Especially in the elderly

       4. Add to glucocorticoid therapy to facilitate steroid tapering

    iii. Other therapies

       1. Reassurance

       2. Patient education

       3. Regular physician monitoring

       4. Range of motion exercises

          a. Especially with atrophy and contracture

       5. Attention to glucocorticoid side effects

          a. Especially osteoporosis

  i. Prognosis

    i. Good

    ii. Majority are self-limiting

    iii. Frequent relapses

       1. 70% of 246 patients on prednisone after 2 years

       2. Some require prednisone up to 10 years

       3. Relapses occur in up to 29%

       4. ESR not as high as with the original presentation

    iv. Those that present with typical symmetrical polyarthritis

       1. May fulfill the criteria for RA

       2. May require DMARDs

4. Takayasu's Arteritis

  a. A vasculitis of the large elastic arteries

    i. Specifically the aorta and its main branches

    ii. "Aortic arch syndrome"

    iii. Coronary and pulmonary arteries

  b. Patchy disappearance of the elastic smooth-muscle layer

    i. Results in stenosis or aneurysm

    ii. Upper extremity artery occlusion results in loss of pulse

    iii. "Pulseless disease"

    iv. "Occlusive thromboaortopathy"

  c. Epidemiology

    i. One case per million persons annually (rare)

    ii. Affects primarily adolescent girls and young women

    iii. Average age 10–30 years

    iv. Can occur in younger and much older individuals

    v. Eight times more common among women than men

    vi. Incidence highest in Asia

       1. Japan

       2. Korea

       3. China

       4. India

       5. Thailand

     vii. Most commonly in Asian females
    viii. Reported worldwide in all racial groups
        1. South American countries have relatively high incidence
  d. Pathogenesis
     i. A granulomatous focal polyarteritis
        1. Granulomas and giant cells predominantly in the media
    ii. Focal "skip lesions" are common (like GCA)
   iii. Adventitia
        1. Characterized by striking thickening
        2. Intense perivascular infiltrates around the adventitia and vasa vasorum
          a. GCA infiltrates are around the inner half of the media
    iv. Media layer
        1. Elastic smooth-muscle cells destroyed in a centripetal direction
        2. Replaced by fibrotic tissue
     v. Intima
        1. Proliferation of the intima
        2. Occlusion of the lumen
          a. Smooth tapering
          b. Narrowing
          c. Complete
        3. Occasionally see thombosis
  e. Etiology
     i. Remains unknown
    ii. No conclusive evidence for infectious organisms
   iii. CD8+ T-cells are a major cell type
        1. Distinguishes these vascular infiltrates from GCA
        2. Smooth-muscle cells damaged by release of pore-forming enzymes
          a. Perforin
          b. Granzyme B
        3. Selective HLA class I molecules are over represented
          a. Specifically HLA-B52
        4. There is **NO** link to HLA-DR4 as seen in GCA
    iv. Role of CD4+ and macrophage effector functions are not understood
  f. Clinical features
     i. Caused by two major components of the disease
        1. Syndrome of generalized inflammation
          a. Fever
          b. Night sweats
          c. Malaise
          d. Anorexia
          e. Weight loss
          f. Diffuse myalgias
          g. Can be misdiagnosed as infection

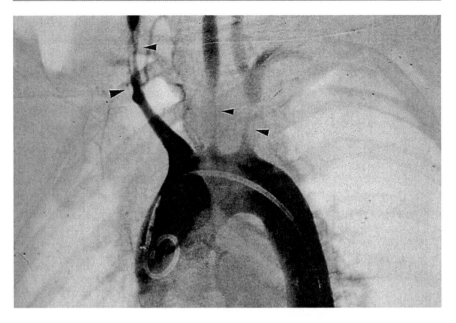

Fig. 10.19 Angiographic findings in Takayasu's arteritis (Reproduced with permission from Cerebrovascular disease. *Atlas of Clinical Neurology*. ImagesMD; 2002-01-24)

        2. Manifestations of vascular insufficiency
           a. Pain over involved arteries
     ii. A triphasic pattern of progression
        1. Phase I
           a. Pre-pulseless inflammatory period
           b. Nonspecific systemic complaints
              i. Fever
              ii. Arthralgia
              iii. Weight loss
           c. Diagnosed as a prolonged viral syndrome
           d. A frequent presentation for <20 years of age
        2. Phase II
           a. Vessel inflammation
           b. Dominated by vessel pain and tenderness
        3. Phase III
           a. Fibrotic stage
           b. Bruits and ischemia predominate
  g. Clinical patterns
     i. No symptoms but incidental findings (10%)
        1. Unequal pulses/blood pressures
        2. Bruits
        3. Hypertension

   ii. Carotid and vertebral arteries
      1. Neurologic and ophthalmologic symptoms
      2. Dizziness
      3. Tinnitus
      4. Headaches
      5. Syncope
      6. Stroke
      7. Visual disturbances
  iii. Inflammatory occlusion of the subclavian
      1. Arm claudication
      2. Pulselessness
      3. Discrepant blood pressures
   iv. Aortitis
      1. Cardiac disease (10%)
         a. Ischemic coronary disease
         b. Coronary arteries directly or indirectly involved
      2. Arrhythmias
      3. Congestive heart failure
      4. Aortic regurgitation
         a. From aortic wall dilation
         b. Occurs in up to 15% of patients
      5. Sudden death
    v. Aortic arch and descending thoracic aorta
      1. Progressively enlarging aneurysms
      2. Possible rupture
   vi. Abdominal aorta including the renal arteries and mesenteric arteries
      1. Renovascular hypertension
      2. More frequent in some ethnic groups
         a. Indians
         b. Chinese
         c. Koreans
      3. GI symptoms
         a. Nausea
         b. Vomiting
         c. Ischemic bowel disease
  vii. The aortic arch and abdominal aorta are most commonly affected
 viii. Pulmonary artery
      1. Up to 70% involved
      2. 25% have symptoms of pulmonary hypertension
   ix. Other common clinical features
      1. Arthralgia (50%)
      2. Asymmetric blood pressure (50%)
      3. Constitutional symptoms (40%)
      4. Erythema nodosum (8%)

Fig. 10.20 Aortic-renal angiography shows multiple small stenoses and dilatations affecting the right renal artery and the abdominal aorta in a milder degree (Reproduced with kind permission from Jarrah Al-Tubaikh. Hypertension. *Internal Medicine.* DOI: 10.1007/978-3-642-03709-2_31. Springer; 2010-01-01)

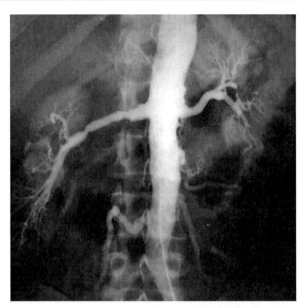

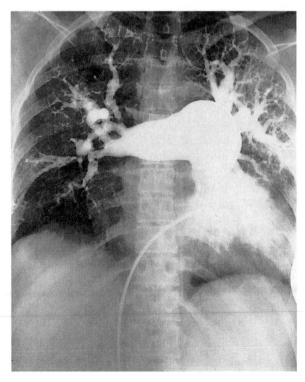

Fig. 10.21 Angiographic findings in Takayasu's arteritis of the pulmonary arteries (Reproduced with permission from Vasculitides. *Atlas of Rheumatology.* ImagesMD; 2002-03-07)

h. Diagnosis
   i. A combination of vasoocclusive disease and systemic inflammation in a young patient
   ii. An age of less than 40 years at disease onset
   iii. Angiography
      1. The gold standard with full aortography
      2. Diagnosis by characteristic findings
   iv. Lesions
      1. Often long-segment stenoses
      2. Arterial occlusions of aorta and visceral vessels at their aortic origins
      3. Aneurysms are uncommon
   v. MRI
      1. Useful for detecting
         a. Vessel wall thickness
         b. Inflammation
         c. Mural thrombus
         d. Pulmonary artery involvement
      2. Can miss lesions in the proximal aortic arch or distal aortic branches
   vi. Biopsy
      1. **Not** necessary if angiogram and clinical symptoms are characteristic
   vii. Laboratory
      1. **NO** specific lab studies useful in the diagnosis
      2. Nonspecific parameters of inflammation
         a. Anemia of chronic disease
         b. Thrombocytosis
         c. Elevated ESR and CRP
            i. ESR may be normal in up to 33% with active disease on biopsy

i. Treatment
   i. Corticosteroids
      1. Remain the therapy of choice
      2. 40–60 mg per day
         a. To control vascular and systemic inflammation
      3. Alternate-day regimens are **not** successful
      4. Taper as clinically indicated and tolerated
         a. 5 mg/day every 2 weeks
         b. Maintenance dose of 10 mg/day
   ii. Low dose aspirin
      1. Or other antiplatelet agents should be added
   iii. Methotrexate
      1. In weekly doses of up to 25 mg
      2. May be useful in sparing steroids
      3. Can induce remission in 80% of patients
   iv. Cytotoxic agents
      1. Cyclophosphamide
      2. Mycophenylate mofetil (MMF)

Requirement	Description
Mandatory criterion	Angiographic abnormalities (conventional, CT or MRI) of the aorta or its major branches
Plus one of these five criteria	Pulse deficit or claudication of the extremities
	Blood pressure discrepancy in four limbs (>10 mmHg)
	Bruit over the aorta and/or its major branches
	Systolic/diastolic hypertension >95th centile for height
	Elevated acute phase reactants (ESR or CRP)
Takayasu arteritis is diagnosed if at least one of the five criteria is present, together with the mandatory criterion	

Fig. 10.22 EULAR classification criteria for Takayasu's arteritis (*CT* computed tomography, *MRI* magnetic resonance imaging, *ESR* erythrocyte sedimentation rate, *CRP* C-reactive protein) (Reproduced with permission from Large vessel vasculitis. *Pediatric Nephrology*. DOI: 10.1007/s00467-009-1312-9. Springer; 2010-04-15)

      3. Overall do not have impressive therapeutic benefit

      4. May use in those who cannot achieve remission

   v. Surgical and angioplastic management

      1. May improve outcome

      2. Treat inflammation prior to intervention

  vi. Other therapies to consider

      1. Antihypertensive

         a. Avoid vasodilators unless the patient has heart failure

      2. Antiplatelet therapy

         a. To prevent thrombosis

      3. Calcium therapy

         a. To prevent osteoporosis

      4. Control hyperlipidemia

 vii. Ways to assess disease control

      1. Monitor acute-phase reactants

         a. ESR, CRP

         b. Helpful in only a subset of patients

         c. 50% of an NIH cohort had active, progressive disease despite normal acute phase reactants

      2. Vascular imaging

         a. May help guide immunosuppression

         b. Adds information beyond laboratory parameters

      3. MRI with gadolinium

         a. Increased uptake in the aortic wall

      4. PET scan

         a. Increased uptake of fluorodeoxyglucose (FDG)

         b. Suggests ongoing inflammation

     5. Vessel wall biopsy
       a. Only with vessel bypass for stenosis
  j. Prognosis
    i. Up to 20% of patients never achieve remission
    ii. Factors that lead to improved prognosis
      1. Early diagnosis
      2. Immunosuppression
      3. Aggressive surgical management
    iii. Sudden death
      1. Myocardial infarction
      2. Stroke
      3. Aneurysmal rupture or dissection
    iv. Renal failure
    v. Cardiac complications
      1. The most common cause of death in Japanese patients
      2. CHF
      3. Ischemic heart disease
      4. Atherosclerotic disease
        a. A critical factor in long-term outcome
    vi. Long-term survival rates 80–90%

Section D: Vasculitis of the Central Nervous System

1. CNS Vasculitis (two forms)
  a. Primary
    i. Primary angiitis of the central nervous system (PACNS)
  b. Secondary conditions that involve the CNS
    i. Infectious diseases
    ii. Drug exposures
    iii. Malignancies
    iv. Systemic vasculitides
    v. Connective-tissue diseases
2. PACNS
  a. A rare and highly heterogeneous clinicopathologic disorder
    i. Can affect any age or sex
    ii. Most common in 30–50 year old
    iii. Statistically more likely to have other conditions that explain the neurologic problem
  b. Defined according to the criteria of Calabrese and Malek
    i. The presence of an acquired neurologic deficit that remains unexplained after a thorough initial basic evaluation
    ii. Classic angiographic evidence consistent with vasculitis or histopathologic demonstration of angiitis within the CNS
    iii. No evidence of systemic vasculitis

      iv. No other secondary conditions
        1. Behcet's disease
        2. Infections
          a. Herpes
          b. HIV
          c. Varicella zoster
          d. Syphilis
          e. Most important conditions to rule out
          f. Angiographic abnormalities similar to angiitis
          g. Similar histologic appearance upon biopsy
          h. Rule out with cultures, special stains, and molecular techniques on CSF and biopsies
        3. Neoplasms
          a. Lymphoma
          b. Lymphomatoid granulomatosis
         4. Drug use
          a. Amphetamines
          b. Cocaine
          c. Heroin
          d. Ephedrine
          e. Phenylpropanolamine
        5. Vasospastic disorders
        6. Connective tissue diseases
          a. SLE
          b. Sjogren's
          c. PAN
          d. Churg-Strauss
          e. Wegener's
        7. Others
          a. Demyelinating disease
          b. Sarcoidosis
          c. Emboli
          d. APS
          e. TTP
          f. Atherosclerosis
          g. Carcinomatous meningitis
    c. Presenting manifestations
      i. Onset can be acute or insidious (over 1–3 months)
      ii. Almost always have a headache
     iii. Chronic meningitis (headache)
     iv. Recurrent focal neurologic symptoms
      v. Unexplained diffuse neurologic dysfunction
        1. Encephalopathy
        2. Behavioral changes
        3. Seizures

      vi. Unexplained spinal cord dysfunction
1. Myelopathy
2. Radiculopathy
3. Subsets of PACNS
  a. Granulomatous angiitis of the central nervous system (GACNS)
     i. About 20% of PACNS fit this category
    ii. Slowly progressive
   iii. Prodrome of 3 or more months
   iv. Additive focal and diffuse neurologic deficits
    v. Minimal or no signs of systemic vasculitis
   vi. Elevated acute-phase reactants and anemia generally absent
  vii. Most frequently encountered clinical findings
1. Chronic headache
2. Focal neurologic defects
3. Alterations in higher cortical functions
4. Spinal-fluid findings consistent with chronic meningitis
5. Inflammatory spinal cord lesions
  viii. Rarer clinical presentations
1. Focal neurological dysfunction only
2. Pure dementia
  ix. Abnormal MRI, angiogram, and CSF
1. Ruled out with a normal LP and MRI
   x. Spinal fluid
1. Mononuclear cell pleocytosis
2. Elevated protein
3. Normal glucose
  xi. Neuroradiographic studies
1. Reflect multifocal vascular insults evolving over time
2. Enhancement of the leptomeninges on MRI
  a. Can increase the diagnostic accuracy of biopsy
  b. Neither sensitive or specific
  xii. Cerebral angiography
1. Inefficient in diagnosis
2. 40% may be normal
3. 40% may show characteristic findings
  a. Multifocal areas of stenosis and ectasia
4. 20% may be nonspecific
  xiii. Biopsies
1. Necrotizing granulomatous angiitis with or without giant cells
2. May be falsely negative in up to one-fifth of patients
  a. Skip-lesions
  xiv. Poor prognosis
1. Highly fatal and progressive
  xv. Treatment
1. Responds to aggressive immunosuppressive therapy
2. Corticosteroids

        3. Cyclophosphamide
        4. Verapamil
        5. Aspirin

b. Benign angiopathy of the central nervous system (BACNS)
   i. Reversible vasoconstrictive disorder
   ii. Diagnosed solely on angiographic grounds
   iii. Usually young women
      1. Present with acute headache or focal neurologic dysfunction
   iv. Normal CSF
   v. Abnormal MRI and cerebral angiograms
   vi. Clinical course
      1. Monophasic
      2. Relatively benign
   vii. Treatment
      1. Usually do not require aggressive and long-term immunosuppression
      2. Corticosteroids
      3. Verapamil
      4. Aspirin
   viii. A form of reversible vasoconstriction
      1. Frequently seen during pregnancy
      2. Angiopathy in the postpartum state
      3. Use of vasoconstricting medications
         a. Diet pills
         b. Sympathomimetic drugs
   ix. Some **do not** have a benign outcome
      1. Significant neurologic sequelae
      2. Fatal cerebral hemorrhage
      3. May require more aggressive therapy

c. Other forms of PACNS
   i. Cases that do not fit neatly into GACNS or BACNS (50%)
   ii. Nongranulomatous pathology
      1. Lymphocytic variant
      2. Leukocytoclastic variant
   iii. Atypical clinical and neuroradiographic features
      1. All clinical features of GACNS
         a. Normal CSF
      2. Presents with mass lesion (15%)
      3. Disease limited to the spinal cord
         a. Majority have granulomatous pathology on biopsy

4. Diagnosis
  a. Biopsy
     i. Modality of choice (gold standard)
     ii. For suspected GACNS
     iii. CSF reveals chronic meningitis
     iv. Granulomatous vasculitis more diagnostic than lymphocytic vasculitis
     v. When contemplating prolonged immunosuppressive therapy

      vi. To rule out mimicking conditions
        1. Infection
        2. Neoplasm
     vii. A superior predictive value over angiography
    viii. Highest yield
        1. Biopsy leptomeninges and cortex from nondominant temporal lobe (if no lesion)
      ix. Sensitivity 75% and specificity 90–100%
  b. Brain MRI
      i. Enhancement of the leptomeninges
     ii. Almost always abnormal
    iii. Nonspecific
    iv. Predictive value of 40–70%
  c. CSF
      i. Pleocytosis
     ii. Elevated protein
    iii. High IgG index
    iv. Oligoclonal bands occasionally seen
  d. Angiogram
      i. Alternating areas of stenosis and ectasia in multiple vessels
     ii. Sensitivity 56–90%
    iii. Predictive value 30–50%
    iv. Other diseases can give similar features (not specific for PACNS)
        1. Severe hypertension
        2. Amyloid angiopathy
        3. Drug induced vasospasm
        4. Syphilis
        5. CNS lymphoma
        6. Thrombotic disorders
     v. Perform initially with a suspected diagnosis of BACNS
        1. An acute presentation
          a. Severe headache
            i. With or without stroke or TIA
          b. Evaluate for emboli and hypercoagulable states
          c. Determine patient drug use
            i. Sympathomimetics
           ii. Cocaine
        2. An acute illness that initially appears nonprogressive
        3. A diffusely abnormal angiogram consistent with vasoconstriction or spasm
        4. Not associated with lesser degrees of angiographic abnormalities
          a. Focal cut-offs
          b. Isolated areas of irregularity
  e. Both angiography and biopsy
      i. Patients with admixtures of GACNS or BACNS
     ii. Atypical presentations

    f. Team approach
       i. Important in obtaining a correct diagnosis
       ii. Neurosurgeon
       iii. Neruoradiologist
       iv. Neuropathologist
       v. Neurologist
       vi. Clinical expert in systemic vasculitides
5. Treatment
    a. No controlled trials for PACNS or BACNS exist
    b. The majority achieve clinical remission
       i. If diagnosed and treated promptly
    c. GACNS
       i. High dose prednisone (1 mg/kg/day) and cyclophosphamide (2 mg/kg/day)
       ii. Corticosteroids tapered
         1. With no further disease progression
       iii. Cyclophosphamide continued
         1. For 6–12 months after the disease has been controlled
       iv. Serial evaluations of disease activity
         1. Repeat lumbar puncture
           a. Ensure improvement or normalization of the CSF
         2. Serial MRI
           a. Ensure no silent progression
         3. Repeat angiogram in 12 weeks
           a. Dramatic improvement with a highly abnormal study
    d. BACNS (reversible vasoconstrictive disease)
       i. A short course of high-dose corticosteroids (1 mg/kg/day)
         1. A period of 2–3 months before taper
       ii. Calcium-channel blockers
         1. Anecdotal evidence for efficacy
    e. Other forms of PACNS
       i. Therapy based on disease severity and the rate of progression
         1. Mild to moderate
           a. High dose corticosteroids alone
         2. Rapidly progressive and profound disease
           a. Regimen similar to GACNS
6. Secondary Forms of CNS Vasculitis
    a. Infections
       i. The most important secondary form of CNS vasculitis to exclude
       ii. Infectious agents
         1. Bacteria
         2. Fungi
         3. Mycobacteria
         4. Viruses
         5. Spirochetes

      6. Atypical agents
      7. Herpes zoster and HIV
        a. Consider in all patients with CNS vasculitis
        b. Especially the immunocompromised
    iii. An angiographic picture indistinguishable from idiopathic PACNS
    iv. Histologically indistinguishable by the presence of necrotizing and granulomatous vasculitis
    v. Obtain detailed history of epidemiologic risk
    vi. Culture all available bodily fluids
    vii. Molecular analysis
      1. For viruses and atypical pathogens
    viii. CNS biopsy
      1. Include special stains and culture for infectious agents
b. Drugs
    i. The most commonly implicated drugs with CNS vasculitis
      1. Cocaine
      2. Amphetamines
      3. Ephedrine
      4. Phenylpropanolamine
      5. Other sympathomimetic agents
    ii. True association has not been established
    iii. Question patients about current or previous drug use
    iv. Therapies similar to those in the treatment of BACNS
c. Neoplasm
    i. Most frequently associated with lymphoproliferative diseases
      1. Hodgkin's and non-Hodgkin's lymphoma
    ii. Often indistinguishable from idiopathic GACNS
    iii. Poor prognosis
      1. A 3 year mortality rate of 90%
d. Connective tissue disease
    i. Two well recognized associations
      1. SLE
      2. Sjogren's
    ii. CNS dysfunction more likely due to other factors
      1. Noninflammatory CNS vascular disease
      2. Drug effects
      3. Infection
    iii. Less than 7% of cases of SLE present with frank vasculitis
e. Systemic vasculitis
    i. CNS vasculitis encountered most often with
      1. Polyarteritis nodosa
      2. ANCA-associated diseases
      3. Behcet's

Section E: Kawasaki Syndrome

1. An acute vasculitis of childhood
2. Occurs predominantly in small and medium-sized muscular arteries
   a. Especially the coronary arteries
3. The primary cause of acquired heart disease in children in the USA and Japan
4. Initially described by Dr. Tomisaku Kawasaki in 1967
5. Morbidity and mortality due to cardiac sequelae
6. Epidemiology
   a. A disease of infants and young children
   b. 80% occur in children younger than 4 years
   c. 50% occur in children younger than 2 years
   d. Peak incidence
      i. Children age 2 years and younger
      ii. 9–12 months
   e. Disease rare after age 11
   f. Boys affected 1.5 times as often as girls
   g. More likely in children of Asian ancestry
      i. 17 times more common among the Japanese
      ii. All races represented
   h. Recurs in 2–4% of cases
   i. Sibling occurrence about 1–2%
   j. Cyclic epidemics
      i. Clusters of cases
      ii. Community wide outbreaks
      iii. Often develop over a 2–4 year period
      iv. Both the USA and Japan
      v. Larger numbers in the late winter to early spring
   1. Cases can occur throughout the year
   k. Epidemiologic factors that adversely affect prognosis
      i. Age < 1 year
      ii. Male sex
      iii. Asian ancestry
      iv. Group more likely to get coronary aneurysms (50%)
7. Etiology
   a. A widespread infectious agent postulated
      i. Age-restricted susceptible population
      ii. Seasonal variations
      iii. Well-defined epidemics
      iv. Acute, self-limited illness
   b. Possible organisms
      i. Staphylococcus
      ii. Streptococcus

       iii. Candida
       iv. Rickettsia
       v. Retroviruses
       vi. EBV
       vii. Exotoxins of staph and strep
          1. Identified in cultures of the rectum and oral pharynx
          2. These toxins may act as superantigens

8. Pathogenesis
   a. Immune activation and cytokine production play a major role
   b. Superantigen theory
      i. Staphylococcal enterotoxins
      ii. Toxic shock syndrome toxin 1
      iii. Streptococcal pyrogenic exotoxins
      iv. Causes T cell expansion
      v. Activation of T cells, B cells, and monocyte/macrophages
   c. Multiple cytokines secreted from activated cells
      i. IL-1
      ii. IL-2
      iii. Soluble IL-2 receptors
      iv. IL-4
      v. IL-6
      vi. IL-10
      vii. TNF-α
      viii. INF-γ
      ix. Soluble CD30 serum antigen
      x. Cause vascular endothelial cell activation
         1. Adhesion molecule up regulation
         2. Vessel wall infiltration by mononuclear cells
      xi. Cytotoxic against stimulated endothelial cells
         1. Endothelial cell damage
         2. Predisposition to aneurysm formation and clot
   d. Immune system activation results in vasculitis
      i. Affects small and medium-sized blood vessels

9. Diagnostic Criteria
   a. Fever
      i. Usually >40°C
      ii. Lasting for ≥5 days
         1. Mean 10 days
         2. Range 5–25 days
      iii. Unresponsive to antibiotic treatment (100%)
   b. Plus four of the following five criteria
      i. Polymorphic rash
         1. Involves trunk and extremities (80%)
         2. Frequently pruritic

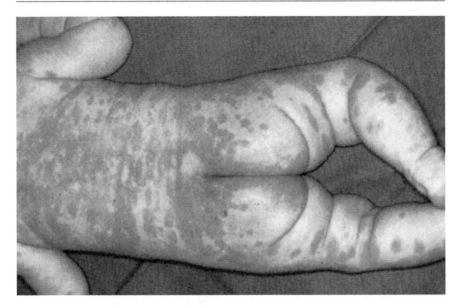

Fig. 10.23 Maculopapular morbilliform rash in Kawasaki disease (Reproduced with permission from Kawasaki disease. *Atlas of Infectious Diseases*. ImagesMD; 2002-01-23)

    ii. Bilateral conjunctival injection (85%)
        1. Nonexudative
        2. Often dramatic
   iii. One or more mucous membrane changes (90%)
        1. Diffuse injection of oral and pharyngeal mucosa
        2. Erythema or fissuring of the lips
        3. Strawberry tongue
   iv. Acute, nonpurulent cervical lymphadenopathy (70%)
        1. Usually a single node, 1.5 cm
    v. One or more extremity changes (70%)
        1. Erythema of the palms or soles
        2. Indurative edema of the hands or feet
        3. Membranous desquamation of the fingertips
        4. Beau's lines
           a. Transverse grooves of the nails
  c. Need meet only four of the five criteria if
    i. Echocardiography demonstrates coronary artery dilation
 d. 90% or greater have
    i. A rash
    ii. Conjunctival injection
   iii. Peripheral extremity changes

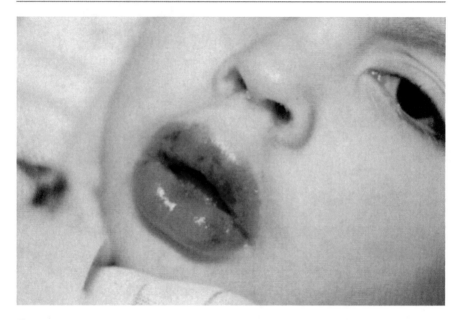

Fig. 10.24 Mucous membrane changes in Kawasaki disease with erythema of the lips (Reproduced with permission from Kawasaki disease. *Atlas of Infectious Diseases*. ImagesMD; 2002-01-23)

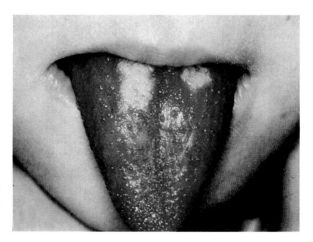

Fig. 10.25 Strawberry tongue in Kawasaki disease (Reproduced with permission from Kawasaki disease. *Atlas of Infectious Diseases*. ImagesMD; 2002-01-23)

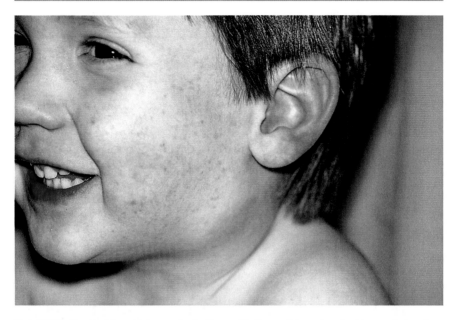

Fig. 10.26 Cervical lymphadenopathy in Kawasaki disease (Reproduced with permission from Kawasaki disease. *Atlas of Infectious Diseases.* ImagesMD; 2002-01-23)

Fig. 10.27 Membranous desquamation of the fingertips in Kawasaki disease (Reproduced with permission from Kawasaki disease. *Atlas of Infectious Diseases.* ImagesMD; 2002-01-23)

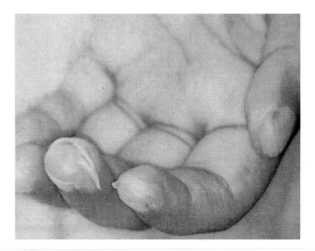

Fig. 10.28 Nail grooves (Beau's lines) in Kawasaki disease (Reproduced with permission from Kawasaki disease. *Atlas of Infectious Diseases.* ImagesMD; 2002-01-23)

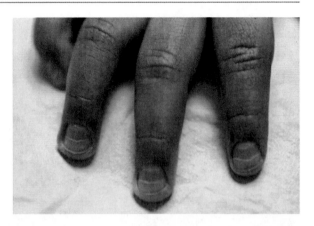

Fig. 10.29 Coronary artery aneurysms in Kawasaki disease (Reproduced with permission from Kawasaki disease. *Atlas of Infectious Diseases.* ImagesMD; 2002-01-23)

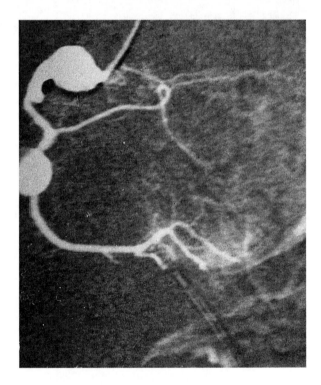

    e. Differential diagnosis
       i. Infection
          1. Scarlet fever shares many of the features
             a. Fever
             b. Conjunctivitis
             c. Mucous membrane involvement
             d. Desquamating skin rash
             e. Rule out by cultures for strep

      ii. Toxicosis
        1. Mercury (acrodynia)
      iii. Allergic/autoimmune
        1. Drug reactions
          a. Antibiotic
          b. Antifungals
          c. Anticonvulsants
        2. Stevens Johnson syndrome
        3. Systemic onset JRA
        4. Other vasculitides
      iv. Malignancies
        1. Leukemia
        2. Lymphoma
10. Clinical Manifestations
    a. Begins acutely with fever
      i. High (100–104°F)
      ii. Prolonged (1–2 weeks)
      iii. Remittent in untreated patient
    b. Early changes (within 1–3 days)
      i. A rash
        1. No distinct morphologic pattern
        2. Most common
          a. Irregular, nonpruritic erythematous plaques
          b. A morbilliform rash
        3. Scarlantiniform rash
        4. Erythema marginatum
        5. Pustules
        6. Not characteristic (suggest another diagnosis)
          a. Diffuse erythema
          b. Crusting
          c. Petechiae
          d. Purpura
          e. Vesicle formation
      ii. Conjunctival injection
      iii. Oral mucosal changes
      iv. Brawny induration of the hands and feet (early)
    c. Late changes (convalescent state at10–14 days)
      i. Characteristic periungual desquamation
        1. May involve the entire hand and foot
      ii. Beau's lines
    d. Ocular findings
      i. Inflammatory, nonpurulent conjunctival injection
      ii. Anterior uveitis
    e. Oral findings (**not** typical-seen in other febrile exanthemas)
      i. Ulcers
      ii. Petechiae
      iii. Exudates

  f. CNS disease
     i. Aseptic meningitis
     ii. Facial palsy
     iii. Subdural effusion
     iv. Symptomatic and asymptomatic cerebral infarction
  g. Sensorineural hearing loss
  h. Pulmonary infiltrates and pleural effusions
  i. Gastrointestinal manifestations
     i. Hepatomegaly
     ii. Hydrops of the gallbladder
     iii. Diarrhea
     iv. Pancreatitis
  j. Renal manifestations
     i. Sterile pyuria
     ii. Proteinuria
     iii. Acute renal insufficiency from interstitial nephritis (rare)
  k. Arthritis
     i. Short lived
     ii. Involve small joints of hands and feet
  l. Cardiac abnormalities
     i. Numerous and varied
     ii. Acute stage manifestations
        1. Pericardial effusions (about 30% cases)
        2. Myocarditis
           a. Frequent tachycardia and gallop rhythms
              i. Disproportionate to degree of fever and anemia
     iii. CHF
     iv. Atrial and ventricular arrhythmias
     v. EKG findings
        1. Decreased R-wave voltage
        2. ST-segment depression
        3. T-wave flattening or inversion
           a. Slowed conduction with PR or QT prolongation
        4. Mitral regurgitation (about 30%)
        5. Pericarditis with friction rubs (less common)
     vi. Coronary artery lesions
        1. Responsible for most of the morbidity and mortality
        2. Aneurysms
           a. More common in patients with pericarditis
           b. Palpable axillary artery aneurysms highly predictive of coronary artery aneurysms in one series
           c. Develop in 15–25% without treatment
           d. Prevalence reduced with IVIG therapy
              i. Fewer than 5%
              ii. Giant coronary aneurysms to fewer than 1%

    e. Risk factors
        i. Male sex
        ii. Age less than 1 year
        iii. Prolonged fever
        iv. Persistently elevated ESR
    f. Usually appear 1–4 weeks after the onset of fever
    g. Rarely appear after 6 weeks of illness
    h. Detected by transthoracic 2-D echo
    i. Description based on size
        i. Small (4 mm)
        ii. Medium (4–8 mm)
        iii. Giant (>8 mm)
    j. Proximal location more common than distal
    k. Most aneurysms regress
        i. Small and medium sizes within 5 years
        ii. 2% present by 1 year
    l. Factors positively associated with regression
        i. Smaller size
        ii. Fusiform morphology
        iii. Female sex
        iv. Age less than 1 year
    m. Giant aneurysms have the worst prognosis
        i. Rarely regress
        ii. Frequent complications
            1. Thromboses
            2. Stenoses
            3. Total occlusion
        iii. Require very close follow-up
        iv. Long-term requirement for anticoagulation
  3. Vessel ectasia
    a. Vessel size larger than age-matched controls
    b. A common finding
vii. Myocardial infarction
  1. Most likely to appear within the first year
  2. 40% occur within the first 3 months
  3. Cases reported more than a decade after initial disease
  4. Symptoms of myocardial ischemia in a preverbal child
    a. Restlessness
    b. Pallor
    c. Weak pulse
    d. Abdominal pain and vomiting
    e. A gallop rhythm with a third heart sound (70%)
m. Other vessel involvement
  i. Abdominal aorta
  ii. Superior mesenteric

       iii. Axillary
       iv. Subclavian
       v. Brachial
       vi. Iliac
       vii. Renal arteries
       viii. Vasculitis of the peripheral extremity
11. Laboratory Findings
    a. **Not** diagnostic
    b. Identify patients at highest risk for coronary involvement
    c. Acute phase
       i. Leukocytosis with a left shift
       ii. Normochromic normocytic anemia
       iii. Elevated acute-phase reactants
       iv. Elevated liver transaminase
       v. Depressed albumin
       vi. Increased platelet turnover
       vii. Marked hypercoagulability
    d. Second week
       i. Profound lymphocytosis
       ii. Marked expansion of the B-cell subset
    e. Third to fourth week
       i. Thrombocytosis
          1. Characteristic
          2. Not often seen in other cases of FUO
          3. Often greater than 1 million ($>106/mm^3$)
    f. Urinalysis
       i. Mild proteinuria
       ii. Sterile pyuria from urethritis
    g. Creatinine rarely elevated
    h. CSF findings with meningeal signs
       i. Non-specific pleocytosis
       ii. Normal protein and glucose
    i. Complement levels normal or increased
    j. ANA and RF negative
    k. ANCA and antiendothelial antibodies
       i. Detected in some patients
       ii. No diagnostic significance
    l. EKG
       i. ST-T wave changes
       ii. Indicative of pericarditis or myocarditis
    m. CXR
       i. Cardiomegaly
    n. ECHO
       i. Recommended in the first week of illness
       ii. Myocardial function

      iii. Valvular regurgitation (rare)

      iv. Coronary artery dilatation and aneurysmal formation

      v. Coronary artery evaluations

         1. Immediately at diagnosis

         2. Within 1 week of illness onset

         3. At 6 and 12 weeks

12. Treatment

  a. Based on preventing aneurysmal formation

  b. Acute phase

      i. Aimed at limiting inflammation

      ii. Aspirin

         1. The most widely used therapeutic agent

         2. 80–100 mg/kg/day split into three doses

            a. Until the fever subsides

      iii. IVIG

         1. The treatment of choice within the first 10 days of illness

            a. Conclusive evidence

            b. Numerous multicenter, double-blinded, placebo-controlled series

         2. Decreases th e incidence of coronary artery aneurysms

            a. ASA plus IVIG

               i. 8% aneurysms at 14 days

               ii. 2% at 30 months

            b. ASA alone

               i. 23% aneurysms at 14 days

               ii. 11% at 30 months

         3. Resolution of acute symptoms

            a. Lessens the fever

            b. Rash regresses

            c. Toxicity improves within 12 h

         4. Reduces myocardial inflammation

         5. Standard of care

            a. 2 g/kg as a single infusion over 10–12 h

            b. Most effective when started within the first 10 days

            c. Aspirin given concurrently

         6. Cost effective

            a. Study by Klassen

            b. Reduced costs of acute care and long-term sequelae (aneurysms, thromboses)

         7. A second dose

            a. For persistent, recurrent fever (10%)

            b. Unknown impact on coronary artery lesions

         8. IVIG resistant subgroup

            a. At greatest risk for developing coronary artery aneurysms and long-term sequelae

      9. Side effects
        a. Acute
           i. Fever
          ii. Chills
          iii. Headache
          iv. Aseptic meningitis (rare)
        b. Long-term
           i. Same risk as other blood products
     10. Mechanism of action
        a. Unknown
        b. Pooled material from 10,000 donors
        c. High titer antibodies
           i. Anti-staphylococcal
          ii. Streptococcal
          iii. Toxic shock toxin
  c. Convalescent phase
    i. Aspirin
      1. Reduce to sslow-doses
        a. 5 mg/kg/day
        b. Sufficient for antiplatelet effect
      2. Continue for an additional 2 months
        a. Until platelet count and indicators of inflammation return to normal
      3. Continue indefinitely in patient with aneurysms
        d. Refractory disease
           i. Steroids
13. Long-Term Follow-up
  a. American Heart Association Guidelines
    i. Multiple aneurysms, giant aneurysms, or known coronary artery obstruction
      1. Close follow-up
      2. Long-term anticoagulation
    ii. History of coronary artery involvement
      1. Stress testing in adolescent years
      2. Follow-up angiography to assess for obstruction or stenosis
      3. Limitations in physical activity

Systemic Sclerosis and Related Syndromes

11

Section A: Epidemiology, Pathology and Pathogenesis

1. Epidemiology
   a. Incidence in the USA
      i. About 19 cases per million per year
      ii. Prevalence of 19–75 cases per 100,000
   b. Peak occurrence in ages 35–65
   c. Greater in females: 7–12:1
   d. Rare in children and men under 30
   e. Ethnic background influences survival and disease manifestation
      i. Caucasians
         1. Less progressive pulmonary interstitial fibrosis
         2. More likely to have anti-centromere antibodies
            a. Associated with HLA-DQB1 molecules
            b. A polar glycine or tyrosine at position 26
         3. Anti-anti-DNA topoisomerase I antibodies
            a. Associated with HLA-DRB1*1101 and *1104
      ii. African Americans
         1. Most common in black women during child-bearing years
         2. Overall no significant predominance
         3. Worse survival rates
         4. More likely to have anti-topoisomerase I (Scl-70) antibodies
            a. Associated with HLA-DRB1*1101 and *1104
      iii. Other ethnic associated haplotypes with Scl-70
         1. Japanese
            a. HLA-DRB1*1502
         2. Choctaw Native American
            a. HLA-DRB1*1602
      iv. Choctaw Native Americans
         1. Highest incidence of cases 469 per 100,000

N.T. Colburn, *Review of Rheumatology*,
DOI 10.1007/978-1-84882-093-7_11, © Springer-Verlag London Limited 2012

      2. 2 cM haplotype on chromosome 15q
         a. Up to 10 generations of prior common ancestors
         b. Region contains the fibrillin-1 gene
         c. Binds TGF-β
         d. The abnormal fibrillarin chain may lead to proteolysis
      3. Associated with HLA-DR2 haplotype
  f. Other disease associations
    i. HLA-DQA
    ii. C4A null allele
    iii. An allele of the Cg2 T-cell antigen receptor
    iv. Low activity of P-450 enzymes
  g. **NO** association with disease
    i. Mutants of the fibronectin gene
    ii. Alleles of pro alpha I, II, or III collagen
    iii. Allotypes of alpha-1 antitrypsin
  h. Environmental factors
    i. Similar concordance rates for monozygotic and dizygotic twins
    ii. Parvovirus B19 detected in bone marrow
    iii. Antibodies to CMV increased
    iv. Homologies between autoantigens and viruses
      1. Scl-70 and p30 gag protein from CMV
      2. Regions of PM-Scl antigen homologous to SV40 large T antigen and HIV tat protein
      3. RNP shares an AA segment with herpes simplex virus (HSV) type II CP4
      4. Fibrillarin homologous to a capsid protein encoded by HSV type 1 and EBV nuclear antigen 1
    v. Occupational exposures
      1. Silica dust with RR of 25
      2. Frank silicosis with RR of 110
         a. None with silicone breast implants
      3. Organic solvents
      4. Trichlorethylene
      5. Perchlorethylene
      6. Biogenic amines
         a. Includes appetite suppressants
      7. Urea formaldehyde
      8. Vinyl chloride
      9. Bleomycin
     10. Tainted rapeseed oil
     11. L-tryptophan
     12. Mercury exposure
     13. Postmenopausal estrogen replacement
     14. Pesticides

2. Pathology
   a. Widespread small-vessel vasculopathy and fibrosis
      i. Affects small arteries, arterioles, and capillaries
      ii. Causes tissue ischemia
      iii. Hypersensitivity of alpha-2 adrenergic receptors on vascular smooth muscle cells
         1. An early event
      iv. **Not** considered a vasculitis
         1. Invasion by mononuclear cells is uncommon
   b. Increased endothelial cell receptor surface expression
      i. HLA class II molecules
      ii. Beta-2 integrins
      iii. ICAM-1
      iv. ELAM-1
         1. Involved in T-cell homing to the skin
      v. P-selectin
   c. Damaged endothelium
      i. Induces platelet activation and thrombosis
      ii. Activated platelets release PDGF and thromboxane A2
         1. Vasoconstriction
         2. Thickened and reduplicated basement membranes
      iii. Occurs in pulmonary and digital arteries
      iv. A lack of new vessel growth
         1. Increased angiogenesis inhibitor (endostatin)
   d. Fibrosis
      i. Increased synthesis of collagen mRNA and proteins
         1. Type I
         2. Type III
         3. Type V
         4. Type VI
      ii. Normal collagen
         1. Normal ratios of type I to III
         2. Normal degradation
      iii. Normal collagenase activity (ECM)
      iv. Increased fibronectin and glycosaminoglycans
   e. Myofibroblasts
      i. Smooth muscle α-actin positive fibroblast cells
      ii. Contribute to ECM production in skin and lungs
      iii. High expression of collagen type I mRNAs
      iv. Enhanced proliferation to PDGF and TGF-β
   f. Dermal infiltrates
      i. Perivascular in early disease
      ii. T-cells
         1. CD4+ more than CD8+
         2. Increased beta 1 and 2 integrins
         3. Increased LFA-1

  iii. Fibroblasts
        1. Increased ICAM-1
  iv. Endothelin-1 and TGF-β
        1. Produced by endothelial cells
        2. Stimulate ECM production by fibroblasts
g. Lung infiltrates
    i. Inflammation with patchy lymphocytes and plasma-cells
   ii. Interstitial fibrosis
  iii. Activated alveolar macrophages
  iv. Fibronectin released in higher amounts
   v. Memory Tcells increased
        1. CD8+ increased in bronchoalveolar lavage (BAL)
        2. Produce IL-4 and IL-5 cytokines
        3. Associated with greater fibrosis
  vi. Intracellular TGF-β1 expression
        1. Alveolar macrophages
        2. Bronchial epithelium
        3. Hyperplastic type II pneumocytes
  vii. Extracellular TGF-β1 expression
        1. In fibrous tissue
        2. Beneath bronchial epithelium
        3. Beneath hyperplastic alveolar epithelium
h. Abnormalities of humoral immunity
    i. Hypergammaglobulinemia
        1. Polyclonal increases in all Igs
   ii. Autoantibody formation
        1. ANA
            a. Seen in 95%
            b. Usually IgG
                i. Especially IgG3
        2. Topoisomerase 1
        3. Centromere
        4. RNA polymerase I and III
        5. U3 RNP systems
        6. All share the ability to be cleaved into fragments
            a. Nonenzymatic metal-dependent
            b. Granzyme B
                i. Serine esterase in cytolytic granules
  iii. **No** evidence for immune complex deposition
3. Pathogenesis
  a. Early
    i. Immune system activation
   ii. Endothelial cell activation and damage
  iii. Fibroblast activation

  b. Late
      i. Structural changes in small blood vessels and tissue fibrosis
      ii. Profibrotic cytokines IL-4 and TGF-β
  c. Unknown antigen specific activation
      i. With oligoclonal expansion
      ii. Vdelta1+ T-cells in blood
      iii. CD8+ in lung
  d. Complement
      i. Not activated
      ii. Serum levels normal
  e. Microchimerism
      i. A graft-versus-host reaction could be an attributing factor
      ii. Microengrafted (fetal-maternal) allogeneic cells
          1. Detected in a higher percentage of scleroderma patients
              a. 45–65%
          2. Found in involved skin and lung
          3. CD34+CD38+ stem cells
          4. CD3
          5. CD19
          6. CD14
          7. CD56/'6
  f. Cytokines and growth factors increased in sera of scleroderma patients
      i. IL-1
      ii. IL-2
      iii. IL-4
      iv. IL-6
      v. IL-8
      vi. Lymphotoxin
      vii. TNF-a
      viii. TGF-b
      ix. PDGF
  g. All skin is abnormal
      i. Presence of procollagen-1 and adherence molecules
      ii. Accumulation of glycosaminoglycan and fibronectin in the ECM
      iii. Loss of sweat glands
      iv. Hair loss in involved areas
  h. Two events responsible for increased production of ECM
      i. Fibroblast proliferation by cytokines
          1. IL-6, IL-4, TGF-β, PDGF, FGF, and endothelin-1
          2. Decreased production of interferon-γ
              a. Reduces collagen synthesis
              b. May contribute to the profibrotic milieu
      ii. Fibroblasts produce higher basal amounts of ECM
          1. Increased levels of TGF-β and pro-alpha1(I) collagen mRNA
          2. Co-localize within inflammatory infiltrates in skin during early events

   3. May be inherently abnormal in their responsiveness to cytokine stimulation

    a. Collagen promoter more active in response to TGF-β

 4. Cancer associations with systemic sclerosis

  a. Breast cancer

   i. Develops in close proximity prior to or at the onset of disease

  b. Lung cancer

   i. Increased 1.8 fold in patient with lung fibrosis ("scar carcinoma")

  c. Esophageal cancer

   i. Incidence **NOT** increased

    1. Despite chronic reflux

   ii. Increased only with the development of Barrett's esophagus

Section B: Clinical Features

1. Initial symptoms nonspecific
   a. Raynaud's
      i. Occurs in about 95%
   b. Fatigue
   c. Musculoskeletal complaints
2. Skin thickening
   a. The first specific clinical clue
   b. Begins as swelling or "puffiness" of the fingers and hands
      i. Involved in virtually all cases
3. Diagnosis requires either
   a. Skin thickening proximal to the MCP joints
   b. Signs of digital ischemia and pulmonary fibrosis
4. ACR requires one major and two minor criteria for the diagnosis
   a. Major criteria
      i. Scleroderma proximal to the MCPs or MTPs
   b. Minor criteria
      i. Sclerodactyly
      ii. Digital pitting scars
      iii. Bibasilar pulmonary fibrosis
5. Expanded ACR criteria for patients with limited systemic sclerosis
   a. Abnormal capillary microscopy
   b. Dilated capillaries
   c. Avascular areas at the nailbeds
   d. Anti-centromere antibodies
6. Scleroderma classified into subsets based on the degree of clinically involved skin
   a. Localized scleroderma
      i. Circumscribed fibrotic areas
      ii. Involves different levels of the skin
         1. Sometimes the underlying soft tissue, muscle, and bone

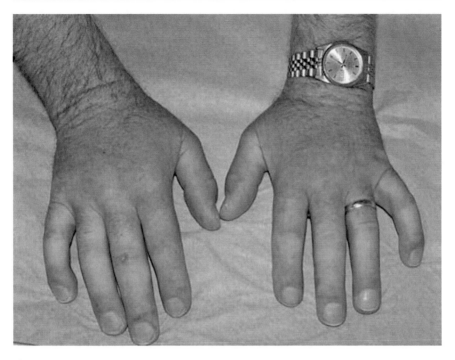

Fig. 11.1 A man with erythema and puffiness of the hands characteristic of early diffuse systemic sclerosis (Reproduced with permission from Systemic sclerosis (scleroderma) and Raynaud's phenomenon. *A Clinician's Pearls and Myths in Rheumatology*. DOI: 10.1007/978-1-84800-934-9_10. Springer; 2009-01-01)

   iii. More common in children and young women
   iv. Benign clinical course
    v. Usually presents as a nonspecific area of erythema and pain
   vi. Expands with a ivory-like fibrotic center
      1. Surrounded by a margin of hyperpigmentation
      2. Lilac in appearance
  vii. Cellular infiltrations
      1. Lymphocytes
      2. Mast cells
      3. Plasma cells
      4. Eosinophils
 viii. Excess collagen deposition
      1. Extends into the dermis
      2. Sometimes deeper
   ix. Lesions distributed asymmetrically
    x. Remain active for weeks to several years
      1. Spontaneous softening leaves a pigmented area
   xi. Cutaneous changes without internal organ involvement

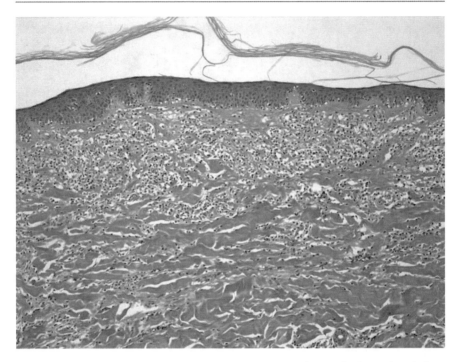

Fig. 11.2 Histology (×100 magnification) shows an interstitial infiltrate of polymorphous inflammatory cells and slight thickening of collagen in early morphea (Reproduced with permission from Differential diagnosis of normal skin. *Dermatopathology: The Basics.* DOI: 10.1007/978-1-4419-0024-1_5. Springer; 2009-01-01)

   xii. Morphea
      1. Isolated
         a. 1–15 cm plaque
      2. Generalized
         a. Multiple plaques commonly on the trunk
  xiii. Linear scleroderma
      1. Bands of skin thickening
      2. Typically follow a linear pattern
      3. Commonly on the legs or arms
         a. More common on the lower extremities
      4. Sometimes on the face (*en coup de sabre*)
         a. May progress
         b. Severe facial hemiatrophy
         c. Linear hair loss
      5. Nondermatomal fibrotic band that infiltrates
         a. Skin
         b. Subcutaneous fat

Fig. 11.3 Localized scleroderma is more common on the lower extremities (Reproduced with permission from Rheumatology. *Atlas of Pediatrics.* ImagesMD; 2006-01-20)

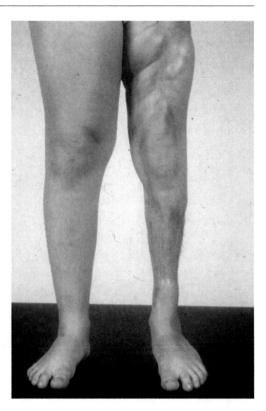

c. Fascia
d. Muscle
6. Bands can disrupt bone growth and cause joint contractures
7. Unknown cause
8. Autoantibodies frequently detected
   a. ANA
   b. Anti-ss-DNA
   c. Anti-histone
9. Treatment does not alter the course but can be helpful
   a. Corticosteroids
   b. Vitamin D
   c. Methotrexate
   d. D-penicillamine
   e. Photochemotherapy
   xiv. Nodular (keloid)
   xv. Localized bullous lesions (rare)
b. Systemic sclerosis
   i. Hallmark characteristics
      1. Thickened skin
      2. Abnormal production of normal type I collagen
         a. A fibroblast subset

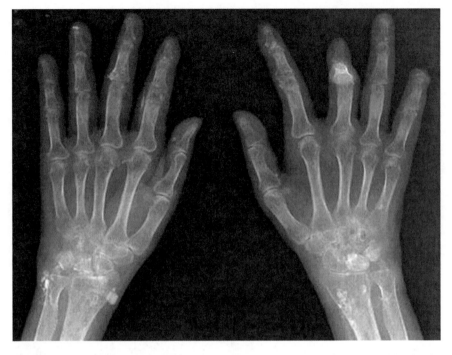

Fig. 11.4 Radiographic examination reveals tissue calcification in the forearms and hands of a patient with systemic sclerosis (Reproduced with permission from Deposition diseases. *Therapy of Skin Diseases.* DOI: 10.1007/978-3-540-78814-0_43. Springer; 2010-01-01)

    3. Accumulation of GAGs and fibronectin in the ECM
    4. A loss of sweat glands
    5. Hair loss
    6. Abnormal involvement of **ALL** skin
        a. Based on the presence of procollagen-1 and adherence molecules
  ii. Demographics
    1. Most commonly seen in women 3:1
        a. Between the ages of 35–64
    2. Rare in children and men under the age of 30
 iii. Limited
    1. Cutaneous thickening of the distal limbs
    2. Also includes the face and neck
    3. No truncal involvement
    4. Late incidence of pulmonary hypertension
        a. Typically in the **absence** of severe pulmonary fibrosis
    5. Arterial occlusive disease
    6. Less likely to develop severe lung, heart, or kidney disease
    7. High incidence of anti-centromere autoantibodies
    8. A >70% 10 year survival rate

9. Raynaud's present for years (1–10) before disease onset
10. CREST syndrome
   a. A subset of limited
   b. Calcinosis
      i. Cutaneous deposits of basic calcium phosphate
      ii. Characteristically in the hands
         1. PIPs and fingertips
      iii. Periarticular tissue
      iv. Over bony prominences
         1. Extensor surface of the elbows and knees
      v. Firm, irregular, and generally nontender
      vi. Range in size from 1 mm to several centimeters
      vii. Can become inflamed, infected, or ulcerated
      viii. Extremely difficult to treat (none consistently successful)
         1. Warfarin
            a. Inhibits vitamin K dependent Gla matrix protein
         2. Aluminum hydroxide
         3. Diltiazem
         4. Probenecid
         5. High doses of bisphosphonates
   c. Raynaud's phenomenon
      i. Episodic self-limited and reversible vasomotor disturbance
      ii. Color changes
         1. Bilateral
            a. Fingers
            b. Toes
            c. Ears
            d. Nose
            e. Lips
         2. Pallor, cyanosis, and then erythema
         3. All three colors not needed to make the diagnosis
            a. Episodic palor
            b. Cyanosis that reverses to erythema
            c. Normal skin
      iii. Occurs in response to environmental cold and/or emotional stress
      iv. Symptoms
         1. Numbness
         2. Tingling
         3. Pain on recovery
      v. Arterial closures
         1. Muscular digital arteries
         2. Precapillary arterioles
         3. Arteriovenous shunts

Fig. 11.5 Skin
manifestations of diffuse
systemic sclerosis
(Reproduced with permission
from Systemic lupus
erythematosus, scleroderma,
and inflammatory
myopathies. *Atlas of
Rheumatology*. ImagesMD;
2005-01-18)

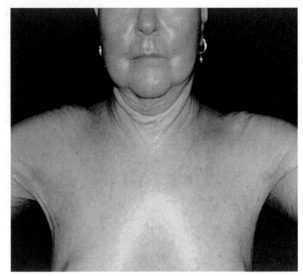

      vi. Rewarming
         1. Reversal of the vasospastic period
         2. Generally occurs 10–15 min after the stimulus has ended
    d. Esophageal dysmotility
    e. Sclerodactyly
    f. Telangiectasia
        i. Dilated venules, capillaries, and arterioles
        ii. Matte, oval, or polygonal macules
        iii. 2–7 mm in diameter
        iv. Hands, face, lips, and oral mucosa
        v. More common in limited SS
        vi. Can bleed if in the GI mucosa
        vii. May disappear spontaneously
        viii. Usually harmless
        ix. A cosmetic problem
  iv. Diffuse systemic sclerosis
    1. Skin thickening over distal and proximal limb sites
    2. Can include the trunk
    3. Raynaud's phenomenon
      a. Occurs within a year
      b. Occurs simultaneously with skin changes
    4. Early stages
      a. Skin thickening begins on the fingers and hands
        i. Virtually all cases
        ii. Consider localized forms if begins elsewhere
      b. Edematous skin

       c. Painful joints and muscles

       d. Tendon friction rubs

       e. Associated esophageal reflux

       f. Rapidly progressive skin changes

          i. Appear over the first months of disease

          ii. Continue for 2–3 years

          iii. May soften, atrophy or return to normal texture

          iv. Skin tethering and contractures with severe fibrosis

    5. More likely to have pulmonary, renal, or cardiac involvement

       a. Cardiopulmonary disease is the leading cause of death

    6. Autoantibodies

       a. To topoisomerase-1 (anti-Scl-70)

       b. To centromere (less likely)

    7. Overall course is highly variable

       a. Relapse is uncommon once remission occurs

    8. Diffuse disease

       a. Worst prognosis

       b. 10-year survival rate of approximately 40–60%

          i. Compared to >70% in the limited form

7. Factors that indicate a poor prognosis

   a. Diffuse skin involvement

   b. Late age of disease onset

   c. African- or Native-American race

   d. The presence of tendon rubs

   e. A diffusing capacity <40% of predicted values

   f. The presence of a large pericardial effusion

   g. Proteinuria

   h. Hematuria

   i. Renal failure

   j. Low Hemoglobin

   k. Elevated ESR

   l. Abnormal EKG

8. Autoantibodies predict clinical features and survival

   a. Anticentromere antibodies

      i. More often in limited disease (50–90%)

      ii. Only 5% in diffuse disease

      iii. Relatively good prognoses

      iv. Associated with

         1. CREST syndrome

         2. Pulmonary hypertension

         3. Primary biliary cirrhosis

         4. Digital amputation

   b. Anti-RNA polymerase III antibodies

      i. Increase the risk of cardiac or renal disease

      ii. Predicts a poor prognosis

      iii. Seen in 25% of diffuse disease

      iv. Only 6% in limited disease

  c. Antifibrillarin antibodies (anti U3 RNP)

      i. Associated with heart and lung involvement

      ii. Predicts a poor prognosis

      iii. Seen in 7% of diffuse disease

      iv. Not seen in limited disease

  d. Anti-topoisomerase and anti-U1 RNP (MCTD) antibodies

      i. Intermediate survival rates

      ii. High risk of pulmonary disease

      iii. Seen in 20–30% of diffuse disease

      iv. 10–15% of limited disease

  e. Anti Th/To

      i. Frequently seen in patients with

         1. Limited disease

           a. Up to 16%

         2. Nucleolar ANA

         3. Negative anticentromere antibody

      ii. Not seen in diffuse

  f. ANA

      i. Equally in both limited and diffuse disease

         1. Up to 95%

      ii. Most likely a nucleolar pattern

9. Raynaud's Phenomenon

  a. 4–5% of the general population have symptoms

  b. Primary Raynaud's phenomenon

      i. No defined underlying cause

      ii. The physical exam and labs are normal

      iii. Onset typically between the ages of 15 and 25 years

  c. Secondary Raynaud's phenomenon

      i. Secondary to an underlying medical condition

      ii. More likely if attacks

         1. Are intense

         2. Begin after the age of 20

      iii. Systemic sclerosis

         1. Enlarged capillary loops

         2. Loss of normal capillaries in the nail fold

         3. Occurs in more than 90%

         4. Associated with

           a. Tissue fibrosis of the finger

           b. Loss of the digital pads (sclerodactyly)

           c. Digital ulceration

           d. Ischemic demarcation

              i. Digital amputation

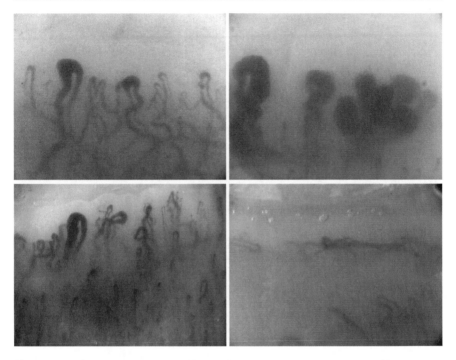

Fig. 11.6 Nailfold capillaroscopy (×200 magnification) demonstrates enlarged capillary loops in systemic sclerosis (Reproduced with permission from Capillaroscopy: questions and answers. *Clinical Rheumatology*. DOI: 10.1007/s10067-007-0681-3. Springer; 2007-11-08)

     iv. "Systemic" Raynaud's
       1. A generalized vasospastic disorder
       2. Vasculopathy of the terminal arterial circulation
         a. Lungs
         b. Kidneys
         c. Heart
       3. Vascular occlusion with
         a. Fibrosis of the intimal layer
         b. Platelet activation
         c. Perturbation of the clotting cascade
         d. Fibrin deposition
  10. Skin Stages
     a. Edematous
       i. Skin mildly inflamed with nonpitting edema and erythema
      ii. Pruritus and swelling associated with
       1. Lymphocyte infiltration
       2. Fibroblast and mast cell activation
       3. Local release of cytokines

        iii. Collagen deposition from activated fibroblasts thickens the dermis

        iv. Varying degrees of hypo- and hyperpigmentary changes

            1. "Salt and pepper" appearance

    b. Fibrotic

        i. Skin becomes more thickened

        ii. Severe drying provokes pruritus

        iii. Persist and worsens over a period of 1–3 years

    c. Atrophic

        i. Inflammation and further fibrosis seem to cease

        ii. Skin atrophic and thinned

        iii. Tethering

            1. Fibrotic tissue binds to underlying structures

        iv. Painful ulcerations at sites of flexion contractures

        v. Late stage

            1. Remodeling appears clinically normal

                a. Especially the trunk and proximal limbs

11. Musculoskeletal

    a. Arthralgias and myalgias

        i. Nonspecific Musculoskeletal complaints

        ii. One of the earliest symptoms of systemic sclerosis

    b. Rheumatoid-like polyarthritis

        i. Joint pain and stiffness out of proportion with objective inflammatory signs

    c. Coarse friction rubs

        i. Caused by inflammation and fibrosis of the tendon sheath or adjacent tissues

        ii. Almost always seen in **diffuse** skin disease

        iii. Predicts a worse overall clinical outcome

    d. Muscle Abnormalities

        i. Noninflammatory benign myopathy

            1. Mild proximal weakness

            2. Atrophy and weakness in late disease from

                a. Disuse

                b. Deconditioning

                c. Malnutrition

            3. Biopsy

                a. Looks normal

                b. Some muscle fiber type 2 atrophy

            4. Normal muscle enzymes

        ii. Mild elevation of muscle enzymes

            1. Waxing and waning of symptoms

            2. Biopsy

                a. Interstitial fibrosis

                b. Fiber atrophy

            3. Minimal inflammatory cell infiltration

      iii. Inflammatory type of myopathy
1. Elevated muscle enzymes
2. Similar to polymyositis and dermatomyositis
3. An overlap syndrome
4. Many fit the definition of mixed connective tissue disease
      iv. Myopathy secondary to medications used in treatment
1. Corticosteroids
2. D-penicillamine
12. Pulmonary
  a. Lung impairment is the leading cause of mortality
  b. Pathology
     i. Fibrosing alveolitis that progresses to interstitial fibrosis
    ii. Loss of lung volume
1. Restrictive ventilatory defect
    iii. Nonprogressive interstitial lung disease (ILD)
1. Typically bibasilar (20%)
2. Seen in limited systemic sclerosis
    iv. Pulmonary vasculopathy
1. Endothelial cell dysfunction
2. Intimal fibrosis
  c. Severe progressive pulmonary fibrosis more common in
     i. Diffuse disease
    ii. African or Native American
    iii. Anti-topoisomerase antibodies
    iv. Advanced late disease

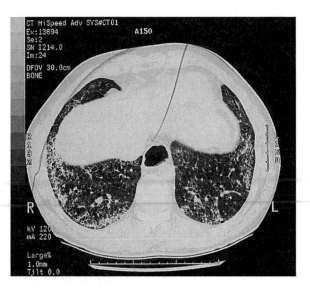

Fig. 11.7 Interstitial lung disease in systemic sclerosis (Reproduced with permission from Systemic lupus erythematosus, scleroderma, and inflammatory myopathies. *Atlas of Rheumatology*. ImagesMD; 2005-01-18)

   d. ILD
       i. Clinical symptoms
           1. Asymptomatic or insidious
           2. Dyspnea on exertion
               a. The most common initial symptom
           3. Easy fatigability
           4. Exertional nonproductive cough
               a. Usually a late symptom
           5. Dyspnea at rest
           6. Pleuritic chest pain (rare)
      ii. Clinical signs (early)
           1. Inspiratory fine or Velcro crackles
           2. PFTs detect reductions in
               a. Lung volumes
               b. Diffusing capacity
     iii. Treatment
           1. Reserved for disease that progresses to the middle and upper lobes
           2. Prednisone and cyclophosphamide
           3. Inflammatory alveolitis
               a. Oral cytoxan (1–2 mg/kg/day)
               b. Monthly IV (800–1,400 mg)
               c. Benefits lung function and survival
           4. Immunosuppressive responders
               a. Evidence of active alveolitis on BAL
                   i. Elevated percentage of neutrophils and/or eosinophils
                       1. >5% of BAL fluid cellularity
               b. Nonspecific interstitial pneumonitis (NSIP) on high resolution CT
                   or lung biopsy
                   i. Ground glass
                  ii. No honey combing
           5. Immunosuppressive non-responders
               a. Progression of lung disease without active alveolitis
               b. Usual interstitial pneumonia (UIP)
                   i. Honey combing
                  ii. Subpleural fibrosis
               c. Fibrosis
                   i. Secondary to fibroblastic foci
                  ii. Similar to idiopathic pulmonary fibrosis
           6. Anti-fibrotic therapy not available
           7. Gamma interferon
               a. Effective in treating some IPF and UIP
   e. Pulmonary hypertension
       i. Usually insidious onset of exertional dyspnea
      ii. Can rapidly become dyspnea at rest with pedal edema
     iii. Isolated without fibrosis

           1. Associated with the CREST syndrome

           2. 8–28%

       iv. 35% of patients with systemic sclerosis by 2D ECHO

        v. Physical exam

           1. An increased pulmonic component of the second heart sound (P2)

           2. Right ventricular gallop

           3. Pulmonic or tricuspid insufficiency murmur

           4. Jugular venous distention

           5. Pedal edema

      vi. CXR and CT scans

           1. Interstitial fibrosis

           2. Predominantly lower lobes

     vii. Clinical signs associated with a high mortality rate

           1. An elevated right ventricular pressure

           2. A low diffusing capacity of less than 40% of predicted

    viii. Treatment

           1. Initially nasal oxygen

           2. Vasodilators such as calcium channel blockers

             a. Nifedipine

             b. Diltiazem

           3. Anticoagulation with warfarin

           4. For severe disease

             a. IV infusions of epoprostenol (PGI2)

             b. Oral nonspecific endothelin antagonist (bosentan)

               i. Contraindications

                 1. Pregnancy

                 2. Cyclosporin

                 3. Glyburide

              ii. Hepatotoxic

  f. Periodic PFTs and 2D ECHO

        i. Most effective methods of early detection of active lung disease

  g. An isolated, low diffusing capacity suggests either

        i. Early restrictive lung disease

       ii. Incipient pulmonary vascular disease

  h. Active alveolitis detected by

        i. High resolution computed tomography

       ii. Bronchoalveolar lavage (BAL)

           1. Abnormally high percentage of neutrophils

           2. Predicts progressive interstitial lung disease

  i. Lung disease can be highly variable

        i. Majority have early, but modest declines in lung function

           1. Stable courses

       ii. About 20% have an insidious decline

           1. Severe impairment of lung function and physical capacity

    j. Less common lung problems
       i. Aspiration
         1. Secondary to esophageal dysfunction or pharyngeal disease
      ii. Chronic cough
     iii. Respiratory distress with muscle disease
     iv. Pulmonary hemorrhage
      v. Pneumothorax
     vi. An increased prevalence of lung cancer
         1. Seen with systemic sclerosis

13. Gastrointestinal
    a. One of the most common problems encountered
    b. Seen in both limited and diffuse disease
    c. Small oral aperture
       i. Periodontal disease
      ii. Poor nutrition
    d. Dysphagia and heartburn
       i. The most common GI symptoms
    e. Esophageal reflux and esophagitis
       i. Loss of secondary peristalsis in the distal esophagus
      ii. Loss of normal esophageal clearance
     iii. Decreased pressures in the lower esophageal sphincter
     iv. Poor gastric emptying
      v. Aspiration
     vi. Unexplained coughing
     vii. Hoarseness
    viii. Atypical chest pain
     ix. Untreated esophagitis leads to
         1. Erosions
         2. Bleeding
         3. Stricture
         4. Barrett's metaplasia
         5. Adenocarcinoma
    f. Pathophysiologic progression of esophageal involvement
       i. Early stages
         1. Neural dysfunction (first)
           a. Abnormal function of the smooth muscle in the distal two-thirds of the esophagus
           b. Due to arteriolar changes of the vasa nervorum
           c. Leads to dysmotility
      ii. Later stages
         1. Smooth-muscle atrophy (second)
         2. Muscle fibrosis (third)
           a. Excess collagen deposition in the lamina propria
    g. Esophageal dysmotility assessed by
       i. Manometry

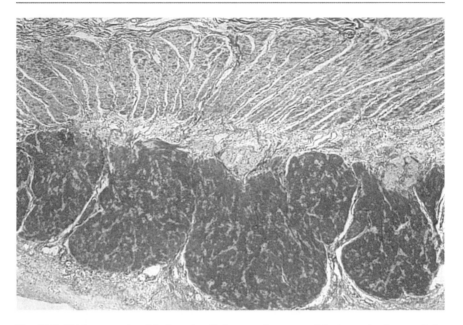

Fig. 11.8 Trichrome stain of the bowel wall shows replacement of the inner circular muscle by collagenous scarring in progressive systemic sclerosis (Reproduced with permission from Pathology of the colon and rectum. *Gastroenterology and Hepatology*. ImagesMD; 2002-01-28)

  ii. Cine esophagraphy
  iii. Routine upper GI with barium swallow
 h. Endoscopy to assess
  i. Reflux esophagitis
  ii. Candidiasis
  iii. Barrett's esophagus
  iv. Stricture of the lower esophageal area
 i. Treatment of esophageal dysmotility
  i. Elevate the head of the bed by 4 in.
  ii. Do not eat for 2–3 h before bedtime
  iii. Decrease acid content in the evening with antacids
   1. H2 blockers
   2. PPI
  iv. Motility agents
   1. Metocloparmide
   2. May help in early disease
 j. "Watermelon stomach"
  i. Seen in scleroderma patients
  ii. Gastric antral venous ectasia
  iii. Can cause upper GI bleeding
 k. Dysmotility of the small intestine
  i. May be asymptomatic

Fig. 11.9 Typical radiographic appearance of small bowel manifestations of systemic sclerosis with distended bowel loops and thickened and seemingly fixed valvulae conniventes (Reproduced with permission from Gastrointestinal manifestations of systemic sclerosis. *Digestive Diseases and Sciences*. DOI: 10.1007/s10620-007-0018-8. Springer; 2008-04-10)

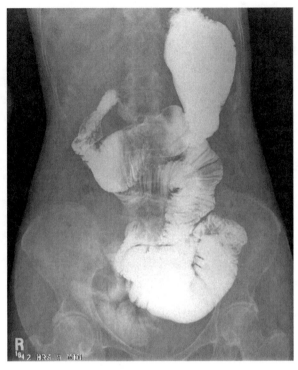

    ii. Serious chronic pseudo-obstruction of the intestine
        1. Severe distension
        2. Abdominal pain
        3. Vomiting
    iii. Malabsorption
        1. Secondary to bacterial overgrowth in stagnant intestinal fluids
            a. Hydrogen breath test
            b. High folate
        2. Low albumin
        3. Low B6/B12/folate/25OH vitamin D
        4. High fecal fat
        5. Low D-xylose absorption
        6. Low carotene
        7. Severe
            a. Vitamin deficiencies
            b. Electrolyte abnormalities
    iv. Pneumatosis cystoids intestinalis
        1. Mimics a ruptured bowel
        2. Air dissects into the bowel wall and peritoneal cavity
        3. No medical or surgical intervention required
        4. A poor prognostic sign

    l. Involvement of the large intestine and rectum
       i. Asymptomatic wide-mouth diverticula
      ii. Muscular atrophy of the large bowel wall
     iii. Unique to systemic sclerosis
     iv. Involves the transverse and descending colon
      v. Fecal incontinence
         1. Secondary to fibrosis of the rectal sphincter
     vi. Barium studies
         1. Relatively contraindicated with poor GI motility
         2. Risk of barium impaction
  m. Management of small and large bowel problems
       i. Stimulation of gut motility in early disease
         1. Metoclopramide
         2. Erythromycin
            a. A motilin agonist
            b. Given half hour before meals
         3. Fiber may help colonic motility
      ii. Diarrhea
         1. Treated as if it were due to bacterial overgrowth
         2. Amoxicillin or cipro for 10 days
         3. Avoid loperamide
         4. If secondary to malabsorption treat with
            a. Vitamins
            b. Minerals
            c. Predigested liquid food supplements
14. Cardiac
  a. Most heart problems are subtle in expression
       i. Rare for clinically significant involvement
      ii. Usually not seen until late in the disease
     iii. Overt cardiac signs correlate with a poor prognosis
  b. Clinical presentations
       i. Dyspnea on exertion
      ii. Palpitations
     iii. Chest discomfort
  c. Sites of involvement
       i. Myocardium
      ii. Myocardial blood vessels
     iii. Pericardium
  d. Myocardial fibrosis
       i. The most common manifestation of scleroderma heart disease
      ii. Characteristic presentation
         1. Equally distributed throughout the right and left heart myocardium
         2. Patchy fibrosis throughout the entire myocardium
         3. Unrelated to extramural coronary artery disease (CAD)
     iii. Usually focal
     iv. An uncommon cause of cardiomyopathy

e. Areas of contraction band necrosis
    i. A consequence of hypoxia/reperfusion injury
    ii. Due to vasospasm of distal coronary vessels
    iii. Seen on thallium during cold provocation of Raynaud's
f. Diastolic dysfunction (frequent)
g. Premature CAD
    i. Secondary to diffuse vasculopathy
    ii. Enhanced by use of high dose corticosteroids
h. Decline in left ventricular ejection fraction
    i. A late manifestation
    ii. CHF
i. Cardiomyopathy
    i. Associated with inflammatory autoimmune myocarditis
j. Pericardial effusion
    i. Small or large
    ii. Up to 40% of asymptomatic patients
    iii. Pericarditis and tamponade rare
k. Conduction defects
    i. EKG demonstrates asymptomatic conduction disease
    ii. Usually not treated unless significant ventricular arrhythmias
15. Renal
a. Kidney disease almost always present in systemic sclerosis

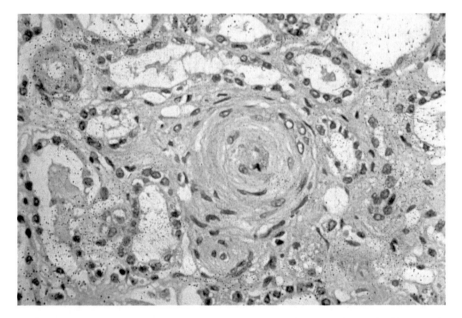

Fig. 11.10 Characteristic vascular lesion of acute systemic sclerosis with mucoid intimal hyperplasia and necrosis of an intralobular artery (Reproduced with permission from Systemic lupus erythematosus, scleroderma, and inflammatory myopathies. *Atlas of Rheumatology*. ImagesMD; 2005-01-18)

b. Renal crisis
  i. Accelerated hypertension and/or rapidly progressive renal failure
  ii. 80% of cases occur early
    1. Within the first 4 or 5 years of disease
    2. Mean 3.2 years
    3. Usually with diffuse disease
  iii. More often occur in fall and winter months
  iv. Blood pressure usually abnormal
    1. >150/90 mmHg
    2. Normotensive crises occur occasionally
  v. Retinopathy
    1. Grade III
      a. Flame-shaped hemorrhages
      b. Cotton-wool exudates
    2. Grade IV
      a. Papilledema
  vi. Rapid deterioration of renal function (within a month)
  vii. Labs
    1. A high creatinine level
    2. Proteinuria

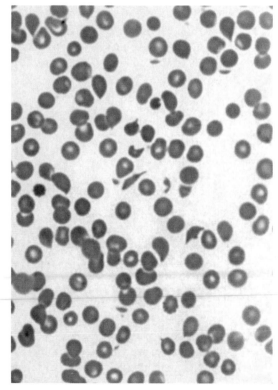

Fig. 11.11 Peripheral blood smear demonstrating evidence of microangiopathic hemolytic anemia and thrombocytopenia seen in renal crisis (Reproduced with permission from Systemic lupus erythematosus, scleroderma, and inflammatory myopathies. *Atlas of Rheumatology*. ImagesMD; 2005-01-18)

         3. Microscopic hematuria
         4. Anemia
         5. Consumptive thrombocytopenia
             a. A microangiopathic process within constricted renal vessels
         6. Elevated renin levels
             a. Twice the upper level of normal (ULN) or greater
     viii. Poor prognoses
         1. Men
         2. Older age of onset
         3. Creatinine levels greater than 3 mg/dl
     ix. Risk factors for renal crisis
         1. Diffuse skin disease
         2. New unexplained anemia
         3. Use of corticosteroids
         4. Pregnancy
         5. Presence of anti-RNA polymerase III antibodies
  c. Renal failure
     i. More likely with prolonged hypertension
     ii. Normotensive renal failure
         1. A minority
         2. No evidence of renal crisis
     iii. High dose corticosteroids increases the risk
  d. Therapeutic interventions
     i. ACE inhibitors
         1. Dramatically changed the incidence and outcome
         2. The most studied ACE inhibitors
             a. Captopril
             b. Enalapril
     ii. Diastolic blood pressure
         1. Keep below 90 mmHg in all scleroderma patients
16. Other Clinical Problems
  a. Major depression
  b. Impotence
  c. Sicca complex with associated Sjogren's syndrome
  d. Carpal tunnel syndrome
  e. Trigeminal neuralgia
  f. Hypothyroidism
  g. Autoimmune thyroiditis

Section C: Other Related Syndromes

1. Diffuse Fasciitis with Eosinophilia
  a. An idiopathic connective tissue disorder first described in 1974
  b. Severe induration of the skin and subcutaneous tissues

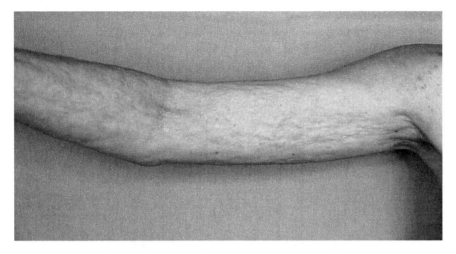

Fig. 11.12 Eosinophilic fasciitis with disseminated scleroderma-like skin changes on the upper extremities (Reproduced with permission from Eosinophilic fasciitis successfully treated with cyclosporine. *Clinical Rheumatology.* DOI: 10.1007/s10067-005-1099-4. Springer; 2005-12-01)

      i. Taut and woody
      ii. A coarse orange-peel appearance ("peau d'orange")
      iii. Mimics systemic sclerosis
  c. Cause unknown
      i. 30% of cases onset following vigorous exercise
      ii. Thought to involve autoimmune mechanisms
      iii. **NO** association with the ingestion of chemicals
  d. Sporadic cases
  e. Simultaneous involvement in all affected areas
      i. Both arms and legs in a symmetrical fashion
  f. Spares the fingers, hands, and face
      i. In contrast to systemic sclerosis
  g. Proximal areas of the extremities generally more affected than distal
  h. Three common early clinical manifestations
      i. Diffuse swelling
      ii. Stiffness
      iii. Tenderness of the involved areas
  i. Clinical manifestations that are **absent**
      i. Raynaud's
      ii. Visceral involvement
      iii. Microvascular disease
      iv. Normal nailfold capillaries
  j. Complications
      i. Vein entrapment
         1. Fibrosis puckers the overlying tissues
         2. Overlying skin will still wrinkle

    ii. Fascial involvement
       1. Carpal tunnel syndrome
       2. Flexion contractures of the digits and extremities
  k. Histologic diagnosis
     i. A deep wedge en bloc full thickness biopsy of an involved area
       1. Skin
       2. Subcutaneous tissue
       3. Fascia
       4. Muscle
    ii. Inflammation
       1. Subcutaneous skin
          a. Mononuclear cell infiltration
             i. Lymphocytes
            ii. Plasma cells
           iii. Histiocytes
          b. Tissue eosinophilia
             i. Striking especially early on
       2. Deeper layer of dermis involved in over 30%
       3. May extend to epi- and perimysial connective tissue

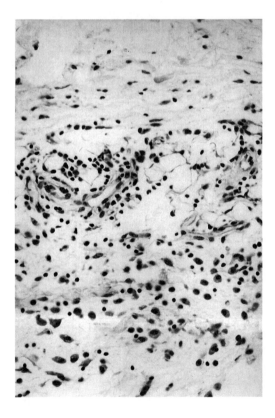

Fig. 11.13 Subcutaneous septa and muscular fascia are infiltrated by lymphocytes, plasma cells, and eosinophils (hematoxylin and eosin, ×400) in eosinophilic fasciitis (Reproduced with permission from Eosinophilic fasciitis successfully treated with cyclosporine. *Clinical Rheumatology*. DOI: 10.1007/ s10067-005-1099-4. Springer; 2005-12-01)

        4. Muscle fiber involvement rare
- l. Clinical diagnosis
  - i. Scleroderma-like skin tightening
  - ii. Peripheral eosinophilia
    1. Often present during early stages only
       a. Tends to decline later
    2. Degree of eosinophilia does not parallel disease activity
  - iii. Skin thickening that spares the digits
  - iv. Hypergammaglobulinemia
    1. Elevations in total gammaglobulin pool
    2. IgG fraction primarily responsible
  - v. **No** Raynaud's phenomenon
  - vi. Autoantibodies usually absent
- m. Temporal association with various hematologic conditions
  - i. Aplastic anemia
  - ii. Myelomoncytic and chronic lymphocytic leukemia
  - iii. Thrombocytopenia
  - iv. Monoclonal gammopathy
  - v. Myeloproliferative syndrome
  - vi. Lymphomas
  - vii. Also GVHD and some solid tumors
  - viii. Monitor closely for hematologic problems
  - ix. May occur at any time in the course of the disease
  - x. Does not correlate with disease severity
- n. Disease course variable
  - i. Self-limited and spontaneous regression (most)
  - ii. Complete remission after 2 years or more
  - iii. Remain unchanged for years
  - iv. Persistent or recurrent disease
- o. Treatment
  - i. 70% respond to corticosteroids
  - ii. Other medications used with variable success
    1. Cimetidine
    2. Hydroxychloroquine
    3. Penicillamine
    4. Immunosuppressive agents
  - iii. Untreated
    1. Fixed joint contractures occur in 85%
    2. Leads to permanent disability
2. Eosinophilia Myalgia Syndrome (EMS)
   - a. First reported in 1989 as an epidemic
     - i. Associated with the use of the amino acid L-tryptopan
     - ii. Treatment for conditions such as insomnia and depression
     - iii. L-tryptophan was contaminated with several potential toxins

        1. 1,1 ethylidenebis (EBT)

        2. 3-(phenyl-amino) alanine

     iv. Initial cases recognized in Los Alamos, New Mexico

  b. Prevalence

     i. Highest in the western USA

     ii. California represents 19% of the US total

  c. Acute phase

     i. Abrupt in onset and lasts weeks to months

     ii. Presents as a multisystem disease

        1. Intense myalgia and arthralgia

        2. Fever

        3. Cough

        4. Fatigue

        5. Weight loss

        6. Peripheral edema

        7. Papular rash associated with eosinophilia

     iii. Subcutaneous edema with woody induration

        1. Similar to eosinophilic fasciitis and systemic sclerosis

        2. Located on the trunk and lower extremities

        3. Spares the face and the acral portions of the body

     iv. Hyperpigmentation

  d. Chronic phase

     i. Last for years

     ii. Scleroderma-like skin changes

        1. Increases 44–82% after 14–36 months from onset

     iii. Xerostomia, and alopecia

     iv. Proximal myopathy

     v. Paresthesias with peripheral neuropathy

     vi. Neurocognitive dysfunction

     vii. Chronic fatigue

  e. The Center for Disease Control established three essential features as surveillance case definitions with more than 1,500 cases and 38 deaths

     i. Blood eosinophil count greater than 1,000 cells/mm^3

     ii. Marked generalized myalgia to limit activity

     iii. Exclusion of neoplasma

  f. EMS generally lacks

     i. Raynaud's

     ii. Digital ischemic lesions

     iii. Tendon friction rubs

     iv. Acral sclerosis

  g. Biopsy

     i. Demonstrates the presence of the prefibrotic cytokines

        1. TGF-β

        2. PDGF-AA

   h. Treatment
      i. Corticosteroids
        1. Helps in the acute inflammatory phase
        2. Does not alter the course of the disease
      ii. Other medications
        1. NSAIDs
        2. D-penicillamine
        3. Methotrexate
        4. Cyclophosphamide
        5. Azathioprine
        6. Cyclosporine

Section D: Treatment

1. Disease-Modifying Interventions
   a. Interventions targeted at
      i. Preventing vascular injury
      ii. Forestalling fibrosis
      iii. Immunosuppression
   b. ACE inhibitors in renal crisis is the best example
   c. The effectiveness of most immunosuppressants not supported in randomized, controlled trials
      i. D-penicillamine
        1. The most studied drug in systemic sclerosis
        2. No difference in skin scores, mortality, or the incidence of renal crisis
        3. Relatively toxic
      ii. Chlorambucil
      iii. Ketanserin
      iv. Interferon-alpha
      v. Photopheresis
   d. Methotrexate
      i. Both positive and negative outcomes
   e. Colchicine
      i. Relatively safe
      ii. Usually ineffective
   f. Cyclosporine
      i. Modest benefit in uncontrolled trials
      ii. Unacceptable renal toxicity
   g. Interferon-gamma
      i. Benefit in skin scores
      ii. Problems with renal crisis
      iii. Considered for interstitial lung disease

   h. Relaxin
      i. A natural hormone made during pregnancy
      ii. A 24 week Phase I/II randomized, placebo-controlled trial
         1. Doses of recombinant drug produce serum levels 3–5 times those of pregnancy
         2. Decreased skin thickening in diffuse cutaneous scleroderma over placebo
      iii. A larger study demonstrated no difference from placebo
   i. Drugs with possible benefits
      i. Minocycline
      ii. Oral bovine collagen type I
      iii. Immunoablation with peripheral-blood stem-cell rescue
      iv. Halofuginone
   j. TGF-β neutralization
      i. Decorin
         1. A small TGF-β binding proteoglycan
      ii. Latency-associated peptide
         1. A potent inhibitor of TGF-β isoforms
      iii. Soluble receptors
      iv. Chimeric antibodies
   k. Corticosteroids
      i. Best to avoid
      ii. May increase the incidence of renal crisis
      iii. Useful for
         1. Comfort with very actively inflamed and tight skin
         2. Inflammatory myositis
2. Symptomatic (Organ-Specific)
   a. Numerous therapies borrowed from other fields of medicine improve the management of organ complications
   b. Skin
      i. Local skin care
         1. Essential
         2. Topical moisturizers
      ii. Pruritus
         1. Troublesome in early diffuse disease
         2. Oral antihistamines
         3. Topical analgesics
         4. Topical corticosteroids
      iii. Ulcers
         1. Keep clean with mild soap and water
         2. Topical antibiotic ointments
         3. Infected treat with antistaphylococcal antibiotics
      iv. Subcutaneous calcinosis
         1. No treatment shown to prevent
         2. A short course of oral colchicine

        a. May reduce inflammation

     3. Surgical debridement with skin breakdown

c. Raynaud's Phenomenon and ischemia

   i. Affects the vast majority

   ii. Avoid cold exposure

   iii. Use layers of warm, loose-fitting clothing

   iv. Stop smoking

   v. Complicated digital-tip ulcers

     1. Vasodilator therapy and analgesics

     2. Nifedipine or other calcium-channel blockers

     3. Prazosin

     4. Topical nitroglycerin paste

   vi. Extended-release nifedipine diminished Raynaud's attacks in a randomized, controlled trial

   vii. Biofeedback ineffective

   viii. Ischemic and/or frankly necrotic fingers and toes require aggressive treatment

     1. IV prostaglandin (PGE1 or alprostadil)

     2. IV prostacyclin (PGE2 or epoprostenol)

     3. Permanent sympathectomies

     4. Medical or surgical sympathetic blocks can determine the potential for reversal vasospasm

     5. Surgical micro-arteriolysis (digital sympathectomy)

     6. Vascular reconstruction

     7. Amputation as a last resort

d. Gastrointestinal

   i. Smooth muscle hypomotility

     1. Primary pathophysiologic abnormality

   ii. Reflux esophagitis and dysphagia

     1. Most common clinical manifestations

   iii. Treatment goals

     1. Suppress acid production

     2. Improve motility

   iv. Nonpharmacologic treatments

     1. Elevate the head of the bed 4–6 in.

     2. Eat frequent small meals (5–6 per day)

        a. Avoid lying down within 3 or 4 h of eating

        b. Abstain from caffeine-containing beverages

        c. Abstain from cigarette smoking

     3. Esophageal strictures may require periodic dilatation

   v. Pharmacologic therapies

     1. Oral antacids

     2. H2 blockers

     3. Proton-pump inhibitors

        a. Omeparazole and lansoprazole

   b. For severe complaints
      i. Esophageal strictures
      ii. Recalcitrant reflux
   c. Controls GI side effects from NSAIDs and calcium channel blockers
   d. Used in management of upper GI bleeding
      i. Watermelon stomach
      ii. Erosive esophagitis
4. Promotility agents
   a. Metoclopramide
   b. For gastroparesis
vi. Small intestinal dysmotility
   1. Postprandial bloating
   2. Diarrhea
   3. Malabsorption
   4. Weight loss
   5. Pseudo-obstruction
   6. Treatment
      a. Broad-spectrum antibiotics given in rotating, 2 weeks courses
         i. Amoxicillin
         ii. Metronidazole
         iii. Doxycycline
         iv. Vancomycin
         v. Trimethoprim-sulfamethoxazole
         vi. Ciprofloxacin
      b. Promotility agents
         i. Metoclopramide
         ii. Erythrmycin
         iii. Octreotide
      c. Supplementation
         i. Fat-soluble vitamins
         ii. Calcium
         iii. Vitamin B12
         iv. Medium-chain triglycerides
      d. Manage pseudo-obstruction medically
         i. Nasogastric suction
         ii. Bowel rest
         iii. Parenteral alimentation
vii. Constipation
   1. Increased fluid intake
   2. Increased dietary bulk
   3. Stool softeners
   4. Recalcitrant cases
      a. Oral osmotic colon cleaners
         i. Polyethylene glycol
      b. Electrolytes

      viii. Fecal incontinence
- 1. Control diarrhea
  - a. Usually secondary to bacterial overgrowth
- 2. Rotating antibiotics
- 3. Low-residue diet
- 4. Antidiarrheal medications
- 5. Bile-acid binding resins (cholestyramine)

  e. Cardiopulmonary
- i. Two primary pulmonary manifestations
  - 1. Interstitial pulmonary fibrosis
    - a. Usually preceded by inflammatory alveolitis
  - 2. Obstructive pulmonary vasculopathy
- ii. Alveolitis
  - 1. Combination therapy
    - a. Cyclophosphamide or azathioprine
    - b. Low dose corticosteroids
  - 2. Stabilizes or improves lung function
- iii. Idiopathic pulmonary fibrosis
  - 1. Interferon-gamma proven effective in a small randomized trial
  - 2. Lung transplantation in end-stage disease
- iv. Pulmonary artery hypertension
  - 1. Conventional management
    - a. Low-flow nasal oxygen (especially at night)
    - b. Rigorous management of right-sided heart failure
    - c. Smoking cessation
    - d. Anticoagulation therapy
  - 2. IV epoprostenol improves
    - a. Exercise capacity
    - b. Hemodynamics
    - c. Dyspnea
- v. Large pericardial effusions
  - 1. Do not require pericardiocentesis
  - 2. May be a harbinger of renal crisis
- vi. Standard care as with any other patient for
  - 1. Pericarditis
  - 2. CHF
  - 3. Serious arrhythmias
- vii. Periodic *Pneumoncoccal* pneumonia vaccines and annual flu shots

  f. Kidneys (renal crisis)
- i. Acute oliguric renal failure associated with malignant hypertension
- ii. ACE inhibitors
  - 1. First choice of drugs for management of acute renal crisis
  - 2. Reverse the hyper-reninemia and hypertension
  - 3. Increased 1 year survival rate from 15% to 76%

      4. Diminish the effects of angiotensin II
      5. Increases levels of bradykinin and angiotensin 1–7
        a. Two potent renal vasodilators
      6. Continued indefinitely
      7. Significant renal function improvement of patients on dialysis
        a. 50% stop within 6–18 months
   iii. Angiotensin II receptor inhibitors (ARBs)
      1. Diminish the effects of angiotensin II
      2. Do **not** increase levels of bradykinin and angiotensin 1–7
      3. Should **NOT** be used to initially manage renal crisis
   iv. Keys to successfully managing renal crisis
      1. Early detection with home blood pressure monitoring
      2. Early introduction of ACE inhibitors and normalization of blood pressure
      3. ACE inhibitors help even those who go on to dialysis (50%)
      4. Renal transplantation if dialysis is required after 18 months
g. Musculoskeletal
   i. Common manifestations in diffuse disease
      1. Arthritis
      2. Tendonitis (often with tendon friction rubs)
      3. Muscle weakness
      4. Joint contractures
   ii. Treatment
      1. Inflammatory myositis
        a. Corticosteroids
        b. MTX
      2. Relieve pain
        a. NSAIDs
        b. Pure analgesics
          i. Acetaminophen
          ii. Propoxyphene
          iii. Tramadol
        c. Narcotics and low dose corticosteroids
          i. <10 mg/day prednisone
          ii. Used if other measures inadequate
      3. Stretch contractures
        a. PT instituted early and aggressively
        b. Especially with diffuse disease
        c. Dynamic splinting **NOT** effective
      4. Strengthen weak muscles

Sjögren's Syndrome

12

Introduction

1. A debilitating autoimmune disorder
   a. A form of "epitheliitis" or an exocrinopathy
2. Henrich Sjogren published a monograph in 1933
   a. Associated dry eyes with arthritis
   b. Introduced the term keratoconjunctivitis sicca (KCS)
3. Prominent salivary and lacrimal gland involvement
   a. Decreased production of saliva (xerostomia) (42%)
   b. Decreased production tears (xerophthalmia) (47%)
4. Other epithelial sites commonly involved
   a. Skin
   b. Urogenital
   c. Respiratory
   d. Gastrointestinal
5. Other systemic autoimmune manifestations
   a. Synovitis
   b. Neuropathy
   c. Vasculitis
   d. Autoantibodies
      i. Anti-SSA/Ro
      ii. Anti-SSB/La
      iii. RF
   e. Immunoglobulins frequently elevated
6. Primary Sjogren's
   a. Diagnosed in the absence of another underlying rheumatic disease
   b. Immunogenetically associated with HLA-B8-DR3
   c. Antinuclear antibodies to Ro/SSA and La/SSB
   d. May be associated with malignancies
      i. Especially non-Hodgkin's lymphoma

N.T. Colburn, *Review of Rheumatology*,
DOI 10.1007/978-1-84882-093-7_12, © Springer-Verlag London Limited 2012

7. Secondary Sjogren's
   a. Diagnosed with evidence of a coexistent autoimmune disease
      i. RA (most frequently)
      ii. SLE
      iii. Scleroderma
      iv. Polymyositis
      v. Polyarteritis nodosa
   b. Immunogenetic and serologic findings usually those of the accompanying disease
      i. HLA-DR4 if associated with RA
8. Epidemiology
   a. Prevalence vary widely
      i. 0.05–4.8% of the population
      ii. Estimated 1–2 million people in the USA
      iii. Primary Sjogren's occurs at a rate of 1/1,000 individuals
         1. Equal in frequency to SLE
      iv. 30% of patients with RA have secondary Sjogren's
   b. Occurs at any age
      i. Appears to increase with age
         1. Diagnosis usually made in midlife
      ii. Mean age at diagnosis is 50 years
      iii. Rare in children
   c. Insidious onset
      i. Diagnosis may be delayed for a number of years
         1. About 9 years
         2. Even after the development of sicca symptoms
      ii. Average duration of symptoms before diagnosis
         1. Varies with organ involvement
         2. 7 years for dyspareunia
         3. 1–5 years for dry mouth
         4. 1 year for dry eyes
   d. Female to male ratio about 9:1
   e. Typical patient is a middle-aged female
9. Classification Criteria and Diagnosis
   a. Dry eyes with keratoconjunctivitis sicca
      i. Schirmer's I test
         1. Place a piece of filter paper under the inferior eyelid and measuring the amount of wetness over a specified time
         2. Wetting of <5 mm in 5 min is a strong indication of diminished tear production
      ii. Schrimer's II test
         1. Put a Q-tip into the nose and stimulate output of major and minor lacrimal glands through the nasolacrimal gland reflex
         2. A 15% false-positive and false-negative rate

Fig. 12.1 Schirmer's test in Sjögren's syndrome (Reproduced with permission from Rheumatoid arthritis, juvenile rheumatoid arthritis, and related conditions. *Atlas of Rheumatology.* ImagesMD; 2002-03-07)

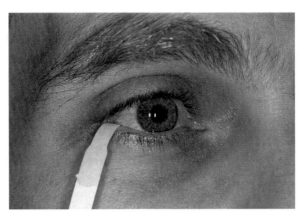

    iii. Rose Bengal (or lissamine green dye)
        1. Used more in the USA and the UK
        2. Applied topically
        3. Taken up by devitalized or damaged epithelium of the cornea and conjunctiva
        4. Documents dryness severe enough to injure corneal tissue
        5. Area of maximum uptake is along the palpebral fissure
        6. 5% false-positive and false-negative rate
    iv. Vital dyes
        1. Detect disturbances in the normal mucin coating of the conjunctival surface
        2. A fluorescein tear film breakup time of less than 10 s suggest dry eyes
           a. Observed on slit lamp examination
    v. Tests used in research studies
        1. Ocular osmolarity
        2. Tear proteins
  b. Dry mouth
    i. Scintigraphy
        1. Utilizes the uptake and secretion of ^{99m}Tc pertechnetate
           a. 60-min period
           b. Quantitates salivary flow rates
        2. A positive result
           a. Delayed uptake
           b. Reduced concentration
           c. Delayed excretion of tracer
    ii. Minor salivary gland biopsy
        1. Focal lymphocytic sialoadenitis
        2. Biopsy through normal appearing lower labial mucosa

3. Adequate yield 5–10 minor glands
4. A focus
   a. An area of >50 lymphocytes per 4 mm^2
   b. Around salivary gland acini or ducts
5. A focus score ≥1 focus/4 mm^{2}supports the diagnosis
6. Findings in minor salivary glands parallel involvement in other organs
7. Biopsy may be abnormal before decreased salivary flow can be documented with scintigraphy
   a. Enough gland destroyed to decrease saliva
   iii. Methods to quantitate saliva production
   1. Lashley cups
      a. Unstimulated whole salivary flow
         i. ≤1.5 ml in 15 min
   2. Dry sponge placed in the mouth
      a. Measure differences between dry and wet weights
   iv. Parotid sialography
   1. An objective test for salivary gland involvement
   2. Typical findings
      a. Diffuse sialectasias
      b. Punctate, cavitary, or destructive pattern
      c. No evidence of obstruction in the major ducts
c. Abnormal serologies and associated autoimmune disease
   i. + RF (usually RA)
   ii. + ANA
   iii. + Anti-SSA or anti-SSB (or both)
10. Differential Diagnosis
   a. Unilateral involvement
      i. Primary salivary gland neoplasms
      ii. Bacterial infection
      iii. Chronic sialadenitis
      iv. Obstruction
   b. Bilateral involvement
      i. Viral infections
      1. Mumps
      2. CMV
      3. Influenza
      4. Coxsackie A
      ii. Granulomatous disease
      1. Sarcoid
      2. TB
      3. Leprosy
      iii. Recurrent parotitis of childhood

    iv. HIV infection

        1. Diffuse infiltrative lymphocytosis syndrome (DILS)

        2. Mimics Sjogren's with common clinical features

           a. Fever

           b. Lymphadenopathy

           c. Weight loss

           d. Bilateral parotid gland enlargement

        3. Contrast to Sjogren's

           a. More xerostomia than xerophthalmia and keratoconjunctivitis sicca

           b. More recurrent sinus and middle ear infections

           c. Multiple areas of lymphocytic infiltration

               i. Interstitial pneumonitis

               ii. Hepatitis

               iii. Gastric mucosa

               iv. Interstitial nephritis

               v. Aseptic meningitis

               vi. Sensorimotor neuropathies

               vii. Uveitis

               viii. Cranial nerve palsies

           d. CD8+ infiltrating lymphocytes

               i. As opposed to CD4+ seen in Sjogren's

           e. Lack antibodies to Ro/SS-A and La/SS-B

  c. Bilateral, symmetric, soft and nontender

      i. Idiopathic

      ii. DM

      iii. Hyperlipoproteinemia (TypeV)

      iv. Hepatic cirrhosis

      v. Anorexia/bulimia

      vi. Chronic pancreatitis

      vii. Acromegaly

      viii. Gonadal hypofunction

      ix. Phenylbutazone ingestion

  d. Other causes

      i. Amyloidosis

11. Pathogenesis

  a. Remains unknown

  b. An unidentified environmental agent (example, virus) may trigger a cascade of events in genetically susceptible hosts

  c. Many viruses investigated, none implicated

      i. Herpes viruses

          1. EBV

          2. CMV

          3. HHV-6, and -8

      ii. Retroviruses

          1. HTLV-1

Fig. 12.2 Salivary gland
histology shows a dense,
diffuse lymphocytic infiltrate
in Sjögren's syndrome
(Reproduced with permission
from Rheumatoid arthritis,
juvenile rheumatoid arthritis,
and related conditions. *Atlas
of Rheumatology*.
ImagesMD; 2005-01-18)

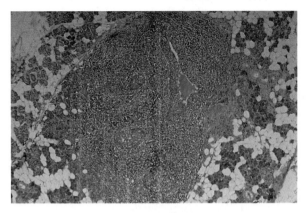

    2. HIV-1
    3. Human retrovirus 5
  iii. Hepatitis C
 d. Hypofunction of the hypothalamic-pituitary-adrenal axis
 e. Genetics
    i. Family members have increased prevalence of Sjogren's
      1. Particularly anti-SSA/Ro autoantibodies
    ii. HLA-DR3 and HLA-DQ2 alleles
      1. More common among Caucasian patients with primary Sjogren's
   iii. Peptide transporter genes TAP1 and TAP2 and microsatellite a2 alleles
      1. Increased frequency in a subset of patients
   iv. Other genetic associations reported outside the HLA
 f. Exocrine tissue infiltrates
    i. T-cells primarily
      1. Mostly CD4+ helper cells
      2. Bear the memory phenotype CD45RO+
      3. Express the alpha/beta TCR and LFA-1
    ii. Macrophages
   iii. Mast cells
   iv. Relatively few B-cells
    v. Adhesion molecules and LFA-1 promotes homing
 g. Periductal lymphocytes
    i. Resistant to apoptosis
    ii. Despite increased expression of Fas
   iii. Apoptosis blocked by the suppressor proto-oncogene Bcl-2
 h. Salivary and lacrimal gland epithelial cells
    i. Express HLA-DR antigens
    ii. Present exogenous antigens and autoantigens to the CD4+ T-cells
   iii. Produce proinflammatory cytokines
      1. IL-1β
      2. IL-6
      3. TNF-α

    i. Activated B cells

       i. Produce increased amounts of immunoglobulin

      ii. Autoantibody reactivity

          1. IgG (rheumatoid factor)

          2. SSA/Ro

          3. SSB/La

     iii. Antibody targets

          1. Muscarinic (acetylcholine) M3 receptor

             a. Blockade in exocrine tissue inhibits secretions

          2. Nerve supply of exocrine tissue

             a. Decreased secretions disproportionate to tissue destruction

     iv. May progress toward B-cell lymphoid malignancy

  j. Infiltrating T-cells produce

       i. IL-10

          1. A role in B-cell proliferation

      ii. IFN-γ

          1. Increases HLA-DR and SSB/La expression by glandular epithelial cells

  k. Complete destruction of salivary tissue is rare

       i. About half of the ducts and acini are destroyed in patients with substantial dryness

  l. Mouse models of Sjogren's

       i. NOD

      ii. NOD.B10

     iii. MRL/lpr

     iv. TGF-β knockout

          1. Develops salivary and lacrimal gland exocrinopathy

          2. TGF-β has a role in acinar cell differentiation

          3. May be important in the early course

12. Ocular Manifestations

  a. KCS or xerophthalmia

       i. Dry or painful eyes

      ii. Foreign-body or gritty sensation

     iii. Burning sensation

     iv. Itchiness

      v. Blurred vision

     vi. Redness

    vii. Photophobia

   viii. Symptoms worsen as the day progresses

          1. Ocular moisture evaporates when the eyes are open

     ix. Complications

          1. Infections

          2. Corneal ulcerations

          3. Visual loss

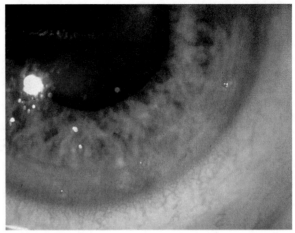

Fig. 12.3 Keratitis in Sjögren's syndrome (Reproduced with permission from Rheumatoid arthritis, juvenile rheumatoid arthritis, and related conditions. *Atlas of Rheumatology.* ImagesMD; 2005-01-18)

b. Ocular symptoms due to aqueous tear deficiency (ATD)
  i. A deficient aqueous middle layer of precorneal tear film
  ii. Normally comprises 90% of tear volume
  iii. Precorneal tear film
    1. Three distinct layers moving outward from the corneal surface
      a. Mucus
      b. Water
      c. Oil
    2. Outer most layer
      a. Covers the hydrated gel
      b. A complex mixture of nonpolar and polar lipids
  iv. Precorneal tear fluid (a complex biochemical mixture)
    1. Water
    2. Electrolytes
    3. Mucins
    4. Antimicrobial proteins
      a. Lactoferrin
      b. Lysozyme
    5. Immunoglobulins
    6. Growth factors
      a. TGF-α
  v. Hydrated gel
    1. Precorneal mucus, protein, and aqueous components
    2. Produced by the meibmian gland
    3. When removed experimentally
      a. KCS occurs
      b. Barrier to fluorescein dye decreases
      c. Contrast sensitivity declines
      d. Irregularity of the corneal surface increases

c. Differential diagnosis of dry eyes
  i. Problems that result in evaporative tear deficiency
  ii. Other lacrimal gland diseases
  iii. Lacrimal duct obstruction
  iv. Loss of reflex tearing
  v. Meibomian gland disease
    1. Blepharitis
      a. A low-grade infection of the meibomian gland
      b. Crusting and discomfort
      c. Most pronounced in the morning on awakening
  vi. Blink abnormality
  vii. Viral infections
  viii. Contact lens irritation
  ix. Medications
    1. Antihistamines
    2. Diuretics
    3. Tricyclic antidepressants
    4. Benzodiazepines
13. Oral Manifestations
  a. Xerostomia
    i. Symptoms and signs of decreased production of saliva
    ii. Burning sensation (up to 40%)
    iii. Change in taste (33%)
    iv. Intolerance of spicy foods
    v. Difficulty swallowing dry food (17%)
    vi. Inability to speak continuously
    vii. Increase in dental caries
      1. At the gingival margins
      2. On the incisal edges of the teeth
    viii. Problems wearing dentures
    ix. GE reflux symptoms
      1. Due to lack of salivary buffering
    x. Disturbed sleep
      1. Due to dry mouth and/or nocturia
    xi. Soft tissue changes on the tongue
      1. May become furrowed
      2. Dry and sticky mucosa
      3. Predisposition to oral candidiasis
        a. Erythematous and covered with white patches
    xii. Swallowing difficulties with esophageal dysmotility
    xiii. Examination
      1. Decreased or absent salivary pooling
      2. Visible enlargement of the major salivary glands

Fig. 12.4 Xerostomia in
Sjögren's syndrome with
absent salivary pooling
(Reproduced with permission
from Rheumatoid arthritis,
juvenile rheumatoid arthritis,
and related conditions. *Atlas
of Rheumatology.*
ImagesMD; 2005-01-18)

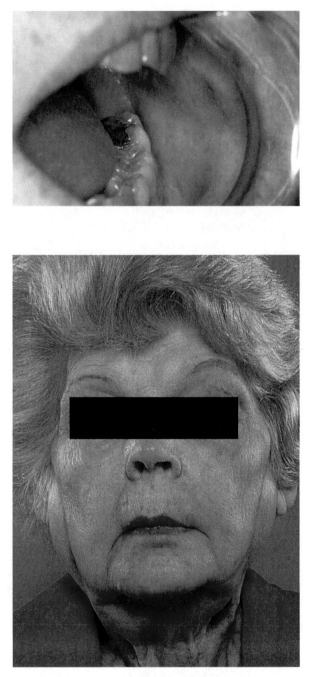

Fig. 12.5 Parotid
enlargement in Sjögren's
syndrome (Reproduced with
permission from Rheumatoid
arthritis, juvenile rheumatoid
arthritis, and related
conditions. *Atlas of
Rheumatology.* ImagesMD;
2002-03-07)

      a. Parotid gland swelling

         i. Displaces the earlobe

         ii. Extends downward over the angle of the jaw

      b. May or may not be tender

      c. May be transient or chronic

      d. Often recurrent

         i. Distinguishes from mumps

   b. Common causes of decreased salivary secretion

      i. Medications

         1. More than 400 implicated

         2. Antihistamines

         3. Anticholinergics

         4. Neuroleptics

         5. Clonidine

         6. Diuretics

      ii. Radiation exposure

         1. Radiation therapy for head and neck tumors

         2. Radioactive iodine for thyroid disorders

            a. Concentrates in exocrine glands

      iii. Psychogenic causes

         1. Fear

         2. Depression

      iv. Dehydration

         1. Thermal

         2. Trauma

         3. Diabetes

      v. Absent or malformed glands (rare)

14. Laboratory Features

   a. ESR (up to 90%)

   b. Hypergammaglobulinemia (80%)

   c. Anemia of chronic disease (25%)

   d. Leukopenia (10%)

   e. Thrombocytopenia (rare)

   f. Autoantibodies

      i. Serologic evidence of autoimmunity

      ii. Rheumatoid factor+ (up to 95%)

      iii. ANA (up to 90%)

      iv. Anti-SS-A/Ro (50–90%)

         1. Antibodies to the 52-kDa Ro antigen

            a. More often associated with Sjogren's

         2. Antibodies to the 60-kDa Ro antigen

            a. More often associated with SLE

      v. Anti-SS-B/La (50–90%)

      vi. Other antigenic targets

         1. Carbonic anhydrase

         2. Pancreatic antigen

Fig. 12.6 Palpable purpura in Sjögren's syndrome
(Reproduced with permission from Rheumatoid
arthritis, juvenile rheumatoid arthritis, and related
conditions. *Atlas of Rheumatology*. ImagesMD;
2005-01-18)

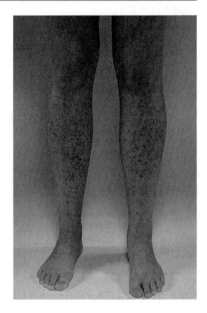

    3. Alpha fodrin
    4. 97-kDa Golgi complex
    5. Mitotic spindle apparatus
    6. M3 muscarinic acetylcholine receptors
    7. Fc-gamma receptors
15. Extraglandular Manifestations
    a. Raynaud's (up to 40%)
    b. Cutaneous
      i. Dry skin and pruritus
        1. Treatment
          a. Decreased frequency of bathing
          b. Mentholated lotions
    c. Vasculitis (5–10%)
      i. Palpable or nonpalpable purpura and petechiae
        1. More frequently on the legs
        2. Histology
          a. Leukocytoclastic vasculitis (seroreactive)
            i. Anti-SSA/Ro and anti-SSB/La antibodies
            ii. RF
            iii. ANA
            iv. Cryoglobulins
            v. Hypocomplementemia
            vi. Hypergammaglobulenemia
            vii. Circulating immune complexes

      b. Mononuclear inflammatory vasculopathy
         i. Usually **NOT** associated with seroreactivity and hypocomplementemia
   ii. Other vasculitic lesions
      1. Urticaria
      2. Erythema multiforme
      3. Erythematous macules
      4. Digital ulcers
d. Thyroid
   i. Hypothyroidism (common)
   ii. **NO** significant differences in the prevalence of autoimmune thyroiditis
      1. Compared with individuals of similar age and gender
e. Respiratory (10–20%)
   i. Nonproductive cough occurs frequently
      1. Tracheal dryness
      2. Diminution in mucus production
   ii. Progressive pulmonary disease is unusual
   iii. Mild interstitial pulmonary disease
   iv. Hyperreactive airways
      1. Obstruction of smaller airways
      2. Lymphocytic infiltrates in bronchiolar walls
      3. Minor abnormalities on PFTs
      4. Bronchodilators may be useful therapy
   v. Mucosal biopsies and BAL
      1. Reveal increased submucosal CD4+ T-cells
   vi. Pleural effusions
      1. Contain lymphocytes and antibodies
         a. SSA/Ro
         b. SSB/La
f. Musculoskeletal
   i. Myalgia, arthralgia, and arthritis (60–70%)
   ii. Arthritis
      1. Distribution similar to RA
      2. Symmetric
         a. Wrists
         b. MCP
         c. PIP joints
      3. Morning stiffness and fatigue (frequent)
      4. Nonerosive
      5. Tends to be mild (in contrast to RA)
      6. Treatment
         a. NSAIDs
         b. Antimalarials
            i. Hydroxychloroquine
         c. Low dose prednisone (≤5 mg)

       7. Secondary Sjogren's and associated RA
g. Neurologic
    i. Peripheral neuropathy not uncommon (2–5%)
       1. Prominent in the lower limbs
       2. Most often sensory
         a. Numbness
         b. Tingling
         c. Burning
    ii. Autonomic neuropathy
    iii. CNS involvement
h. Hematologic (lymphoid malignancy)
    i. 44-fold increase in the frequency of B-cell lymphomas than age matched controls
    ii. 5–8% overall frequency of lymphoma
    iii. Usually non-Hodgkin's lymphoma of mucosa-associated lymphoid tissues (MALT)
    iv. Cervical lymph nodes and salivary glands also involved
    v. Signs and symptoms of lymphoma
       1. Significantly or prominently swollen salivary glands
       2. Preceded by the development of a monoclonal gammopathy
       3. Loss of a previously positive rheumatoid factor
       4. Loss of the monoclonal gammopathy
       5. Development of hypogammaglobulinemia
       6. Clues of excessive lymphoproliferation
         a. Regional or generalized lymphadenopathy
         b. Hepatosplenomegaly
         c. Pulmonary infiltrates
         d. Renal insufficiency
         e. Purpura
         f. Leukopenia
    vi. Evaluations
       1. CT scans
       2. Fine-needle aspirates for cytology
       3. Flow cytometric analyses
       4. Biopsy
i. Reproductive
    i. Obstetrical complications
       1. More likely related to concomitant autoimmune disease in secondary Sjogren's
       2. Does not appear to be increased in primary disease
    ii. A low risk of congenital heart block in mothers with anti-SSA/Ro antibodies
    iii. Vaginal dryness
       1. Commonly associated with dyspareunia

    2. Treatment
      a. Water-soluble lubricants
      b. Vaginal estrogen preparations in postmenopausal women
  j. Urinary Tract
    i. Irritable bladder not uncommon
    ii. Increased urinary frequency
    iii. Renal abnormalities
      1. Diminished ability to concentrate urine (about half of all cases)
      2. Distal renal tubular acidosis (RTA) (about 15%)
        a. Urine pH generally above 5.5
        b. Associated with systemic acidosis
        c. Results in mobilization of calcium from bone
          i. Osteoporosis
          ii. Hypercalciuria
        d. Treatment
          i. Oral alkaline preparations
            1. Sodium and potassium citrate
            2. 1–2 mEq/kg/day
          ii. Corrects acidosis
          iii. Decreases the risk of stones
      3. Nephrocalcinosis
        a. Low urinary citrate
          i. Normally complexes urine calcium
        b. Increased calcium phosphate stones
      4. Tubular proteinuria (about half of cases)
      5. Interstitial nephritis
      6. Glomerular disease (about 2%)
        a. Especially with longer disease duration
        b. Tends to be associated with cryoglobulins
        c. Glomerulonephritis
          i. Mixed cryoglobulinemia
          ii. Low C4 levels in the serum
16. Treatment of Sjogren's Syndrome
  a. Patient education and self-management strategies
  b. Keratoconjunctivitis sicca symptoms (xerophthalmia)
    i. Tear replacement and conservation
    ii. Artificial tears
      1. Derivatives of cellulose
      2. Instilled frequently to ameliorate symptoms
      3. Preservative-free preparations are superior
      4. Small dispensers minimize the risk of bacterial growth and infection
    iii. Discourage eye rubbing and rinsing the ocular surface with tap water
    iv. Duration and benefit of artificial tears insufficient
      1. Concentrated viscous solutions
        a. Refresh and Celluvisc

          b. Provide longer benefit

          c. May blur vision

     2. Hydroxypropylcellulose pellets

          a. Insert under the lower eyelids

          b. Dissolve by absorbing water

          c. Prolong the retention of moisture in the eye

     3. Viscous ointments at night

          a. Refresh PM

          b. Lacrilube

  v. Treat and prevent blepharitis

     1. Wash the lashes with baby shampoo

  vi. Humidifiers

     1. Useful in arid climates and at high altitudes

  vii. Evaporation of tears slowed by the use of glasses with side shields

  viii. Cholinergic drugs

     1. Systemic pilocarpine and cevimeline

     2. Stimulate functioning glands to produce more tears

          a. Only 30–50% of lacrimal glands are destroyed

     3. M3 muscarinic receptors stimulated on lacrimal and salivary acinar glands

          a. Stimulates ATPase needed for secretion

     4. Pilocarpine

          a. 5 mg orally 4 times a day

          b. Adverse effects

             i. Increased perspiration

            ii. Feeling hot and flushed

           iii. Increased bowel and bladder motility

          c. Caution in the presence of bronchospasm

     5. Cevimeline

          a. Longer half life (4 h vs. 1.5 h)

          b. 30 mg orally 3 times daily

          c. Higher specificity for the M3 receptor

          d. Lessens cardiac and pulmonary toxicity

            i. Heart and lungs have M2 receptors

     6. Patients with some tear production on Schirmer's II testing

          a. More likely to respond to these drugs

     7. Avoid or use with caution in patients with

          a. Narrow-angle glaucoma

          b. Asthma

          c. On beta-blockers

     8. Common side effects

          a. Sweating

          b. Gastrointestinal disturbances

  ix. Other therapies

     1. Topical corticosteroids

      2. Cyclosporine

      3. Intraocular androgens

   x. Severe ocular surface disease (scleritis, inflammatory nodules, corneal ulcers)

      1. Autologous serum

      2. Topical steroids

      3. Topical cyclosporine

  xi. Punctal plugs

      1. May be used in refractory cases

      2. Obstructs the normal lacrimal drainage system

      3. Collagen plugs dissolve and last about 2 days

      4. Silicon plugs are durable

      5. Permanent punctual occlusion

        a. If eye surface is improved without excessive tearing

 xii. Systemic treatments

      1. Role remains unclear

c. Xerostomia

   i. Frequent dental care is important

      1. Daily topical fluoride use

      2. Antimicrobial mouth rise

  ii. Avoid medications that promote mouth dryness

 iii. An appropriate diet and limited sugar intake

  iv. Artificial saliva and lubricants

      1. MouthKote

      2. Salivart

   v. Stimulants for salivary secretions

      1. Sugar-free chewing gum

      2. Mints

      3. Candy

  vi. Oral moisturizers and lubricants

 vii. Secretagogues

      1. Such as pilocarpine

      2. Increase secretions in patients with sufficient exocrine tissue

viii. Oral candidiasis

      1. Antifungal oral troches or vaginal suppositories

        a. Nystatin

          i. Nystatin vaginal tablets preferred

         ii. Other oral preparations contain glucose or sucrose

        b. Clotrimazole

      2. Oral fluconazole

        a. 2 weeks for resistant cases

      3. Dentures should be removed during treatment course

  ix. Angular cheilitis

      1. Topical antifungal agents

    x. Bacterial parotitis should be treated with
      1. Warm compresses
      2. Massage of the parotid gland
      3. Antibiotics, if necessary
    xi. Avoid alcohol
    xii. Frequent water ingestion
    xiii. Removal of nasal polyps
17. Treatment of Systemic Manifestations
  a. Hydroxychloroquine
    i. Commonly used for milder systemic manifestations
      1. Fever
      2. Rashes
      3. Arthritis
  b. Patients with prominent systemic manifestations
    i. Methotrexate
    ii. Prednisone
    iii. Azathioprine
    iv. Other immunomodulatory drugs
    v. Approach similar to treatment of SLE
  c. Desipramine
    i. Best tricyclic antidepressant
    ii. Treats poor sleep and symptoms of fibromyalgia
    iii. Low anticholinergic effects
  d. Superficial vasculitis and dermatitis
    i. Treated with steroids
  e. Lymphoma
    i. Treated in consultation with an oncologist
    ii. Based on the type and stage of disease

Behcet's Disease

13

1. Behcet's disease (BD)
   a. A chronic inflammatory vascular disorder
   b. Unknown etiology
2. Epidemiology
   a. Prevalence
      i. Countries with highest incidence
         1. Eastern Mediterranean
         2. The Middle East
         3. East Asia
      ii. Named the "Silk Road Disease"
         1. Trade trail of Marco Polo
         2. Extends from the Orient (Japan) through Turkey and into the Mediterranean basin
   b. Recognized world wide
   c. Occurs primarily in young adults
      i. Mean age at onset 25–30 years (40 years)
      ii. Juvenile cases infrequent (1–2%)
   d. Male to female ratio
      i. 1:1 along the Silk Road
      ii. Females predominate in
         1. Japan
         2. Korea
         3. Western countries
3. Pathogenesis
   a. Strong association with HLA-B51
      i. 3–6 times increased incidence in Japanese and eastern Mediterranean
      ii. A more complete expression of manifestations
      iii. A more severe clinical course
      iv. Not increased in BD patients in the USA

N.T. Colburn, *Review of Rheumatology*,
DOI 10.1007/978-1-84882-093-7_13, © Springer-Verlag London Limited 2012

    b. HLA-DRB1*04
       i. An association reported in Caucasians
    c. Neutrophil hyperreactivity
       i. Increased migration during attacks
       ii. Normal during remissions
    d. Major histocompatibility complex class I chain-related gene A (MICA)
       i. Linkage dysequilibrium with HLA-B51
       ii. Gene products expressed on fibroblasts and endothelial cells
       iii. A role in the presentation of antigen to NK cells or $\gamma\delta+$ cells
       iv. Activated $\gamma\delta+$ T-cells
          1. Increased in the circulation
          2. Increased in mucosal lesions
          3. Exact role uncertain
    e. Th1 response by lymphocytes
       i. Elevated levels of IL-12
  f. Molecular analysis
       i. Herpes simplex viral RNA and DNA
       ii. Streptococcal antigens
       iii. Mycobacterial heat shock proteins
          1. Specifically stimulate $\gamma\delta+$ T-cells
    g. Antigen-driven immune mechanisms
       i. Cross-reactivity and molecular mimicry postulated
       ii. Peptides from strep or viral HSP
       iii. Homologous human HSP
       iv. Mucosal antigens
4. Clinical Features (frequency of occurrence)
    a. Aphthous oral ulcers (97–100%)
       i. The first and most persistent clinical feature
          1. The initial manifestation in 25–75% of patients
       ii. 2–12 mm red-rimmed lesions
          1. Round or oval
          2. Discrete
          3. Painful

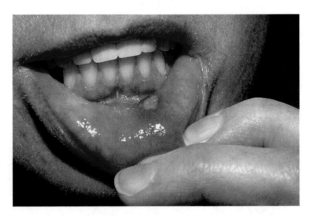

Fig. 13.1 Buccal mucosa oral ulcer of Behçet's disease (Reproduced with permission from Infections of the vulva. *Atlas of Infectious Diseases.* ImagesMD; 2003-01-23)

   iii. Sites of ulceration
      1. Mucous membranes (preferential)
         a. Lips
         b. Gingiva
         c. Cheeks (buccal mucosa)
         d. Tongue
      2. Rarely involved
         a. Palate
         b. Tonsils
         c. Pharynx
   iv. Characteristically occur in crops
      1. Six or more of various size
    v. Most heal without scarring within 10 days
   vi. Differential diagnosis of aphthous stomatitis
      1. Idiopathic (70%)
      2. B12/folate deficiency (22%)
      3. Gluten-sensitive enteropathy (2%)
      4. Menstrually related (2%)
      5. IBD (2%)
      6. Behcet's (1%)
      7. Complex aphthosis
         a. Recurrent oral and genital aphthous ulcers
         b. Multiple (>3)
         c. Without systemic manifestations
 b. Genital ulcers (80–100%)
    i. Vulva
      1. Painful
      2. Often develop during the premenstrual stage
      3. A frequent site
   ii. Vagina
      1. May be asymptomatic
  iii. Scrotum
      1. A frequent site

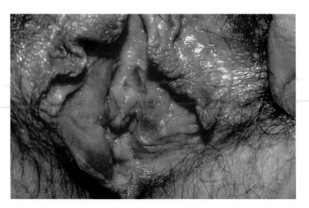

Fig. 13.2 Vaginal ulcers of Behçet's disease (Reproduced with permission from Infections of the vulva. *Atlas of Infectious Diseases.* ImagesMD; 2003-01-23)

     iv. Penis

     v. Perianal

    vi. Deeper than oral lesions

    vii. Lesions in men tend to be more painful than those in women

   viii. Leave scars after healing

    ix. Differential diagnosis of genital ulcers

       1. Behcet's is a rare cause of genital ulcers

       2. Venereal ulcers are the most common type

          a. HSV

          b. Syphilis

          c. Chancroid

          d. Lymphogranuloma venereum

          e. Granuloma inguinale (donovanosis)

       3. Nonvenereal causes

          a. Trauma

             i. Mechanical

            ii. Chemical

          b. Adverse drug reactions

          c. Nonvenereal infections

             i. Nonsyphylitic spirochetes

            ii. Pyogenic

           iii. Yeast

          d. Vesiculobullous skin diseases

          e. Neoplasms

             i. Precarcinoma

               1. Bowen's disease

            ii. Carcinoma

               1. Basal cell

               2. Squamous cell

          f. Rheumatic diseases

             i. Reiter's

            ii. Crohn's

  c. Skin lesions (35–65%)

     i. Common

     ii. Erythema nodosum

    iii. Pseudofolliculitis

     iv. Papulopustular

     v. Acneiform nodules

    vi. Pyoderma gangrenosum-like lesions

    vii. Thrombophlebitis

   viii. Neutrophilic inflammation

       1. Similar to Sweet's syndrome

  d. Pathergy

     i. An excessive skin response to trauma

     ii. A result of neutrophil hyperreactivity

iii. Highly specific for BD (pathognomonic)

iv. Unknown mechanism

    1. Related to increased neutrophil chemotaxis

v. A positive test

    1. Insert a sterile, sharp, 20-gauge needle perpendicular at the volar forearm to a depth of about 0.5 cm

    2. Assess after 24–48 h

    3. An erythematous papule or pustule >2 mm in diameter

    4. More likely positive at times of active disease

vi. Rate of a positive reaction

    1. More common in Japan and Turkey

    2. Less common in England and the USA

vii. Pathergy equivalents (sterile abscesses or pustules)

    1. After therapeutic injections

    2. At intravenous injection sites

    3. Skin trauma

e. Ocular Inflammation (50–79%)

  i. Typically follows mucocutaneous symptoms by a few years

  ii. Often progresses

    1. A chronic, relapsing course

    2. Affects both eyes

  iii. The leading cause of acquired blindness in Japan

    1. 11–12% in or before middle age

  iv. Hypopyon uveitis

    1. The presence of inflammatory cells in the anterior chamber

    2. Finding in the original Behcet's patients

      a. Initially believed to be pathognomonic

    3. Infrequent among patients in Western countries

  v. Anterior/posterior uveitis

    1. Blindness limited mostly to patients with posterior uveitis

    2. Occurs on an average of 4 years after onset of Behcet's

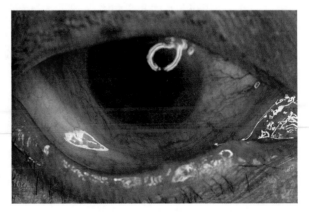

Fig. 13.3 Anterior uveitis with hypopyon in Behçet's disease (Reproduced with permission from Vasculitides. *Atlas of Rheumatology.* ImagesMD; 2002-03-07)

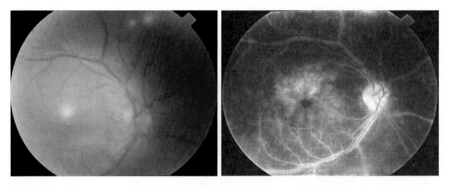

Fig. 13.4 Fundus photograph of the right eye in a patient with Behçet's disease showing retinal infiltrates (*left*) and the multilobular pattern of cystoid macular edema (*right*) (Reproduced with permission from A clinical approach to the diagnosis of retinal vasculitis. *International Ophthalmology*. DOI: 10.1007/s10792-009-9301-3. Springer 2010-03-31)

      vi. Panuveitis with posterior chamber involvement
     vii. Conjunctivitis
    viii. Corneal ulceration
     ix. Retinal vasculitis
        1. Episodes of retinal occlusion and areas of ischemia
        2. Neovascularization
        3. Vitreous hemorrhage and contraction
        4. Glaucoma
        5. Retinal detachment
      x. Cerebral venous thrombosis
        1. Leads to optic disk edema
     xi. Papillitis
        1. Seen with ocular inflammation and CNS disease
     xii. Cranial nerve palsies
        1. Result from brain-stem lesions
    xiii. Visual field defects
        1. Result from intracranial lesions
  f. Vascular Involvement (10–37%)
      i. Large vessel involvement of both arterial and venous systems
     ii. Thrombotic tendency is a feature of the disease
        1. Thrombosis in one-fourth of all patients
        2. Factor V Leiden mutation in up to one-third of patients
    iii. Deep venous thrombosis
        1. The most common vascular complication
        2. Risk for chronic venous stasis
          a. Especially patients with recurrences
     iv. Other thrombotic complications
        1. Occlusion of the superior or inferior vena cava
          a. A high risk of mortality

Fig. 13.5 A T2-weighted image showing thrombosis of the posterior part of the superior sagittal sinus thrombosis in a patient with neuro-Behçet's syndrome (Reproduced with permission from Behçet's syndrome and the nervous system. In: *Behçet's Syndrome* DOI: 10.1007/978-1-4419-5641-5_6. Springer 2010-01-01)

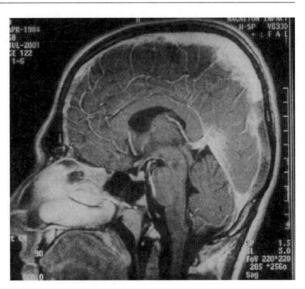

   2. Budd-Chiari syndrome
   3. Cerebral venous thromboses
   4. Cavernous transformation of the portal vein
   5. Varices
      a. Chest wall
      b. Abdomen
      c. Esophagus
 v. Arterial lesions
   1. Systemic circulation
   2. Pulmonary arterial bed
   3. Stenoses
   4. Occlusions
   5. Aneurysms
      a. Aorta or its branches at high risk for rupture
      b. Pulmonary artery
         i. Pulmonary artery-bronchial fistula with hemoptysis
         ii. Fatal aneurysms
            1. Behcet's disease is a frequent cause among vasculitides (virtually alone)
   6. CAD and MI
      a. Uncommon
      b. No significant difference in the prevalence of cardiac abnormalities among Behcet's and controls
      c. Sporadic reports of
         i. Valvular lesions
         ii. Myocarditis
         iii. Pericarditis

Fig. 13.6 Pulmonary artery
aneurysm in Behçet's disease
(Reproduced with permission
from Vasculitides. In: *Atlas of
Rheumatology* Images MD;
2002-03-07)

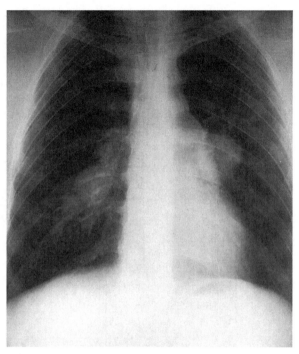

g. CNS disease (10–30%)
 i. More common in Europe and the USA than in Asia
  1. 30% of patients in Western countries
 ii. 41% mortality
 iii. A late manifestation
  1. 1–7 years after the initial onset of disease
 iv. Diagnostic presentation (a combination)
  1. Stroke
  2. Aseptic meningitis with CSF pleocytosis
  3. Mucocutaneous lesions
 v. Predilection for
  1. Small vessels in the brain stem
  2. Periventricular white matter
  3. Brainstem
   a. The most commonly involved region
 vi. Neurologic manifestations
  1. Headaches (52%)
  2. Meningoencephalitis (28%)
  3. Cranial nerve palsies (16%)
  4. Seizures (13%)
  5. Cerebellar ataxia
  6. Hemiplegia/paraparesis

       7. Pseudobulbar palsy

       8. Extrapyramidal signs

       9. Intracranial hypertension

          a. From dural sinus thrombosis

          b. 25% of patients

      10. Recur during flares of oral, genital, and joint lesions

  h. Gastrointestinal Involvement (0–25%)

     i. Melena

    ii. Abdominal pain

   iii. Single or multiple ulcerations

       1. Primarily involving the distal ileum and cecum

       2. Tendency to perforate or bleed

       3. May recur postoperatively

       4. Differentiate from IBD and mucosal changes of NSAIDS

  i. Arthritis (30–50%)

     i. Intermittent, migratory, monoarticular, or oligoarticular asymmetric

       1. Knees

       2. Ankles

       3. Elbows

       4. Hands or wrists

    ii. Less frequently involved

       1. Shoulders

       2. Spine

       3. Hips

       4. Small joints of the hands and feet

       5. Polyarticular

          a. Resembles rheumatoid arthritis

   iii. Arthralgia is common

       1. Lacks diagnostic value

   iv. Ankylosing spondylitis or radiographic sacroiliitis

       1. Increased frequency

    v. Destructive arthropathy unusual

   vi. Synovial findings

       1. Fluid

          a. Increased WBC count

             i. Primarily neutrophil

          b. Cell counts average 5,000–10,000/mm^3

       2. Biopsies

          a. Superficial neutrophilic infiltration

  j. Other less frequent clinical features

     i. Glomerulonephritis

    ii. Peripheral neuropathy

   iii. AA-type amyloidosis

       1. Presents as nephrotic syndrome

       2. Reported primarily in Mediterranean countries

     iv. Epididymitis (5%)

     v. MAGIC syndrome

       1. Mouth and genital ulcers with inflamed cartilage

       2. Features of both BD and relapsing polychondritis

       3. Name proposed in 1985 by Firestein and colleagues

5. Laboratory Features

  a. Nonspecific

  b. Common findings

     i. Acute phase reactants

       1. Increased especially in patients with large vessel vasculitis

       2. Increased CRP and ESR

       3. Leukocytosis

       4. May be normal with active eye disease

     ii. Normal or negative

       1. RF

       2. Cryoglobulins

       3. Complement components

     iii. Increased immunoglobulins

       1. IgG

       2. IgA

       3. IgM

     iv. Increased alpha-2 globulin

     v. Elevated CSF protein and cell count

       1. Especially in patients with neurologic involvement

     vi. Findings most often occur during disease exacerbation

     vii. Return to normal during remission

  c. HLA-B51

     i. Areas of high prevalence

     ii. Patients with eye disease

6. Diagnosis

  a. Diagnostic criteria based on the 1990 International Study Group (ISG) for Behcet's Disease

     i. Recurrent oral ulcerations

       1. Minor aphthous, major aphthous, or herpetiform ulceration, which occurred at least three times in one 12 month period

     ii. Plus any two of the following

       1. Recurrent genital ulceration

         a. Aphthous ulceration or scarring

       2. Eye lesions

         a. Anterior or posterior uveitis

         b. Or cells in vitreous on slit lamp examination

         c. Or retinal vasculitis

      3. Skin lesions
        a. Erythema nodosum
        b. Pseudofolliculitis
        c. Papulopustular lesions
        d. Acneiform nodules
     i. In a post-adolescent patients not on corticosteroid treatment
      4. Positive pathergy test
        a. 2 mm erythema 24–48 h after #25 needleprick to depth of 5 mm
  b. Suggestive diagnosis
    i. Western countries
      1. In the setting of aphthosis
        a. Large-vessel disease
        b. Or acute central nervous system infarction
    ii. Patient with complex aphthosis
      1. In the presence of other characteristic lesions
      2. Exclusion of other systemic disorders associated with mucocutaneous involvement
  c. Differential diagnoses
    i. Sprue
    ii. Hematologic disorders
    iii. HSV
    iv. IBD
      1. Virtually all the features of BD can be seen in Crohn's colitis
      2. Considered especially in patients with
        a. Iron deficiency
        b. Markedly elevated ESR (>100 mm/h)
        c. Even minor bowel complaints
    v. Cyclic neutropenia
    vi. Acquired immunodeficiency syndrome (AIDS)
    vii.   Other oral-genital-ocular syndromes
      1. Erythema multiforme
      2. Reactive arthritis
        a. Mucocutaneous lesions nonulcerative and painless
        b. Uveitis usually limited to the anterior chamber
      3. Mucous membrane pemphigoid
      4. Vulvovaginal-gingival form of erosive lichen planus
    viii. Other oral-ocular-arthritis syndromes
      1. SLE
      2. Reiter's syndrome
      3. Systemic vasculitis

7. Disease Activity
   a. Monitor mucocutaneous manifestations
      i. Record the number, size, and location of lesions
      ii. Percentage of time that lesions are present since the last evaluation
   b. Ocular disease
      i. Frequent ophthalmologic examinations
      ii. Periodic monitoring for those at risk
   c. Careful history and physical examination
      i. Attention to vascular and neurologic systems
   d. Standardized forms to score disease activity and ocular inflammation (BSAS)
8. Treatment
   a. Aphthous lesions (mucocutaneous manifestations)
      i. Topical or intralesional corticosteroids
      ii. Dapsone
         1. 100 mg/day
      iii. Colchicine
         1. 0.6 mg 2–3 times per day
         2. Also used in the treatment of more serious manifestations
      iv. Thalidomide
         1. 100–400 mg/day
         2. Used in the prevention and treatment of mucosal and follicular lesions in males
         3. Toxicity is a concern
      v. Methotrexate
      vi. Levamisole
         1. 150 mg/day for 3 days every 2 weeks
      vii. Interferon alpha
         1. 9×10^6 units 3 times a week for 3 months
         2. Followed by 3×10^6 units 3 times a week
   b. Ocular/CNS disease
      i. Aggressive treatment warranted in young males who are at greatest risk of eye complications
      ii. Azathioprine
         1. 2.5 mg/kg/day orally
         2. Improves long-term prognosis
         3. Beneficial effects on the development and progression of
            a. Mucosal ulcers
            b. Arthritis
            c. Deep venous thrombosis (DVT)
      iii. Cyclosporine
         1. 5–10 mg/kg/day
         2. For uveitis

    iv. Interferon-alpha
      1. Useful for mucocutaneous lesions and arthritis
      2. Considered as a treatment for ocular disease
    v. Chlorambucil
      1. 0.1–0.2 mg/kg/day
      2. Drug of choice for severe, uncontrolled ocular disease
        a. Loss of useful vision reduced from 75% to 20%
      3. Drug of choice for severe, uncontrolled CNS disease
      4. Large-vessel vasculitis
      a. Including DVT
    vi. Cyclophosphamide
      1. 0.5–1.0 g/m^2 month IV
      2. 1–2 mg/kg/day oral
      3. Uncontrolled ocular disease
      4. CNS disease
      5. Large-vessel vasculitis
        a. Including DVT
    vii. Corticosteroids
      1. 1–2 mg/kg/day oral
      2. 1 g/day for 3 days IV
      3. Suppresses inflammation in acute phases of the disease
      4. A limited role in chronic management of CNS or ocular complications
    viii. Levamisole
    ix. Methotrexate
      1. 7.5–15 mg/week oral
    x. Tacrolimus (FK506)
      1. 0.1 mg/kg/day
c. Antibiotics
    i. Based on the rationale that streptococci may play a role in the pathogenesis
    ii. Benzathine penicillin
      1. Useful for treating mucocutaneous lesions
      2. Prevention of arthritis
    iii. Minocycline
      1. Useful for mucocutaneous lesions
d. Thrombotic disease
    i. Cerebral venous thrombosis
      1. Heparin
      2. Colchicine
      3. Corticosteroids
    ii. Progressive and recurrent venous thrombosis
      1. Corticosteroids and immunosuppressive agents
        a. Inflammation underlies the thrombosis

      iii. Budd-Chiari syndrome
  1. Anticoagulants
  2. Colchicine
  3. Corticosteroids
  4. Combination of anti-aggregants
  5. Portocaval shunting
     a. If the inferior vena cava is patent
  e. Surgical treatment
     i. Systemic arterial aneurysms at risk for rupture
     ii. Pulmonary arterial aneurysms with uncontrolled bleeding
     iii. Arterial vasculitis with aneurysms of the systemic or pulmonary circulation
  1. Treat with alkylating agents first prior to surgery
  2. High risk of anastomotic recurrences or continued disease
9. Prognosis
  a. Mortality up to 16% in 5 years
  b. Major causes of mortality
     i. CNS involvement
     ii. Vascular disease
     iii. Bowel perforation
     iv. Hemoptysis with pulmonary disease
     v. Serious cardiac disease

Relapsing Polychondritis

14

1. Relapsing polychondritis (RPC)
   a. An uncommon episodic systemic disease characterized by widespread and progressive inflammation of cartilaginous structures
   b. Term first used by Pearson and associates to describe the episodic nature
2. Etiopathogenesis
   a. Unknown inciting agent
      i. Infectious
      ii. Toxic
      iii. Immunologic
   b. Considered an autoimmune disorder
      i. Cellular and humoral responses to cartilaginous structures
         1. Collagen types II, IX, and XI
      ii. Lymphocytes exposed to cartilage mucopolysaccharides
         1. Induce lymphoblast transformation
         2. Macrophage migration responses
      iii. Activated lymphocytes and macrophages secrete mediators
         1. Induce the release of lysosomal enzymes
         2. Especially proteases
      iv. Attempts at repair of the inflammatory damage leads to
         1. Formation of granulation tissue
         2. Fibrosis
      v. Humoral immunity involved
         1. Antibodies to native type 2 collagen
         2. Circulating immune complexes
      vi. Degree of immune response correlates with clinical disease activity
   c. HLA-DR-4
      i. 60% increased frequency compared with 25% in normal controls
      ii. About 20% have disease associated with RA
3. Epidemiology
   a. Predominantly Caucasian
   b. Occurs in all age groups

N.T. Colburn, *Review of Rheumatology*,
DOI 10.1007/978-1-84882-093-7_14, © Springer-Verlag London Limited 2012

        i. Range 20–60 years

        ii. Peaks between 40 and 50 years

    c. Both genders equally affected

        i. Women more often have serious airway involvement

    d. Frequently unrecognized

        i. Mean delay in diagnosis of 2.9 years

4. Pathology

    a. Histopathology of involved cartilage is highly characteristic

        i. Regardless of location

    b. Cartilage matrix

        i. Acidophilic (pink) rather than the normal basophilic (blue)

    c. Inflammatory cell infiltrates

        i. Initially PMNs

        ii. Later lymphocytes and plasma cells

        iii. Invade cartilage form the periphery inward

        iv. Granulation tissue and fibrosis develop adjacent to the infiltrates

            1. Results in sequestration of cartilage segments

    d. Chondrocytes

        i. Increased lipids and lysosomes as demonstrated by EM

5. Clinical Features

    a. Auricular chondritis (89%)

        i. The most frequent and characteristic clinical feature

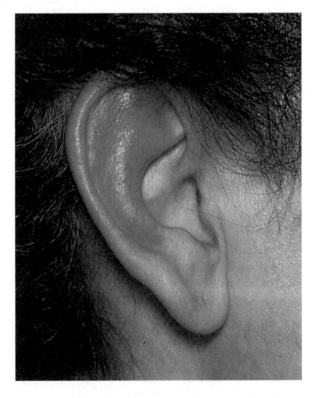

Fig. 14.1 Auricular chondritis of relapsing polychondritis (Reproduced with permission from Joint infections and rheumatic manifestations of infectious diseases. *Atlas of Infectious Diseases*. ImagesMD; 2002-01-23)

    ii. The most common presenting symptom (26%)

    iii. Characterized by sudden onset of pain and swelling

       1. Redness and warmth with purplish-red discoloration

       2. Attacks may last from a few days to several weeks

    iv. Involves the cartilaginous portion of the external ear

       1. Spares the lobule

       2. Distinct to cellulites

    v. Inflammation may subside spontaneously or with treatment

    vi. Repeated attacks lead to a soft and floppy external ear

       1. "Cauliflower ear"

b. Nasal chondritis (72%)

    i. Third most common presenting symptom (13%)

    ii. Develops suddenly as a painful fullness of the nasal bridge

    iii. May see epistaxis with inflammation

    iv. Less recurrent than auricular chondritis

    v. Cartilage collapse may occur

       1. Even in the absence of clinical inflammation

       2. Results in a "saddle nose" deformity

c. Respiratory tract chondritis (56%)

    i. Initial presenting symptom in 15% of cases

    ii. Inflammatory involvement of laryngeal and tracheobronchial tract

       1. Hoarseness

       2. Choking sensation

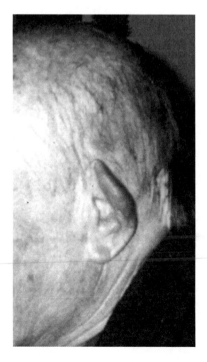

Fig. 14.2 Repeated attacks of relapsing polychondritis lead to a soft and floppy external ear (Reproduced with permission from Relapsing polychondritis with features of dementia with Lewy bodies. *Acta Neuropathologica.* DOI: 10.1007/s00401-006-0098-0. Springer 2006-07-24)

3. Tenderness over the thyroid cartilage
4. Nonproductive cough
5. Stridor
6. Wheezes
7. Dyspnea
8. Tracheobronchial wall thickening and stenosis
   a. May be asymptomatic
   b. May lead to stenosis
   c. May cause major airway collapse
      i. Secondary to dissolution of the tracheal and bronchial carti-laginous rings
      ii. Requires emergency tracheostomy
   iii. Inflammatory involvement of first- and second-order bronchi
      1. Late in the disease
   iv. Respiratory tract infections may complicate the clinical course
d. Involvement of organs of special sense
   i. Eyes
   ii. Audiovestibular apparatus (46%)
      1. The initial presentation in 6%
      2. Sudden onset hearing loss and vertigo
      3. Tinnitus
      4. Fullness in the ear
         a. Due to serous otitis media
      5. Inflammatory edema or cartilage collapse of
         a. Auricle
         b. External auditory canal
         c. Eustachian tube
         d. Leads to conductive hearing loss
      6. Inflammation of the internal auditory artery
         a. Leads to sensorineural hearing loss
e. Polyarthritis (81%)
   i. The second most common presenting symptom (23%)
   ii. Migratory, asymmetric, episodic, nonerosive, and nondeforming
   iii. Involves large and small joints of the peripheral and/or axial skeleton
   iv. A predilection for
      1. Large joints
      2. Sternoclavicular
      3. Costochondral
      4. Sternomanubrial
   v. May mimic seronegative RA
      1. Involvement of the small joints of the hands and feet
   vi. Flail chest
      1. Secondary to inflammatory lysis of the costosternal cartilage
      2. Can interfere with ventilatory efforts

f. Ocular inflammation (65%)
   i. The initial presenting symptom 14% of the time
   ii. Virtually every structure of the eye and surrounding tissues may be affected
   iii. Common presentations
      1. Scleritis/episcleritis
      2. Uveitis
      3. Conjunctivitis
      4. Iritis/chorioretinitis
      5. Keratitis
   iv. Less common presentations
      1. Optic neuritis
      2. Scleromalacia
      3. Retinal detachment
      4. Proptosis
      5. Exophthalmos
      6. Extraocular muscle palsy
      7. Glaucoma
   v. Other complications
      1. Cataracts
      2. Corneal ulcerations and thinning
      3. Loss of visual acuity
      4. Blindness
g. Vascular involvement
   i. Vasculitis
      1. Up to 30% of cases
      2. Involved vessels range in size
         a. Capillaries
            i. Leukocytoclastic vasculitis
         b. Large arteries
            i. Aortitis
         c. Internal auditory artery
            i. Sudden onset hearing loss and vertigo

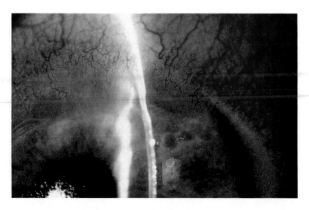

Fig. 14.3 A patient with relapsing polychondritis demonstrating peripheral ulcerative keratitis in the absence of scleritis (Reproduced with permission from Scleritis, ocular manifestations of immunologic disease, and noninfectious keratitis. In: *Atlas of Ophthalmology.* ImagesMD; 2002-02-01)

      ii. Aortic aneurysms
        1. Occur in multiple sites
        2. Sudden rupture can occur without active disease
      iii. Arterial thrombosis
        1. Due to vasculitis or coagulopathy
      iv. Medium vessel disease
        1. Presents as polyarteritis
      v. Small vessel disease
        1. Presents as leukocytoclastic vasculitis
  h. Cardiovascular involvement (24%)
      i. Aortic regurgitation (insufficiency)
        1. The most common cardiac manifestation
        2. The second most serious complication
          a. After respiratory involvement
        3. Due to progressive dilatation of the aortic root
          a. Distinguishes it from aortic insufficiency of other common rheumatic diseases
        4. Acute aortic valve cusp rupture
          a. Can occur early in the course
        5. Aortic and mitral valve replacement
          a. Limited success
          b. 24% require repeat valvuloplasty
          c. 50% mortality during the first 4 post-operative years
      ii. Mitral regurgitation
      iii. AV block and conduction defects
      iv. Pericarditis
      v. Cardiac ischemia
      vi. Arrhythmias
 i. Cutaneous Manifestations (17%)
      i. Erythema nodosum
      ii. Panniculitis
      iii. Livedo reticularis
      iv. Urticaria
      v. Cutaneous polyarteritis nodosa
      vi. Aphthous ulcer
      vii. Alopecia
     viii. Abnormal nail growth
 j. Other Clinical Manifestations
      i. Neurologic (infrequent)
        1. Cranial neuropathies
          a. Cranial nerves II, III, IV, VI, VII, and VIII
        2. Headaches
        3. Seizures (rarely)
        4. Encephalopathy

        5. Hemiplegia

        6. Dementia

        7. Meningoencephalitis

        8. Ataxia

    ii. Renal disease

        1. Indicates a worse prognosis

        2. Usually focal GN

        3. Wide variety of GN reported

          a. Segmental

          b. Proliferative

          c. Crescenteric

6. Associated Disorders

  a. 40% have other autoimmune, rheumatologic, inflammatory, or hematologic disorders

  b. RPC follows the associated disorder by several months to years

  c. The most common diseases associated with RPC

    i. SLE

    ii. Systemic vasculitis

    iii. RA

    iv. Sjogren's

    v. Spondyloarthropathy

  d. Other diseases associated with RPC

    i. Systemic sclerosis

    ii. Overlap connective tissue disease

    iii. Behcet's

    iv. Essential mixed cryoglobulinemia

    v. Thyroid disease

    vi. IBD

    vii. Spondyloarthropathies

    viii. Myelodysplastic syndrome

        1. Transformation to or concurrent findings of leukemia or myeloma reported

    ix. Malignancy

7. Diagnosis

  a. Based on clinical features

  b. Biopsy not always necessary

  c. Diagnostic criteria set forth by McAdam in 1976 requires the presence of three or more clinical features

    i. Recurrent chondritis of both auricles

    ii. Nonerosive and seronegative inflammatory polyarthritis

    iii. Chondritis of nasal cartilages

    iv. Inflammation of ocular structures

        1. Conjunctivitis

        2. Keratitis

        3. Scleritis/episcleritis

        4. Uveitis

      v. Chondritis of the respiratory tract
        1. Laryngeal cartilages
        2. Trachea
     vi. Cochlear and/or vestibular damage
        1. Neurosensory hearing loss
        2. Tinnitus
        3. Vertigo

8. Differential Diagnosis
  a. Exclude other causes of chondritis (especially infectious perichondritis)
     i. Fungal diseases
     ii. Syphilis
     iii. Leprosy
     iv. Bacterial infections
     v. Frostbite
     vi. Midline granuloma
  b. Most other disorders do not present as multifocal chondritis
  c. Other causes of saddle nose deformities
     i. Wegener's granulomatosis
     ii. Syphilis
  d. Inherited degenerative chondropathy
     i. Autosomal dominant disease
     ii. Caused by myxoid degeneration of thyroid and cricoid cartilage
     iii. Characteristics
        1. Saddle nose deformity at birth
        2. Laryngeal stenosis at 9–12 years of age

9. Laboratory Diagnostics
  a. Abnormal results generally nonspecific
  b. Anemia of chronic disease
  c. Mild leukocytosis
  d. Thrombocytosis
  e. Elevated ESR
  f. Hypergammaglobulinemia
     i. Increased alpha and gamma globulins
  g. UA typically normal
  h. Autoantibodies
     i. Rheumatoid factor (10–20%)
     ii. ANA (15–25%)
     iii. ANCA (about 25% during active disease)
     iv. Antibodies to collagen type II, IX, and XI
        1. Type II found in about 20% of patients
        2. Not prognostic of disease activity
  i. Serum complements usually normal or high
  j. Cryoglobulins found in a small number

10. Radiographic Abnormalities
    a. Soft tissue radiographs of the neck
        i. Demonstrate narrowing of the tracheal air column
        ii. Suggest tracheal stenosis
    b. Tomography or axial CT
        i. More accurately define the degree of tracheal narrowing
    c. Radiographs of the joints
        i. Periarticular osteopenia
        ii. Joint space narrowing occasionally
    d. Cartilaginous calcifications of the pinnas
        i. From repeated inflammation
11. Diagnostic modalities useful in detecting and following disease activity
    a. ESR
        i. An accurate predictor of disease activity in most patients
    b. Radiographic imaging
        i. Demonstrates functional complications
    c. PFTs with flow volume loops
    d. Patients with prominent symptoms and signs of cardiovascular disease
        i. Echo
            1. Also should be used routinely to detect silent disease
        ii. Cardiac cath
        iii. Angiography
12. Treatment
    a. NSAIDS
        i. May be adequate for patients with mild polychondritis
        ii. Arthralgia
        iii. Nasal or auricular chondritis
    b. Corticosteroids
        i. Considered the pharmacologic mainstay of therapy
        ii. Patients with more severe disease
            1. Scleritis/uveitis
            2. Systemic symptoms
        iii. 30–60 mg/day of prednisone
            1. With an immunosuppressive agent
                a. Azathioprine
                b. Cyclophosphamide
            2. Taper soon after clinical improvement
        iv. IV pulse methylprednisolone
            1. For acute airway obstruction unresponsive to oral corticosteroids
    c. MTX and dapsone
        i. Used successfully as steroid-sparing agents
        ii. Especially with continued inflammation or an inability to taper steroids
        iii. Dapsone (50–200 mg/day) for patients without major organ involvement

    d. Cyclosporin A
      i. Used with good success
    e. Cyclophosphamide
      i. For severe disease
        1. Control manifestations with corticosteroids and cyclophosphamide
        2. Later switch to less toxic medications such as MTX
      ii. 6 months of monthly pulse IV shows improvement in renal function
    f. Combination therapy
      i. Oral prednisone, dapsone, and cyclophosphamide used with variable response
    g. Tracheostomy
      i. May be required in acute airway obstruction
    h. Surgery
      i. Severe cardiac valvular involvement
        1. Aortic insufficiency may require valve replacement
      ii. Large-vessel aneurysms
      iii. Airway obstruction caused by tracheal stenosis or tracheomalacia
      iv. Dynamic airway collapse
        1. Intrabronchial stent placement
      v. NOT recommended for nasal septal collapse
        1. Further collapse frequently occurs postoperatively
13. Prognosis
    a. In 1976 McAdam reported
      i. Survival rate
        1. 74% at 5 years
        2. 55% at 10 years
      ii. Infection the major cause of death
      iii. Cardiovascular disease the second most common cause of death
        1. Systemic vasculitis
        2. Rupture of large-vessel aneurysms
        3. Cardiac valvular disease
      iv. 15% died as a direct consequence of cardiovascular or respiratory tract RPC
      v. Airway obstruction
        1. The cause of death in 10%
        2. Plus superimposed infection the cause of death in 28%
      vi. Poor prognostic indicators
        1. Coexistent vasculitis
        2. Early saddle nose deformity in younger patients
        3. Presence of anemia in older patients
    b. In 1998 Trentham reported
      i. Average disease duration 8 years
      ii. Survival rate significantly improved at 94%
      iii. Due to improved medical and surgical management respiratory and cardiovascular complications
    c. Malignancy is an uncommon cause of death

Antiphospholipid Syndrome

15

1. Major clinical features of antiphospholipid syndrome (APS)
   a. Recurrent arterial or venous thromboses
   b. Pregnancy morbidity
      i. Including fetal loss
   c. The persistent presence of antiphospholipid antibodies
      i. Anticardiolipin antibodies
      ii. Lupus anticoagulant
      iii. B2-glycoprotein I
      iv. Anti-prothrombin antibodies
2. Minor clinical features
   a. Thrombocytopenia
   b. Hemolytic anemia
   c. Livedo reticularis
   d. Cardiac valve disease
   e. Transient cerebral ischemia
   f. Transverse myelopathy
   g. Multiple sclerosis-like syndromes
   h. Chorea
   i. Migraine
3. APS may be primary or secondary
   a. Primary
      i. The presence of antiphospholipid antibodies (aPL) and one of the following
         1. Thrombosis
         2. Recurrent fetal loss
         3. Thrombocytopenia
         4. No underlying disorder as cause
            a. Up to 10% with primary disease will evolve into SLE within 10 years

N.T. Colburn, *Review of Rheumatology*,
DOI 10.1007/978-1-84882-093-7_15, © Springer-Verlag London Limited 2012

b. Secondary
   i. To an underlying disease process
   ii. SLE
      1. 50% have aPL
      2. Presence of aPL part of the immunology diagnostic criteria
   iii. Other autoimmune diseases
   iv. HIV infection
   v. Vasculitis
   vi. Thrombosis and SLE
      1. 50% with both SLE and aPL will develop an event
      2. Avascular necrosis increased in SLE and aPL
      3. Odds ratio for risk of thrombosis with different aPLs
         a. 5.6 with lupus anticoagulant
         b. 3.02 with anti-β2-GP1
         c. 2.2 with anticardiolipin antibody
4. Epidemiology
   a. More frequent in adults
      i. Although children are affected
   b. More frequent in women than men
   c. Relatives of affected patients have anticardiolipin antibodies or the lupus anticoagulant without clinical complications
   d. An association with the HLA-DQB locus
5. Etiology and Pathogenesis
   a. Many of the antigens involved in the production of aPL are components of the clotting cascade
   b. Antibody postulates
      i. May directly interfere with normal anticoagulation
      ii. Pathogenesis may relate to antibody specificity or host susceptibility
         1. Not all people with antiphospholipid antibodies experience clinical complications
      iii. Animal studies support antibody involvement
         1. Mice passively immunized with human anticardiolipin antibodies suffer pregnancy wastage or fetal resorption
         2. Mice infused with either purified immunoglobulins or anticardiolipin antibodies from APS developed increased thrombus size and delayed thrombus disappearance
   c. Two-hit hypothesis
      i. aPL plus another prothrombotic factor
      ii. Both necessary for the thrombotic clotting cascade
   d. aPL and thrombosis
      i. 3–7% of patients per year with aPL experience a new thrombotic event
      ii. 10% and 25% overall positive predictive value of aPL in predicting
         1. Future stroke
         2. Venous thrombosis
         3. Recurrent fetal loss

    iii. Positive aPL
       1. Does **NOT** correlate statistically with the development of thrombosis
       2. Seen in up to 8% of the normal population
       3. Associated with a variety of chronic infections
         a. HIV
         b. Hepatitis C
       4. Present in about 20% of patients with systemic vasculitis

e. Antiphospholipid antibodies
    i. Heterogeneous with specificities for target plasma proteins and an affinity for phospholipid surfaces
       1. Prothrombin
       2. Phospholipids
         a. Cardiolipin
         b. Phosphatidylserine
       3. Phosphatidylethanolamine
       4. Protein-phospholipid complexes
       5. Lupus anticoagulant
    ii. Activates endothelial cells and upregulates adhesion molecules
    iii. Antibody-mediated platelet activation
    iv. Selective inhibition of the protein C anticoagulant pathway

f. β_2-glycoprotien 1 (β_2GP1)
    i. A lipid-binding anticoagulant plasma protein
    ii. A natural anticoagulant
       1. Inhibits coagulation reactions catalyzed by negatively charged phospholipids
         a. Prothrombin-thrombin conversion
       2. Antiphospholipid antibodies induce thrombosis by neutralizing the anticoagulant effects of B_2GP1
    iii. Binds negatively charged molecules and becomes antigenic
       1. Undergoes a conformational change
       2. Exposes a cryptic antigen
       3. Leads to clustering of molecules
       4. Provides a high antigen density
    iv. Binds to phosphatidylserine on activated or apoptotic cell membranes
    v. Markedly enhances binding of antiphospholipid antibodies
       1. Anticardiolipin antibodies bind to B_2GP1 directly
       2. B_2GP1-phospholipid complex
       3. Bind epitopes on phospholipids in phospholipid- B_2GP1complexes
    vi. Mice immunized with B_2GP1 result in antibodies specific for B_2GP1and cardiolipin
    vii. anti-B2-glycoprotein 1 antibody
       1. Binds an octapeptide in the fifth domain of B_2-glycoprotein

6. Clinical Features
   a. Clinical syndromes associated with antiphospholipid antibodies
      i. **C** – Clot:
         1. Recurrent arterial and/or venous thromboses
      ii. **L** – Livedo reticularis:
         1. Lace-like rash over the extremities and trunk exaggerated by cold
      iii. **O** – Obstetrical loss:
         1. Recurrent fetal loss
      iv. **T** – Thrombocytopenia
   b. Thrombosis
      i. Venous and arterial
         1. Occurs anywhere in the body
         2. Leads to a variety of clinical presentations
         3. Two-thirds of thrombotic events are venous
         4. One-third of thrombotic events are arterial
      ii. Factors which increase thrombotic risk
         1. Antibody characteristics
            a. IgG with anti-B_2-glycoprotein 1 reactivity
            b. High titers of antibody
            c. Lupus anticoagulant
         2. Increased tissue factor release
            a. Infection
            b. Surgery
         3. Abnormal endothelium
            a. Active vasculitis/inflammatory disease
            b. Atherosclerosis and associated risk factors (DM)
            c. Catheterization for arteriography/IV access
         4. History of previous thrombosis or fetal loss
         5. Other prothrombotic risk factors
            a. Smoking
            b. Oral contraceptives
            c. Pregnancy
            d. Homocystinemia
            e. Hereditary hypercoagulable disorders
               i. Factor V Leiden (APC resistance)
               ii. Protein C or S deficiency
               iii. Prothrombin gene mutation (20210 G)
               iv. Antithrombotin III deficiency
      iii. Characteristics of patients presenting with their first DVT
         1. The incidence of aPL was 15%
         2. The incidence of Factor V Leiden was 10–30%
         3. The incidence of prothrombin gene polymorphism (20210 G) was 6%
      iv. Sites of thombosis
         1. The site of initial thrombosis often predicts the site of recurrent thrombosis

Fig. 15.1 Pulmonary embolism in a lupus patient with antiphospholipid syndrome (Reproduced with permission from Systemic lupus erythematosus, scleroderma, and inflammatory myopathies. *Atlas of Rheumatology.* ImagesMD; 2005-01-18)

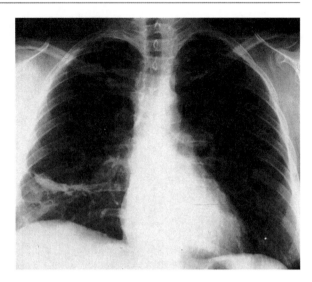

2. Deep veins of the leg
   a. Site most frequently affected in the venous circulation
3. Pulmonary vessels
   a. Pulmonary emboli occur in 30% of patients
   b. Pulmonary hypertension in 5%
4. Inferior vena cava
5. Renal
   a. Renal artery or vein thrombosis and a thrombotic microangiopathy can cause renal insufficiency
6. Hepatic (Budd-Chiari syndrome)
   a. Venous thrombosis of the liver
7. Axillary
8. Cavernous or sagittal veins
v. Arterial thrombosis
   1. Strokes and TIAs
      a. The most common presentations of arterial thrombosis
   2. aPL found in 5–10% of unselected patients with stroke
      a. A relative risk of 2.3
   3. aPL found in 45–50% of patients <50 years old with stroke
      a. A relative risk of 8.3
   4. Described as infarctions
      a. Myocardial
      b. Adrenal
      c. Gastrointestinal
      d. Gangrene of the extremities
         i. Digital gangrene

Fig. 15.2 Gangrene in antiphospholipid antibody syndrome (Reproduced with permission from Rheumatology. *Atlas of Pediatrics.* ImagesMD; 2006-01-20)

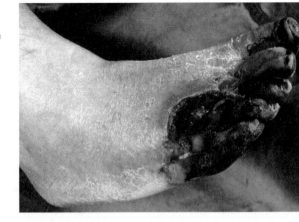

c. Catastrophic antiphospholipid syndrome
   i. Widespread thromboses with life-threatening consequences
   ii. Multiple thromboses of medium and small arteries
      1. Three or more organs
      2. Occurs over a few days
   iii. Exclude TTP and diffuse DIC
d. Pregnancy morbidity
   i. Contributions of antiphospholipid antibodies to morbidity
      1. Recurrent miscarriage
         a. 15% have positive aPL
         b. 2% of normal pregnancy have aPL
      2. Preeclampsia
      3. Placental insufficiency
      4. Intrauterine growth retardation
      5. Preterm birth
      6. Maternal thrombosis
   ii. Recurrent pregnancy loss can occur at any stage of gestation
      1. Characteristic fetal death in the second or third trimester
      2. Pregnancy usually lost before the tenth week
      3. Aborted fetus small for gestational age but normal
   iii. Causes of fetal death
      1. Placental vessel thrombosis
      2. aPL antibodies displace annexin V from placental trophoblast surfaces and vascular endothelial cells
         a. Annexin V is an anticoagulant protein
            i. Thromboregulatory role at the vascular-blood interface in the placenta
            ii. Shields anionic phospholipids that induce thrombus formation

1. Rapid development of predominant small vessel occlusions following an identifiable trigger factor in 50% of cases
2. Unusual organs affected (e.g., ovaries, uterus, testes, bone marrow)
3. High frequency of pulmonary complications such as acute respiratory distress syndrome or diffuse alveolar hemorrhage (uncommon)
4. Patients often present with abdominal pain because of intraabdominal vascular complications affecting bowel, gall bladder, pancreas, adrenal glands, or spleen
5. Early loss of consciousness complicating systemic inflammatory response syndrome
6. Serologic evidence of disseminated intravascular coagulation without hemorrhagic manifestations in one fifth of patients. This may cause problems in differential diagnosis.
7. Severe thrombocytopenias, which may result in hemorrhage (particularly cerebral)

Fig. 15.3 Catastrophic antiphospholipid syndrome (Reproduced with permission from Update on the diagnosis, treatment, and prognosis of the catastrophic antiphospholipid syndrome. *Current Rheumatology Reports.* DOI: 10.1007/s11926-009-0073-6. Springer; 2010-02-01)

    e. Other clinical features of APS
        i. Thrombocytopenia

            1. May occur alone
            2. Frequently mild to moderate
                a. Platelet counts range 100,000–150,000 cells/mm^3
            3. Does **not** protect patients from thrombosis
            4. Anticoagulation with thrombocytopenia may increase the risk for bleeding
        ii. Livedo reticularis
        iii. Cardiac valvular disease
            1. Cardiac valvular vegetations (Libman-Sacks endocarditis)
            2. Valvular insufficiency
                a. Mitral > aortic
                b. Up to 50% of patients with aPL and SLE
                c. Can cause embolic strokes
                d. 5% need valve replacement
        iv. Accelerated atherosclerosis (controversial)
        v. Leg ulcers
            1. Skin thrombosis cause cutaneous ulceration
        vi. Migraine headaches
        vii. Variety of neurologic complications
            1. Chorea
            2. Memory loss
            3. Dementia

       4. Multiple sclerosis (MS)-like syndromes
         a. MS misdiagnosed based on MRI finding
         b. Patients with aPL usually have
           i. A normal IgG index
           ii. Negative oligoclonal bands
       5. Transverse myelopathy
       6. Seizures
         a. Even with a normal brain MRI
     viii. Hemolytic anemia
       1. Positive Coombs' test
      ix. Ischemic optic neuropathy
       x. Retinal artery or vein occlusion
      xi. Sensorineural hearing loss
     xii. Pseudotumor cerebri
7. Diagnosis
  a. None of the clinical features of APS are confined to this disorder
  b. Clinical features strongly diagnostic of APS
     i. Unexplained arterial or venous thrombosis
     ii. Thrombosis at unusual sites
       1. Renal or adrenal veins
     iii. Thrombosis in a person younger than 50 years
     iv. Recurrent thrombotic events
     v. Recurrent spontaneous abortions
     vi. Second or third-trimester losses
     vii. More than one of these clinical features in the same individual
     viii. A patient with SLE
  c. Laboratory confirmation
     i. An unequivocally positive test for lupus anticoagulant
     ii. Medium-to-high titers of anticardiolipin antibodies
       1. Preferably the IgG isotype
       2. Present for more than 6 weeks
8. Differential Diagnosis
  a. With unexplained venous thrombosis
     i. Factor V Leiden (activated protein-C resistance)
     ii. Protein C, S, or antithrombin III deficiency
     iii. Antifactor VIII
     iv. Dysfibrinogenemias
     v. Abnormalities of fibrinolysis
     vi. Nephrotic syndrome
     vii. Polycythemia vera
     viii. Behcet's disease
     ix. Paroxysmal nocturnal hemoglobinuria
     x. Thrombosis associated with oral contraceptives

    b. With unexplained arterial occlusions
       i. Hyperlipidemia
      ii. Diabetes mellitus
     iii. Hypertension
     iv. Vasculitis
      v. Sickle cell disease
     vi. Homocystinuria
    vii. Buerger's disease
   c. With pregnancy wastage
       i. Fetal chromosomal abnormalities
      ii. Anatomic anomalies of the maternal reproductive tract
     iii. Maternal disorders
        1. Endocrine
        2. Infectious
        3. Autoimmune
        4. Drug-induced disease
   d. Other causes for elevated levels of aPL
       i. Chronic immune stimulations
      ii. Primary conditions (**MAIN**)
        1. **M** – Medications
          a. Most common are phenothiazines and other drugs associated with drug-induced lupus
            i. Chlorpromazine (a phenothiazine)
           ii. Hydralazine
          iii. Phenytoin
          iv. Procainamide
           v. Quinidine
        2. **A** – Autoimmune diseases
        3. **I** – Infectious diseases
          a. Chronic infections
            i. HIV
              1. 60% have elevated aPL
           ii. Hepatitis C
          b. aPL induced by infections are **not** associated with increased thrombotic risk
            i. Not directed against B_2-glycoprotien I
        4. **N** – Neoplasms
          a. The most common is lymphoma
9. Laboratory
   a. Anticardiolipin (aCL) antibody test
       i. Use a standardized ELISA technique
      ii. Reported according to
        1. Isotype (IgG, IgM, or IgA)
        2. Level of positivity

  iii. Semiquantitative
    1. High (>80 units)
    2. Medium (20–80 units)
    3. Low (10–20 units)
  iv. Medium-to-high positive IgG and IgM (rarely IgA)
    1. Most specific for the diagnosis of APS
  v. Usually due to binding by anti-B2 glycoprotein 1 antibodies
  vi. A positive aCL but negative anti-B2-glycoprotien 1
    1. Usually those with infections
    2. **Not** at increased risk for clotting
  vii. Measurement **unaffected** by anticoagulation
  viii. Used to determine aPL levels in a patient on heparin or warfarin
 b. Lupus anticoagulant test (LA)
  i. Associated with a higher risk of thrombosis than aCL
  ii. Prolongation of clotting times by antiphospholipid antibodies in vitro
  iii. Prolongation of PTT in about one-half of patients
    1. Presence not excluded with a normal PTT
  iv. Also affects prothrombin time (PT)
    1. Indicates an extremely high level of lupus anticoagulant
    2. Indicates the presence of a prothrombin (factor II deficiency)
     a. Associated with excessive bleeding rather than hypercoagulability
     b. Rarely associated with autoimmune disorders
      i. Including SLE
    3. If both PTT and PT are prolonged
     a. Measure prothrombin level directly to exclude a deficiency
  v. Identified by the following criteria
    1. An abnormal phospholipid-dependent screening test of homeostasis
     a. Activated prothrombin time
     b. Russell viper venom time
      i. A confirmatory test for the lupus anticoagulant
      ii. Directly activates factor X and bypasses factors required in the intrinsic pathway
      iii. Performed like PTT, except
       1. Intrinsic coagulation factors proximal to factor X are not required
       2. Less phospholipids present in the reaction
      iv. Not affected by factor deficiencies
      v. More sensitive than prolongation of the PTT
     c. Kaolin clotting time
     d. Dilute prothrombin time
     e. Textarin time
    2. **Failure to correct** the prolonged screening coagulation test value upon 1:1 mixing with normal platelet-poor plasma
     a. With a factor deficiency is present or induced by warfarin the assay **corrects** with addition of normal plasma

       3. Shortening or **correction** of the prolonged screening test value upon the
          addition of excess phospholipids or hexagonal-phase phospholipids
          a. Phenomenon seen only with the lupus anticoagulant
       4. Exclusion of other coagulopathies
    vi. Not reliable in patients on oral anticoagulants or heparin
       1. When initiating coumadin therapy
          a. Check an assay insensitive to the lupus anticoagulation test at the
          same time INR is drawn
          b. Tests whether the lupus anticoagulant is interfering with the reli-
          ability of the INR
          c. Two tests not affected
            i. Chromogenic factor X
            ii. Prothrombin-proconvertin time
       2. Patients on heparin
          a. Treat plasma with heparinase
          b. Removes heparin prior to coagulation tests
c. The B_2-glycoprotein I antibody test
   i. Measured by ELISA
d. aPL test
   i. LA and aCL both positive (70%)
   ii. LA negative and aCL positive (15%)
   iii. LA positive and aCL negative (15%)
   iv. LA negative and aCL negative (<1%)
   v. Negative results
      1. Large clots will consume aPL
         a. Leads to false negatives
         b. Repeat the test 6 weeks after the event
   i. May show a positive result
      2. Pathogenic aPL directed against other targets not detected by LA and
         aCL assays
         a. Prothrombin
         b. Phosphatidylserine
         c. Thrombomodulin
         d. Annexin V
         e. Protein C and S
         f. Specifically directed against B_2-glycoprotein I
         i. Not detected by the aCL ELISA
      3. Evaluate for other causes of thrombosis
      4. **NO** "seronegative" APS
e. Anti-prothrombin antibodies
   i. Measured by ELISA
   ii. Responsible for a positive lupus anticoagulant
      1. Increases risk for thrombosis
   iii. Depletes prothrombin leading to hemorrhage

f. aPL levels
  i. Fluctuate widely over time
    1. Spontaneous
    2. In response to clinical events
      a. A lupus flare
      b. Change in pregnancy status
      c. Thrombosis
    3. In response to therapy
      a. Immunosuppression or anticoagulation
      b. May or may not change
g. False-positive VDRL
  i. A clue to the presence of an antiphospholipid antibody
    1. Up to 50% of subjects with aCL antibodies
    2. Not a good test for the presence of aPL
  ii. Measures agglutination (flocculation) of lipid particles
    1. Contain cholesterol and the negatively charged phospholipid cardiolipin
    2. aPL binds to cardiolipin to cause flocculation
      a. Indistinguishable from that seen with syphilis
  iii. Patients with only a false-positive VDRL and no other aPL
    1. **Not** at increased risk for clot or fetal loss
10. Treatment
  a. Thrombosis
    i. Active clots
      1. Control initial clot with unfractionated heparin
      2. Then switch to warfarin
    ii. Prophylaxis
      1. Oral anticoagulants
        a. Most lifelong
      2. High risk of recurrence
        a. Between 44% and 69%
      3. Target INR 3.0
        a. Usually effective in preventing thrombosis
      4. Use an assay insensitive to the lupus anticoagulant to ensure a reliable INR
        a. Chromogenic factor X
        b. Prothrombin-proconvertin time
      5. Adequate anticoagulation
        a. Factor X level less than 15% of normal
    iii. Recurrent thrombotic events
      1. Occurs despite adequate anticoagulation with coumadin
      2. Treat with twice daily subcutaneous heparin
        a. Achieve a PTT of 1.5–2 times normal

   iv. Immunosuppressive therapy
    1. Little or no role in the treatment of this syndrome
    2. Hydroxychlorquine has been used
   v. Treatment of catastrophic APS (remains unproved)
    1. High dose corticosteroid (taper over a few months)
    2. IV cyclophosphamide pulses
    3. Plasma exchange
    4. Heparin followed by warfarin
 b. Pregnancy morbidity
  i. Subcutaneous heparin
   1. 5,000–10,000 units twice a day (or every 8 h)
  ii. Low dose aspirin
   1. One daily
   2. Prescribe prior to conception
  iii. Heparin
   1. Stopped prior to delivery
   2. Continued 6–12 weeks post delivery
  iv. Some clinicians report a 100% success rate (average 80%)
  v. Coumadin
   1. Contraindicated during pregnancy
   2. Can lead to fetal malformations
  vi. Osteoporosis prevention with prolonged heparin therapy
   1. Calcium
   2. Vitamin D
  vii. Pregnancy loss despite heparin
   1. 4 or 5 day pulses of IVIG (0.4 g/kg/day) given monthly
   2. One low dose aspirin
  viii. High-dose corticosteroids
   1. Unsatisfactory therapeutic option because of side effects
  ix. Children born to mothers with APS
   1. Develop normally
   2. Low risk of developing APS
  x. Examine the placenta for evidence of infarction
   1. Even if no problems occurred during the pregnancy
 c. Prolonged PTT due to the lupus anticoagulant
  i. Monitor heparin levels directly
  ii. Monitor thrombin time
   1. Measures the clotting system distal to the effects of aPL
 d. Elevated levels of aPL with no history of thrombosis or recurrent fetal loss
  i. Most clinicians prescribe an aspirin daily
 e. Low molecular weight heparin (LMWH)
  i. No controlled trials in patients with APS
  ii. Several reported cases of failure
   1. To prevent extension of clots
   2. To prevent a new episode of thrombosis

        iii. Used in patients subtherapeutic on warfarin
             1. Until INR ≥ 3
        iv. Use caution with creatine clearance (CrCl) < 20–30 cc/min
             1. Cleared by the kidney
    f. Heparin-induced thrombocytopenia (HIT)
        i. Develops in patients with aPL
        ii. Anticoagulate until warfarin therapeutic
        iii. Substitute thrombin inhibiting medications for heparin
             1. Argatroban
                a. Given IV
                b. Cleared by the liver
                c. Monitor with PTT
             2. Lepirudin
                a. Given IV
                b. Cleared by the kidney
                c. Monitor with PTT
             3. Danaparoid
                a. Given subcutaneously
                b. Cleared by the kidney
                c. Monitor with heparin levels
        iv. Do **NOT** use LMWH as a substitute
    g. Antiplatelet agents may be useful
        i. Ticlopidine
11. Clinical Presentation
    a. Patient with APS on warfarin presents with dangerously high INR
        i. Bleeding risk greatest when INR 5 or higher
        ii. Hold warfarin until INR decreases to the desired range
        iii. For a more rapid decrease
             1. 1 mg of vitamin K orally or IV
                a. Decreases excessive anticoagulation within 12 h
                b. Do not give subcutaneous
                    i. Increases warfarin resistance for several days
        iv. For severe bleeding
             1. Fresh frozen plasma
             2. Replace coagulation factors acutely
12. Prognosis
    a. Variable clinical courses for APS
        i. Some have one clinical complication but no others
        ii. Some experience all of the major complications
    b. Patient subsets where the risk of thrombosis are unknown
        i. Women who have only a history of pregnancy loss
        ii. Patients with aCL or lupus anticoagulant but no clinical symptoms
    c. Risk of recurrent thrombosis
        i. Small in patients treated appropriately with oral anticoagulants
    d. Prolonged anticoagulation
        i. Associated with a significant risk of hemorrhage

Adult Still's Disease

16

1. The clinical features of adult Still's disease resemble the systemic form of JRA
   a. Seronegative chronic polyarthritis associated with a systemic inflammatory illness
   b. Initially described in 1897 by George F. Still (pathologist)
   c. Subsequently detailed in adults in 1971 by Eric Bywaters
2. Epidemiology
   a. Rare
   b. Affects both genders equally
   c. Exists worldwide
   d. Majority present at age 16–35 years
      i. 75% before age 35
3. Pathogenesis
   a. Etiology unknown
   b. Principal hypothesis implicates a virus or other infectious agent
   c. Linkage to HLA antigens inconclusive
   d. Immune complexes may play a pathogenic role (not confirmed)
   e. **NO** association with pregnancy and use of hormones
   f. Stress may play a role as inducer (not confirmed)
   g. Circadian release of proinflammatory cytokines
      i. Accounts for many clinical features
      ii. IL-6
      iii. IL-18
         1. Elevated
         2. Stimulates ferritin synthesis in monocytes/macrophages
4. Clinical Findings
   a. Preceded by a prolonged course of nonspecific signs and symptoms
   b. A prodromal sore throat occurs days to weeks before other symptoms
      i. Occurs in 70% (50–92%)
   c. The most striking manifestations
      i. Severe arthralgia (98–100%) and myalgia (84–98%)
      ii. Malaise

N.T. Colburn, *Review of Rheumatology*,
DOI 10.1007/978-1-84882-093-7_16, © Springer-Verlag London Limited 2012

    iii. Weight loss (19–76%)
    iv. Fever (83–100%)
  d. Less common clinical manifestations
    i. Lymphadenopathy (48–74%)
    ii. Splenomegaly (45–55%)
    iii. Pleuritis (23–53%)
    iv. Abdominal pain (9–48%)
    v. Hepatomegaly (29–44%)
    vi. Pericarditis (24–37%)
    vii. Pneumonitis (9–31%)
  e. Unusual manifestation (numerous)
    i. Alopecia
    ii. Sjogren's
    iii. Subcutaneous nodules
    iv. Necrotizing lymphadenitis
    v. Acute liver failure
    vi. Pulmonary fibrosis
    vii. Cardiac tamponade
    viii. Aseptic meningitis
    ix. Peripheral neuropathy
    x. Proteinuria
    xi. Microscopic hematuria
    xii. Amyloidosis
    xiii. Hemolytic anemia
    xiv. DIC
    xv. TTP
    xvi. Orbital pseudotumor
    xvii. Cataracts
    xviii. Sensorineural hearing loss
    xix. Hemophagocytic syndrome
  f. Patients appear severely ill
    i. Often receive numerous courses of antibiotics
    ii. Presumed septic with negative cultures
  g. Fever
    i. Initial symptom
    ii. Usually sudden onset high and spiking
    iii. Spikes once daily (rarely twice daily)
      1. Usually early morning and/or late afternoon/evening
      2. Quotidian or diquotidian pattern
    iv. Lasts 2–4 h
    v. Temperature elevation marked
      1. 66% with fever >40°C
    vi. Returns to normal in 80% of untreated patients
      1. Can return below normal

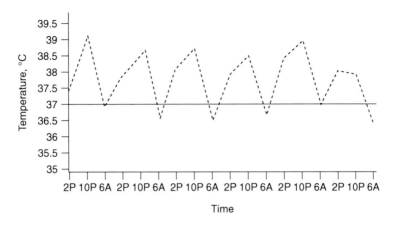

Fig. 16.1 Fever pattern in adult-onset Still's disease (Reproduced with permission from Rheumatoid arthritis, juvenile rheumatoid arthritis, and related conditions. *Atlas of Rheumatology*. ImagesMD; 2002-03-07)

    vii. Very ill when febrile
        1. Feels well with normal body temp
   viii. Pattern contrasts with that seen with infection
        1. Baseline elevation in body temperature
        2. Episodic fever spikes
     ix. Patients evaluated for FUO
        1. 5% eventually diagnosed with Still's
  h. Arthritis (88–84%)
     i. Initially affects only a few joints
     ii. Evolves to polyarticular disease
   iii. Most commonly affected joints
        1. Knee (84%)
        2. Wrist (74%)
        3. Ankle, shoulder, elbow, and PIP joints (50%)
        4. MCP (33%)
        5. DIP (20%)
    iv. Other joints affected
        1. MTPs
        2. Hips
        3. Tempromandibular joint (TMJ)
     v. Neck pain (50%)
    vi. Arthrocentesis yields
        1. Class II inflammatory synovial fluid
        2. Neutrophil predominance
   vii. Destructive arthritis (20–25%)

Fig. 16.2 Wrist involvement in adult-onset Still's disease (Reproduced with permission Rheumatoid arthritis, juvenile rheumatoid arthritis, and related conditions. *Atlas of Rheumatology.* ImagesMD; 2005-01-18)

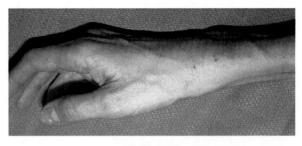

Fig. 16.3 Rash in adult-onset Still's disease (Reproduced with permission from Rheumatoid arthritis, juvenile rheumatoid arthritis, and related conditions. *Atlas of Rheumatology.* ImagesMD; 2002-03-07)

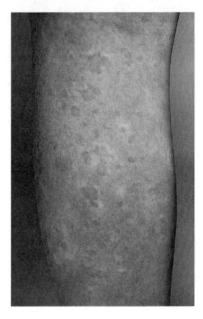

   i. Still's rash
      i. Present in more than 85% of patients
      ii. Almost pathognomonic
      iii. Salmon pink
      iv. Macular or maculopapular
      v. Frequently evanescent
      vi. Often occurs with the evening fever spike
         1. Evening rounds may detect this near-diagnostic finding
      vii. More common on the trunk and proximal extremities
      viii. Precipitated by
         1. Mechanical irritation
            a. Clothing
            b. Rubbing
            c. Koebner's phenomenon (up to 40%)

        2. Heat
           a. Hot bath
           b. Applying a hot towel
      ix. May be mildly pruritic
       x. Skin biopsies and immunofluorescent studies
           1. Neurivascular mononuclear cell infiltrate
           2. Nondiagnostic
5. Laboratory Findings
    a. **No** diagnostic tests
    b. Serum ferritin
      i. An acute-phase reactant that reflects inflammation
      ii. An extremely elevated level suggest the diagnosis
     iii. A value of ≥1,000 mg/dl in the proper clinical setting
         1. Confirmatory
         2. Especially associated with a low glycosylated ferritin
     iv. Values >4,000 mg/dl seen in <50%
      v. Reason for such elevations unknown
    c. CRP
      i. Frequently greater than 10 times upper limit of normal
    d. ESR
      i. Universally elevated >50 (96–100%)
    e. Leukocytosis
      i. Range 12–40,000/mm^3 present in 90% (71–97%)
      ii. 80% have WBC count > 15,000/mm^3
     iii. Neutrophils ≥ 80% (55–88%)
    f. LFT
      i. Elevated in up to three-quarters of patients (35–85%)
    g. Anemia
      i. Common (59–92%)
      ii. Sometimes profound
    h. Thrombocytosis (52–62%)
    i. Hypoalbuminemia (44–88%)
    j. RF and ANA
      i. Generally negative or low titer
    k. Synovial and serosal fluids
      i. Inflammatory
      ii. Predominance of neutrophils
6. Radiographic Findings
    a. Early
      i. Soft-tissue swelling
      ii. Effusions
     iii. Periarticular osteoporosis (occasionally)

Fig. 16.4 Radiographic changes in adult-onset Still's disease include periarticular osteopenia and loss of joint space (Reproduced with permission from Rheumatoid arthritis, juvenile rheumatoid arthritis, and related conditions. *Atlas of Rheumatology*. ImagesMD; 2002-03-07)

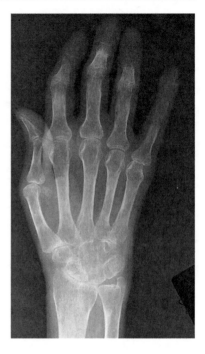

 b. Late
  i. Joint erosions
  ii. Fusions
   1. Carpal bones (50%)
   2. Tarsal bones (20%)
   3. Cervical spine (10%)
 c. Characteristic radiographic findings
  i. Typically found in the wrist
  ii. Nonerosive narrowing of carpometacarpal and intercarpal joints
  iii. Progresses to bony ankylosis
7. Diagnosis
 a. Diagnosis one of exclusion
  i. With the proper clinical and laboratory abnormalities
  ii. With the absence of another explanation (infection or malignancy)
 b. Criteria of Cush (practical guide)
  i. Diagnosis requires the presence of all of the following
   1. Fever >39°C (102.2°F)
   2. Arthralgia or arthritis
   3. RF < 1:80
   4. ANA < 1:100

      ii. In addition, any two of the following
         1. WBC count ≥ 15,000 cells/mm³
         2. Still's rash
         3. Pleuritis or pericarditis
         4. Hepatomegaly or splenomegaly or generalized lymphadenopathy
  c. Most do not present with the full-blown syndrome
  d. Typical presentation for adult Still's disease
      i. High, daily fever spikes
      ii. Severe myalgia, arthralgia, and arthritis
      iii. Still's rash
      iv. Leukocytosis
  e. Markedly elevated serum ferritin highly suggestive
8. Differential Diagnosis
  a. Granulomatous disorders
      i. Sarcoidosis
      ii. Idiopathic granulomatosis hepatitis
      iii. Crohn's disease
  b. Vasculitis
      i. Serum sickness
      ii. PAN
      iii. Wegener's
      iv. TTP
      v. Takayasu's
  c. Infection
      i. Viral
         1. Hepatitis B
         2. Rubella
         3. Parvovirus
         4. Coxsackie
         5. EBV
         6. CMV
         7. HIV
      ii. Subacute bacterial endocarditis
      iii. Chronic meningococcemia
      iv. Gonococcemia
      v. TB
      vi. Lyme
      vii. Syphilis
      viii. Rheumatic fever
  d. Malignancy
      i. Leukemia
      ii. Lymphoma
      iii. Angioblastic lymphadenopathy

     e. Connective tissue disease
        i. SLE
       ii. Mixed connective tissue disease
  9. Disease Course and Outcome
     a. Median time to achieve clinical and laboratory remission
        i. 10 months while receiving therapy
       ii. 32 months requiring no therapy
     b. Can remit years after onset
     c. Course generally follows one of three patterns (one-third of patients each)
        i. Self-limited disease
           1. Remission within 6–9 months
           2. One-fifth to one-third
       ii. Intermittent flares
           1. One recurrence
             a. Two-thirds
             b. 10–36 months from the original illness
           2. Multiple flares
             a. Up to ten flares reported
             b. Intervals of 3–48 months
             c. Recurrent episodes generally milder than the original
             d. Respond to lower doses of meds
             e. Timing of relapse unpredictable
      iii. Chronic Still's disease
           1. Chronic arthritis is the principle problem
           2. Severe involvement of the knees and hips
             a. Require total joint replacement
           3. Most common in the hip
     d. Markers of chronic disease or poor prognosis
        i. Presence of polyarthritis (four or more joints involved)
       ii. Root joint involvement (shoulders or hips)
      iii. A childhood episode
           1. Occurs in about one of six patients
      iv. More than 2 years of therapy with systemic corticosteroids
     e. A controlled study of patients 10 years after the diagnosis of Still's
        i. Significant higher levels of pain, physical disability, and psychologic disability than unaffected siblings
       ii. Levels of pain and disability lower than other chronic rheumatic disease
      iii. No difference in Still's patients and controls in overcoming handicaps
           1. Educational attainment
           2. Occupational prestige
           3. Social functioning
           4. Family income
     f. 5 year survival rate 90–95%
        i. Similar to the survival rate for lupus
       ii. Vast majority lead remarkably full lives after disease onset

g. Premature death may be slightly increased
h. Causes of mortality
   i. Hepatic failure
   ii. DIC
   iii. Amyloidosis
   iv. Sepsis
   v. Acute respiratory distress syndrome (ARDS)
   vi. Heart failure
   vii. Carcinoma of the lung
   viii. Status epilepticus

10. Acute Treatment
  a. NSAIDs
    i. About one-fourth respond (20–40%)
    ii. A commonly used regimen
      1. High dose enteric-coated aspirin
      2. Achieve a serum salicylate level of 15–25 mg/dl
      3. Sometimes combined with indomethacin (150 mg/day)
    iii. Side effects
      1. Hepatotoxicity
        a. Elevated LFTs usually return to normal
        b. Despite continued NSAID therapy
      2. Increased risk of DIC
  b. Systemic corticosteroids
    i. Patients who fail to respond to NSAIDs
    ii. For severe disease
      1. Pericardial tamponade
      2. Myocarditis
      3. Severe pneumonitis
      4. DIC
      5. Rising LFTs during NSAID treatment
    iii. Prednisone in a dose of 0.5–1.0 mg/kg/day
    iv. About one-third require at least 60 mg of prednisone daily
    v. Relapses occur during tapering
      1. Add one of the slow-acting antirheumatic drugs
        a. Methotrexate
    vi. IV pulse methylprednisolone used for life-threatening disease

11. Chronic Treatment
  a. Medications used to treat arthritis (the most common cause of chronicity)
    i. IM gold
    ii. Hydroxychloroquine
      1. Mild chronic systemic disease may respond as well
        a. Fatigue
        b. Fever
        c. Rash
        d. Serositis

      iii. Sulfasalazine
         1. Increased toxicity may occur
      iv. Penicillamine
      v. Methotrexate
         1. Low doses (similar to those used in RA)
         2. Used in both chronic arthritis and chronic systemic disease
  b. Immunosuppressive agents
      i. Used in resistant cases
      ii. Azathioprine
      iii. Cyclophosphamide
      iv. Cyclosporine
      v. IVIG (controversial)
      vi. Mycophenolate mofetil
      vii. Leflunomide
  c. Biologics
      i. TNF-α elevated in Still's disease
      ii. Etanercept and infliximab beneficial
         1. Especially articular manifestations
      iii. Anakinra
         1. Successful in refractory disease
  d. Therapy after a decade of disease
      i. About one-half of patients will require second-line agents
      ii. One-third will require low-dose corticosteroids
  e. Multidisciplinary approach
      i. Physiotherapists
      ii. Occupational therapists
      iii. Psychologists
      iv. Arthritis support groups

Therapeutic Injections for Rheumatic Diseases

17

1. In 1951 Hollander demonstrated that hydrocortisone salts could be effective when injected into arthritis joints
2. Major objectives of local injections
   a. Enter a painful structure
   b. Remove excess fluid
   c. Instill corticosteroids likely to provide the longest duration of relief
3. Indications for therapeutic injections
   a. When only one or a few joints are inflamed
      i. Infection must be excluded
   b. As an adjunct to systemic drug therapy in systemic polyarthritis
   c. To assist in rehabilitation and prevent deformity
   d. To relieve pain in OA exhibiting local inflammatory signs
   e. Recurrent joint effusion
   f. Soft-tissue regional disorders
      i. Bursitis
      ii. Tenosynovitis
      iii. Periarthritis
      iv. Nodules
      v. Epicondylitis
      vi. Ganglia
      vii. Soft-tissue trigger point injection
      viii. Intra-articular injection for synovitis
4. Rheumatic diseases where corticosteroid injections are indicated
   a. RA
   b. OA
   c. SLE
   d. Crystal deposition disease
   e. Spondyloarthropathies
   f. Tietze's
   g. Entrapment neuropathies

N.T. Colburn, *Review of Rheumatology*,
DOI 10.1007/978-1-84882-093-7_17, © Springer-Verlag London Limited 2012

5. Effectiveness of an injection
   a. Ranges from 50% to 90%
   b. Lasts days to months
6. Contraindications for corticosteroid injections
   a. Absolute
      i. Established infections
      ii. Either regional (cellulitis) or systemic (bacteremia)
   b. Inaccessible joints
   c. Intra-articular fracture
   d. Excessive patient anxiety
   e. Joint instability
   f. Bleeding diatheses
      i. Proceed with caution
      ii. Possible induction of a hemearthrosis
      iii. Decompress established joint swelling due to bleeding
   g. Joint or soft-tissue injection in patients on warfarin
      i. Low risk if INR < 4.5
   h. Previous failure to respond to local injection
      i. Precludes a repeat attempt
      ii. Unless suboptimal technical situation
7. Complications that can follow injections
   a. A transient increase in pain
      i. The most common
   b. Post-injection flare (2%)
      i. Steroid crystal induced synovitis
         1. A local reaction to corticosteroid crystals
      ii. 6% of injections in a large series of patients with RA
      iii. Particularly with injections of the lateral epicondyle
      iv. Usually occurs within 6–18 h after an injection
         1. Distinguishes from an infection
         2. Infections manifest after 2–4 days
      v. Generally subsides within 24 h
      vi. Intracellular steroid crystals seen with joint aspiration
         1. Look like CPPD crystals
         2. Polarize with the first order red compensation like gout crystals
         3. Bacteria seen with an infection
      vii. Management
         1. Rest
         2. Analgesia
         3. NSAIDs
         4. Cold packs
      viii. Provoked by the less-soluble (long-acting) corticosteroid preparations
         1. Use one of the more soluble corticosteroids with a history of post-injection flare

    c. Skin and subcutaneous atrophy at the site of injection
    d. Skin hypopigmentation
       i. Forewarn dark skinned patients about potential loss of pigmented cells
    e. Systemic effects of the injection
       i. Mild and transient
      ii. Flushing
     iii. Slight agitation
     iv. Exacerbation of diabetic tendencies
    f. Repeated injections
       i. Signs of exogenous hypercortisolism
      ii. Adrenal suppression
         1. Possible with more than twice per month
         2. One corticosteroid injection can suppress cortisol levels (HPA axis) by 30% for up to 7 days
         3. Test adrenal reserve prior to major physiologic stress
            a. Such as abdominal surgery
            b. May need supplemental corticosteroid
    g. Structural damage
       i. One corticosteroid injection transiently weakens a tendon
         1. Up to 40%
         2. For 3–12 weeks
      ii. Tendons, ligaments, and their attachments can be disrupted when injected directly
         1. Confine injections to adjacent synovial sheaths and bursae
         2. Never inject Achilles tendon
    h. Injection limits
       i. A minimum of 4–6 weeks between injections
      ii. Weight bearing joints should not be injected more frequently than every 6–12 weeks
     iii. The same joint or tendon sheath should not be injected more than three times yearly
     iv. Three or four injections per year for large nearly normal weight-bearing joints
         1. More frequent in established arthritis for which few therapeutic alternatives exist
    i. Induction of infection
       i. Incidence rates reported
         1. 1:1,000
         2. 1:16,000
         3. 1:50,000 in experienced hands
      ii. Risk factor
         1. Injected within the previous 3 months (up to 20%)
    j. Rare association with osteonecrosis
    k. Erythroderma

8. Injection Technique
   a. Be familiar with the regional anatomy
   b. Mark the area to be entered
   c. Position so that structures on either side of the injection target are relaxed
   d. Skin-cleansing and hand-washing are sufficient asepsis
   e. Sterile gloves and sterile draping reserved for
      i. Immunocompromised patients
      ii. A probable lengthy or difficult procedure
   f. Anesthetize
      i. Spray the site with ethyl chloride solution
      ii. Infiltrate the skin and subcutaneous tissues with lidocaine
         1. Delivered through an ultra thin needle
      iii. Track lidocaine to the structure of interest
         1. May leave the smaller needle in place
         2. Puncture same site with a larger needle
   g. Obtaining fluid assures that the needle has entered the synovial space
   h. Evacuate all obtainable synovial fluid
      i. Prolongs relief for knee synovitis in RA patients injected with triamcinolone compared with no aspiration (prospective trial)
9. Corticosteroid preparations
   a. Less-soluble compounds preferred for joint-space injections
      i. Reducing the solubility increases the duration of the local effect
      ii. Slower diffusion of the medication will occur
      iii. Less soluble preparations have greater potency
      iv. More likely to result in adverse consequences
   b. Use short- or long-acting corticosteroids for injections into tendon sheaths
      i. More soluble
      ii. Less soft tissue atrophy
      iii. Less chance of tendon rupture
   c. Use the longest acting, least-soluble preparations for injections into inflamed joints
      i. Tend to be more effective
   d. Fluorinated compounds
      i. Used for peritendon and bursal injections
      ii. A propensity to cause soft-tissue atrophy
   e. Short-acting, soluble
      i. Dexamethasone (Decadron)
         1. Prednisone equivalent 40 mg
      ii. Hydrocortisone acetate (Hydrocortone)
         1. Prednisone equivalent 5–10 mg
   f. Long-acting, less soluble
      i. Methylprednisolone acetate (Depo-Medrol)
         a. Prednisone equivalent 25–100 mg
      ii. Dexamethasone acetate (Decadron LA)
         1. Prednisone equivalent 80 mg

    g. Longest-acting, least soluble
        i. Triamcinolone acetonide (Kenalog)
            1. Prednisone 12.5–50 mg
       ii. Triamcinolone hexacetonide (Aristospan)
            1. Prednisone equivalent 25 mg
    h. Combination steroids
        i. Longest-acting and short-acting steroid combined
       ii. Betamethasone sodium phophate/acetate (Celestone)
            1. Prednisone equivalent 50 mg
    i. Dose and volume
        i. 1 to 2 cc to large joints (knees, hips, shoulders)
       ii. ½ to 1 cc to medium sized joints (wrists, elbow, ankles)
      iii. ¼ to ½cc to small joints (interphalangeal, metaphalangeal) and soft-
            tissue sites
       iv. Optimal dose depends on
            1. Size of the joint
            2. Degree of inflammation
            3. Amount of fluid present
                a. Aspirate effusions dry before injections
            4. Concentration of corticosteroid used
        v. Bursa
            1. Prednisone equivalent 10–20 mg
       vi. Tendon sheath
            1. Prednisone equivalent 10–20 mg
      vii. Small joints of the hands and feet
            1. Prednisone equivalent 5–15 mg
     viii. Medium sized joints (wrist, elbow)
            1. Prednisone equivalent 15–25 mg
       ix. Large joints (knee, shoulder, ankle)
            1. Prednisone equivalent 20–50 mg
            2. 1 mg/kg dose for injection of a child's knee
    j. Dilute with lidocaine
        i. Provides immediate temporary relief
       ii. Assures the clinician that the desired structure was entered
      iii. Provides a vehicle to deliver corticosteroid to all reaches of the joint
            space
    k. Flocculation of corticosteroid suspensions can occur
        i. Especially if a paraben compound is used as a preservative
       ii. Shake the syringe vigorously immediately prior to injecting
      iii. Minimizes joint precipitation
10. Methods to Promote Drug Delivery
    a. Move an injected joint through its physiologic range
    b. Gently massage an injected soft-tissue structure
    c. Period of rest after injection
        i. Triamcinolone-injected knees with 24 h of rest after injection fared bet-
            ter 6 months later compared with injected knees not rested

11. Injections in Specific Disorders
    a. RA
        i. Be careful not to over rely on intraarticular therapy
        ii. Certain extra-articular features respond well to local injections
            1. Entrapment neuropathies due to synovial proliferation
                a. Carpal tunnel
                b. Cubital tunnel
                c. Tarsal tunnel (medial aspect of the ankle)
            2. Rheumatoid nodules
                a. Usually shrink in response to corticosteroid delivered nearby
    b. OA
        i. Features of local inflammation often present
            1. Predicts response to injection
        ii. Pain often arises from structures exterior to the joint
            1. Inject irritated pes anserine bursa
            2. Pain relief greater and longer lasting with soft-tissue injections compared with intra-articular in OA patients
    c. Crystalline arthropathy
        i. Joint entry important for diagnosis and treatment
        ii. Intra-articular injection avoids the toxicities of systemic therapy
        iii. Concomitant gout and infection a negligible possibility
        iv. Local injection immediately after obtaining synovial fluid
            1. The treatment modality of choice
    d. Glenohumeral joint
        i. Affected by primary OA, infection, and adhesive capsulitis
        ii. Adhesive capsulitis
            1. Treat by injecting a large volume of diluted corticosteroid-anesthetic mixture

Nonsteroidal Anti-inflammatory Drugs

18

1. NSAIDs are used in many different forms of arthritis
   a. Reduce pain
      i. Analgesic as narcotics (in therapeutic doses) in acute pain
   b. Decrease gelling
   c. Improve function
   d. Anti-inflammatory
      i. Achieved by a number of mechanisms
   e. Antipyretic agents
      i. Inhibit prostaglandins in the CNS which reduces fever
   f. Antiplatelet
      i. Most decrease platelet aggregation by preventing thromboxane A2 production
      ii. Prevents the first step in coagulation
2. NSAIDs can not alter the natural history of any disease
3. One of the most commonly used classes of drugs in the world
   a. In some countries there are up to 40 NSAIDs from which to choose
4. Frequency of use
   a. Prescriptions for the elderly exceeds that for younger patients by 3.6 fold
      i. 50% of regular users are over the age of 60
   b. In the USA there are 17 million regular uses
   c. Estimated cost > $1.7 billion in annual costs
5. Clinical efficacy and tolerability of NSAIDS are similar at equipotent doses
   a. Individual responses are highly variable
   b. If no response to an NSAID of one class switch to another
6. Sodium salicylic acid
   a. Discovered in 1763 but probably used for centuries
      i. Hippocrates, Celsus, and Galen recorded the use of willow bark known to contain salicylates to treat fever and pain
   b. The acetyl derivative (acetylsalicylic acid (ASA)) has anti-inflammatory activity
   c. 1853 – Acetylsalicylate (aspirin) first synthesized

N.T. Colburn, *Review of Rheumatology*,
DOI 10.1007/978-1-84882-093-7_18, © Springer-Verlag London Limited 2012

d. 1899 – Aspirin introduced to the USA (Bayer Company)
  i. Felix Hoffman gave this to his arthritic father which helped
7. Indoleacetic acid derivatives
  a. Phenylbutazone
    i. Introduced in 1949
    ii. The first nonsalicylate NSAID developed for use
    iii. Bone-marrow toxicity was seen
      1. Particularly in women over the age of 60
    iv. Rarely prescribed
  b. Indomethacin
    i. Developed in the 1960s (1965) to substitute for phenylbutazone
  c. COX-2 inhibitors
    i. Introduced in the 1990s
8. Eight major structural classifications of NSAIDs
  a. Drugs in each class tend to have similar side effects
  b. Salicylate
    i. ASA
    ii. Nonacetylated sodium salicylate and choline salicylate
    iii. Tinnitus as a consistent side effect
  c. Acetic acid
    i. Indole derivatives (indomethacin, tolemtin, sulindac)
    ii. Phenylacetic acid (diclofenac)
    iii. Pyranocarboxylic acid (etodolac)
  d. Propionic acids
    i. Ibuprofen, naproxen, fenoprofen, and ketoprofen
    ii. Generally a very safe group
  e. Enolic acids
    i. Oxicams (piroxicam, meloxicam)
    ii. Pyrazolones (phenylbutazone)
      1. Removed from market
      2. Associated with aplastic anemia
  f. Pyrrolo-pyrrole
    i. Ketorolac
  g. Nonacidic compounds
    i. Nabumetone
  h. Diaryl substituted pyrazole
    i. Celecoxib, rofecoxib
    ii. Thought to be safe for the stomach
9. Mechanisms of Action
  a. Primary mechanism of action
    i. Inhibition of prostaglandin (PG) synthesis
    ii. Some are potent inhibitors of PG synthesis
    iii. Others prominently affect biologic events not mediated by PG
  b. Differential affects attributed to
    i. Variations in the enantiomeric state of the agent

      ii. Pharmacokinetics

      iii. Pharmacodynamics

      iv. Metabolism

10. Inhibition of Prostaglandin Synthesis

    a. NSAIDs inhibit the production of prostaglandins of the E series

    b. Prostaglandins of the E series

      i. Proinflammatory

      ii. Increase vascular permeability

      iii. Increase platelet aggregation

      iv. Inhibit apoptosis

    c. Other effects of prostaglandin inhibition

      i. Reestablish normal cell-cycle responses without effecting apoptosis

      ii. Reduce PGH synthase gene expression

    d. NSAIDs specifically inhibit cyclooxyenase (COX)

      i. Reduces conversion of arachidonic acid to prostaglandins

11. Inhibition of Cyclooxyenase

    a. ASA acetylates the COX enzyme

    b. Nonsalicylate NSAIDs are reversible inhibitors of the COX enzyme

      i. Effect based on serum half-life

    c. Two major isoforms of the COX enzymes

      i. Each differ in regulation and expression

      ii. 70-kd molecular weight

      iii. Similar but slightly different active sites

      iv. 60% C-DNA homology

      v. On different genes

    d. COX-1

      i. On chromosome 9

      ii. Lacks a TATA box and upstream transcriptional start sites

        1. Suggests a continuously transcribed stable message

      iii. Expressed constitutively in most tissues

        1. Stomach

        2. Intestine

        3. Kidney

        4. Platelets

      iv. Inhibited by all NSAIDs to varying degrees

      v. Maintains the integrity of the gastric and duodenal mucosa

      vi. Modulates renal plasma flow in patients with

        1. Relative dehydration

        2. Clinically significant CHF

        3. Cirrhosis with or without ascites

        4. Intrinsic kidney disease

          a. SLE

          b. DM

    e. COX-2

      i. On chromosome 1

      ii. Contains a TATA box and bases upstream of the transcriptional start sites

           1. Binding sites

              a. NF-κB

              b. SP-1

              c. GRE

              d. PEA-3

              e. AP2

              f. Nuclear factor IL-6

              g. E-box

              h. cAMP response elements

     iii. An inducible enzyme

     iv. Found constitutively in the kidney and brain

      v. Usually undetectable in most tissue

     vi. Expression increased

           1. During states of inflammation

           2. In response to mitogenic stimuli

    vii. Expression inhibited

           1. By corticosteroids

   viii. Important for

           1. Modulating glomerular blood flow

           2. Renal electrolyte and water balance

f. All NSAIDs inhibit the activity of both COX-1 and COX-2

      i. Clinical effectiveness due to effects on COX-2

     ii. Toxic effects secondary to inhibition of COX-1

g. COX nonselective

      i. Ibuprofen

     ii. Naproxen

    iii. Meclomen

    iv. Indomethacin

h. COX-1 selective

      i. Low dose aspirin

           1. Binds to serine 530 on COX-1

i. COX-2 selective

      i. Low dose etodolac and meloxicam

           1. Ten fold inhibition of COX-2 compared to COX-1 in vitro

           2. Effect mitigated at higher doses

     ii. Diclofenac

    iii. Nabumetone

j. Specific COX-2 inhibitors (or COX-1 sparing agents)

      i. 300 times more effective at inhibiting COX-2 than COX-1

     ii. Valdecoxib

    iii. Celecoxib

    iv. Rofecoxib

           1. Removed from market due to safety concerns

    2. VIGOR (Vioxx GI Outcomes Research) study
      a. Four-fold increased risk of acute heart attack in rofecoxib compared with naproxen (0.4% vs. 0.1%, RR 0.25)
  v. Various studies of celecoxib and rofecoxib
    1. Effective at inhibiting
      a. OA pain
      b. Dental pain
      c. RA pain and inflammation
    2. Compared to
      a. Naproxen 500 mg BID
      b. Ibuprofen 800 mg TID
      c. Diclofenac 75 mg BID
    3. Twofold to threefold decreased incidence of GI
      a. Bleeding
      b. Perforation
      c. Obstruction
12. Other Mechanisms of NSAIDs
  a. Lipophilic
    i. Incorporate in the lipid bylayer of cell membranes
    ii. Interrupts protein-protein interactions important for signal transduction
      1. Inhibits stimulus–response coupling
      2. Critical for recruitment of phagocytic cells to sites of inflammation
  b. Disrupts neutrophil activity
    i. Decreased endothelial cell adherence
    ii. Decreased expression of L-selectins
    iii. Inhibits activation and chemotaxis
    iv. Reduces toxic oxygen radical production
  c. Inhibits NF-κB dependent transcription
    i. Inhibits inducible nitric oxide synthetase
  d. Scavenges superoxide radicals
  e. Affects T-lymphocyte function
    i. Inhibits rheumatoid factor production
  f. Specific NSAIDs and mechanisms of action
    i. Salicylates
      1. Inhibit phopholipase C activity in macrophages
      2. Inhibit the arachidonic cascade earlier than COX enzymes
    ii. ASA
      1. Inhibits expression of inducible nitric-oxide synthetase
      2. Decreases production of nitrite in vitro
    iii. Nonacetylated salicylates and indomethacin
      1. Inhibit neutrophil function
        a. Aggregation
        b. Adhesion
        c. Enzyme release

      iv. Indomethacin and piroxicam
         1. Inhibit superoxide formation
      v. Salicylates
         1. Depress lymphocyte transformation
         2. Inhibit cytokine production by inhibiting NF-κB
      vi. Salicylates, piroxicam, ibuprofen, fenoprofen, and tolmetin
         1. Suppress proteoglycan production in cartilage
     vii. Sulindac, meclofenamate, and diclofenac
         1. Inhibit effects on lipooxygenase products
    viii. Piroxicam
         1. Inhibits rheumatoid factor production

13. Pharmacology
   a. General properties of NSAIDs
      i. Weak organic acids with acidic properties
         1. Sequester preferentially in inflamed joints
         2. A longer synovial half-life than plasma half-life
      ii. Bind avidly to serum proteins (> 95%)
         1. Mainly albumin
         2. Results in higher delivery levels
            a. Localized inflamed sites increase vascular permeability
         3. Salicylates are the least highly protein-bound (68%)
     iii. Increased serum free component secondary to
         1. A decrease in serum albumin
         2. Institution of other highly protein-bound medications
         3. Other hypoalbuminemic states
            a. Elderly
            b. Chronically ill
      iv. Ionization constants (pKa) ranging from 3 to 5
         1. Un-inonized in the acidic environment of the stomach
         2. Can lead to mucosal damage
   b. Absorption
      i. All absorbed completely after oral administration
      ii. Absorption rates vary
         1. Altered GI blood flow or motility
         2. When taken with food
         3. Enteric coating
   c. Metabolism
      i. Metabolized **predominantly in the liver**
         1. Most metabolized through the P450 CYP2C9 isoenzyme
      ii. Inactive metabolites excreted in the urine
     iii. Caution in patients with hepatic or renal dysfunction
         1. Renal dysfunction
            a. Some inactive metabolites may be resynthesized to the active compound

    b. Prostaglandins important in maintaining adequate glomerular flow and pressure with dysfunction
       i. Vasodilates renal arteries
      ii. Increase sodium loss
     iii. Increase renin release
  2. Liver dysfunction
    a. Elevated aminotransferases (ALT and AST)
       i. Can occur with all NSAIDs
    b. NSAID induced hepatotoxicity
       i. Evident during the first 6 months
      ii. Obtain LFTs during the first month
     iii. Every 3–6 months thereafter
    c. Special NSAIDS metabolized in the liver
       i. Diclofenac
      ii. Flurbiprofen
     iii. Celecoxib
     iv. Rofecoxib
    d. Use lowest possible doses with
       i. Clinically significant liver disease
      ii. Cirrhosis with or without ascites
     iii. Prolonged PTT
     iv. Low serum albumin levels
    e. Idiosyncratic severe hepatitis
       i. Indomethacin
      ii. Diclofenac
     iii. Sulindac
     iv. Phenylbutazone
    f. Fatal hepatotoxicity
       i. Children using indomethacin
         1. Not for children < 11 years with arthritis
    g. Cholestasis
 iv. Oxaprozin has two metabolic pathways
   1. Some portion secreted directly into the bile
   2. Another part further metabolized and excreted in the urine
 v. Salicylates have zero-order kinetics
   1. Narrow range of effectiveness
   2. Incremental dose increases lead to very high serum levels once the metabolism is saturated
   3. Caution when changing chronic steady state levels
    a. Especially with altered renal or hepatic function
vi. Enterohepatic circulation
   1. Indomethacin
   2. Sulindac
   3. Piroxicam
   4. Results in a prolonged half-life

vii. "Prodrugs"
  1. Sulindac and nabumetone
  2. Active compound produced after first-pass metabolism through the liver
  3. Decreases exposure of the GI mucosa to local effects
  4. Also inhibits COX-1
    a. A risk for an NSAID-induced upper GI event
  5. Sulindac
    a. Reversibly metabolized to sulindac sulfide
      i. A potent COX inhibitor
    b. Converted back to the parent compound in the gut and kidney
    c. Undergoes extensive enterohepatic recirculation
    d. Long half life of 16–18 h
  6. Nabumetone
    a. Non-acidic
    b. A poor inhibitor of prostaglandin synthesis
    c. 6-methoxy-2-naphthylacetic acid
      i. The active metabolite
      ii. A potent inhibitor of prostaglandin synthesis
    d. Hepatically not renally cleared
    e. Does not undergo enterohepatic circulation
d. Plasma half-life
  i. Differences in plasma half-life explains the diverse clinical effects
    1. Long half-lives
      a. Clinical responses are delayed
      b. **Piroxicam**
        i. The longest serum half-life
        ii. About 57 h
      c. Others with long half-lives (>10 h)
        i.   Diflunisal
        ii.   Nabumetone
        iii. Naproxen
        iv.   Oxaprozin
        v.   Phenylbutazone
        vi.   Meloxicam
        vii. Salicylate (up to 15 h with SR)
        viii. Sulindac
        ix.   Celecoxib
        x.   Rofecoxib
    2. Shorter half-lifes
      a. Clinical responses are more prompt
      b. Unwanted side effects disappear rapidly when discontinued
      c. ASA
        i. A short half-life
        ii. 0.25 h

      d. **Diclofenac**
        i. A short half-life
        ii. About 1.1 h
      e. Others with short half-lives (<6 h)
        i. Etodolac
        ii. Fenoprofen
        iii. Flurbiprofen
        iv. Ibuprofen
        v. Indomethacin
        vi. Ketoprofen
        vii. Tolmetin
    ii. Synovial-fluid concentrations
      1. Do not vary greatly once plasma steady-state achieved
    iii. Highly lipid-soluble NSAIDs
      1. Penetrate the central nervous system more effectively
      2. Produces changes in mentation, perception, and mood
        a. Associated with indomethacin
        b. Particularly in the elderly
14. Adverse Effects
  a. Hepatotoxicity
    i. Elevation in hepatic transaminase levels
      1. More often in patients with JRA or SLE
      2. Clinically significant when
        a. Elevations exceed 2 or 3 times ULN
        b. Serum albumin altered
        c. Prothrombin times altered
    ii. Overt liver failure
      1. Diclofenac
      2. Flurbiprofen
      3. Sulindac
    iii. Cholestasis
      1. Highest incidence with sulindac
  b. Prostaglandin-related adverse effects
    i. Due to inhibition of PG synthesis in local tissues
    ii. Hypersensitivity reaction
      1. Increased risk for anaphylaxis with PG inhibition
      2. Seen in patients with
        a. Allergic Rhinitis
        b. Nasal polyposis
        c. History of asthma
        d. Chronic urticaria
      3. Acute bronchospasm and shortness of breath
      4. Severe asthmatic with nasal polyps
        a. Highest risk patient
        b. Up to 78% may react to ASA

     5. Exact mechanism unclear
       a. A sensitivity, not an allergy
         i. **NOT** IgE mediated
       b. Inhibition of COX activity leads to decreased E prostaglandins
         i. Important in maintaining bronchodilation
       c. Arachidonate shunted into the leukotriene pathway
         i. Large stores of arachidonate leads to excess substrate for leukotriene metabolism
         ii. 5-fold increase in bronchial expression of leukotrienes C4 synthetase
         iii. Excessive production of leukotrienes C, D, E (slow reacting substance of anaphylaxis (SRSA))
         iv. Release of highly reactive products
         v. SRSA pathway stimulates anaphylaxis
     6. Mechanistic theories
       a. Salsalate does not inhibit COX
         i. Does **not** cause asthma attacks
         ii. NSAID of choice for ASA-sensitive asthma patients
       b. Leukotriene inhibitors block bronchospasm provoked by NSAIDs in ASA-sensitive patients
       c. NSAID-induced asthma attacks
         i. Acute in onset
         ii. Severe and prolonged
         iii. Can be resistant to glucocorticoids
c. Platelet effects
   i. Platelet aggregation
     1. Induced primarily by thromboxane A2 production
     2. Platelet COX-1 activation
     3. No COX-2 in platelets
   ii. Nonsalicylate NSAIDs effect on platelets
     1. Reversible
     2. Related to the half-life of the drug
   iii. ASA effect on platelets
     1. Acetylates the COX-1 enzyme
     2. Permanently inactivates the platelet
       a. Platelet cannot make new COX enzyme
       b. Lacks normal platelet aggregation after ASA exposure
     3. Normal platelet function returns only with repopulation of platelets not exposed to ASA
   iv. Pre-surgical management
     1. Discontinue NSAIDs at a time determined by 4 or 5 times their serum half-life
     2. ASA should be discontinued 1–2 weeks prior
       a. Allows a normal platelet population to re-establish

    v. Thrombosis prophylaxis

       1. Numerous thrombotic events reported to the FDA since approval of the coxibs

       2. Abnormal blood vessels

          a. Require COX-2

          b. Produce antithrombotic prostaglandin I2 (prostacyclin)

          c. Inhibiting COX-2 tips the balance toward prothrombotic thromboxane A2

       3. For patients at risk for thrombosis

          a. Low-dose ASA given concomitantly with either

             i. Nonselective NSAIDs

            ii. Specific COX-2 inhibitors

d. Gastrointestinal effects

    i. The most clinically significant adverse effects occur in the GI tract

   ii. E prostaglandins effect the gastric mucosa by

       1. Inducing a protective superficial mucous barrier

          a. NSAIDs decrease mucous secretion

       2. Inducing bicarbonate output

          a. NSAIDs decrease bicarbonate output

       3. Increasing mucosal blood flow in the superficial gastric cell layer

          a. NSAIDs decrease mucosal blood flow

       4. Inhibiting gastric acid secretion

          a. NSAIDs increase gastric acid secretion

   iii. A wide range of GI problems

       1. Abdominal pain, dyspepsia, nausea, vomiting and diarrhea

          a. Especially with meclofenamate

          b. Cause unknown

       2. Gastroesophageal reflux

       3. Esophagitis

       4. Esophageal stricture

       5. Gastritis

       6. Mucosal erosions

       7. Hemorrhage

       8. Peptic Ulcer Disease (PUD)

          a. One of the most common side effects of NSAID therapy

          b. Ulcer structural changes due to systemic inhibition of prostaglandin synthesis

          c. NSAIDs in the presence of stomach acid

             i. Leads to oxidative uncoupling of cellular metabolism

            ii. Formation of local tissue injury

            iii. Cell death

            iv. Ultimate ulcer formation

          d. Affects gastric, duodenal, large and small bowel mucosa

e. Relative risk (summarized in clinical trials)
   i. 4.0–5.0 for the development of gastric ulcer
   ii. 1.1–1.6 for the development of duodenal ulcer
   iii. 4.5–5.0 for the development of clinically significant gastric ulcer with
       1. Hemorrhage
       2. Perforation
       3. Death
f. Routine stool guaiac testing insensitive in detection
g. Endoscopic studies
   i. Shallow erosions or submucosal hemorrhages
      1. More common in the stomach
         a. Prepyloric area
         b Antrum
      2. Typically asymptomatic
         a. Half of all patients who develop significant peptic ulcers do **NOT** develop symptoms
      3. Prevalence data difficult to determine
   ii. NSAID-induced ulcers > 3 mm with obvious depth
      1. Found in 15–31%
      2. Unknown how many heal or progress
   iii. Those treated with COX-2 specific inhibitors
      1. Induction of ulcers occurs at the same rate as patients who received placebo (4–8%)
      2. Ulcer complications 2–3 times less when compared with active comparators
      3. Delayed healing in ulcers secondary to low-dose ASA
   iv. After 1 week of treatment, ulcers > 3 mm with obvious depth were seen in
      1. 15% of healthy volunteers taking diclofenac or ibuprofen at standard doses
      2. 19% of healthy volunteers taking naproxen
   v. After 12 weeks of treatment
      1. 26% of patients with OA and RA taking naproxen or ibuprofen at standard doses
9. Perforation
   a. Dysfunction in GI mucosal permeability
   b. Colonic diverticuli
10. Obstruction
   a. Induce stricture formation that precipitates small- or large-bowel obstruction
   b. May be hard to detect on contrast radiographic studies
11. Death
   a. Responsible for greater than 16,000 deaths annually in the USA

      iv. Hospitalization for adverse GI effects

         1. Risk 7–10-fold greater in people with RA treated with NSAIDs

         2. Responsible for greater than 100,000 hospitalizations in the USA annually

         3. Medical cost estimated at $3.9 billion per year

      v. Risk factors for developing GI toxicity

         1. Age > 60

         2. History of PUD

         3. Prior use of anti-ulcer therapies for any reason

         4. Concomitant use of corticosteroids

            a. ≥10 mg/day

            b. Especially in patients with RA

         5. Comorbidites with a chronic disease state

            a. Significant cardiovascular disease

            b. Severe RA

            c. COPD

         6. History of abdominal pain of unclear etiology

            a. With or without NSAIDs

         7. Anticoagulant therapy

         8. Increased doses of specific and singular NSAIDs

         9. Tobacco and alcohol use

      vi. The safest NSAIDs

         1. Nonacetylated salicylates

     vii. The least safe NSAIDs

         1. Those with prominent enterohepatic circulation

         2. Significantly prolonged half-lives

         3. Increased GI toxicity due to re-exposure of gastric and duodenal mucosa to bile reflux and the active drug moiety

         4. Examples

            a. Sulindac

            b. Piroxicam

15. Management of Patients at Risk for GI events

   a. Superficial erosions by endoscopy

      i. Patients present with dyspepsia or upper-GI distress

      ii. Typically on nonselective NSAID

     iii. Often heal spontaneously without change in therapy

   b. Gastric or duodenal ulcer while taking NSAIDs

      i. Treatment should be discontinued

      ii. Therapy for ulcer disease instituted

         1. H2-antagonist

         2. PPIs

     iii. Determine if H. pylori antibodies are present

         1. Treat if necessary

   c. Prevention of NSAID-induced gastric and duodenal ulcers
     i. Misoprostol
       1. Strongest evidence for prevention of NSAID-induced gastric ulceration and its complications
       2. A prostaglandin E1 analog
       3. Locally replaces the prostaglandin normally synthesized in the gastric mucosa
       4. Usual dose 200 μg qid
       5. Inhibits by 40% the development of complications compared with placebo
         a. Bleeding
         b. Perforation
         c. Obstruction
       6. An 87% reduction in risk for HAQ scores > 1.5 (worse disease)
       7. Proven pharmacoeconomic utility
       8. The most common adverse event is diarrhea
         a. Up to 30%
         b. Caused study withdrawal in up to 10%
     ii. PPIs
       1. Prevents NSAID-induced duodenal ulcers
       2. Those proven protective for NSAID induced ulcers
         a. Omeprazole
         b. Esomeprazole
         c. Rabeprazole
         d. Lansoprazole
         e. Pantoprazole
     iii. H2 blockers
       1. Controversial whether protective
         a. Simetidine
         b. Aanitidine
         c. Famotidine
         d. Nizatidine
         e. Sucralfate
         f. Antacids
       2. Not recommended for GI protection
       3. May reduce NSAID-induced GI discomfort
     iv. Other measures to decrease NSAID-induced side effects
       1. Use the lowest dose possible
       2. Use alternative analgesics
16. Renal Adverse Effects
   a. Effects of NSAIDs on renal function
     i. Sodium retention
       1. Increased blood volume
       2. Important in patients with borderline CHF
     ii. Changes in tubular function

   iii. Papillary necrosis
   iv. Acute tubular necrosis
   v. Hyperkalemia
   vi. Hyponatremia
   vii. Interstitial nephritis
   viii. Reversible renal failure due to
     1. Alterations in GFR
     2. Renal plasma flow
 b. Prostaglandins and prostacyclins
   i. Maintain intrarenal blood flow
     1. Vasodilates renal arteries
   ii. Maintain tubular transport of electrolytes and water
     1. Increase sodium loss
     2. Increase renin release
   iii. Little effect on the normal kidney with euvolemia
   iv. Maintains GFR and pressure in renal insufficiency or hypovolemia
 c. NSAID reversible impairment of GFR
   i. All NSAIDS have the potential except
     1. **Nonacetylated salicylates**
     2. **Poor prostaglandin inhibitors**
   ii. Occurs more frequently in people with
     1. CHF
     2. Established renal disease with altered intrarenal plasma flow
      a. Hypertension
      b. Diabetes
      c. Artherosclerosis
     3. Induced hypovolemia
      a. Salt depletion
      b. Significant hypoalbuminemia
     4. Triamterene-containing diuretics
      a. Increase plasma renin levels
      b. Together with NSAIDs may develop acute renal failure
 d. NSAID-induced interstitial nephritis
   i. Typically manifests as nephrotic syndrome
     1. Edema or anasarca
     2. Proteinuria
     3. Hematuria
     4. Pyuria
   ii. **Absent** stigmata of drug-induced allergic nephritis
     1. Eosinophilia
     2. Eosinophiluria
     3. Fever
   iii. Histology
     1. Interstitial infiltrates of mononuclear cells
     2. Relative sparing of the glomeruli

  iv. Associated with the following NSAIDs

   1. Phenylpropionic acid derivatives

    a. Fenoprofen (acute allergic interstitial nephritis)

    b. Naproxen

    c. Tolmetin

   2. Indoleacetic acid derivative

    a. Indomethacin

   3. A.P.C. compounds (ASA, phenacetin, and caffeine)

 e. NSAID-induced acute tubular necrosis

  i. Associated with phenylbutazone

 f. NSAID-induced hyperkalemia

  i. NSAIDs decrease renin release

   1. Produces a state of hyporeninemic hypoaldosteronism

   2. May be amplified in patients taking potassium-sparing diuretics

 g. NSAID-induced salt retention with peripheral edema

  i. Inhibition of intrarenal prostaglandin production

   1. Decreases renal medullary blood flow

  ii. Increased tubular reabsorption of sodium chloride

  iii. Direct tubular effects

  iv. 2–3% frequency with standard doses of both nonselective NSAIDs and the COX-2 specific inhibitors

 h. NSAID-induced hyponatremia

  i. Increased effect of antidiuretic hormone

   1. Reduces excretion of free water

  ii. May be potentiated by thiazide diuretics

 i. NSAID-induced hypertension

  i. All NSAIDs associated with increases in mean blood pressure except nonacetylated salicylates

  ii. Check hypertensive patients routinely for changes in blood pressure

  iii. Inhibit the clinical effects of hypertensive medications

   1. ACE inhibitors

   2. Beta-blockers

   3. Diuretics

 j. NSAID-induced acute renal failure

  i. Prostaglandin mediated

  ii. Both COX-1 and COX-2 involved

   1. COX-1

    a. More dominant role in the maintenance of GFR

   2. COX-2

    a. Found in the glomeruli and renal vasculature

    b. Dominant contributor to salt and water homeostasis

    c. Selective COX-2 inhibitors similar effects on blood pressure and induction of edema

  iii. Monitor all patients at risk for renal complication carefully

      iv. No patient with a creatinine clearance of <30 cc/min should be treated with an NSAID or a COX-2 specific inhibitor

      v. Sulindac

         1. Described as having less renal effects

         2. "Prodrug" activated to sulindac sulfide

            a. The active compound

         3. The kidney reverts the active compound back to sulindac

         4. Behaves as other NSAIDs in patients with renal compromise

            a. Offers no advantage

            b. Should not be used preferentially

17. Other Adverse Effects

   a. Nonspecific reactions associated with NSAIDs

      i. Skin rash

      ii. Photosensitivity

   b. Phenylpropionic acid derivatives

      i. Induce aseptic meningitis

         1. Especially in SLE

         2. Underlying mechanism of action unknown

      ii. Associated with a reversible toxic amblyopia

   c. Auditory complications

      i. Tinnitus

         1. A common problem with higher doses of salicylates

         2. Associated with a wide range of plasma levels

         3. Indicates the plasma level is above therapeutic range

         4. Used as a "poor man's" way of monitoring salicylate levels

         5. Mechanism unknown

         6. Reversible with discontinuation of medication

      ii. Hearing deficit

         1. Seen with higher levels of salicylates in children and the elderly

         2. Reversible with decreasing the dose

   d. CNS side effects

      i. Phenylpropionic acid derivatives (particularly ibuprofen)

         1. Aseptic meningitis

            a. Especially in patients with SLE

      ii. Psychosis

      iii. Indomethacin (to a lesser extent tolmetin)

         1. Cognitive dysfunction

            a. More common in elderly patients

         2. Headaches

            a. Probenecid may be co-administered to reduce the dose of indomethacin by half

            b. Works as a uricosuric and renal tubular blocking agent

            c. Increases the mean plasma elimination half-life

            d. May also interfere with indomethacin's passage through the blood–brain barrier

        3. Dizziness
        4. Loss of concentration
        5. Depersonalization
        6. Tremor
        7. Psychosis

e. Bone marrow failure
    i. Particularly with phenylbutazone and indomethacin
    ii. 4.2 adjusted odds ratio of neutropenia for patients treated with an NSAID (using Medicaid claims data)
        1. 3.5 OR excluding phenylbutazone or indomethacin
        2. Incidence of neutropenia quite small
    iii. Aplastic anemia reported with most NSAIDs
        1. Particularly phenylbutazone
    iv. Neutropenia and thrombocytopenia associated with most NSAIDs
    v. Hemolytic anemia particularly associated with
        1. Mefenamic acid
        2. Ibuprofen
        3. Naproxen
    vi. Pure red cell aplasia associated with
        1. Phenylbutazone
        2. Indomethacin
        3. Fenoprofen

f. ASA
    i. Associated with smaller babies and neonatal bruising
    ii. Prostaglandin inhibition may result in premature closure of the ductus arteriosus

g. Pulmonary adverse effects
    i. Pulmonary infiltrates with eosinophilia
        1. Presents with pneumonia-like symptoms
            a. SOB
            b. High fever
        2. Peripheral blood eosinopilia also noted
        3. Corticosteroids and discontinuance of the drug required to reverse the process

18. Drug-Drug Interactions (concomitant therapy with NSAIDs)
a. Warfarin
    i. Seen with nonselective NSAIDs (except the nonacetylated salicylates) and those that inhibit COX-1
    ii. Displaces warfarin from its albumin-binding sites
    iii. Increased risk for bleeding due to antiplatelet effects
    iv. PT may be prolonged
    v. Increased risk of bleeding from gastroduodenal ulcers
    vi. Less risk for a significant GI bleed when treated with COX-2-specific inhibitors

      vii. Phenylbutazone inhibits metabolism of warfarin
         1. Increases anti-coagulation effect
  b. Competitive binding effects
     i. Seen with other highly protein-bound drugs
        1. Antibiotics
           a. Aminoglycosides
              i. Seen with most NSAIDs
              ii. May increase aminoglycoside level
         2. Phenytoin
           a. NSAIDs displaces phenytoin from plasma protein
              i. Reduces total concentration for the same active concentration
           b. Phenylbutazone inhibits metabolism
              i. Increasing plasma concentration and risk of toxicity
  c. Lithium
     i. NSAIDs inhibit renal excretion
     ii. Increases plasma lithium level
     iii. Use NSAIDs with caution
  d. Cholestyramine
     i. An anion-exchange resin
        1. Binds NSAIDs in the gut
        2. Reduces the rate of NSAID absorption and bioavailability
     ii. Seen with naproxen
  e. Sulfonylurea
     i. Interaction with two major NSAIDs
        1. Phenylbutazone
           a. Inhibits sulfonylurea metabolism
           b. Increases risk of hypoglycemia
        2. High-dose salicylate
           a. Potentiates hypoglycemia by different mechanism
  f. Beta-blocker
     i. Interaction with all prostaglandin-inhibiting NSAIDs
     ii. Blunts hypotensive effect
        1. No negative chronotropic or inotropic effect
  g. Hydralazine
     i. Interaction with all prostaglandin-inhibiting NSAIDs
     ii. Loss of hypotensive effects
  h. Diuretics
     i. Interaction with all prostaglandin-inhibiting NSAIDs
     ii. Furosemide
        1. Loss of natriuretic, diuretic, hypotensive effects
     iii. Spironolactone
        1. Loss of natriuretic effect
     iv. Thiazide
        1. Loss of hypotensive effect
           a. No natriuretic or diuretic effects

    i. Digoxin
       i. Interaction with most NSAIDs
      ii. May increase digoxin levels
    j. Methotrexate
       i. Interaction with most NSAIDs
      ii. May increase MTX plasma concentration
    k. Sodium valproate
       i. Interaction with ASA
      ii. Inhibits valproate metabolism
         1. Increases plasma valproate concentration
    l. Antacids
       i. Interaction with indomethacin, salicylates, and other NSAIDs
         1. Aluminum-containing antacids
           a. Reduces rate and extent of absorption
         2. Sodium bicarbonate
           a. Increases rate and extent of absorption
   m. Cimetidine
       i. Interaction with piroxicam
         1. Increases plasma concentrations and half-life
    n. Probenecid
       i. Interaction with most NSAIDs
      ii. Reduces metabolism and renal clearance of NSAIDs
    o. Caffeine
       i. Interaction with ASA
      ii. Increases rate of absorption of ASA
    p. Metoclopramide
       i. Interaction with ASA and probably others
      ii. Increases rate and extent of absorption in patients with migraines
19. Other Rarer Adverse Reactions
    a. Febrile reactions
       i. Ibuprofen
    b. Drug-induced lupus
       i. Phenylbutazone
    c. Vasculitis
       i. Indomethacin
      ii. Naproxen
    d. Pericarditis, myocarditis
       i. Phenylbutazone
    e. Stomatitis
       i. Most NSAIDs
    f. Cutaneous effects (photosensitivity, erythema multiform, urticaria, toxic epidermal necrolysis)
       i. Most NSAIDs
      ii. Especially piroxicam
    g. Porphyria cutanea tarda
       i. Naproxen

    h. Sulfa allergy
       i. Celecoxib
20. Other Benefits of NSAIDs
    a. Decreases heterotopic bone formation after joint replacement
       i. Pretreatment with NSAIDs
    b. Treatment of familial adenomatous polyposis
       i. Celecoxib approved at 400 mg BID
    c. Treatment of colon cancer and Alzheimer's

Corticosteroids

19

1. The dramatic anti-inflammatory effects of corticosteroids first described in RA
   a. Discovered in 1949
   b. Drs. Hench and Kendall won the Nobel Prize in 1950
2. Long-term supraphysiologic therapy results in devastating side effects
3. Short-term efficacy of corticosteroids remains unsurpassed
4. Corticosteroid Physiology
   a. Corticosteroid hormones are essential for normal development and homeostasis maintenance during basal and stress conditions
   b. A product of
      i. The hypothalamic-pituitary-adrenal (HPA) axis
      ii. The central stress response system
   c. Basal conditions
      i. Levels fluctuate with a circadian rhythm that follows the light–dark cycle
   d. Stressful conditions
      i. Central stress response system is stimulated
      ii. "Fight or flight"
      iii. Enhances the production and secretion of adrenal corticosteroids
   e. Inflammatory stress
      i. Associated with production of cytokines such as
         1. TNF-α
         2. IL-1
         3. IL-6
      ii. Normally proinflammatory cytokines stimulate the HPA axis
         1. Feedback suppression of cytokine production and the inflammatory response
      iii. Abnormal low level corticosteroid production facilitates unchecked amplification of inflammation and tissue injury
      iv. Two possible pathogenetic mechanisms in rheumatic diseases
         1. Defects in the bi-directional feedback loop
            a. Between CNS and peripheral inflammatory pathways
         2. Tissue resistance to the actions of corticosteroids

5. Cellular and Molecular Effects of Corticosteroids
    a. Corticosteroid effects mediated by two types of receptors
        i. Type I
            1. Mineralocorticoid receptors
            2. Located mainly in the kidneys and various parts of the CNS
            3. Critical in the basal regulation of circadian adrenocortical activity
        ii. Type II
            1. Corticosteroid receptors
            2. Present in virtually all cells of the body
            3. Produced in two alternatively spliced forms
                a. Alpha
                    i. Mediates classic anti-inflammatory activities
                b. Beta
                    i. Inhibits corticosteroid action
                    ii. Competes with the alpha form
                c. Ratio of alpha to beta Type II receptors hypothesized to modulate cellular actions
                    i. Beta forms confer "resistance" to corticosteroid action if predominate
            4. Mediate the anti-inflammatory and metabolic actions
            5. In the absence of corticosteroid ligands
                a. These receptors exist in association with several classes of heat shock proteins (HSP)
                    i. HSP 90
                    ii. HSP 70
                    iii. HSP 56
                    iv. HSP 26
            6. Upon corticosteroid binding
                a. Heat shock proteins disassociate from the receptor
                b. Corticosteroid-receptor complex migrates to the nucleus
                c. Regulates gene expression and other cellular activities
    b. Major intracellular activities of the corticosteroid-receptor complex
        i. Competitive**inactivation** of c-fos:c-jun complexes
        ii. Inhibition of NF-κB activity
            1. Mediated through enhanced**induction** of the inhibitory factor IκB
        iii. Alter gene transcription
            1. Hinders nearby gene promoter-enhancer sequences that reside near corticosteroid receptor binding sites
        iv. Enhances production of cyclic AMP
        v. Destabilizes several classes of messenger RNA
            1. Including cytokine mRNA
        vi. Contributes to apoptosis of mature and activated lymphocytes
    c. Corticosteroid **suppression** at the cellular level
        i. Inflammatory and immune mechanisms at virtually all levels
        ii. NF-κB
            1. Due to transcriptional activation of the inhibitor IκB

      iii. AP-1 and NFAT activity
         1. Mediated through glucocorticoid (GC) binding to an intracellular GC receptor in the cytoplasm
         2. In turn promotes nuclear translocation and binding to GC response elements in gene promoters
         3. Ap-1 activity inhibited through physical interference of GC receptor with Ap-1 binding
      iv. Phospholipase A2
         1. Through induction of lipocortin-1
         2. Results in decreased arachidonic acid synthesis
         3. Corresponding decrease in prostaglandin and leukotriene production
      v. Metalloproteinases production
      vi. COX-2
      vii. Neutrophil and monocyte migration to inflamed sites
     viii. Endothelial cell functions
         1. Including expression of adhesion molecules
            a. ICAM-1i
      ix. Neutrophil and macrophage phagocytosis and enzyme release
      x. Antigen processing and presentation to lymphocytes
      xi. T-cell proliferation and IL-2 synthesis and secretion
      xii. Fibroblast proliferation
     xiii. DNA and collagen synthesis
     xiv. Osteoblast growth and osteoprotegerin production
      xv. Cellular activation and differentiation
     xvi. Proinflammatory cytokines through destabilization of mRNA
         1. TNF-α
         2. IL-1
         3. IL-12
         4. INF-γ
    xvii. Related mediators
         1. Prostaglandin E2
         2. Leukotrienes
  d. Corticosteroid cellular suppression
      i. Immature T cells
      ii. Activated T-effector lymphocytes
      iii. Natural killer cells
      iv. Immature B cells
         1. Minimal suppression on mature antibody producing B cells
  e. Corticosteroid suppression of Type I responses
      i. *Suppresses* macrophage activation and cellular immunity or Type 1 responses
         1. Diseases such as RA
         2. Respond dramatically to corticosteroid therapy
      ii. **Biases** immune responses toward humoral immunity or Type 2 responses
         1. Diseases such as lupus glomerulonephritis
         2. Require supraphysiologic levels of corticosteroid for disease suppression

      iii. **Minimal** suppression on the production of anti-inflammatory cytokines
        1. IL-4
        2. IL-10
   f. Corticosteroid suppressive effects on hormonal synthesis and release
      i. Hypothalamus
        1. Corticotropin
        2. Gonadotropin-releasing hormones
      ii. Pituitary
        1. Adrenocorticotropic
        2. Thyroid-stimulating
        3. Growth hormone
      iii. Adrenal gland
        1. Cortisol
        2. Androgens
      iv. Gonads
        1. Estrogen
        2. Testosterone
        3. Decreases hormonal action on target cells
  g. Other molecular and cellular effects of corticosteroids
      i. Enhance B-adrenergic receptor expression
      ii. Enhance cyclic AMP production
      iii. Alter adipocyte activity
        1. Changes in adipose tissue distribution
      iv. Promote type IIb skeletal muscle fiber atrophy
      v. Increase muscle catabolic activity
      vi. Alter neuronal activities in many parts of the brain
        1. Neuropeptide and neurotransmitter
        2. Catecholamines
        3. Gamma-aminobutyric acid
        4. Prostaglandins
      vii. Enhance activity of detoxifying enzymes
      viii. Promote insulin resistance
      ix. Increase blood glucose and liver glycogen
  h. Other physiologic effects of corticosteroids
      i. Alterations in mood or behavior
        1. Enhance behavioral arousal and euphoria
        2. Emotional lability
        3. Insomnia
        4. Depression
        5. Increased appetite
      ii. Impaired wound healing
6. Corticosteroid Pharmacology
  a. 17-hydroxy-21 carbon steroid molecules
      i. The principal, naturally occurring form
        1. Cortisol (hydrocortisone)

      ii. The most widely used synthetic compounds
         1. Prednisone
         2. Prednisolone
         3. Methylprednisolone
         4. Dexamethasone
            a. One of the most potent synthetics
  b. Dose
      i. Potency roughly correlates with the duration of hypothalamic-pituitary axis suppression
      ii. Dosing from the least to most suppressive
         1. Intermittent oral
         2. Alternate day
         3. Single daily AM dose
         4. Intermittent IV pulse therapy
            a. Initial treatment of severe life-threatening disease
            b. No role in long term therapy
            c. As a second agent with a cytotoxic drug
         5. Multiple daily
      iii. Usually given orally in doses of 1–2 mg/kg/day in divided doses
         1. Divided doses
            a. Immunologic effects of prednisone typically last 8–12 h before dissipating
            b. Especially in the first 2–4 weeks
         2. Single daily doses
            a. Consolidate to single dose before starting a taper
      iv. Low dose
         1. <15 mg/day
      v. Medium dose
         1. 15 to <40 mg/day
      vi. High dose
         1. >40 mg/day
  c. Biological equivalency (glucocorticoid potency)
      i. Correlates with the duration of biologic activity
      ii. Determined with cortisol as a reference value of 1
  d. Biological half-life (three major groups)
      i. Short-acting (half-life 12 h)
         1. Hydrocortisone
            a. Glucocorticoid potency = 1
            b. Mineralocorticoid potency = 1
         2. Cortisone
            a. Glucocorticoid potency = 0.8
            b. Mineralocorticoid potency = 0.8
      ii. Intermediate-acting (half-life 12–36 h)
         1. Prednisone
            a. Glucocorticoid potency = 4
            b. Mineralocorticoid potency = 0.25

     2. Prednisolone
       a. Glucocorticoid potency = 4
       b. Mineralocorticoid potency = 0.25
     3. Methylprednisolone
       a. Glucocorticoid potency = 5
       b. Mineralocorticoid potency = insignificant in usual doses
     4. Triamcinolone
       a. Glucocorticoid potency = 5
       b. Mineralocorticoid potency = insignificant in usual doses
   iii. Long-acting (half-life 48 h)
     1. Paramethasone
       a. Glucocorticoid potency = 10
       b. Mineralocorticoid potency = insignificant in usual doses
     2. Betamethasone
       a. Glucocorticoid potency = 25
       b. Mineralocorticoid potency = insignificant in usual doses
     3. Dexamethasone
       a. Glucocorticoid potency = 30–40
       b. Mineralocorticoid potency = insignificant in usual doses
e. Biologic effects influenced by
   i. Mineralocorticoid effects
     1. Determines the amount of sodium retention
     2. Insignificant in usual doses of
       a. Methylprednisolone
       b. Triamcinolone
       c. Paramethasone
       d. Betamethasone
       e. Dexamethasone
     3. Potency expressed in milligrams
       a. Comparisons to cortisol reference value of 1
  ii. Scheduling
 iii. Route of administration
  iv. Formulation of the preparation
   v. Patient
  vi. Tissue
 vii. Cortisol-binding globulin (transcortin)
     1. Influences corticosteroid availability
     2. Found in
       a. Plasma
       b. Various tissues at different levels
viii. Disease
     1. Steroid responsive rheumatic diseases
     2. Selective complications of connective tissue diseases
       a. RA
       b. SLE

        c. PM/DM

        d. Sjogren's

     3. Vasculitis disorders (initial treatment)

     4. Polymyalgia rheumatica

7. Corticosteroid Therapy

  a. Dosing regimens

     i. Non standardized

     ii. Usually individualized

     iii. Maximize therapeutic effects

     iv. Minimize side effects

  b. High dose schedules

     i. Used when urgent control of the disease process is required

     ii. High-dose IV bolus treatment

        1. 1,000 mg methylprednisolone daily for 3 days

        2. Treatment of acute glomerulonephritis in SLE

     iii. Produces sustained clinical effects for weeks or even months

     iv. Profound effects on lymphocyte function and number

  c. Daily or alternate-day high-dose oral treatment

     i. 60 mg of prednisone daily for up to 1 month

        1. Followed by tapering to the lowest possible dose that maintains disease control

        2. A more rapid taper achieved with a steroid sparing drug

        3. Minimizes consequences of prolonged therapy

     ii. For severe but less threatening disease

        1. Thrombocytopenia

        2. Pleurisy in SLE

  d. Intermittent low oral doses

     i. In the physiologic range

     ii. <7 mg of prednisone daily on an as needed basis

     iii. Used for symptomatic control in RA

     iv. Unlikely to see rapid development of side effects

     v. Gives control over drug withdrawal

  e. Alternate day therapies

     i. Preferred to minimize side effects

     ii. Many conditions cannot tolerate alternate-day schedules (RA)

  f. Local injections or topical therapy

     i. Target the area specifically involved

     ii. Intrasynovial therapy

     iii. Needle injections into joint, bursa, or tendon sheath

     iv. Toxicity minimized

     v. Formulations available for these indications

        1. Triamcinolone acetonide

        2. Hexacetonide

  g. Parental

     i. Intramuscular

     ii. Intravenous

8. Side Effects of Corticosteroid Therapy
   a. Likelihood of developing side effects depends on
      i. The type of corticosteroid
      ii. Dose
      iii. Duration of exposure
      iv. Host, tissue, and cell variables
   b. Therapy that supplements an endogenous deficiency
      i. Less likely to produce side effects
   c. Therapy that exceeds physiologic need
      i. Produces a syndrome that resembles Cushing syndrome
         1. Truncal obesity
         2. Moon facies
         3. Supraclavicular fat deposition
         4. Posterior cervical fat deposition (buffalo hump)
         5. Mediastinal widening (lipomatosis)
         6. Weight gain
      ii. Suppresses adrenal production of corticosteroids and androgens
   d. Adverse consequences of corticosteroid therapy
      i. Glucose intolerance
         1. Uncommon
         2. Diabetic ketoacidosis
         3. Hyperosmolar, nonketotic diabetic coma
      ii. Growth suppression
         1. Less if dose $\leq$ 0.5 mg/kg
      iii. Acne
      iv. Osteonecrosis
      v. Cataract formation
         1. Even at prednisone 5 mg/day
         2. Posterior subcapsular cataracts
      vi. Skin disorders
         1. Bruising
         2. Striae
         3. Delayed wound repair
      vii. Peptic ulcer disease
         1. Doses > 10 mg/day with NSAIDs
         2. Usually gastric
         3. Gastric hemorrhage
      viii. Obesity
      ix. Infection
      x. Hirsutism or virilism
      xi. Abnormal menstruation or impotence
      xii. Depressed hormone levels
         1. TSH
         2. Testosterone
         3. FSH/LH

      xiii. Mental disturbance
          1. Doses ≥ 30 mg/day
          2. Uncommon
          3. Can see psychosis
      xiv. Muscle weakness
          1. Doses > 10–20 mg/day
       xv. Osteoporosis
          1. Doses ≥ 5–7.5 mg/day
          2. Uncommon
          3. Can see spontaneous fractures
      xvi. Hyperlipoproteinemia
     xvii. Atherosclerosis
    xviii. Suppressed delayed-type hypersensitivity reactions
      xix. Negative nitrogen balance
          1. Uncommon
          2. Can see metabolic alkalosis
       xx. Benign intracranial hypertension (pseudotumor cerebri)
  e. Osteoporosis
       i. All corticosteroid preparations inhibit bone formation
          1. More often at doses ≥ 5–7.5 mg/day
      ii. Vertebral compression fractures
          1. A frequent and devastating complication
     iii. Likelihood linked to maximum dose and cumulative duration
          1. Anticipate with any extended period of therapy
     iv. High risk patients
          1. Men
          2. Postmenopausal women
          3. A disease process which itself causes bone loss (RA)
      v. Mechanisms by which corticosteroids induce osteoporosis
          1. Inhibits ovarian and testicular sex steroid hormones
          2. Inhibits intestinal calcium absorption
            a. Secondary hyperparathyroidism
            b. Leads to osteoclast activation and inhibition
      vi. Therapeutic and preventive measures
          1. Adequate intake of calcium (1,500 mg/day) and vitamin D (400–800 IU/day)
          2. Estrogen replacement for postmenopausal women
          3. Androgen replacement therapy for men
          4. Bisphosphonate therapy in high-risk patients
          5. Education in the standards of care
            a. Both patients and health-care professionals
          6. Bone mineral densitometry
            a. Assess risk for osteoporosis-related problems
  f. Infections
       i. Laboratory findings

           1. Neutrophilia

           2. Monocytopenia

           3. Lymphopenia

    ii. Susceptible conditions

           1. Corticosteroid deficiency

              a. Leads to an unrestrained inflammatory response

              b. Severe, even life-threatening tissue injury

           2. Corticosteroid excess

              a. Impaired host defense

              b. Increased incidence and severity of infections

   iii. Likelihood of developing infection depends on

           1. Maximum dose

              a. Doses ≥ 0.3 mg/kg

              b. Prednisone 2–10 mg/day

                 i. Rarely associated with infectious complications

              c. Prednisone 20–60 mg/day

                 i. Pronounced suppressive effects on host defense mechanisms

               ii. Progressive increase in infection risk after 14 days of treatment

           2. Cumulative duration of therapy

              a. Cumulative doses greater than 700 mg

                 i. Progressive increased risk of infection

    iv. Organisms that pose greatest risk

           1. Facultative intracellular microbes

              a. Mycobacteria

              b. Pneumocystis carinii

              c. Fungi

           2. Severe cases of acute pyogenic infections

           3. Herpes virus

              a. Viral infections in general **NOT** a major problem

    v. High dose corticosteroids mask symptoms of infectious disease

           1. Abscess formation

           2. Bowel perforation

           3. High degree of suspicious required to make the diagnosis

    vi. Chronic infections

           1. Not apparent and progress rapidly on corticosteroid therapy

           2. Obtain a baseline

              a. CXR

              b. Tuberculin skin test

                 i. Suppression of the cellular response within 2 weeks of continuous corticosteroid therapy

               ii. Negative tuberculin test

                    1. Not totally reliable after starting corticosteroid therapy

                    2. Even with a positive control

  g. Adrenal Insufficiency

    i. Exogenous corticosteroids suppress endogenous HPA axis

            1. Produces secondary adrenal deficiency
              a. The most common cause
              b. Results from suppression of ACTH
            2. Adrenal cortex atrophies in 1 week without ACTH

         ii. Short course therapy
            1. Suppression can occur with as little as 5 days of prednisone at 20–30 mg/day
            2. HPA axis function returns rapidly after stopping

       iii. Prolonged periods of treatment (weeks to months)
            1. More than 20 mg of prednisone per day for 1 month
            2. Greater than 3–5 mg daily for more than a year
            3. HPA axis function requires up to 12 months to return
              a. 6–8 months average
            4. Adrenal responsiveness to ACTH is the last limb to recover
            5. If stressed unable to respond with the usual cortisol output
              a. Up to 200–300 mg/day

       iv. Patients at increased risk for acute adrenal insufficiency
            1. Corticosteroid taper
            2. Acute stress
              a. General anesthesia
              b. Surgery
              c. Trauma
              d. Acute infections

       v. Patients with suspected adrenal insufficiency
            1. Provide supplemental corticosteroid therapy
              a. Mimics the normal cortisol response
            2. Obtain an ACTH (Cortrosyn) stimulation test
              a. Give 0.25 mg IM
              b. Measure baseline and 60 min plasma cortisol
              c. Normal response
                i. Double baseline cortisol
                ii. 60 min level > 18 (g/dl)

       vi. Morning corticosteroid therapy
            1. Minimizes the risk of HPA axis suppression
            2. Taken daily before 10:00 a.m.
            3. Natural cortisol secretion has a circadian rhythm
              a. Peak levels in the morning
            4. Less suppressive effects on the release of cortisol-releasing factor

   h. Rare adverse side effects
      i. Sudden death
            1. Rapid administration of high-dose pulse therapy
      ii. Cardiac valvular lesions
            1. Patients with SLE
      iii. CHF
            1. Predisposed patients

      iv. Panniculitis
          1. Follows withdrawal
       v. Pancreatitis
      vi. Convulsions
     vii. Epidural lipomatosis
    viii. Exophthalmos
      ix. Allergic reaction
          1. Urticaria
          2. Angioedema
  i. Establish a clinical baseline before instituting therapy
       i. Infections
          1. Baseline CXR
          2. TB skin test
      ii. Glucose intolerance
          1. Baseline fasting glucose
          2. Periodic glucose monitoring
             a. For longer courses of therapy
     iii. Gastrointestinal erosive disease
          1. Baseline stool guaiac test
          2. CBC with mean cell volume
      iv. Cardiovascular disease and hypertension
          1. Aggravated by corticosteroid medications
          2. Baseline physical exam
             a. Blood pressure determination
             b. Presence of peripheral edema
               3. Periodic reevaluation
       v. Mental disturbance
          1. Baseline MiniMental status examination
          2. Especially with a history of mental disorders
  j. Corticosteroid withdrawal syndromes
       i. Classically presents in Addisonian crisis
          1. Fever
          2. Nausea and vomiting
          3. Hypotension
          4. Hypoglycemia
          5. Hyperkalemia
          6. Hyponatremia
      ii. Develop an exacerbation of the underlying inflammatory disease
     iii. Withdrawal symptom complex
          1. Diffuse muscle and joint pain
          2. Weight loss
          3. Fever
          4. Headache
          5. Changes in plasma cortisol levels
             a. Frequently higher than normal
             b. Do not correlate with symptoms

      iv. Therapeutic approach
         1. Slow careful taper over a period of weeks to months
         2. For doses greater than 40 mg/day
            a. Taper at a rate of about 10 mg/week
         3. For doses between 20 and 40 mg/day
            a. Taper at a rate of about 5 mg/week
         4. Below 20 mg/day and especially less than 5 mg/day
            a. Withdrawal symptoms are common
            b. Dose changes within the normal physiologic range
               i. rapid reduction from 5 to 2.5 mg/day represents a 50% reduction
               ii. Severe withdrawal symptoms
         5. Reduction management
            a. Patient-dictated schedule
               i. Close follow-up
            b. Alternate-day schedule
               i. First step before reducing the average daily dose
               ii. Works well in SLE
              iii. Rarely tolerated in RA
                   1. Symptoms worsen on the "off day"
9. Glucocorticoid Drug Interactions
   a. Corticosteroid metabolism
      i. Hepatic cytochrome P450 enzymes
         1. Particularly CYP3A4
   b. Drugs that up-regulate CYP3A4 levels
      i. Reduce levels of corticosteroid and decrease effectiveness
      ii. Anticonvulsants
         1. Carbamazepine
         2. Phenobarbital
         3. Phenytoin
      iii. Rifampin
         1. Double the dose of corticosteroid to get the same immune modulating effect
      iv. Phenylbutazone and sulfinpyrazone
         1. No longer used or marketed
   c. Drugs that inhibit metabolism
      i. Increase corticosteroid effectiveness
      ii. Ketoconazole
      iii. Macrolide antibiotics
         1. Erythromycin
         2. Triacetyloleandomycin
10. Routine Measures for Patients on Corticosteroid Therapy
   a. Prescribe at the lowest possible dose
      i. Discontinue as soon as disease activity permits
   b. Encourage physical activities
      i. Avoid immobilization
      ii. Helps to prevent myopathy

    c. Implement fall/fracture prevention program
    d. Calcium supplements
        i. Minimum intake of 1,500 mg/day
    e. Vitamin D supplements
        i. Minimum of 400 IU/day
    f. Bisphosphonate therapy
        i. Implement if >7.5 mg/day for >3 months
    g. Patient education concerning adverse effects

Disease-Modifying Antirheumatic Drugs 20

1. Disease-Modifying Antirheumatic Drug (DMARD) Designations in RA
   a. A drug must change the course of the disease for at least 1 year
   b. Change evidenced by one of the following
      i. Sustained improvement in physical function
      ii. Decreased inflammatory synovitis
      iii. Slowing or prevention of structural joint damage
   c. Drugs conventionally classified as DMARDs
      i. Hydroxychloroquine (HCQ)
      ii. Auranofin
      iii. Not shown to retard radiologic damage
   d. Biologic agents
      i. Considered as DMARDs
      ii. Favorable impact on structural damage
2. Therapeutic Onset of Action
   a. Delayed onset of action
      i. Distinguishes older DMARDs
      ii. 3–6 months to achieve a significant response
   b. Rapid onset of action
      i. Biologic agents
      ii. Loading dose strategies
         1. Leflunomide
      iii. Rapid dose escalation
         1. Methotrexate (MTX)
3. Therapeutic Principles
   a. Initiate DMARD therapy early and aggressively
      i. At the time of diagnosis
      ii. With evidence of active disease
         1. Synovitis
         2. Morning stiffness

N.T. Colburn, *Review of Rheumatology*,
DOI 10.1007/978-1-84882-093-7_20, © Springer-Verlag London Limited 2012

        3. Bony erosions or deformities
          a. Develop within the first 3–12 months of RA
        4. Extra-articular disease manifestations
    b. Target disease remission
      i. Often not achieved with standard DMARD monotherapy
      ii. Substitute or add another DMARD to improve clinical response
        1. With intolerable side effects
        2. With no evidence of clinical efficacy
4. DMARDs Available for RA Treatment
    a. IM gold (Solganal, Myochrysine)
    b. Hydroxychloroquine (Plaquenil)
    c. Sulfasalazine (Azulfidine)
    d. D-penicillamine (Cuprimine, Depen)
    e. Oral gold/auranofin (Ridaura)
    f. Methotrexate (Rheumatrex)
    g. Leflunomide (Arava)
    h. Azathioprine (Imuran)
    i. Cyclosporine (Sandimmune, Neoral)
    j. Minocycline (Minocin, Dynacin)
    k. Etanercept
    l. Infliximab
    m. Prednisone
5. Methotrexate
    a. Commonly employed as the initial DMARD
    b. For the treatment of moderate to severe RA
    c. Considered the most effective
    d. Blocks DNA synthesis
      i. A folate analogue
      ii. Inhibits dihydrofolate reductase
      iii. Reduces tetrahydrofolate formation
        1. A single-carbon donor
        2. Essential for purine and pyrimidine synthesis
      iv. Decreases metabolically active reduced folates
      v. Leads to a suppression of lymphocyte proliferation
      vi. Not the major mechanism of action at low doses used in RA
    e. Anti-inflammatory effects
      i. Forms polyglutamates inside the cell
      ii. Inhibits the enzyme 5-aminoimidazole-4-carboxamidoribonucleotide (AICAR) transformylase
      iii. Increases the intracellular concentration of the substrate AICAR
      iv. Stimulates the release of adenosine
        1. Binds specific receptors on the surface of
          a. Lymphocytes
          b. Monocytes
          c. Neutrophils
            i. Potent inhibitor of neutrophil function
        2. Down-regulates inflammatory pathways

f. Other*inhibitory* mechanisms of action
   i. Neovascularization
   ii. Neutrophil adherence
   iii. IL-1 and IL-8 production by stimulated PBMCs
   iv. TNF production by stimulated peripheral T cells
g. Clinical efficacy and safety
   i. Firmly established by prospective, controlled trials
   ii. Long-term efficacy and tolerability
      1. Long-term benefits for up to 11 years
      2. Nearly 50% of patients remain on therapy for at least 5 years
   iii. Generally preferred over other DMARDS
      1. Acts relatively quickly
         a. Often within several weeks
      2. Suppresses disease activity in long-standing RA where other treatments have failed
      3. Combination therapy with methotrexate results in improved efficacy over methotrexate alone
         a. Without additive increase in side effects
   iv. Favorably impacts RA at early stages
      1. 2,000 NEJM study of RA of less than 3 years duration
         a. MTX associated with an ACR-20 response rate of 60%
         b. Not significantly different from the etanercept comparison group
      2. Retards the appearance of new erosions in involved joints
h. Side Effects
   i. Generally well tolerated
   ii. Dose related side effects
      1. Nausea and vomiting
      2. Anorexia
      3. Stomatitis
         a. Oral ulcers
      4. Bone-marrow suppression
         a. Leukopenia
         b. Thrombocytopenia
         c. Pancytopenia
         d. Megaloblastic anemia
   iii. Concurrent treatment with folic or folinic acid
      1. Lowers the frequency and severity of dose related side effects
   iv. Other side effects
      1. Fatigue
      2. Flu-like symptoms
      3. Headache
         a. Can worsen migraine headaches
      4. Photosensitivity
      5. Increased risk of infections
      6. B-cell lymphoma (rare)
         a. Some related to EBV
         b. May resolve if MTX stopped

     v.   Idiosyncratic toxicities
        1. Pneumonitis
          a. Stop MTX
          b. **DO NOT** rechallenge
          c. Rule out opportunistic infections
             i. *Pneumocystis carinii* pneumonia
        2. Hepatic fibrosis and cirrhosis
     vi.   Toxicities that require monitoring
        1. Myelosuppression
        2. Liver fibrosis
        3. Pneumonitis
     vii.   Obtain prior to starting MTX therapy
        1. CBC with platelets
        2. Hepatitis B and C serologies
        3. LFTs with AST, ALT, alkaline phosphatase
        4. Albumin
        5. Creatinine
        6. CXR dated within the past year
     viii.   Every 4–8 weeks
        1. CBC with platelets
        2. LFTs with AST, ALT, alkaline phosphatase
        3. Albumin
        4. Creatinine
 i. Pharmacology
     i. Major clearance by the kidney
        1. Contraindicated in the setting of significant renal insufficiency
          a. Serum creatinine levels > 2.0–2.5 mg/dl
     ii. Liver metabolism
        1. Should not be given in the setting of significant liver disease
        2. Use with caution in patients with hepatitis B or C infections
        3. Alcohol consumption increases risk for liver damage
          a. More than 2 drinks per week
        4. Avoid trimethoprim-sulfamethoxazole
          a. Decreases excretion
        5. Liver biopsy recommended in the following settings
          a. As a baseline with risk factors for cirrhosis
             i. Significant alcohol use
             ii. Positive hepatitis serology
             iii. Elevated liver transaminase levels
          b. During therapy if
             i. Persistently elevated (>3 months) AST or ALT
             ii. Albumin levels decrease
        6. **Routine** liver biopsy **not** recommended

    iii. Pulmonary
        1. MTX accumulates in pleural effusions
        2. Can cause neutropenia if reabsorbed
    iv. Dosing
        1. Initial starting dose
          a. Usually 7.5–10 mg/week
        2. Maintenance dose
          a. 7.5–25 mg/week
        3. Advance up to 25 mg/week
          a. For maximum clinical efficacy
          b. Limited by tolerability
        4. Routes of administration
          a. The most convenient
            i. Oral route
          b. The most predictable absorption
            i. Parenteral route
          c. Easiest and less painful
            i. SQ route
            ii. Bioavailability similar to IM
          d. Enhanced clinical efficacy
            i. After 20 mg no further absorption orally
            ii. Switch from oral to parenteral administration
            iii. Parenteral serum levels 30% higher than oral
        5. Folic acid
          a. 1 mg/day
          b. Should always be given with MTX
          c. Increase dose to 2–5 mg/day
            i. With symptoms of toxicity (mouth sores)
        6. Folinic acid
          a. 5 mg
          b. One dose 24 h after the weekly dose of MTX
          c. Helps mouth sores even if folic acid fails
    v. Contraindicated in pregnancy
        1. Use a reliable form of contraception at the child-bearing age
        2. Stop for 3 months in both males and females before conception
  j. Rheumatic conditions in which MTX is indicated
    i. RA and JRA
    ii. Psoriatic arthritis
    iii. Reactive arthritis (Reiter's syndrome)
    iv. Ankylosing spondylitis (peripheral arthritis)
    v. Polymyositis/dermatomyositis
    vi. Wegener's granulomatosus
    vii. Adult-onset Still's disease

       viii. SLE
        ix. Polymyalgia rheumatica/giant cell arteritis
         x. Sarcoidosis
       xi. Uveitis

6. Sulfasalazine (SSZ)
   a. Pharmacology
      i. Synthesized in 1942
     ii. Links an antibiotic (sulfapyridine) with an anti-inflammatory agent (5-aminosalicylic acid (5-ASA))
    iii. About 30% absorbed from the GI tract
    iv. About 70% degraded in the gut into
       1. Sulfapyridine
         a. The bulk of which is absorbed from the gut
       2. 5-ASA
         a. The majority of which is excreted in the feces
      v. Dosing
       1. Initial dose
         a. 500 mg BID
         b. Start at 500 mg
         c. Increase by 500 mg each week
       2. Maintenance dose
         a. 1–1.5 g BID
         b. Increase up to 3 g/day in divided doses
       3. 3 months of treatment
         a. Usually required to achieve maximum clinical effect
         b. A measurable result can be seen in 4 weeks
   b. Mechanism of action
      i. Suppresses various lymphocyte and leukocyte functions
     ii. Inhibits AICAR transformylase (like MTX)
       1. Results in extracellular adenosine release
    iii. Reduces the activation of NF-κB
       1. Decreases certain genes associated with inflammation
   c. Clinical efficacy and safety
      i. Effective for the treatment of early mild to moderate RA
       1. 24 week randomized, double-blind, placebo-controlled trial
         a. SSZ treatment with an ACR-20 response rate of 56% compared with 29% for placebo
         b. Less radiographic progression of joint damage than placebo
     ii. For many years the first and most commonly used DMARD in Europe
    iii. Generally well tolerated
    iv. Often combined with other DMARDs
     v. Does not increase the risk for infection
    vi. Should not be used in patients with
       1. Sulfa allergies
       2. Glucose 6-phosphate dehydrogenase deficiency

d. Side effects
   i. Low potential for toxicity
   ii. Most common
     1. Nausea and vomiting
       a. Titrate up slowly
       b. Take with meals
       c. Enteric-coated tablets
     2. Diarrhea
     3. Abdominal pain
     4. Dyspepsia
     5. Rash
       a. 1–5%
     6. Neutropenia
       a. 1–5%
       b. Severe agranulocytosis (rare)
   iii. Myelosuppression
     1. Requires monitoring
     2. Prior to starting SZS obtain
       a. CBC
       b. LFTs with ALT
       c. G6PD
     3. Every month during the first 3 months obtain
       a. CBC
       b. LFTs with ALT
       c. Creatinine (at the first month)
     4. Every 3 months obtain
       a. CBC
       b. LFTs with ALT
       c. Creatinine
   iv. Other side effects
     1. Headache and dizziness
     2. Azoospermia
       a. Reversible on stopping drug
     3. Pulmonary infiltrates with eosinophilia
     4. Hepatic enzyme elevation ± fever
     5. Adenopathy
     6. Rash
e. Rheumatic conditions in which SZS is indicated
   i. RA
   ii. Reactive arthritis (Reiter's syndrome)
   iii. Psoriatic arthritis
   iv. Ankylosing spondylitis (peripheral manifestations)
   v. Enteropathic arthritis
7. Antimalarials
  a. Hydroxychloroquine (HCQ), chloroquine, and quinacrine
   i. HCQ main antimalarial used in the USA

b. Pharmacology
   i. Absorbed efficiently from the GI tract
   ii. Extended serum half-lives
      1. Due to tissue depot effects
   iii. Dosing
      1. HCQ
         a. Usual doses 200–400 mg/day
         b. <6.5 mg/kg of ideal body weight
            i. Patients <66 in. in height should get 300 mg
            ii. Patients <60 in. in height should get 200 mg
         c. 6–12 months of therapy
            i. Generally required to achieve a clinical effect
      2. Chloroquine
         a. Usual dose 250 mg/day
         b. ≤3.5 mg/kg of ideal body weight
            i. Patients <66–70 in. in height should get less than 250 mg
      3. Quinacrine
         a. Usual dose 100–200 mg/day
      4. Decrease all doses further if there is renal or liver dysfunction
   iv. Drug interactions
      1. Cimetidine decreases the clearance of antimalarials
      2. Antimalarials antagonize
         a. Anticonvulsants
         b. Amiodarone
      3. Smoking induces hepatic cytochrome P-450 enzymes
         a. Results in accelerated metabolism of antimalarials
c. Mechanism of action
   i. Weak bases that concentrate principally within acidic cytoplasmic vesicles (lysosomes)
   ii. Raises intravesical pH
      1. Interferes with the processing of autoantigenic peptides
      2. Disrupts the normal assimilation of peptides with class II MHC molecules
   iii. Increase lipoprotein (LDL) receptors
      1. Helps to lower lipid levels
   iv. Decrease degradation of insulin
      1. Helps to prevent diabetes mellitus
   v. Inhibit platelet aggregation and adhesion
      1. Helps to prevent thrombosis
d. Clinical efficacy
   i. Antimalarials are the **least** toxic of all DMARDS
   ii. Can be safely combined with other DMARDs
   iii. Hydroxychloroquine
      1. Indicated primarily for the early treatment of mild to moderate RA or seronegative disease

2. Treatment superiority over placebo in a randomized, controlled trial involving 125 patients with mild disease of <5 years

e. Side effects
  i. Most common
    1. Nausea and vomiting
      a. Start at half dose
      b. Titrate up over 2–4 weeks
    2. Abdominal pain
    3. Headache and dizziness
  ii. Other less common side effects
    1. Myopathy
      a. Seen with high doses
      b. Seen with renal insufficiency
    2. Rash
      a. Hyperpigmentation of skin
        i. Gray-black with chloroquine
        ii. Yellow with quinacrine
      b. Bleaching of hair
    3. Blurred vision
    4. Aplastic anemia
      a. Rare
      b. Associated with quinacrine
      c. Especially if lichen planus rash develops
  iii. Retinal toxicity
    1. Seen mostly with therapy longer than 10 years
    2. Seen with doses exceeding 400 mg/day or >6.5 mg/kg/day
    3. Corneal deposits
      a. **Not** an indication to stop antimalarials
      b. Chloroquine causes more corneal deposits and retinopathy
        i. Binds more avidly to corneal and retinal pigmented epithelium than HCQ
    4. Retinopathy
      a. An **absolute** indication to stop therapy
      b. Very uncommon
      c. Less than 1–2% of those on antimalarials for more than 2 years
      d. Extremely rare if dosed according to ideal (lean) body weight
      e. Quinacrine does not cause retinopathy
        i. Add with HCQ or chloroquine without added retinal toxicity
      f. Loss of red light perception
        i. The first evidence of toxicity
        ii. Stop the antimalarial if detected
          1. There will be no loss of vision
      g. Decrease in visual acuity and/or macular pigmentary changes
        i. Progressive changes
        ii. Stop the antimalarial if detected
          1. May not stop further vision loss

      iv. Macular damage requires monitoring
        1. Obtain eye exam prior to starting an antimalarial
          a. For those >40 years
          b. For those with prior eye disease
        2. Obtain eye exam at 6 months
          a. After starting an antimalarial
          b. Every 6 months exams
            i. Patients on chloroquine
        3. Obtain eye exam every year
          a. Patients on hydroxychloroquine
        4. More frequent eye exams (every 3–6 months)
          a. Patients on higher than recommended doses
          b. Patients who have coexistent eye disease
          c. Patients who have renal or liver dysfunction
        5. Amsler grid
          a. An added inexpensive safety measure
          b. Instruct in its use
          c. Patients should use each day at home
          d. If the lines become blurry
            i. Patient should be examined immediately
    f. Rheumatic conditions in which antimalarials are indicated
      i. SLE
        1. Conditions especially responsive
          a. Skin manifestations
          b. Serositis
          c. Fatigue
          d. Joint disease
        2. Maintains remissions and prevents flares of disease
          a. Flares of lupus nephritis or CNS manifestations
          b. Maintain therapy while at high risk for flares
        3. Mild antithrombotic effect
          a. May decrease risk of thrombosis
          b. Especially those with antiphospholipid antibodies
      ii. RA
      iii. Palindromic rheumatism
      iv. Psoriatic arthritis (controversial)
        1. Use with caution
          a. Antimalarials may exacerbate psoriatic skin lesions
        2. Sjogren's syndrome
        3. Sarcoidosis
  8. Minocyline
    a. Principally for the treatment of mild RA
    b. Rational for use
      i. Based on an old (and still unsubstantiated) theory
      ii. Infection may be a triggering event for RA

c. Dosing
   i. Usual dose 100 mg BID
d. Mechanism of action
   i. Unknown
   ii. Biologic activities that confer antirheumatic properties
      1. Inhibits collagenase activity
      2. Inhibits the expression of nitric oxide synthase type 2
      3. Up-regulates the synthesis of IL-10
         a. An anti-inflammatory cytokine
e. Clinical efficacy and safety
   i. Several placebo-controlled trials showed decreased signs and symptoms in RA
f. Side Effects
   i. Dizziness
   ii. GI symptoms
      1. Dyspepsia
   iii. Skin rash
   iv. Skin hyperpigmentation
      1. Reverses after stopping the drug
      2. A problem with long-term drug use
   v. Headache
   vi. Rare associations
      1. SLE-like symptoms
      2. Autoimmune hepatitis
      3. pANCA positivity
   vii. Toxicities requiring monitoring
      1. None
9. Gold Compounds
   a. A steady decline in the use of gold compounds for the treatment of RA
   b. Pharmacology
      i. Two parenteral gold formulations
         1. Sodium malate
         2. Myochrysine
      ii. One oral gold compound
         1. Auranofin
            a. Limited use in clinical practice
            b. Lack of sustained clinical efficacy
            c. Slow onset of action
            d. Poor GI tolerability
            e. Limited use
               i. Early mild RA
               ii. Combination with other medications
      iii. Dosing
         1. Initiated with a test dose of 10 mg IM
         2. Followed by 25–50 mg 1 week later
            a. If no untoward reactions occur

3. Weekly injections
   a. If an excellent response obtained
      i. Give every 2 weeks for several months
   b. If remission maintained
      i. Give every 3–4 weeks
   c. Proceed until 1 g given
      i. 1 g given without improvement
         1. Therapy abandoned
         2. Lack of efficacy
4. IM gold continued as long as it works
   a. Less than 10% remain on therapy 5 years after initiation
      i. Side effects
      ii. Inefficacy

c. Clinical efficacy and safety
   i. Established for the treatment of RA with gold injections
   ii. Documented in several prospective clinical trials
   iii. Injectable gold and MTX therapy produce similar rates of clinical response
   iv. IM gold preparations result in short-term remissions
   v. Long-term studies show that erosions continue to develop

d. Side effects
   i. Gold has a higher incidence of toxicity than MTX
      1. Requires drug discontinuation
   ii. Oral gold has fewer side effects than gold injections
   iii. Oral gold's most notable side effects
      1. GI intolerance
      2. Diarrhea
         a. Usually does **not** cause colitis like IM gold
   iv. Other side effects
      1. Dermatitis, stomatitis, and/or pruritus
      2. Nitritoid reaction
         a. Flushing and hypotension
         b. Occurs 15–30 min after receiving gold
         c. Especially Myochrysine
      3. Proteinuria
         a. Due to membranous glomerulonephritis
      4. Hematologic reactions
         a. Eosinophilia
         b. Leukopenia
         c. Thrombocytopenia (ITP)
         d. Aplastic anemia
      5. GI intolerance
         a. IM gold can cause severe colitis
         b. Usually seen early in therapy

      v. Toxicities requiring monitoring
        1. Myelosuppression
        2. Proteinuria
     vi. Baseline evaluation obtain
        1. CBC with platelets
        2. Creatinine
        3. Urinalysis
    vii. Every 2 weeks for 20 weeks obtain
        1. CBC with platelets
        2. UA
   viii. After 20 weeks at each injection obtain
        1. CBC with platelets
        2. UA
  e. Rheumatic conditions in which gold is indicated
      i. RA and JRA
     ii. Psoriatic arthritis
    iii. Palindromic rheumatism
    iv. Reactive arthritis (Reiter's syndrome)

10. Leflunomide (LEF)
  a. A novel DMARD indicated for the treatment of moderate to severe RA
  b. Used in most of the disease where MTX is used with similar results
  c. Not FDA approved
  d. Mechanism of Action
      i. A77 1726 (the active metabolite) selectively inhibits dihydroorotate dehydrogenase
        1. A key enzyme in the de novo **pyrimidine** synthesis pathway
     ii. Leads to a decrease in de novo synthesis of uridine
        1. Resultant decrease in the synthesis of **pyrimidines**
        2. Uridine lowered below a critical level
          a. Tumor suppressor p53 activated
          b. Lymphocyte cell division arrested in the G1 stage
    iii. Lymphocytes *(B cells > T cells)* have low pools of pyrimidine nucleotides
        1. Increases drug sensitivity
  e. Pharmacology
      i. A pro-drug rapidly converted to its active metabolite, A77 1726
     ii. A77 1726
        1. Extensively bound to plasma proteins
        2. Long plasma half-life
          a. 15–18 days
          b. May take up to 2 years to reach undetectable plasma concentrations
    iii. Dosing
        1. Load with 100 mg po daily for 3 days

      2. To decrease side effects
        a. Load with 100 mg 1 day a week for 3 weeks
      3. 10–20 mg daily
        a. 20 mg every other day
          i. Works as well as 10 mg daily
          ii. Can save money
   iv. Drug Interactions
      1. Rifampin
        a. Increases serum level of active metabolite
        b. Increases toxicity
f. Clinical Efficacy and Safety
   i. Superior clinical efficacy to placebo
   ii. Benefits comparable to those of low dose MTX or SSZ
   iii. Retards radiologic progression of joint disease
   iv. Improves quality of life
   v. May be used in combination with MTX or in place of it
      1. When MTX is contraindicated or not tolerated
      2. Added in those with benefit from MTX but still with active disease
g. Side Effects
   i. Nausea, vomiting, and diarrhea
      1. Occurs in up to 17%
      2. Can lead to significant weight loss
   ii. Skin rash
      1. Occurs in up to 8%
      2. Allergic reaction usually at higher doses
   iii. Neutropenia > thrombocytopenia
   iv. Alopecia
   v. Mouth ulcers
   vi. Elevated serum transaminases
      1. Several reports of severe hepatotoxicity
        a. Liver failure
        b. Death
      2. Risk associations
        a. First months of therapy initiation
        b. Additional hepatotoxic medications (MTX)
        c. Reactivation of coexistent hepatitis B
   vii. Teratogenicity
      1. Contraindicated in pregnancy
   viii. Does **NOT** cause pneumonitis like MTX
   ix. Mild toxic reactions
      1. Resolves with halfing the maintenance dose
   x. Moderate or serious toxicity
      1. Drug should be discontinued
      2. May need to clear A77 1726 from the body

   xi. Drug elimination procedure
     1. Cholestyramine
      a. 8 mg 3 times daily for 11 days
      b. Or 4 g tid for 5 days
      c. Does not have to be consecutive days
      d. Rapidly reduces plasma concentrations
     2. Indications
      a. Cases of overdose
      b. Toxicity
      c. Desire for pregnancy (both males and females)
       i. Active metabolite plasma level must be less than 0.02 μg/ml on 2 occasions 14 days apart
   xii. Toxicities requiring monitoring
     1. Thrombocytopenia
     2. Hepatotoxicity
   xiii. Baseline evaluation obtain
     1. Hepatitis B and C serology
     2. Creatinine
     3. CBC
     4. LFTs including ALT and AST
   xiv. Every 4–8 weeks obtain
     1. CBC
     2. LFTs including ALT and AST
   xv. Precautions to decrease the chance of hepatotoxicity
     1. Limit use of other drugs with potential for additive liver toxicity
     2. Do not use in patients with hepatitis B or C
     3. Continue monthly monitoring of ALT and AST even after 6 months if
      a. Also on MTX
      b. Minor elevations of liver associated enzymes
     4. Recommendations with elevated liver enzymes
      a. Minor sporadic elevation [>1× and <2× ULN]
       i. Follow with repeat testing
      b. Elevated liver enzymes >2 times ULN or persistent minor elevations
       i. Dose reduction
      c. Elevated liver enzymes >3 times ULN
       i. Stop leflunomide
       ii. Consider drug elimination protocol
   xvi. Use with caution in patients with renal impairment
 11. Azathioprine (AZA)
  a. Used primarily for treating RA not been managed with other DMARDs
  b. Pharmacology
   i. Available formulations
    1. 50 mg tablets
    2. 100 mg/20 ml vial

    ii. Dosing
       1. 50–200 mg/day (1–2.5 mg/kg/day)
       2. Start 50 mg/day
       3. Increase by 25 mg every 1–2 weeks to desired dose
  c. Clinical efficacy and safety
    i. Evidence from small controlled studies
       1. More effective than placebo for RA therapy
    ii. Larger trials
       1. Less efficacy for RA therapy than MTX
       2. Similar efficacy as D-penicillamine and cyclosporine
    iii. After 4 years of follow-up
       1. Greater radiologic progression of joint damage than MTX
  d. Mechanism of action
    i. An orally administered purine analogue
    ii. A prodrug converted in the liver to 6-mercaptopurine (6-MP)
    iii. 6-MP
       1. Active metabolite
       2. Converted to thiopurine nucleotides
       3. Decreases de novo synthesis of purine nucleotides
       4. Thiopurine nucleotides incorporated into nucleic acid
       5. Results in both cytotoxicity and decreased cellular proliferation
    iv. Two enzymes necessary for 6-MP metabolism
       1. Xanthine oxidase
         a. Inhibition by allopurinol results in
           i. Accumulation of 6-MP
           ii. Increased toxicity
       2. Thiopurine methyl-transferase (TPMT)
         a. Inhibition by sulfasalazine results in
           i. Accumulation of 6-MP
           ii. Increased toxicity
         b. TPMT's activity affected by genetic polymorphism
           i. 90% have high activity
           ii. 10% have intermediate activity
             1. More frequent adverse side effects
               a. Particularly GI
           iii. 0.3% have low activity
             1. At risk for sudden onset of severe myelosuppression
               a. Occurs between 4 and 10 weeks after starting azathioprine
         iv. Blacks have less TPMT activity than whites
         v. Erythrocyte mean corpuscular volume
           1. Should increase by 5 cu μ
           2. A measure of maximum effect

  e. Side effects
     i. Patients with RA more frequently intolerant of AZA than MTX
       1. More than 25% stopped drug because of GI distress and other side effects
         a. Nausea, vomiting, and diarrhea
    ii. Other side effects
      1. Skin rash
      2. Hepatitis
      3. Pancreatitis
      4. Myelosuppression
      5. Increased risk for lymphoproliferative disorders
        a. Lymphoma increased 2–5 times
        b. More significant in organ transplant patients than RA
      6. Infections
        a. Herpes zoster
      7. Hypersensitivity syndrome
        a. Within first 2 weeks of use
    iii. Monitoring
      1. Within 2 weeks of a dose change
        a. CBC
        b. LFTs
        c. Creatinine
      2. Every 3 months
        a. CBC
        b. LFTs
    iv. Avoid in pregnancy
    v. Avoid live vaccines
  f. Drug–drug interactions
     i. With allopurinol
       1. Reduce azathioprine dose by 75%
       2. Or do not use at all
    ii. With sulfasalazine
      1. Increases risk of leukopenia
    iii. With Bactrim/Septra
      1. Increases risk of leukopenia
    iv. With warfarin
      1. May cause warfarin resistance
  g. Rheumatic conditions in which azathioprine is indicated
     i. RA
    ii. SLE
      1. Particularly lupus nephritis
    iii. Polymyositis/Dermatomyositis
    iv. Behcet's syndrome

       v. Other rheumatic diseases
          1. In an attempt to decrease corticosteroid dosages
12. Cyclosporine (CsA)
   a. Controlled trials of CsA in RA
      i. Reduced signs and symptoms
      ii. Slowed progression of joint erosions
   b. Mechanism of action
      i. A potent immunomodulating agent
         1. Originally developed as an antifungal agent
         2. Primary use to prevent organ transplant rejection
      ii. Inhibits IL-2 production and the proliferation of activated T-cells
         1. CsA binds to a cytoplasmic protein (immunophilin)
         2. Immunophilin in turn binds to calcineurin
         3. Blocks calcineurin's interaction with calmodulin
         4. Calmodulin necessary to dephosphorylate NFAT
            a. Nuclear factor of activated T-cells
            b. Transcription factor activates IL-2 and other T-cell activation genes
   c. Pharmacology
      i. Dosing
         1. Doses of 5–10 mg/kg/day
            a. Cause unacceptable renal toxicity
         2. Doses of 2.5–5 mg/kg/day
            a. Similar clinical benefits as the higher doses
            b. Lower incidence of renal toxicity
            c. Recommended starting dose
         3. Maximum dose
            a. 5 mg/kg/day
         4. Two doses commonly used in practice
            a. For patients less than 60 kg
               i. 75 mg twice daily
            b. For patients greater than 60 kg
               i. 100 mg twice daily
         5. If no clinical response after 3 months of treatment
            a. Check a serum-trough level
            b. Serum trough level below 100 mg/ml
               i. Not absorbing CsA adequately
      ii. Conventional oil-based CsA formulation
         1. Individual variability in pharmacokinetic properties
         2. Mean oral bioavailability is 30%
     iii. Microemulsion-based formulation (Neoral)
         1. Higher oral bioavailability
         2. More predictable absorption
         3. Dosed at lower levels than the oil-based
         4. Achieves the same blood concentration and therapeutic effect

    iv. Both formulations equivalent in clinical efficacy and toxicity
      1. In patients with RA
    v. When changing from the conventional to the microemulsion formulation
      1. A 1:1 dose-conversion recommended
      2. Serum trough level for those receiving >4 mg/kg/day
      3. If >100 mg/ml
        a. Initial dose of Neoral no higher than 4 mg/kg/day
    vi. Bioavailability affected by food
      1. High fat diet
        a. Increases CsA absorption
        b. Decreases metabolism
      2. Grapefruit juice and marmalade from Seville oranges
        a. Contains dihydroxy-bergamottin
        b. Inhibits cytochrome P450 enzyme in the small intestine
        c. Increases CsA absorption (levels)
        d. Decreases metabolism
d. Side effects
    i. Toxicity a limiting factor in the use of CsA
    ii. Nephrotoxicity
      1. Commonly leads to hypertension
      2. A rise in the serum creatinine
      3. Contraindicated in
        a. Uncontrolled hypertension
        b. Renal insufficiency
    iii. Other side effects
      1. GI distress
      2. Hypertrichosis
      3. Tremors and headaches
      4. Paresthesias
      5. Gum hyperplasia
      6. Increased risk of infection
      7. Hyperpigmentation
      8. Anorexia
      9. Hepatotoxicity (rare)
     10. Anemia
        a. CsA does**not** decrease white blood cell count
     11. Cancer risk
        a. Studies implicate cyclosporine in causing lymphomas
          i. EBV-associated lymphomas reportedly regress when CsA is stopped
        b. A retrospective case-controlled study (1998 A&R) found no increased risk of lymphoproliferative disease or skin cancer in RA
     12. Hyperuricemia and tophaceous gout

      a. Switch to tacrolimus
        i. Causes less hyperuricemia
        ii. Similar immunomodulatory properties
    13. Bone pain
      a. Treat with calcium channel blockers
      b. Lower CsA dose
  iv. Monitoring
    1. Baseline evaluation
      a. CBC
      b. UA
      c. Creatinine
    2. Every 2 weeks for the first 3 months
      a. Creatinine
      b. BP monitoring
    3. Every month
      a. Creatinine
        i. Increases 30% over baseline
          1. Stop CsA
          2. Decrease daily dose by 0.5–1.0 mg/kg
      b. Blood pressure (BP) monitoring
        i. If diastolic BP rises above 95 mm Hg
          1. Treat with medications that do not interfere with CsA metabolism
          2. Most recommended in order of use
            a. Dihydropyridine calcium antagonist
              i. Nifedipine
            b. Beta-blocker
            c. Diuretic
              i. Do not use potassium sparing agents
            d. ACE
            e. Amlodipine
      c. Magnesium
      d. CBC
      e. LFTs
      f. Potassium
      g. Lipid levels
  v. Drug-drug interactions
    1. Medications that increase cyclosporine levels
      a. Ketoconazole
      b. Calcium antagonists
        i. Diltiazem
        ii. Verapamil
      c. H2 antagonists
      d. Statins
      e. ACE inhibitors

      2. Medications that increase cyclosporine levels
        a. Anticonvulsants
        b. Antibiotics
          i. Rifampicin
          ii. Nafcillin
        c. St. John's wort
          i. Induces cytochrome P450 3A4
          ii. Induces duodenal P-glycoprotein
          iii. MDR-1 gene
          iv. Causes marked reduction in CsA levels with subsequent loss of transplant
      3. Concomitant use
        a. NSAIDs
          i. May contribute to renal insufficiency
          ii. Lower dose or stop with an increase in creatinine or BP
          iii. Renal toxicity more manageable in RA in protocols where CsA is used without NSAIDs
        b. Colchicine
          i. Causes neuromyopathy
          ii. CsA may reduce the clearance of colchicine
    e. Rheumatic diseases in which CsA is indicated
      i. Those refractory to other therapies
      ii. RA
        1. More effective when combined with MTX
        2. Studies in treating RA
          a. CsA more effective than placebo
          b. CsA has similar efficacy to that of other DMARDs
      iii. PM/DM
        1. Refractory disease
        2. Interstitial lung disease
      iv. Psoriatic arthritis
      v. SLE
        1. Membranous glomerulonephritis
      vi. Uveitis
13. D-Penicillamine
  a. An approved DMARD for the treatment of RA
  b. Rarely used today
    i. High incidence of toxicity
    ii. Conflicting data on prevention of joint erosions
    iii. Takes 6 or more months for a significant response
  c. Useful in RA patients who have extra-articular manifestations
    i. Vasculitis
    ii. Felty's syndrome
  d. Mechanism of action
    i. Unknown

e. Pharmacology
   i. Effective in RA in doses of 600–1,500 mg daily
   ii. Initial doses between 125 and 250 mg/day
   iii. Stepwise increase
      1. By 125–250 mg every 3 months
      2. To a maximum of 750–1,000 mg/day
   iv. Higher doses associated with a significant increase in side effects
      1. The dose can be reduced when the disease is controlled
      2. Most patients suffer an exacerbation if the drug is stopped
f. Side effects
   i. More than 25% discontinue the drug within the first 12 months because of side effects
   ii. Major adverse reactions
      1. Skin rashes and/or pruritus
      2. Anorexia, nausea, dysgeusia
      3. Proteinuria
         a. Membranous nephropathy
      4. Hematuria
      5. Myelosuppression
         a. Neutropenia
         b. Thrombocytopenia (ITP)
      6. Autoimmune phenomena
         a. Induction of ANA
         b. Drug-induced lupus
         c. Goodpasture's syndrome
         d. Myasthenia gravis
         e. Pemphigus
   iii. Adverse reactions occur more frequently in
      1. Patients who demonstrate slow sulfoxidation
      2. Patients with HLA-DR3 and B8 haplotypes
   iv. Monitoring
      1. Baseline evaluation
         a. CBC
         b. Creatinine
         c. UA
      2. Every 2 weeks until stable dosage
         a. CBC
         b. UA
      3. Every month
         a. CBC
         b. UA
g. Rheumatic diseases in which D-penicillamine is indicated
   i. RA
   ii. Systemic sclerosis
   iii. Wilson's disease

    iv. Cystinuria

    v. Primary biliary cirrhosis

14. Protein A Column

  a. Staphylococcal protein A column (Prosorba)

    i. Approved as a medical device for the treatment of moderate to severe RA

    ii. Used in conjunction with plasmapheresis

      1. Apheresis of 1,250 ml of blood through the column once a week for 12 weeks

  b. Indications

    i. Reserved for treatment of the most refractory RA cases

    ii. Also used to treat idiopathic thrombocytopenia purpura

  c. Mechanism of action

    i. Unclear

    ii. Uses staphylococcal protein A covalently bound to an inert silica matrix

    iii. Removes immunoglobulin G and IgG-containing circulating immune complexes

  d. Studies have shown

    i. 12 weekly treatments afford modest benefits over a sham treatment

  e. Costly

    i. Each column costs $1,000 plus the cost of the pheresis

  f. Precautions

    i. Patients on ACE inhibitors can experience severe hypotension

15. Combination DMARD therapy

  a. MTX is the anchor drug for most combination regimens

    i. Most clinical trials of combination therapy have included MTX

  b. Partial responders to MTX require further DMARD therapy

  c. "Step-up" approach

    i. Add 1 or 2 DMARDs to background MTX to improve clinical response

    ii. Studies support the clinical efficacy and safety of this strategy

      1. MTX and HCQ

      2. MTX, HCQ, and SSZ

      3. MTX and leflunomide

      4. MTX and azathioprine

      5. MTX and CsA

      6. MTX and etanercept

      7. MTX and infliximab

  d. Most commonly used DMARD combinations

    i. "Triple therapy"

      1. MTX+SSZ+HCQ

    ii. MTX+CsA

    iii. MTX+a TNF inhibitor

      1. Trials have shown superior efficacy both symptomatically and in decreasing radiographic damage versus MTX alone

        2. Can be cost-prohibitive
          a. Etanercept costs \$1,200–\$1,600 per month
          b. Inflixamab costs \$900–\$3,000 per month
        3. Long-term consequences of TNF-α suppression is unknown
     e. A 56-week clinical trial
       i. Compared 2 g/day SSZ alone to a regimen of SSZ 2 g/day, prednisolone 60 mg/day, and MTX 7.5 mg/week
       ii. Combination regimen had significantly less joint damage than those receiving SSZ alone

16. Dapsone
    a. Antimicrobial effects
      i. Used as treatment of leprosy
      ii. Used as *Pneumocystis carinii* prophylaxis in patients allergic to sulfa antibiotics
    b. Anti-inflammatory effects
      i. Dermatoses
        1. Particularly useful in those involving PMNs
      ii. Rheumatic diseases
        1. Skin vasculitis
          a. Leukocytoclastic
          b. Urticarial
          c. Erythema elevatum diutinum
          d. Cutaneous PAN
        2. Skin lesions of Behcet's disease
        3. SLE rashes
          a. Bullous disease
          b. Panniculitis
        4. Relapsing polychondritis
        5. Pyoderma gangrenosum
    c. Pharmacology
      i. A sulfone
      ii. Poorly water soluble
      iii. Poorly absorbed through the GI tract
      iv. Metabolized by the liver
      v. Dosing
        1. Range from 50 to 200 mg
        2. Average 100 mg a day
      vi. Drug interactions
        1. Probenecid
          a. Slows renal excretion
    d. Mechanism of action
      i. A free oxygen radial scavenger
      ii. Impairs the myeloperoxidase system
    e. Side effects
      i. Hemolysis and methemoglobinemia

          1. Hemolysis due to a metabolite of dapsone
             a. Causes oxidation of glutathione
                i. Glutathione essential for erythrocyte membrane integrity
             b. G6PD necessary to produce NADPH
                i. NADPH is a cofactor for glutathione reductase
                ii. Glutathione reductase reduces the oxidized glutathione back to an active form
          2. All patients have some degree of hemolysis
          3. Supplement with 1 mg of folate daily
       ii. Other side effects
          1. Leukopenia
          2. Hypersensitivity syndrome
          3. Liver toxicity
          4. Nausea
          5. Peripheral neuropathy (on high doses)
       iii. Monitoring
          1. Every month for 3 months
             a. CBC
             b. Reticulocyte count
          2. Every 3 months
             a. CBC
             b. Reticulocyte count
             c. LFTs
             d. Creatinine
          3. All patients should be screened for G6PD deficiency
             a. Deficient patients will have severe hemolysis
             b. Especially those of Mediterranean or African descent
17. Thalidomide
   a. Anti-inflammatory, immunomodulatory, and anti-angiogenic properties
   b. Mechanism of action
       i. Reduces TNF-α production by 40%
          1. A major effect
       ii. **Not** immunosuppressive
          1. Not associated with opportunistic infections
   c. Dosing
       i. 50–300 mg a day
   d. Side Effects
       i. Sedation
       ii. Constipation
       iii. Rash
       iv. Sensory polyneuropathy
          1. Frequency up to 50%
          2. More common in women
          3. Not related to daily or cumulative dose
          4. Often progressive and nonreversible

        5. A baseline EMG/NCV should be performed
          a. Repeat every 6 months
        6. Discontinue the drug if
          a. A 50% decline in the sensory nerve action potential (SNAP)
          b. Development of subjective complaints at monthly follow-ups
      v. Teratogenicity (phocomelia)
      vi. FDA requirements
        1. Registration for its use
        2. Stringent regulations and guidelines
   e. Conditions in which thalidomide is used
      i. Inflammatory skin diseases associated with
        1. SLE
        2. Behcet's
      ii. Useful for severe oral and/or genital ulcerations
18. DMARD therapy should be*continued indefinitely* in patients who are doing well
   a. Spontaneous remissions in RA that requires DMARDs are very uncommon
   b. Continued efficacy requires maintenance therapy
   c. Severe flares may occur with discontinuation of most of these drugs

Cytotoxic and Immunoregulatory Agents

21

1. Precautions for patients on immunosuppressant medications
   a. Should not receive live attenuated virus vaccines
      i. Yellow fever
      ii. Measles
      iii. Mumps
      iv. Rubella
      v. Oral polio
      vi. Varicella
   b. Avoid contact with children recently vaccinated with oral polio vaccine
      i. Virus shed in stool
   c. Other vaccinations tolerated without an increased risk of flare
   d. May have blunted protective antibody titers
2. Mycophenylate mofetil (MMF) (Cellcept)
   a. Pharmacology
      i. Available formulation
         1. Capsules 250 and 500 mg
         2. Oral suspension 200 mg/ml
         3. IV form 500 mg/20 ml
   b. Dosing
      i. 500–1,500 mg 2 times/day
   c. Mechanism of action
      i. An inactive prodrug
      ii. Hydrolyzed to the active mycophenolic acid (MPA)
         1. Inhibits lymphocyte proliferation and migration
      iii. MPA
         1. A reversible inhibitor of inosine-5′-monophosphate dehydrogenase (IMPDH)
            a. IMPDH
               i. An enzyme necessary for the de novo synthesis of the purine guanosine

N.T. Colburn, *Review of Rheumatology*,   533
DOI 10.1007/978-1-84882-093-7_21, © Springer-Verlag London Limited 2012

      ii. Guanosine initiates a proliferative response to antigen in T and B cells

      iii. Cytokine production **NOT** affected

   2. Inhibits carbohydrate (fucose, mannose) transfer to glycoproteins

     a. Results in less production of adhesion molecules

       i. VLA-4

       ii. ICAM-1

d. Side effects

  i. GI

   1. Especially diarrhea (25%)

   2. Enterohepatic recycling of glucuronide-conjugated MPA contributes to GI toxicity

    a. GI mucosal cells are 50% dependent upon de novo synthesis of purines inhibited by MPA

  ii. Leukopenia

  iii. Anemia

  iv. Hepatotoxicity

  v. Infections

  vi. Lymphoproliferative malignancies

   1. Less likely to cause than azathioprine

e. Monitoring

  i. Weekly with dose change

   1. CBC

   2. LFTs

  ii. Every 1–3 months

   1. CBC

   2. LFTs

  iii. Avoid in pregnancy

  iv. Avoid live viruses

f. Interactions

  i. Decreases bioavailability

   1. Cholestyramine

   2. Administration with food or antacids

  ii. Tacrolimus

   1. Potentiates effects

g. A good alternative to azathioprine

  i. Patients with gout who need allopurinol

   1. Allopurinol inhibits xanthine oxidase

   2. Results in accumulation of 6-MP

    a. The active metabolite of azathioprine

  ii. Patients who need warfarin

   1. Azathioprine causes warfarin resistance

h. Rheumatic diseases treated successfully with MMF

  i. SLE (in particular)

   1. Lupus nephritis

          a. Alternative therapy
             i. Reduced proteinuria and improved creatinine in 13 people with cyclophosphamide-resistant nephritis over a mean 12.8 months
            ii. Combination MMF and prednisolone as effective as cyclophosphamide and prednisolone with follow-up azathioprine and prednisolone at inducing complete and partial renal remission in 42 SLE DPGN for 12 months
          b. DPGN
          c. Membranous
        2. Cutaneous lupus
          a. Discoid
          b. Subacute cutaneous lupus
     ii. Vasculitis
    iii. Renal allograft rejection
3. Cyclophosphamide (Cytoxan)
    a. Mechanism of action
       i. One of the most potent immunosuppressive drugs available
      ii. An inactive prodrug
     iii. Activated by hepatic cytochrome P-450 enzymes
     iv. Phosphoramide mustard
        1. The major active metabolite
        2. Alkylates DNA
          a. Cross-linking of DNA
          b. Breaks in DNA
          c. Decreased DNA synthesis
          d. Apoptosis
        3. Marked effect on rapidly dividing cells
        4. Alterations in humoral and cellular immunity (B > T cells)
       v. Acrolein
        1. Another major metabolic product
        2. Hemorrhagic cystitis
        3. Bladder cancer
    b. Pharmacology
       i. Available formulations
        1. 25- and 50-mg tablets
        2. 100-, 200-, 500-, and 1,000-mg vials
      ii. Dosing
        1. Lower doses in elderly
          a. Less bone marrow reserve
          b. Cellularity = 100% − age
        2. Liver disease does **NOT** increase toxicity
        3. Decrease initial dose in renal insufficiency
          a. 25% if creatinine clearance less than 50 cc/min
          b. 50% if creatinine clearance less than 25 cc/min

4. Administer after dialysis
   a. Drug is dialyzable
5. Oral
   a. 50–150 mg daily
   b. 0.7–3 mg/kg/day
6. Monthly IV (typical protocol)
   a. Prior to cyclophosphamide
      i. Premedicate 15–30 min
         1. Dexamethasone 10 mg
         2. Lorazepam 1 mg
         3. Ondansetron 8 mg
      ii. Mesna
         1. 25% of cyclophosphamide dose in milligrams in 500 cc normal saline
   b. Cyclophosphamide infusion
      i. Initial dose
         1. 0.75 g/m^2 of body surface area in 1,000 cc NS
         2. Creatinine clearance less than 35–40 cc/min
            a. Decrease initial dose to 0.50 g/m^2 of BSA
      ii. Subsequent monthly doses depend on WBC counts at 10–14 days
         1. If nadir <3,000/mm^3
         2. Reduce dose by 0.25 g/m^2
         3. If nadir >4,000/mm^3
         4. Increase dose to max of 1 g/m^2
   c. Post-cyclophosphamide infusion
      i. Mesna
         1. 25% of cyclophosphamide dose in mg in 500 cc normal saline
      ii. Compazine SR
         1. 15 mg BID for 2–3 days
   d. Dosing interval
      i. Monthly for six doses, then
      ii. Every 2 months for three doses, then
      iii. Every 3 months for four doses, then
      iv. Maintenance with azathioprine or MMF
c. Side effects
   i. Bone marrow suppression
      1. WBC nadir 8–14 days after a dose
      2. Keep WBC nadir above 3,000/mm^3
   ii. Infections
      1. All types
      2. Especially herpes viruses
      3. Prior to therapy screen for
         a. Hepatitis B and C

  b. HIV

  c. TB

 4. Decrease prednisone dose to less than 20–25 mg/day as soon as possible

 5. Prophylaxis for *Pneumocystis carinii* pneumonia

  a. Bactrim/septra

  b. Dapsone

  c. Inhaled pentamidine

 6. Pneumococcal vaccine

iii. Hemorrhagic cystitis and bladder cancer

 1. Non-glomerular hematuria

  a. Up to 50% of patients

 2. Bladder cancer

  a. Develops in 5%

  b. 31-fold decrease

 3. Methods to decrease risk

  a. Use monthly IV pulse therapy

   i. Instead of daily oral therapy

  b. Use Mesna

   i. A sulfhydryl compound

   ii. Binds and inactivates acrolein in the urine

  c. Stop smoking

   i. Increases risk of bladder cancer

  d. Give daily oral therapy in the morning

   i. Force fluids (> 2 l/day)

iv. Malignancy

 1. Risk increased 2–4 fold

 2. The higher the cumulative dose, the greater the risk

 3. Non-Hodgkin's lymphomas

  a. Small percentage with Wegener's granulomatosis

v. Infertility risk

 1. Ovarian failure

  a. Ranges from 45% to 70%

  b. Slightly less with monthly IV than daily oral dosing

  c. Unlikely with less than 6 monthly doses

  d. Common with over 15 monthly pulses

 2. Varies depending on age and cumulative dose

  a. Less than 20 years

   i. 13% risk

  b. 20–30 years

   i. 50% risk

  c. Greater than 30 years

   i. 100% risk of premature ovarian failure

 3. Azoospermia found in 50–90% of men

    4. Strategies to limit toxicity
       a. Bank ova and sperm
       b. Gonadotropin-releasing hormone analogue
          i. Lupron depot
            1. 3.75 mg IM monthly
            2. 11.25 mg IM every 3 months
          ii. Plus estradiol
            1. 0.3 mg/day
            2. Biweekly patch
              a. If patient hypercoagulable
            3. Reduces hot flashes
            4. Protects bone
       c. Testosterone
          i. 100 mg IM every 15 days
   vi. Pulmonary
      1. Pneumonitis or pulmonary fibrosis
       a. Less than 1%
  d. Other side effects
    i. Reversible alopecia
    ii. Syndrome of inappropriate antidiuretic hormone secretion
    iii. Nausea
    iv. Teratogenicity
  e. Monitoring
    i. Daily dosing
      1. Every 1–2 weeks until stable
       a. CBC
      2. Monthly
       a. CBC
       b. UA
      3. After cessation of therapy
       a. Every 6–12 months
         i. UA
         ii. Urine cytology
    ii. Monthly dosing
      1. Before each dose
       a. CBC
       b. UA
      2. 10–14 days after each dose
       a. CBC
       b. UA
    iii. Avoid in pregnancy
    iv. Avoid live vaccines
  f. Interactions
    i. Increased frequency of leukopenia
      1. Cimetidine
      2. Allopurinol

g. Rheumatic diseases in which cyclophosphamide is indicated
  i. Successful where less potent and less toxic medicines have failed
    1. Almost all rheumatic diseases
  ii. Wegener's granulomatosis
    1. Considered the cornerstone of therapy
    2. Otherwise a fatal disease process
  iii. SLE
    1. Especially in lupus nephritis
      a. Superior efficacy in preservation of renal function
    2. Difficult to demonstrate overall improvements in mortality
  iv. Systemic vasculitic syndromes
4. Chlorambucil
  a. Dosing
    i. 0.1 mg/kg/day (2–8 mg/day)
  b. Indications
    i. Behcet's disease
      1. Primary use
      2. Eye disease
      3. Neuropsychiatric complications
    ii. Cryoglobulinemia
    iii. Refractory polymyositis
    iv. Lupus nephritis
    v. Amyloidosis secondary to chronic inflammatory arthritis
      1. RA
      2. JRA
      3. AS
  c. Side effects
    i. Myelosuppression
    ii. Induction of leukemia and other malignancies
      1. Great risk as an alkylating agent
5. Tacrolimus
  a. A macrolide produced by a fungus
  b. Mechanism of action
    i. Immunosuppressive effects similar to cyclosporin
      1. At a dose 10–100 times lower
    ii. Potent inhibitors of T-cell activation
      1. Inhibits transcription of early T-cell inducible activation genes (IL-2)
        a. Interferes with the binding of NF-AT to the enhancer region
    iii. Causes less increase in uric acid (than cyclosporine)
      1. Useful in transplant patients with tophaceous gout
6. Sirolimus
  a. Mechanism of action
    i. Inhibits T cell proliferation by binding to cytoplasmic immunophilin
    ii. Immunophilin
      1. Inhibits IL-2 receptor transduction events
      2. Prohibits the T cell from responding to IL-2

7. IVIG
   a. Available in solutions which vary from 3% to 12% Ig
   b. Dosing
       i. 1–2 g/kg administered over 1–5 days
   c. Side effects
       i. Headache (2–20%)
       ii. Flushing
       iii. Chest tightness
       iv. Back pain/myalgias
       v. Fever, chills
       vi. Nausea
       vii. Diaphoresis
       viii. Hypotension
       ix. Aseptic meningitis
       x. Clot
       xi. Methods to avoid side effects
           1. Premedication
               a. Tylenol
               b. Benadryl
               c. Solu-Cortef
           2. Slow the infusion rate
               a. Start rate at 30 ml/h
               b. Increase to a maximum of 250 ml/h
   d. Monitoring
       i. 24 h after infusion
           1. Creatinine
   e. Precautions
       i. Anaphylactic reactions in patients with hereditary IgA deficiency
       ii. Transmission of infectious agents (rare)
   f. Rheumatic diseases in which IVIG is indicated
       i. Autoimmune thrombocytopenia
           1. Acts by Fc receptor blockade
           2. Reduces the efficacy of the reticuloendothelial system to remove antibody-coated platelets
           3. Reduces autoantibody production
           4. Decreases autoantibody binding to platelets
       ii. Kawasaki's disease
           1. Reduces expression of adhesion molecules on endothelial cells
           2. Binds cytokines that cause inflammation
           3. Reduces the number of activated T cells
           4. Binds staphylococcal toxin superantigens
       iii. Dermatomyositis and polymyositis
       iv. Wegener's granulomatosis
           1. Reduces the level of ANCA autoantibodies
       v. Antiphospholipid antibody syndrome

8. Plasmapheresis
   a. Theoretically removes pathogenic immune complexes and autoantibodies
   b. Diseases treated
      i. Hepatitis B–associated polyarteritis nodosa
         1. In combination with antiviral agents (alpha-interferon)
      ii. Hepatitis B or C associated cryoglobulinemia
      iii. Severe lupus pneumonitis and neuropsychiatric lupus with coma
         1. Used in combination therapy
            a. Corticosteroids and cytotoxic medications
            b. Decreases risk of rebound flare when pheresis is stopped
   c. Exchange protocols
      i. Most remove 2–4 l (40 mg/kg) of plasma over a 2-h period daily
      ii. Replacement fluid
         1. Albumin-saline
         2. Protein-containing solution
         3. Fresh-frozen plasma
            a. 1–2 units as part of the replacement solution
            b. Decreases risk of infection and bleeding
      iii. Monitoring
         1. Coagulation studies
         2. Immunoglobulin levels
            a. Hypogammaglobulinemia may develop
               i. Treat with IVIG
9. High-Dose Immunoablative Therapy
   a. Used with or without autologous hematopoietic stem cell transplantation
   b. With autologous stem cell transplantation
      i. A method of increasing the intensity of chemotherapy
      ii. Stem cells (CD34+) collected prior to chemotherapy
      iii. Higher doses of cyclophosphamide (200 mg/kg) given to ablate the immune system
      iv. Rescue from bone marrow failure by reinfusion of the patient's own stem cells
      v. Allows reconstitution of the immune system without redeveloping autoimmune disease
   c. Without autologous stem cell transplantation
      i. High-dose immunoablative therapy (50 mg/kg for 4 days)
      ii. CD34+ stem cells express high levels of aldehyde dehydrogenase
         1. Responsible for cellular resistance to cyclophosphamide
      iii. Bone marrow repopulates without reinfusion of harvested stem cells
      iv. Less expensive
      v. Potentially more effective
         1. Reinfused harvested stems cells develop autoimmune lymphocytes
   d. For the treatment of severe autoimmune disease in patients failing standard therapy
      i. RA

    ii. SLE
    iii. Systemic sclerosis
    iv. Multiple sclerosis
  e. Varying success rates
      i. 5–10% mortality
  f. High cost (up to $100,000)

Biologic Agents

22

1. Distinct from traditional antirheumatic drugs
   a. Often large molecules
   b. Derived from or resemble naturally occurring effector molecules
      i. Antibodies
      ii. Soluble cell-surface receptors
   c. Target-specific components of the immune response
2. Factors in the development of biologic agents
   a. The chronic progressive pathophysiology of rheumatic diseases
   b. Toxicities or ineffectiveness of DMARDs used long-term
   c. Progress in understanding the immune response underlying rheumatic diseases
   d. Advances in biotechnology, molecular biology, and pharmaceutical development
3. Goals of therapy
   a. The induction of immunologic tolerance
   b. Disease remission
4. Immunological signaling
   a. The first signal
      i. Antigen presented in the context of the appropriate MHC molecule to specific TCRs
      ii. Inhibition
         1. No signal occurs
   b. The second signal
      i. Additional stimulation occurs
         1. Costimulatory cell-surface molecules
         2. Cytokines
      ii. Inhibition
         1. Ignorance
            a. No immune reaction to antigen
         2. Tolerance
            a. Specific anergy to antigen

    c. Propagation and shaping of the response
        i. Depends on overall activity of mediators
           1. Cytokines
           2. Chemokines
    d. Drug mechanism
        i. Interrupts a dysregulated immune response
        ii. Re-establishes normal immune homeostasis
5. Classification of biologic agents
    a. Monoclonal antibodies
        i. Against T-cell surface molecules
           1. CD4 (anti-CD4)
        ii. Against B-cell surface molecules
           1. CD20 (anti-CD20)
        iii. Activation antigens
           1. CD25 (anti-TAC)
        iv. Against adhesion molecules
           1. ICAM-1/LFA-1 interaction (anti-CD11α receptor)
        v. Against complement
           1. C5 (anti-C5)
        vi. Against costimulatory molecules
           1. CD40L (anti-CD40L)
    b. Biologics targeting T-/B-cell collaboration molecules
        i. CD28/B7 (CTLA-4 Ig)
    c. Biologics targeting inflammatory cytokines
        i. Cytokine receptor antagonist proteins (IL-1 Ra)
        ii. Soluble receptors (TNFα receptor)
    d. Methods targeting antigen/TCR/MHC interaction
        i. Oral tolerance (Type II collagen in RA)
        ii. TCR Vβ peptide vaccine
        iii. MHC peptide vaccine
    e. Other
        i. Antisense oligonucleotides (against ICAM-1)
        ii. T-cell vaccination
        iii. Gene therapy
           1. IL-1 Ra
           2. Fas ligand
        iv. IL-10
           1. An anti-inflammatory cytokine
6. Monoclonal antibodies and soluble receptors are immunogenic large proteins
    a. Decreases half-life
    b. Decreases clinical utility
    c. Leads to adverse effects
7. Factors that determine whether an agent elicits an immune response
    a. Route of administration
        i. Subcutaneous more immunogenic than IV
        ii. Oral doses tend to be the least immunogenic

    b. Immunosuppressive effects of the agent or concomitant medications
       i. Minimizes immune responses
    c. Dose and dosing frequency
       i. Minimized with regular administration of larger doses
    d. Modification to the compound
       i. Reduced immunogenicity
          1. Polyethylene glycol treatment
          2. Glycosylation of proteins
    e. Foreign proteins
       i. More likely to induce an immune response
       ii. Fully human compounds though can be immunogenic
8. Antigen-/TCR-/MHC-Specific Therapies
    a. Therapy targets
       i. Agents causing the disease
       ii. Clones of T- or B-cells programmed to respond to the etiologic antigens
    b. Advantages
       i. Obviates many adverse effects seen with nonspecific agents
       ii. Prevents further reactivity to the etiologic antigen
       iii. Induces remission
    c. Biologic agents targeting the trimolecular complex (Ag/TCR/MHC)
       i. Used successfully in animal models of autoimmune disease
          1. Induces tolerance and completely abrogates disease
          2. Most successful when administered before or soon after disease initiation
       ii. Use hindered in human rheumatic diseases
          1. Specific antigens in humans remain largely undefined
          2. Particular TCR/MHC interactions remain unknown
          3. Usually present for treatment long after the disease initiated
          4. "Antigenic drift" in chronic immune reactions
       iii. Specific interventions tested in human disease
          1. Vaccination with TCR-derived peptides
             a. TCR Vβ
          2. Vaccination with MHC fragments or with relevant peptides linked to MHC fragments
             a. Cartilage protein gp39/DR4 in RA
          3. Administration of antibodies to MHC molecules
             a. Tolerated well
             b. Efficacy awaits further testing
    d. Induction of bystander tolerance
       i. Antigens distinct from the etiologic agent but relevant to the disease
          1. Oral ingestion of type II collagen in RA
       ii. No conclusive proof of efficacy of oral tolerance in human disease

9. T-Cell-Directed Therapies
   a. CD4
      i. One of the earliest targets chosen for study
      ii. A key role in the inflammation of RA and other rheumatic diseases
      iii. Success in animal models of autoimmune disease
         1. Long-term clinical benefit
         2. Specific immunologic tolerance
         3. Induced tolerance to the treating agent
      iv. In patients with RA
         1. Uncontrolled studies
            a. Decreases in the number of circulating CD4+ T-cells
            b. Suggested clinical benefit
         2. Rigorous, double-blind placebo-controlled trials
            a. Clinical efficacy no greater than that of placebo
            b. Induction of long-term decreases in CD4+ T-cells
            c. Antibodies used elicited an immune response
         3. Use of anti-CD4+ antibodies failed in RA
            a. Efficacy varies with particular patient subsets or stages of disease
            b. Characteristics of the biologic agent must be well-defined
               i. Some anti-CD4 antibodies preferentially target naïve CD4 T-cells
               ii. Memory Th1 CD4 T-cells have the greatest relevance to rheumatic disease
10. Inhibition of Costimulatory Molecules
    a. Cell surface molecules that provide the second signal in immune responses
    b. Some of the most important pairs of costimulatory molecules
       i. CD28 and CTLA-4
          1. Bind B7-1 (CD80) and B7-2 (CD86)
             a. Present on antigen-presenting cells
          2. Essential for T-cell-driven immune responses
             a. Initiation
             b. Sustenance
             c. Regulation
          3. Affect Th1/Th2 balance
          4. Effective in several animal models of RA and SLE
       ii. CD40 ligand (CD40L; CD154)
          1. Binds CD40
          2. Essential for the formation of lymph node germinal centers
          3. Essential for the production of antibodies
          4. Affect Th1/Th2 balance
          5. Effective in several animal models of RA and SLE
11. Inhibition of Adhesion Molecules
    a. Roles of adhesion molecules in autoimmune responses
       i. Regulates inflammatory cells at sites of active disease
          1. Recruitment
          2. Retention
          3. Activation

     ii. Costimulatory signals to T-cells

     iii. Mediate functions (angiogenesis)

  b. Adhesion molecules as targets for biologic therapies

     i. Interaction of LFA-1 (CD11a/CD18) with ICAM-1 (CD54)

       1. Anti-adhesion therapy with anti-ICAM-1 antibody

     ii. The interaction of VLA-4 (CD49d/CD29) with VCAM-1 (CD106)

     iii. Inhibition in animal models of autoimmune diseases led to

       1. Clinical improvement

       2. Immunologic tolerance

     iv. Other adhesion molecule targets

       1. E-selectin

       2. CD44

  c. Immune-mediated conditions with trials of anti-adhesion therapy

     i. Psoriasis

     ii. Ulcerative colitis

     iii. Multiple sclerosis

12. Inhibition of Proinflammatory Cytokines

  a. Inhibitors of TNF for the treatment of RA have achieved the greatest success

  b. Etanercept (Enbrel)

     i. A dimeric soluble p75-TNF-receptor/Fc fusion protein

     ii. A bioengineered molecule derived from Chinese hamster ovary cells

     iii. Created by linking the extracellular binding regions from two p75 (TNF-RII) receptors to the Fc portion of human IgG1

     iv. Binds **soluble** TNFα and lymphotoxin (TNFβ)

     v. Half-life 72 h

     vi. Dosing

       1. 25 mg subcutaneous twice a week

     vii. Monitoring

       1. PPD prior to use

       2. Monthly for 3 months

         a. CBC

       3. Every 3 months

         a. CBC

  c. Infliximab

     i. A chimeric mouse-human anti-TNF monoclonal antibody

       1. Constant regions of human IgG1 heavy and partial kappa light chain domains (IgG1κ Fc)

       2. Coupled to the variable region (Fv) of a mouse light chain

       3. Chimeric antibodies

         a. About 70% human

           i. The Fc fragment

           ii. Constant regions

         b. About 30% murine

           i. The antigen-binding variable regions

     ii. High-affinity for human TNF-α

      iii. Binds **both soluble and cell bound** TNFα
         1. Ability to kill cells with TNFα bound to its surface
         2. Does **NOT** bind lymphotoxin
      iv. Dosing
         1. 3–10 mg/kg IV every 4–8 weeks
      v. Monitoring
         1. PPD prior to use
         2. Monthly for 3 months
            a. CBC
         3. Every 3 months
            a. CBC
      vi. Precaution
         1. Do not use in patients with CHF
   d. Adalimumab
      i. Fully humanized anti-TNF monoclonal antibody
         1. Produced by repertoire cloning of phage libraries
      ii. Given subcutaneously every other week
      iii. Do not see neutralizing antibodies
   e. Variability in clinical efficacy with anti-TNF therapy
      i. Heterogeneity in synovial TNF expression
      ii. Genetic polymorphisms encoding TNF
      iii. Differences in TNF target specificity and binding avidity
   f. Side effects with anti-TNFα biologic agents
      i. Hypersensitivity reactions
         1. Etanercept
            a. Injection site reaction (50%)
               i. Last 3–5 days
               ii. Usually resolves by 3 months of use
               iii. Treat with topical steroid or antihistamine
               iv. Rotate the injection sites
         2. Infliximab
            a. Infusion reactions
               i. Hypotension or hypertension
               ii. Headache
               iii. Dyspnea and nausea
               iv. Rash
               v. Rarely a severe allergic reaction
               vi. Treatment
                   1. Stop the infusion
                   2. Restart at slower rate
            vii. Premedicate
               1. If patients has had a prior reaction
               2. If patient has a history of ≥3 drug allergies
               3. Allegra 180 mg
                   a. 45 min prior to infusion
               4. ASA (better than acetaminophen)
               5. Solu-Cortef

    ii. Pancytopenia/aplastic anemia
       1. Usually seen with other medications being used
         a. MTX
   iii. Demyelinating syndromes
       1. Reversible when agent is stopped
       2. Do **NOT** use in patients with
         a. Multiple sclerosis
         b. Optic neuritis
   iv. Opportunistic infections
       1. TB
       2. Fungal
       3. Pneumocystis
       4. *Listeria*
       5. Infliximab > etanercept associated TB and fungal infections
         a. Cause maybe demographics of patients treated
            i. Many outside the USA
           ii. Many Crohn's patients
       6. PPD prior to starting
         a. Get CXR
            i. If risk factors present
           ii. If positive PPD present
       7. Patients with latent TB
         a. Prophylactic therapy with isoniazid (or equivalent) for 9 months
         b. Do **not** start anti-TNF therapy until antituberculous therapy given at least 2 weeks
    v. Infections
       1. Serious infections occur in 2–3%
       2. Do **not** use if predisposed to serious infections
       3. Hold anti-TNF therapy during active infection
   vi. Autoimmune phenomenon
       1. Etanercept
         a. Non-neutralizing antibodies (16%)
         b. Positive ANA (11%)
         c. Lupus-like syndrome
         d. Usually resolves after stopping the agent
         e. Treat with a brief course of corticosteroids
       2. Infliximab
         a. Human anti-chimeric antibodies (HACA) (17%)
         b. Use with MTX or other immunosuppressant
         c. Positive ANA (20–30%)
         d. Antiphospholipid antibodies
         e. Lupus-like syndrome
         f. Usually resolve after stopping the agent
         g. Treat with a brief course of corticosteroids

      vii. Malignancy
         1. Lymphoma
            a. May be more common with high-dose (10 mg/kg) monthly infliximab
         2. Treatment not recommended if less than 5 years from any cancer
     viii. Others
         1. Seizures
         2. Colonic perforations
  g. Diseases treated with anti-TNFα therapies
     i. Etanercept
        1. RA
            a. 2 placebo-controlled trials
               i. Produced ACR-20 response rates in the range of 60–70%
            b. Combination therapy with MTX
               i. Incremental clinical benefits
            c. Early RA
               i. Proved similar to MTX in clinical efficacy
              ii. More effective than MTX for preventing joint damage
        2. Polyarticular JRA
        3. Ankylosing spondylitis
        4. Psoriatic arthritis
     ii. Infliximab
        1. RA (large clinical trial)
            a. 428 patients
            b. Active RA despite MTX therapy
            c. Maintained on constant dose of MTX
            d. Randomly treated with placebo or 3 mg/kg or 10 mg/kg of infliximab
            e. Treated at week 0, 2, and 6, and then every 4 or 8 weeks for 30 weeks
            f. Infliximab treated achieved ACR-20 response rates of 50–58% compared with 20% for placebo
            g. Infliximab plus MTX significantly reduced radiologic progression of joint damage compared with MTX alone
        2. Crohn's disease
        3. Ankylosing spondylitis
        4. Psoriatic arthritis
     iii. Considered contraindicated in lupus-like diseases
  h. IL-1 as a cytokine target
     i. A proinflammatory cytokine
     ii. Exists in two forms transcribed from closely related but distinct genes
        1. IL-1α
            a. Located in the cytosol
            b. Membrane bound
        2. IL-1β
            a. Secreted into the extracellular space

        b. ProIL-1β cleaved by interleukin-1β-converting enzyme (ICE)

        c. The predominant form that binds to the IL-1 receptor

        d. Triggers intracellular signaling leading to a proinflammatory response

           i. Synergistic to that induced by TNFα

          ii. Leads to B-cell activation

         iii. Rheumatoid factor production

         iv. Induces synoviocyte/chondrocyte enzyme production

           v. Cartilage degradation

         vi. Stimulates osteoclasts

        vii. Bone resorption

    iii. Il-1 Ra (Anakinra, Kineret)

       1. Inhibitor of IL-1

       2. A recombinant nonglycosylated version of the naturally occurring human IL-1 receptor antagonist

       3. Blocks the biologic activity of IL-1

         a. Competitively inhibits IL-1 binding to the IL-1 type I receptor

         b. No signal transduced

       4. For patients with inflammatory synovitis (such as RA)

         a. Insufficient amount of IL-Ra produced to neutralize the amount of locally produced IL-1

       5. Half-life 4–6 h

       6. Dosing

         a. 100 mg subcutaneous daily

       7. Monitoring

         a. Monthly for 3 months

           i. CBC

         b. Every 3 months

           i. CBC

       8. Side Effects

         a. Serious infections (2%)

         b. Neutropenia (3%)

         c. Injection site reactions (70%)

       9. Precautions

         a. Do **not** use in patients with active infection

  i. Other cytokine targets

      i. IL-6

     ii. IL-17

    iii. IL-2

    iv. IL-15

     v. Interferons [β,γ,α]

    vi. TGF-β

13. Modification of Th1/Th2 Balance

  a. Th1 T-cell subset

    i. Functions primarily in cell-mediated immunity

    ii. Play a dominant role in RA

     iii. Development driven by
        1. IL-12
        2. IL-18
        3. IFN-gamma
  b. Th2 T-cell subset
     i. Development driven by
        1. IL-10
           a. Exerts additional anti-inflammatory effects
           b. Assessed in RA studies
        2. IL-4
        3. Inhibit Th-1
  c. Factors that modulate the Th1/Th2 balance
     i. Relative strength or timing of costimulation
     ii. Specific chemokines or other mediators in the local milieu
        1. TNF substance P
     iii. Therapeutics (especially RA)
14. Inhibition of Other Inflammatory Mediators
  a. Chemokines
     i. Direct trafficking of leukocytes to inflammatory sites
     ii. Inhibitors have potential utility in allergic and infectious diseases
     iii. Targets
        1. IL-8
        2. MCP-1
        3. RANTES
        4. MIP-1α
  b. Interferons [β,γ,α]
     c. Components of the complement cascade
     i. Antibodies to C5
  d. Others
     i. PAF
     ii. Substance P
     iii. Nitric oxide
     iv. Matrix metalloproteinase inhibitors
     v. Il-1 converting enzyme (ICE) inhibitors
     vi. Gene-based strategies
        1. Targeting factors that control transduction and translation
        2. Antisense oligonucleotides
        3. Gene transfer of regulatory factors
     vii. Ribozyme treatment
     viii. Specific protease and peptidomimetic inhibitors
        1. p38 MAP kinase inhibitor
        2. Small orally bioavailable molecules
        3. Cheaper to produce than macromolecules

15. Potential Targets for TNF Biologic Therapy
    a. TNF expressed as a transmembrane molecule on the surface of macrophages
    b. mRNA assembled into an active trimer at the cell surface
    c. Transcription, translation, and mRNA stability modulated by
        i. Gene therapy
        ii. Kinase inhibitors
    d. Protease TNF-converting enzyme (TACE)
        i. Cleaves the extracellular portion of TNF
        ii. Inhibition of TACE prevents TNF from being secreted
    e. Cleaved TNFα (TNF-β from T-cells)
        i. A soluble molecule
        ii. Circulates as a homotrimer
        iii. Binds to specific cell-surface receptors found on most cells
            1. TNF-RI (p55 or CD120a)
            2. TNF-RII (p-75 or CD120b)
    f. Inhibitors of TNF cell-surface receptor binding
        i. Small molecule peptides or peptidomimetics of TNF/TNF-R
        ii. Monoclonal antibodies that specifically bind TNF
            1. Prevent signal transduction
        iii. Soluble forms of the TNF receptor that bind TNF
            1. TNF-RI and TNF-RII secretion increased by
                a. Gene therapy
                b. Cytokines
    g. Signal transduction leads to
        i. Production of prostaglandins and proinflammatory cytokines
        ii. Endothelial cell expression of adhesion molecules
        iii. Recruitment of neutrophils and monocytes into synovial fluid
        iv. Synoviocyte/chondrocyte production of collagenase
            1. Destroys cartilage and bone

Osteoporosis

23

Section A: Epidemiology, Pathology and Pathogenesis

1. Osteoporosis
   a. A skeletal disease
   b. Marked by low total or regional bone mass
   c. Microarchitectural deterioration
   d. Both hydroxyapatite and osteoid reduced proportionately
   e. Leads to an increased susceptibility to fracture
2. Osteoporotic Fracture
   a. The single most important clinical consequence
   b. A major health problem in the elderly
   c. Risk determinants
      i. Low bone mass
      ii. Skeletal fragility
      iii. Propensity to fall
3. Bone Density
   a. A measure of bone mass
   b. Measured noninvasively using densitometric techniques
   c. Main focus of risk assessment and therapy
   d. Fracture risk and mortality correlate strongly with bone density
      i. At any given age
      ii. 50-year-old white woman
         1. 19% lifetime risk of hip fracture if radial bone mass at the tenth percentile for age
         2. 11% lifetime risk if radial bone mass at the 90th percentile
4. Fracture Morbidity and Costs
      i. Population at greatest risk for fracture
         1. Older white women
      ii. Lifetime risk for hip, wrist, or clinical vertebral fracture (age 50)
         1. 40% in white women
         2. 13% in white men

Fig. 23.1 A highly unstable
intertrochanteric fracture (five pieces)
in a 92-year-old patient with severe
osteoporosis (Reproduced with
permission from A physiological
approach in stabilization and
consolidation of unstable femoral neck
fracture in osteoporotic elderly patients:
a retrospective review. *European
Journal of Orthopaedic Surgery &
Traumatology.* DOI: 10.1007/s00590-
003-0084-3. Springer; 2003-09-01)

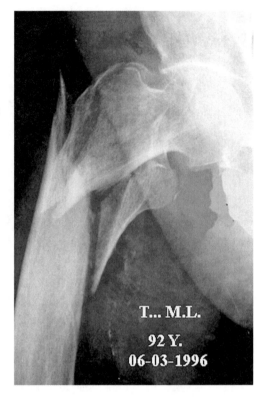

b. The most common types of fracture
   i. Vertebral
   ii. Wrist
c. Osteoporotic fractures in white women aged 65–84
   i. Hip and spine (90%)
   ii. Wrist (70%)
   iii. All other (30–50%)
   iv. All sites (70%)
5. Hip Fractures
   a. More strongly associated with bone density than any other site
   b. Risk factors
      i. Rises exponentially with age
      ii. Three times as great in women than men at most ages
         1. 16% lifetime risk of hip fracture for Caucasian women
         2. 5% lifetime risk of hip fracture for men
         3. 2–3% per year in men and women by age 85
      iii. Factors independent of bone density
         1. Falls
            a. Responsible for 90% of all hip fractures in the elderly
            b. 75% are falls within the home

Fig. 23.2 Osteoporosis of the lumbar spine. Lateral radiograph shows diminished bone density, thinning, and accentuation of cortical density compared with the medullary portion of vertebrae ("empty box"). Arrows point to the coarse trabecular markings due to osteoporotic loss of secondary trabeculae (Reproduced with permission from Systematic approach to metabolic diseases of bone. *Diagnostic Imaging of Musculoskeletal Diseases.* DOI: 10.1007/978-1-59745-355-4_2. Springer; 2009-01-01)

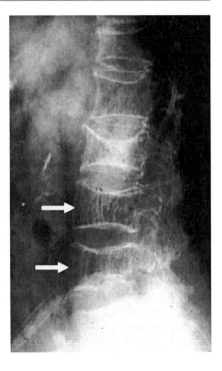

  2. Neuromuscular impairment
  3. Poor vision
  4. Low body weight
  5. Weight loss
  6. A positive family history
  7. Sedative use
  8. Previous vertebral fracture
 c. Mortality and morbidity
   i. In the first 6 months after fracture
    1. Greatest time for mortality
    2. Acute complications of the fracture
    3. Severe coexisting medical conditions
   ii. In the first year after fracture
    1. 12–20% higher mortality than the general population
    2. Higher mortality in men and African Americans
   iii. After 12 months
    1. 50–70% show decreased physical function
    2. 20–30% previously noninstitutionalized patients require nursing home care
6. Vertebral Fractures
 a. The most common osteoporotic fracture
 b. The strongest risk factor for additional fractures

   c. A common hallmark of osteoporosis that requires treatment

   d. 20% lifetime risk for Caucasian women

      i. Majority are asymptomatic or not diagnosed

   e. 6% lifetime risk for vertebral fracture for men

   f. Radiographically identified

      i. Three times the incidence of **clinically** diagnosed vertebral fractures

      ii. 5–10% of white women at age 55

      iii. 30–40% at age 80

      iv. Risk of a new vertebral fracture

         1. 0.5% per year at age 55

         2. 2–3% per year at age 80

   g. Risk factors

      i. Low bone density

         1. Strongly related

         2. Incidence in women exceeds men at older age

      ii. Occupation and/or sports trauma

         1. Incidence in men aged 50–65 same as women

      iii. Falls

         1. 25% of the elderly

   h. Clinical manifestations

      i. 30% asymptomatic

      ii. Less than 15% ever come to medical attention

      iii. Refracture is common

      iv. Anatomical changes with 1.5 in. loss of height

         1. In the thoracic spine leads to progressive kyphosis

         2. In the lumbar spine leads to flattening of the lordotic curve

         3. Scoliosis may develop

         4. Paraspinal musculature progressively shortens

            a. Prolonged contracture leads to back pain

            b. Paraspinal muscle pain greatest

            c. Minimum vertebral body pain

      v. Increase in number and severity of fractured vertebrae

         1. Increase in kyphosis and scoliosis

         2. Lowest thoracic ribs lowered to the pelvic rim

         3. Loss of truncal shape and abdominal protrusion

         4. Postprandial abdominal pain

            a. Prevented by consumption of smaller meals

   i. Clinical diagnosis

      i. Severe back and physical disability

         1. Only one-third diagnosed due to acute pain

      ii. Kyphosis

      iii. Chronic pain and interference with ADLs (50%)

      iv. Depression (40%)

   j. Radiographically identified (undiagnosed)

      i. Increased back pain

ii. Disability with activities
1. Bending
2. Putting on socks
3. Getting in and out of an automobile

k. Increased mortality
  i. Survival decreases 20–60% of age adjusted norms
  ii. Causes
    1. Pulmonary infections
    2. Each vertebral fracture decreases forced vital capacity by 9%
    3. Comorbid conditions

l. Treatment
  i. Acute
    1. Analgesics as needed
      a. Intense, localized pain
      b. Reduced spine motion
    2. Reduce activity or immobilization for several days
    3. Pain generally lasts 4–6 weeks
      a. Seek other causes of a vertebral fracture if longer
        i. Metastatic disease
        ii. Myeloma
        iii. Thyroid disease
    4. Radicular pain syndromes
      a. **UNCOMMON** with osteoporotic fracture
      b. Consider other diseases

  ii. Chronic
    1. Education is essential
      a. Instructions on performing ADLs
        i. Bending
        ii. Lifting
        iii. Stooping
      b. Avoid increased loads on a brittle skeleton
    2. Goals of therapy
      a. Reduce pain
      b. Restore function
      c. Improve quality of life
      d. Prevent additional fractures
    3. Major targets
      a. Rehabilitation
      b. Appropriate analgesia
        i. Reduce chronic back pain
    4. Avoid constipation
      a. Occurs with drugs such as
        i. Narcotic analgesics
        ii. Some anti-inflammatory meds
        iii. Generic calcium supplements
      b. Stool softeners should be prescribed

7. Wrist Fractures
   a. 90% due to falls
   b. Four times more common in women than in men
   c. Risk greater in healthier, more active women with low bone density
   d. Incidence plateaus among women around age 65
      i. A change in the falling pattern with advancing age
         1. A fall on the hip more likely than on an outstretched arm
         2. Slower gait
         3. Decreased reflexes
8. Risk Factors for Fracture
   a. Bone mass
      i. One of the strongest determinants of fracture risk
         1. Both men and women
      ii. Primary focus of risk assessment and treatment
   b. Different risk factors for fractures of different bones
   c. Women with an existing vertebral fracture (compared with the risk without)
      i. Four-fold increased risk of having another vertebral fracture
      ii. Two-fold increased risk of subsequent hip fracture
      iii. 50% greater risk of a nonvertebral fracture
      iv. Risks independent of bone density
         1. Vertebral fractures are a marker for general skeletal fragility
   d. History of any nonspine, low-trauma fracture after 50
      i. Increased risk of subsequent fractures
         1. Hip
         2. Vertebral
         3. Nonspine
   e. Familial history as a risk factor for fracture
      i. Strong genetic component to bone mass
      ii. Possible genetic influence on fracture risk
      iii. Family predisposition
         1. Site-specific
         2. Independent of bone density
      iv. Daughters of women who have had a vertebral or hip fracture
         1. Lower bone mass in the spine and hip
      v. Women whose mothers or siblings have had hip fractures
         1. Increased risk of hip fracture
9. Health Care Cost of Osteoporosis
   a. Substantial and increasing
   b. Medical expenditures for osteoporotic fractures estimated at $14 billion
      i. 60% account for treatment of hip fracture
      ii. Women account for 80% of all hospitalizations for fracture
         1. 77% for hip fractures
10. Prevalence of Osteoporosis and Osteopenia
    a. World Health Organization (WHO) definitions
       i. Osteopenia in women

         1. A bone mineral density (BMD) between 1.0 and 2.5 standard deviations below the mean for young adult women

      ii. Osteoporosis in women

         1. A BMD equal to or greater than 2.5 standard deviations below the young adult mean

         2. Established osteoporosis

            a. Women in the above group who already have experienced one or more fractures

  b. Prevalence

      i. Estimates in white women using a combination of BMD at the hip, spine, and radius

         1. 30% US postmenopausal aged 50 or older have osteoporosis

         2. 54% have low bone mass

         3. Risk of fracture due to low BMD approaches or exceeds

            a. Hypertension

            b. Diabetes

            c. High blood cholesterol

      ii. Using a BMD value derived from young males for the total hip

         1. 4% of all US males over 50 have osteoporosis

         2. 33% have low bone mass

         3. About 10 million men affected

         4. 40–50% higher if BMD of the femoral neck used

      iii. Estimated prevalence varies by

         1. The measurement technique or skeletal site used

         2. The selection of a normal reference population

         3. The variability of the measurement technique

      iv. T-scores

         1. Useful for estimating and comparing prevalence among populations

         2. Arbitrary cut-off points

         3. Little evidence for a BMD threshold at which fractures occur

11. Pathophysiology

  a. Bone remodeling

      i. Maintains biomechanical integrity of the adult skeleton

      ii. Formation and resorption are coupled temporally

         1. Occur at remodeling sites on the surfaces of cancellous bone

         2. Occur in proximity to the Haversian systems of cortical bone

      iii. Remodeling balance

         1. Quantity of bone replaced equal to the quantity removed

      iv. Remodeling imbalance (osteoporosis)

         1. A reduction in bone mass

         2. Bone resorption exceeds bone formation leading to net bone loss

            a. Periosteal resorption exceeds endosteal apposition

            b. Seen with an increase in remodeling sites

         3. Remaining tissue is normal

  b. Causes of age-related declines in bone strength
       i. A decline in mass
      ii. Alterations in geometry
     iii. Qualitative changes in bone
  c. Bone strength
       i. Bone density strongly related to the strength of bone
      ii. A correlation ($r=0.6–0.8$) between bone density and in vitro fracture
          loads
     iii. Affected by changes that accompany bone loss and aging
          1. Geometric
          2. Microarchitectural
          3. Qualitative
      iv. Older bones are weaker
          1. Independent of their lower mass
       v. Changes seen in cortical bone
          1. Decreases in thickness
          2. Increases in the porosity
          3. Microfractures accumulate
          4. Partially compensated by periosteal bone apposition
             a. Increases bone size and strength
      vi. Changes seen in trabecular bone
          1. Thinning
          2. Perforation
          3. Reduction in the number and connectivity of the trabecular plates
          4. Microfractures accumulate
     vii. Disproportionately large loss of strength as bone mass declines
          1. Loads generated during normal activities can exceed fracture loads
  d. Bone loss
       i. A gradual age-related process
          1. Begins by the fourth or fifth decade
          2. By age 80
             a. Women have lost 40% of their peak adult bone mass
             b. Men have lost 25% of their peak adult bone mass
          3. Changes in mineral metabolism and bone-cell function
      ii. Accelerates after menopause for a period of 5–15 years
          1. Due to a cessation of ovarian function and estrogen deficiency
          2. Bone loss seen in up to 25 years after menopause
     iii. Triggers for bone loss
          1. Increased local production of bone-resorbing cytokines
          2. Accelerated turnover
          3. A remodeling imbalance
          4. Low serum estradiol levels
             a. Levels <5 pg/ml (mean age 72)
                i. Increased risk of hip and vertebral fracture

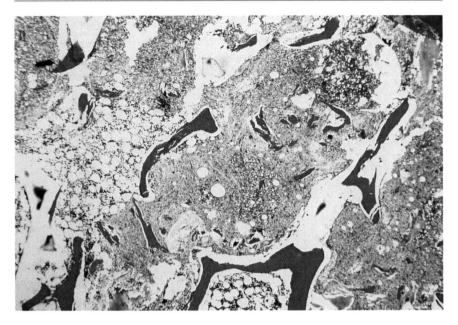

Fig. 23.3 The two cardinal features of the histopathology of osteoporosis are decreased bone mass from thinning of the trabeculae and loss of microarchitectural connectivity (Reproduced with permission from Diseases of bone and connective tissue. *Atlas of Rheumatology*. ImagesMD; 2005-01-18)

    b. Increases fracture risk in late postmenopausal women
    c. Effects calcium homeostasis
    d. Downregulates bone growth factors
    e. Strong associations
        i. Low bone mineral density
        ii. High bone turnover
        iii. Increased fracture risk in elderly men
            1. No association with testosterone deficiency
    iv. Other age-related changes
        1. Decreases in vitamin D production
        2. Changes in vitamin D metabolism
        3. Deficiencies in calcium intake and absorption
        4. Secondary hyperparathyroidism
            a. Stimulates bone resorption
        5. Decreased osteoblast function and bone formation
12. Genetic, Gender, and Racial/Ethnic Differences
    a. Bone mass at age 70 is a combination of
        i. Peak bone mass achieved as a young adult
        ii. Subsequent bone loss

b. Peak bone mass
   i. Determined largely by genetics
      1. Accounts for 70–80% of the interindividual variation
         a. Twin studies
      2. Specific genes undefined
   ii. Impacted by environmental factors
      1. Especially diet and mechanical load
      2. Calcium supplementation
         a. Increases bone accretion in adolescent females
         b. Gains do **not** persist after supplements stopped
c. Bone size and mass
   i. Gender differences do not appear until the onset of puberty
   ii. By young adulthood most males have larger and thicker bones than females
      1. A bone strength advantage
      2. Part of the lower fracture risk among men later in life
   iii. Age-related bone loss at the hip greater in women than in men
d. Osteoporosis in men
   i. **NOT** a rare disease
   ii. Fracture risk
      1. A 60-year-old man has a 25% lifetime risk of developing an osteoporotic fracture
      2. About 30% of all hip fractures worldwide occur in men
      3. There are no adequate data available to determine what level of bone loss significantly increases a man's risk of developing fragility fractures
   iii. Diagnosing osteoporosis in men
      1. Use the same diagnostic criteria in men as women
      2. T-score of −2.5 or less have osteoporosis
   iv. Treatment
      1. Use the same non-pharmacologic and pharmacologic measures in men as women
      2. Treat hypogonadal males with androgen replacement therapy
e. Geographic variability in hip fracture rates
   i. Highest incidence
      1. >6 per 1,000 per year
      2. White populations of Northern Europe and North America
   ii. Intermediate rates
      1. 4–6 per 1,000 per year
      2. Great Britain, New Zealand, and Finland
   iii. Lowest rates
      1. 2–3 per 1,000 per year
      2. Hong Kong, China, Japan, and Asia
   iv. Other contributions to geographic variability
      1. Lifestyle factors
      2. Level of economic development

13. Risk factors for osteoporosis
    a. Non-modifiable
       i. Age
       ii. Race
          1. Caucasian
          2. Asian
       iii. Female gender
       iv. Early menopause
          1. <45 years old
       v. Slender build
          1. <127 lb
       vi. Positive family history
    b. Modifiable
       i. Low calcium intake
       ii. Low vitamin D intake
       iii. Estrogen deficiency
       iv. Sedentary lifestyle
       v. Cigarette smoking
       vi. Alcohol excess
          1. >2 drinks/day
       vii. Caffeine excess
          1. >2 servings/day
       viii. Medications
          1. Excess thyroxine
          2. Glucocorticoids
             a. Supraphysiologic doses (>7 mg/day)
                i. Directly inhibit osteoblastic bone formation
                ii. Impair intestinal calcium absorption
                iii. Promote renal calcium excretion
                   1. Lowers serum calcium levels sufficiently to increase the secretion of PTH
                      a. PTH stimulates bone resorption
                iv. Impair secretion of gonadal steroids
                   1. Further increases bone resorption
             b. Bone formation and bone resorption both affected
                i. Significant bone loss and fracture within 6 months of therapy initiation
                ii. Fracture at T-scores lower than senile osteoporosis
                   1. T-Score < −1.5
                      a. 30–50%
                      b. 15% within the first year
             c. Inhaled corticosteroids
                i. Doses greater than 1,200 ug of triamcinolone acetonide or equivalent
                   1. Mild increases in bone turnover markers
                   2. **Insignificant** changes in spine and femoral neck BMD

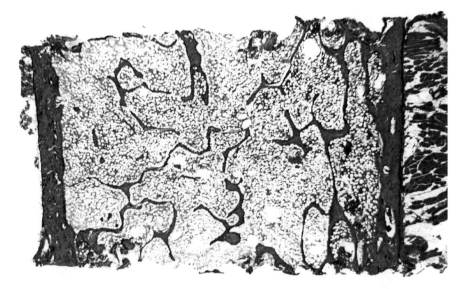

Fig. 23.4 This histological section from a patient with corticosteroid-induced osteoporosis demonstrates thin trabeculae with a well-preserved distribution and connectivity within the marrow spaces (Reproduced with permission from Bone microarchitecture in males with corticosteroid-induced osteoporosis. *Osteoporosis International.* DOI: 10.1007/s00198-006-0278-8. Springer; 2007-02-28)

Section B: Clinical and Laboratory Features

1. Diagnostic Studies in Osteoporosis
   a. Low bone mass
      i. Association with risk of future fracture
         1. Greater than elevated cholesterol or hypertension in predicting MI or stroke
         2. Regardless of race or gender
      ii. Bone densitometry
         1. Identifies individuals with low bone mass
         2. Historical and lifestyle risk factors not reliable
   b. Rule out other causes osteoporosis
      i. Hyperparathyroidism
      ii. Hyperthyroidism
      iii. Hypogonadism
      iv. Cushing's syndrome
      v. Liver disease
      vi. Multiple myeloma
      vii. RA
      viii. Renal Failure
      ix. Alcoholism

      x. COPD

     xi. IBD

    xii. Osteomalacia

   xiii. Osteogenesis imperfecta

   xiv. Medications

        1. Corticosteroids

        2. Cyclosporine

        3. Dilantin

        4. Antiseizure meds

        5. Heparin

        6. Thyroxine

c. Normal lab tests with osteoporosis as the primary reason for low BMD

       i. CBC

      ii. ESR

     iii. Alkaline phosphatase

     iv. Serum calcium and phosphorus

      v. Serum creatinine

     vi. Serum CO_2 and chloride

    vii. TSH

   viii. Testosterone

     ix. 24-hour urine calcium and creatinine

        1. Phosphorus if osteomalacia

d. WHO Criteria for the Diagnosis of Osteoporosis (1994)

       i. Based on comparisons to peak adult bone mass (PABM) from a population of Caucasian postmenopausal women

        1. T-scores

          a. Number of SD the patient's value is below or above the mean value for young normal subjects' PABM

            i. T-score of −2.0

              1. 2 SDs below normal

            ii. T-score of > -1.0

              1. Normal

          b. Major strength of the WHO criteria

            i. Young, normal BMD as the comparison level

            ii. Recognizes the prevalence of the problem

        2. Does **NOT** compare to individuals of similar age and gender

          a. Not everyone loses bone as they age

        3. Z scores

          a. Comparison of bone mass to age-matched subjects

          b. Number of SDs below or above the mean value for age-matched normal subjects

          c. Indicates whether bone mass is appropriate for age or other factors may account for low bone mass

            i. Useful for the growing child or adolescent

            ii. Prior to the acquisition of PABM

      d. Age-similar standards in the diagnosis of osteoporosis
         i. Prevalence would not increase with age
         ii. Osteoporosis would be underestimated
    4. Absolute BMD
      a. Actual bone density value expressed in g/cm^2
      b. Best parameter for percent changes during longitudinal follow-up
ii. WHO definition of osteoporosis
    1. 2.5 standard deviations below PABM
    2. T-score of −2.5 (even in the absence of a fracture) with a normal Z-score
      a. Indicates that age (and menopause) are the most important factors causing the low BMD
    3. A characteristic osteoporotic fracture
    4. Identifies certain individuals with high fracture risks
iii. WHO criteria for osteopenia
    1. T-score between −1.0 and −2.5
    2. A lower risk for fracture than those with osteoporosis
    3. Requires evaluation and possible treatment
    4. Identifies certain individuals
      a. Vertebral fractures occur at osteopenic BMD
         i. Corticosteroid treatment
      b. High bone turnover
         i. Identified by biochemical markers
      c. Increased risk of falling
      d. Advanced age
iv. Shortcomings of the WHO criteria
    1. Criteria based entirely on BMD
    2. Does not consider other components of fracture risk
    3. Low BMD does not necessarily indicate on-going bone loss
    4. Imperfect in predicting a given individual's risk
    5. Does not account for changes in bone microarchitecture
      a. Also influences bone strength and fracture risk
      b. Low bone mass not always osteoporosis
    6. Disparities among values at different sites with different methods
      a. T-scores
         i. Calculations based on inconsistent reference population databases
         ii. Differences observed from 11 FDA-approved peripheral BMD/US devices
    7. Bone densitometry cannot distinguish among causes of low bone mass
    8. Applies only to Caucasian postmenopausal women
v. WHO criteria provides the clinician with
    1. An objective number for the diagnosis of osteoporosis
    2. Objective thresholds for the institution of treatment
      a. Regardless of the presence of other risk factors
    3. The National Osteoporosis Foundation recommends treatment at a T-score of −2 and below

      vi. The National Health and Nutrition Examination Survey III (NHANES III)
- 1. Reference population established by WHO for osteoporosis of the total hip and femoral neck
- 2. Composed of men and women from many ethnic groups
- 3. Data useful for
  - a. Diagnosing osteoporosis at the hip
  - b. Standardized results
    - i. Incorporated into software for the three major manufacturers of dual energy x-ray absorptiometry (DEXA) machines
  - c. The relationship between BMD and hip fracture risk for elderly Caucasian women

   vii. WHO criteria in **premenopausal** women
- 1. Low bone mass
  - a. **DO NOT** have an increased risk of fracture
    - i. Even when compared to age-matched controls with normal bone mass
  - b. Probably never reached PABM
  - c. Generally healthy
  - d. Normal rates of bone remodeling
  - e. With menopause
    - i. Bone turnover usually increases
    - ii. Remodeling space increases
    - iii. Fracture risk may increase with changes
- 2. Consider secondary causes for exceptionally low bone mass
  - a. Not standard of care to obtain a bone mass measurement

2. Bone Mass Measurements
- a. Indications for bone mass measurements
  - i. To diagnose osteopenia or osteoporosis
  - ii. Predict fracture risk
  - iii. Monitor the response of BMD to therapy
- b. Recommendations by the National Osteoporosis Foundation for screening
  - i. Women age 65 and older
  - ii. Postmenopausal women under age 65 with other risk factors
  - iii. Postmenopausal women with fractures
  - iv. Women considering therapy for osteoporosis
  - v. Women on hormone replacement therapy for prolonged periods
- c. Medicare indications for bone densitometry utilization
  - i. Estrogen deficiency plus one risk factor for osteoporosis
  - ii. Radiographic findings
    - 1. Vertebral deformity
    - 2. Fracture
    - 3. Osteopenia
  - iii. Primary hyperparathyroidism
  - iv. Glucocorticoid therapy
    - 1. ≥7.5 mg/day of prednisone for ≥3 months
  - v. Monitoring the response to an FDA-approved osteoporosis medication

d. Two major categories of bone densitometry devices based on sites evaluated
   i. Central skeleton
     1. Spine and hip
       a. Best predictors of fracture risk
       b. L2-L4 most frequently evaluated
       c. Best precision for longitudinal monitoring
     2. DEXA measurement
       a. Total body bone mass
       b. Body composition
       c. Vertebral morphometry
   ii. Peripheral skeleton
     1. Finger
     2. Heel
     3. Tibia
     4. Wrist/forearm
     5. Measured by
       a. Quantitative ultrasound (QUS)
       b. Peripheral quantitative computed tomography (pQCT)
       c. Peripheral DEXA (pDEXA)
     6. Peripheral devices
       a. Precise and accurate
       b. More widely available
       c. Less expensive
       d. Popular as a screening tool
          i. Adequate in many patients
          ii. Technique less sensitive in diagnosing osteoporosis than central densitometry
       e. Consider follow-up central densitometry if
          i. History of fragility fractures
          ii. Two or more risk factors for bone loss
          iii. Medical conditions associated with bone loss
          iv. Medications that cause bone loss
          v. Postmenopausal women not on estrogens being considered for treatment
e. Bone densitometry devices
   i. Most accurate and widely used
     1. DEXA
       a. Best accuracy and precision with the least radiation exposure
          i. Radiation exposure
             1. About 2 μSv per site
             2. CXR = 100 μSv
          ii. Precision error
             1. Ranges from <1–3% CV
             2. Total body (<1% CV)
             3. Lateral spine (2–3% CV)

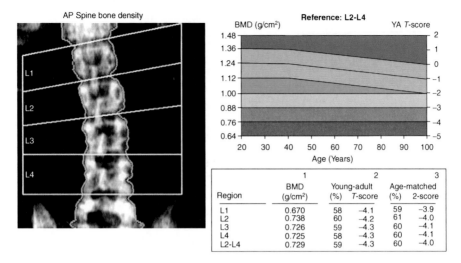

AP Spine bone density

Reference: L2-L4

Region	BMD (g/cm²)	Young-adult (%)	T-score	Age-matched (%)	2-score
L1	0.670	58	−4.1	59	−3.9
L2	0.738	60	−4.2	61	−4.0
L3	0.726	59	−4.3	60	−4.1
L4	0.725	58	−4.3	60	−4.1
L2-L4	0.729	59	−4.3	60	−4.0

Fig. 23.5 DEXA scan of spine with severe osteoporosis (Reproduced with permission from Presentation and diagnosis of primary hyperparathyroidism. *Endocrine Surgery.* DOI: 10.1007/978-1-84628-881-4_16. Springer; 2009-01-01)

  b. NOT recommendations for BMD screening

  c. Medicare indications for bone densitometry utilization

 2. CT

 3. US

ii. Least radiation dose exposure

 1. QUS (0 μSv)

  a. Calcaneus

  b. Tibia

 2. Single-energy x-ray absorptiometry (SEXA) (<1 μSv)

  a. Radius

  b. Calcaneus

 3. pDEXA (<1 μSv)

  a. Forearm

   i. Less than pQCT of the forearm (<5 μSv)

 4. Radiographic absorptiometry (RA) (<1 μSv)

iii. Least precision error (% CV, percentage coefficient of variation)

 1. QUS of tibia (0.5% CV)

  a. Higher with calcaneus at 2–4% CV

 2. DEXA of total body (<1% CV)

 3. RA of phalanges (1.0% CV)

 4. pQCT of forearm (1.0% CV)

iv. Utility for detecting osteopenia or osteoporosis depends on

 1. Age of the patient

  a. Discrepancies more often in early postmenopausal women (50–55 years) than in women older than 65

2. Site measured
  a. Overestimation of bone mass in the spine
    i. Degenerative changes (osteophytes or facet hypertrophy) in the elderly
      1. More accurate measurement obtained from the hip
    ii. Vertebral fractures
    iii. Aortic calcification
  b. Bone mass measurement in the hip affected by
    i. Hip malposition
    ii. Including the ischium in the field of measurement
3. Bone Mass Measurements to Predict Fracture Risk
  a. Fracture risk reduction expressed as
    i. Current fracture risk within 3–5 years of BMD measurement
    ii. Lifetime fracture risk
  b. Current fracture risk increases 1.5–3.0 times for each SD reduction in BMD
    i. T-score of –1.0
      1. 12% bone loss
      2. Fracture risk two times increased
    ii. T-score of –2.0
      1. 24% bone loss
      2. Fracture risk four times increased
    iii. T-score of –3.0
      1. 36% bone loss
      2. Fracture risk eight times increased
    iv. T-score of –4.0
      1. 48% bone loss
      2. Fracture risk 16 times increased
    v. A previous fragility fracture
      1. Risk of subsequent fracture doubles again
      2. If T-score was –3
        a. Fracture risk is $2 \times 8 = 16$
  c. For osteopenia to be seen on routine radiographs
    i. 30% BMD loss
  d. In the elderly
    i. BMD correlates at different sites
    ii. Fracture risk prediction uniform
      1. Regardless of skeletal site measured or device used
        a. Except for the hip
      2. Prediction from femoral neck BMD greater than any other site
  e. In perimenopausal women
    i. Current fracture risk should not be used with or without low BMD
    ii. Fracture risk does not increase in the same way as with elderly women
  f. Lifetime risk of fracture
    i. Risk estimates of hip, wrist, or vertebral fracture
      1. 50-year-old white woman
        a. 40%

      2. 50-year-old white man

        a. 13%

      3. Not validated in longitudinal studies

    ii. Low bone mass at menopause increases the lifetime risk

4. Repeat Bone Mass Measurements

  a. Bone densitometry ideal for serial measurements of BMD

    i. Ease

    ii. Precision

    iii. Accuracy

  b. Typically use central measurement devices

    i. Areas of the skeleton rich in trabecular bone

    ii. Trabecular bone has a large surface area and high turnover rate

    iii. Responses to therapy detected over a short period of time

      1. Areas of the spine and hip

      2. Estrogen or bisphosphonate therapies

    iv. Peripheral skeletal sites composed mainly of cortical bone

  c. Significant changes in precision error for repeated measurements

    i. Beyond the least significant change represent real BMD changes

    ii. $\geq 3\%$ in the spine

    iii. $\geq 6\%$ in the femur

  d. Scans should not be performed more frequently than every 2 years

    i. "Regression to the mean"

      1. Phenomenon seen during controlled trials of antiresoptive therapies

        a. Used to assess the reduction in new vertebral and hip fractures

      2. Rates of change in BMD differed among study subjects

        a. Some subjects improved during the first year while other did not

        b. Some that improved during the first year actually lost bone mass during the second year

  e. Standardized BMD (sBMD)

    i. Developed by the Bone Densitometry Standards Committee

    ii. Serial BMD measurements on different manufacturers' instruments are difficult to compare

    iii. Improves comparisons between different instruments

    iv. For spine or total hip serial measurements

      1. Include an additional 1% precision error in calculations of the percentage change

Section C: Treatment

1. Less than 25% of patients sustaining an osteoporotic fragility fracture are evaluated for and/or placed on medical therapy for osteoporosis

2. US National Osteoporosis Foundation guidelines

  a. T-score below -2.5

    i. With no other risk factors present

    b. T-score below −2.0

       i. With one or more strong risk factors

          1. Prior fracture

3. Agents that treat osteoporosis work by reducing bone resorption

    a. Increase BMD

    b. Reduce biochemical markers of bone turnover

    c. Some show fracture reduction after 1 year of treatment

4. Bone health determinants

    a. Adequate intake of calcium

       i. 1,000 mg/day

          1. Premenopausal women and men

       ii. 1,200 mg/day

          1. Men and women over the age of 50

       iii. 1,500 mg/day

          1. Postmenopausal women

             a. Ingests only 500 mg and 600 mg from dietary sources

          2. Men ≥65 years of age

       iv. Only one-third of ingested calcium is absorbed

       v. To check absorption of a particular calcium supplement

          1. Place in vinegar to see if it dissolves in 30 min

       vi. Supplement shortfalls in dietary calcium intake

          1. MVI

          2. Calcium tablets

          3. Elixirs

    b. Adequate intake of vitamin D

       i. 400–800 units/day

    c. An active lifestyle

       i. Regular weight bearing exercise

          1. Stimulates bone formation

          2. Inhibits resorption

       ii. May reduce the incidence and severity of falls

       iii. Improves muscular strength and coordination

       iv. Walking

          1. 40 min or more

          2. Four times a week

          3. Carry light weights (1 or 2 lb)

       v. Aerobic and resistance exercise

       vi. Spinal resistance exercises

    d. Avoid cigarette smoking

    e. Avoid factors that negatively impact BMD

       i. Limit alcohol consumption to two drinks/day or less

       ii. Limit caffeine consumption to two servings/day or less

    f. Fall prevention

       i. Counsel patients to reduce their risk of falling

       ii. Avoid activities that produce undesirable forces on the skeleton

          1. High impact

          2. Pushing

        3. Pulling

        4. Bending

        5. Lifting

     iii. Institute a fall reduction program

     iv. Major risk factors for falls

        1. Use of sedatives

        2. Sensorium-altering drugs

        3. Antihypertensive medication

        4. Visual impairment

        5. Proprioceptive loss

        6. Lower-extremity disability

     v. Modifiable risk factors

        1. Remove obstacles to ambulation in the home

        2. Carpet slick surfaces and stairs

        3. Remove throw rugs and children's toys

        4. Install railings

        5. Install night lights

  g. Encourage consumption of low-fat dairy products

     i. Safest way to increase calcium intake without increasing risk of kidney stones

     ii. Major bioavailable sources

        1. Dairy products

           a. Milk 300 mg/cup (8 oz)

           b. Cheese 300 mg/oz

           c. Yogurt 300 mg/cup (8 oz)

        2. Calcium-fortified drinks

        3. General non-dairy diet contains about 300 mg

5. Calcium Supplementation

  a. Calcium carbonate

     i. Least expensive form of calcium supplement

     ii. Examples

        1. OS Cal

        2. Caltrate

        3. Tums

     iii. Divided doses of no more than 500 mg per dose (500 mg tid)

        1. With food for reliable absorption

           a. Acid buffering capacity

        2. Needs acidification for best absorption

     iv. 20% of patients experience gastrointestinal distress

        1. Upper GI gas

        2. Constipation

  b. Calcium citrate

     i. Example

        1. Citracal

     ii. Usually does not cause GI upset

      iii. Better in patients with
         1. Achlorhydria
         2. On medications that limit acid in the stomach
      iv. More expensive
   c. For patients with constipation due to calcium
      i. A calcium/magnesium preparation
      ii. Magnesium stimulates bowel motility
6. Vitamin D
   a. Essential
      i. Absorbs calcium from the GI tract and assimilates into bone
      ii. Direct effect on bone remodeling
      iii. Direct or indirect effect on muscle strength and balance
   b. Need adequate intake
      i. 400–800units/day
      ii. Assures adequate serum levels of 25-hydroxyvitamin D
   c. Sources of vitamin D
      i. Multivitamins
         1. 400 units of vitamin D per tablet
      ii. Calcium supplements
         1. 100 IU or 200 IU of vitamin D
      iii. Foods supplemented with vitamin D
         1. Milk
         2. Orange juice
   d. Vitamin D metabolism and action
      i. Two sources
         1. 90% produced in the skin by UV sunlight exposure
            a. Cutaneous precursor of vitamin D (7 dehydrocholesterol) converted into vitamin D3 (cholecalciferol)
               i. Takes only 20–30 min to start this process
               ii. Sunblock filters out the wavelength of light required for vitamin D synthesis
         2. 10% from dietary intake
            a. Dietary sources from animal and plant products
               i. D3
                   1. Main vitamin D from animal source
               ii. D2 (ergocalciferol)
                   1. Main vitamin D from plant source
               iii. Both D2 and D3
                   1. Equal potency
                   2. Equal bioavailability
      ii. A fat-soluble vitamin
         1. Absorption dependent on emulsification by bile acids
         2. Rule out malabsorption in patients with vitamin D deficiency
      iii. Metabolism in the liver
         1. Vitamin D transported to the liver by vitamin D binding protein
         2. Converted by 25 hydroxylase to 25 hydroxyvitamin D (25 OH vit D) (calcifediol)

      3. Process interfered with by
        a. Severe liver disease
        b. Isoniazid
        c. Anticonvulsants and antituberculous drugs
          i. Accelerate the inactivation of 25 OH vit D after formation
      4. The best test to determine **total body vitamin D** stores
        a. Measurement of **25 OH vitamin D**
        b. Levels less than 15 ng/ml
          i. Secondary hyperparathyroidism develops
        c. Levels less than 8 ng/ml
          i. Vitamin D deficient
    iv. Metabolism in the kidney
      1. 25 OH vitamin D hydroxylated by 1-alpha hydroxylase to 1, 25 hydroxyvitamin D (1, 25 OH vit D) (calcitriol)
        a. Hydroxylation increased by
          i. Increased parathyroid hormone levels
          ii. Hypophosphatemia
        b. Hydroxylation decreased by
          i. Renal insufficiency
            1. CrCl <30–40 ml/min
          ii. Ketoconazole
      2. 1, 25 hydroxyvitamin D **not** a good indicator of total body vitamin D stores
  e. Vitamin D deficiency
    i. 16% of healthy, ambulatory, postmenopausal women in the Southeastern USA
    ii. 50% of hip fracture patients in Boston
    iii. In recently menopausal women
7. Pharmacological intervention for at-risk patients
  a. In older women
    i. Calcium and vitamin D
      1. Shown to prevent bone loss
      2. Reduces the risk of spine and nonspine fractures
  b. In patients taking glucocorticoid therapy
    i. Calcium (1,500 mg/day) and vitamin D (800 units/day)
    ii. If urinary calcium excretion exceeds 300 mg/day
      1. Add a thiazide diuretic
    iii. For patients on 7.5 mg/day for at least 3 months
      1. Particularly postmenopausal women
      2. Individuals who have T-scores of −1.0 or less
      3. Those who have had fragility fractures
    iv. Bisphosphonates
      1. The agents of choice for the prevention and treatment of glucocorticoid induced osteoporosis
      2. Alendronate, risedronate, and etidronate
      3. Significantly increase bone mass

     v. Calcitonin
       1. Also used
       2. Effects less than those seen with bisphosphonates
     vi. Associated hypogonadism
       1. Gonadal steroid replacement
8. Two major categories of pharmacologic agents for osteoporosis
  a. Bone resorption–inhibiting agents
    i. Estrogen
    ii. Bisphosphonates
    iii. Raloxifene
    iv. Calcitonin
    v. Widely used
    vi. Repeatedly demonstrated efficacy and safety
    vii. Characteristically increase bone mass during the first 12–24 months
    viii. Stabilize at a constant level thereafter
    ix. Reduce bone resorption without affecting bone formation
      1. Bone formation temporarily exceeds resorption
        a. Bone mass increases
        b. Referred to as the bone remodeling transient
      2. Bone formation gradually declines to the level of resorption
        a. After 12–24 months
        b. Bone mass stabilizes
  b. Bone formation–stimulating agents
    i. Fluoride
    ii. Androgens
    iii. Growth hormone
    iv. Parathyroid hormone
    v. Typically a progressive linear increase in bone mass
9. Markers to assess bone remodeling
  a. Bone formation
    i. Serum alkaline phosphatase
    ii. Serum osteocalcin
  b. Bone resorption
    i. Urine N-telopeptides (NTX)
      1. Provides an estimate of bone turnover
      2. A breakdown product of type I collagen in bone
      3. 24-hour urine or second voided morning spot urine
        a. 15% average value difference between the two methods
      4. Normal urine NTX
        a. 20–65 BCE/mmol Cr
      5. Predicts loss of bone mineral density over the next year
        a. > 50 BCE/mmol Cr
      6. Represents good control on present therapy
        a. Between 20 and 35 BCE/mmol Cr
    ii. Serum N-telopeptides
    iii. Urine pyridinoline crosslinks

10. Bisphosphonates
    a. Share a common chemical structure
        i. Two phosphonic acids joined to a carbon
        ii. Bind avidly to hydroxyapatite crystals on the surfaces of bone
    b. Mechanism of action
        i. Resist metabolic degradation
        ii. Reduce the ability of individual osteoclasts to resorb bone
        iii. Reduce the total number of osteoclasts
        iv. Accelerate osteoclast apoptosis
        v. Remarkably free from systemic toxicity
        vi. Very poor intestinal absorption
            1. Further inhibited by the presence of food or medications
    c. Major side effect
        i. Esophageal/GI pain
            1. Contains nitrogen which can be irritating to the esophagus
            2. Avoid reflux
            3. Minimize by taking the medications first thing each morning on an empty stomach with a full glass of water
            4. Remain upright and take nothing by mouth for at least 30 min after ingestion
        ii. Do not give to patients
            1. With active upper GI disease
            2. Who develop upper GI complaints
            3. Who are unable to be upright after ingestion
    d. FDA-approved for the prevention and treatment of postmenopausal osteoporosis
        i. Alendronate
        ii. Risedronate
        iii. Both have proven anti-fracture efficacy at both the spine and the hip
    e. Alendronate
        i. First bisphosphonate approved by the FDA
        ii. Study results
            1. Early Postmenopausal Intervention Cohort (EPIC)
                a. 2,357 patients in early 50s without osteoporosis
                b. 5-mg alendronate daily
                c. Effective in preventing accelerated bone loss that occurs in the early postmenopausal period
            2. Phase III trial
                a. 1,000 women in late 60s with established osteoporosis
                b. 10-mg alendronate daily
                c. Increased spinal bone density by 10% after 3 years
                d. About 4% average change in BMD at the femoral neck with no change at the forearm
            3. Fracture Intervention Trial (FIT)

      a. 2,000 women with low femoral neck BMD and prevalent vertebral fractures

      b. Significantly reduced the frequency of vertebral, hip, and wrist fractures

    4. Bone mass increments reported over a 2–3-year period

      a. Spine (7–8%)

      b. Hip (5–6%)

    5. Observed reduction in fracture incidence

      a. Spine (47–50%)

      b. Hip (51–56%)

  iii. FDA-approved dosing

    1. For treatment of bone loss in recently menopausal women

      a. 5 mg/day

      b. 35 mg once weekly

    2. For treatment of postmenopausal osteoporosis

      a. 10 mg/day

      b. 70 mg once weekly

    3. For treatment of corticosteroid-induced osteoporosis

      a. 5 mg/day for men and estrogen-replete women

      b. 10 mg daily for estrogen-deficient women

    4. Once-a-week preparations

      a. Provide a more convenient dosing regimen

      b. Similar to the daily dose regimen in

        i. Efficacy

        ii. Toxicity

        iii. Cost

f. Risedronate

  i. A nitrogen-containing pyridinyl bisphosphonate

  ii. Two pivotal studies

    1. More than 3,600 women with low BMD and prevalent vertebral fractures

      a. Primary endpoint new vertebral fractures

        i. Reduced by 41–49% after only 1 year

      b. Secondary endpoint nonvertebral fractures

        i. Reduced by 33–39%

      c. Significantly increased BMD at the spine and hip

    2. Nearly 9,500 postmenopausal women who had low BMD

      a. One of the largest trials of osteoporosis

      b. Produced a significant reduction in hip fractures

      c. A subgroup of elderly women did **not** show benefit

        i. With clinical risk factors for fracture

        ii. Without low BMD

  iii. Clinical trials

    1. Almost 16,000 subjects

    2. Well tolerated

        3. Adverse events no different from those of placebo

        4. Good GI tolerability

        5. Approved for prevention and treatment of

           a. Postmenopausal osteoporosis

           b. Corticosteroid-induced osteoporosis

        6. Reported bone mass increments observed over a 2–3 year period

           a. Spine (4–5%)

           b. Hip (2–3%)

        7. Observed reductions in fracture incidence

           a. Spine (33–46%)

           b. Hip (8–58%)

    iv. Dosing

        1. Essentially the same as for alendronate

        2. 5 mg daily for all indications

        3. Similar levels compared with an overnight fast when

           a. Taken 2 h before or after a meal

           b. At least 30 min before retiring in the evening

g. Other bisphosphonates

    i. Not approved by the FDA

    ii. Used "off-label" for osteoporosis

    iii. Etidronate

        1. Shown to increase BMD in two prospective, randomized, controlled trials of women with postmenopausal osteoporosis

        2. Administered in an intermittent cyclic regimen

           a. 200 mg BID 14 days every 3 months

           b. Must be taken on an empty stomach

           c. Between meals, at bedtime, or during the night

    iv. Pamidronate

        1. Given by IV infusion

        2. Typical regimen

           a. Initial dose of 90 mg

           b. Subsequent doses of 30 mg every third month

           c. Infuse over 60 min

        3. Useful for those who cannot tolerate oral bisphosphonates

11. Calcitonin

a. A peptide hormone secreted by specialized cells in the thyroid

b. Acts directly on osteoclasts to reduce bone resorption

    i. Binds to specific osteoclast receptors

c. Salmon calcitonin

    i. More potent and longer duration of action than human

    ii. Available since 1984

    iii. Dosing

        1. 50–100 IU daily

        2. Subcutaneous injections

      iv. Results in slight gains in BMD
          1. Less than that achieved with estrogen or bisphosphonates
          2. Greatest effect in those with rapid bone turnover
      v. Effects compromised by
          1. Development of neutralizing antibodies
          2. Downregulation of receptors
      vi. Not widely used
          1. Limited and transient effectiveness
          2. Inconvenience and discomfort of injections
          3. Relatively high cost
          4. Limited tolerance
             a. 20% develop nausea or flushing
             b. Skin irritation with injections
  d. Nasal calcitonin
      i. Introduced in 1995
      ii. Better tolerated than the subcutaneous form
      iii. Recommended daily dose
          1. 200 IU
          2. One spray
      iv. Clinical study
          1. 5 year, multicenter, double-blind, placebo-controlled
          2. 1,255 women with postmenopausal osteoporosis
          3. Modest improvement in spinal bone mass
          4. 36% reduction in the incidence of spinal fractures
          5. No effect on the incidence of
             a. Hip fracture
             b. Other nonvertebral fracture
             c. Not sufficient power to show this difference
      v. Extremely well tolerated
      vi. No concerns regarding long-term safety
      vii. Mild to moderate analgesic effect
          1. An important side benefit
          2. Particularly those with acute painful vertebral fractures
  e. Reported bone mass increments observed over a 2–3 year period
      i. Spine (0–1%)
      ii. Hip (0%)
  f. Observed reductions in fracture incidence
      i. Spine (33%)
      ii. Hip (0%)
12. Estrogen
  a. An effective agent for preventing bone loss in recently menopausal women
  b. Postmenopausal Estrogen and Progestin Intervention (PEPI)
      i. 875 recently menopausal women
      ii. Randomized to groups receiving estrogen (with or without progestin) or placebo
      iii. Women receiving estrogen showed approximately 5% increase in spinal BMD over 3 years

   c. Shown to increase bone mass
      i. 5–10% when started after age 65 years
     ii. 5–6% observed in the spine over a 2–3-year period
    iii. 3–4% observed in the hip over a 2–3-year period
    iv. Must be continued to maintain benefits
        a. Once stopped bone mass levels drop quickly
   d. Shown to reduce fracture risk
      i. Small prospective and large cross-sectional studies
     ii. 25–50% fewer spine and hip fractures
    iii. 42% fewer in the spine over a 2–3-year period
   e. A variety of extraskeletal effects
      i. Relieves symptoms of estrogen deficiency
        1. Hot flashes
        2. Vaginal dryness
     ii. Increased risk of cardiovascular events in women with established coronary disease
    iii. A decreased risk for Alzheimer's disease and colon cancer
        1. Cross-sectional studies
    iv. Small but significant risk of venous thromboembolic events
     v. Slight increase risk for breast cancer
   f. Dosing
      i. Esterified estrogens show a typical dose response
        1. 0.3 mg daily effective for preventing bone loss
        2. 0.625 mg daily provide gains in BMD
        3. 1.25 mg daily provide further gains
     ii. Hormone preparations commonly used
        1. Conjugated estrogens (Premarin and Estratabs)
          a. Premarin 0.625–1.25 mg a day or days 1–25
        2. Estradiol (Estrace)
          a. 0.5–1.0 mg a day or days 1–25
        3. Estradiol patch (Estraderm, Vivelle, Climara)
          a. 0.05–0.1 mg patch twice a week
        4. Combination pills (Prempro, Premphase)
          a. 0.625/2.5 or 5.0 mg (Premarin/Provera) a day
          b. Or 0.625 (Premarin) days 1–14
            i. Then 0.625/5.0 mg (Premarin/Provera) days 15–25
        5. Combination patch (Combipatch)
          a. 0.05/0.14 mg or 0.05/0.25 mg patch twice a week
        6. Medroxyprogesterone (Provera)
          a. 2.5–5 mg a day or 5–10 mg days 15–25
    iii. Adding a progestin to estrogen protects the endometrium from the effects of unopposed estrogen
        1. Women with an intact uterus must take estrogen in combination with progesterone (either cyclically or daily)
        2. Progestins may increase the risk of breast cancer more than estrogen alone

iv. Poor long-term compliance to estrogen
  1. Only 15% of women who would benefit from estrogen are actually taking the medication
  2. 30–50% of prescriptions are never filled
  3. Only 20% who are taking estrogen are still taking it 3–5 years later
v. Contraindicated in
  1. Those who might be pregnant
  2. Those with undiagnosed genital bleeding
  3. Known or suspected cancer of the breast
  4. Known or suspected estrogen-dependent neoplasm
  5. Active thrombophlebitis or thromboembolic disorder

13. Selective Estrogen-Receptor Modulator (SERM)
  a. Agents that function as estrogen agonists in some tissues and estrogen antagonists in other tissues
    i. Different expression of estrogen-regulated genes in different tissues
  b. Raloxifene
    i. Example of a SERM
    ii. Dosed at 60 mg a day
    iii. Shown to improve bone mass and to reduce spine fractures
    iv. FDA-approved for the treatment of postmenopausal osteoporosis
      1. Study of 607 recently menopausal women
      2. Prevented bone loss
      3. Generally well tolerated
    v. Side effects
      1. Increase in leg cramps
      2. Increase in hot flashes
      3. Increased risk of thromboembolic disease
        a. Similar to hormone replacement therapy
    vi. MORE Study (Multiple Outcomes of Raloxifene Evaluation)
      1. 7,705 women
      2. Bone density slightly but significantly increased in the spine and hip
      3. Risk of new vertebral fractures reduced by 30–50%
      4. No effect on hip fracture or other nonvertebral fracture
        a. Not powered to show this effect
    vii. Extraskeletal effects
      1. Favorable changes in lipids
        a. Decreases LDL
        b. Neutral effects on HDL and triglycerides
      2. Small but significant increased risk of venous thrombosis
        a. Similar to that of estrogen
      3. Associated with 70% fewer cases of breast cancer
        a. Known anti-estrogen effect on breast tissue

14. Combinations Therapy for Osteoporosis
  a. Produces increment in bone mass greater than those observed when the drugs are used alone

  i. Bisphosphonates and estrogens
  ii. Bisphosphonates and raloxifene
 b. Leads to normal bone histomorphometry
 c. Likely to reduce fractures to a greater degree than that seen with single drug therapy
 d. Coherence Therapy
  i. Anti-resorptive medication used in combination with or alternating with a bone formation–stimulating agent
  ii. Increases bone mass significantly more than any single agent alone
  iii. Anti-fracture efficacy not demonstrated
  iv. Combinations
   1. Alendronate with parathyroid hormone (PTH)
   2. Estrogens with PTH
15. PTH
 a. A bone formation–stimulating agent
 b. Stimulates both bone formation and bone resorption in humans
 c. Hyperparathyroidism
  i. Persistently elevated serum PTH levels
  ii. Stimulates bone resorption more than formation
  iii. Causes bone loss
 d. As single daily injections
  i. Transient PTH bursts disproportionately enhance bone formation
  ii. Bone mass increments over 1–2-year study periods
   1. 15% in the lumbar spine
   2. 5% in the hip
  iii. Decreased vertebral fracture risk
   1. Reported as much as 65%
  iv. No data sufficiently powered to assess hip fractures
   1. Likely reduced based on normal histomorphometry reports
16. Sodium Fluoride
 a. Directly stimulates osteoblasts
 b. Reported to increase bone mass by 16–24% over a 4 year period
 c. Fracture reduction efficacy disappointing
 d. Not FDA-approved for osteoporosis
  i. Lack consistent anti-fracture efficacy
  ii. No long-term safety data
 e. Side effects
  i. Symptomatic gastritis
   1. 20–30% of patients on 50 mg/day
   2. 50% of patients on 75 mg/day
  ii. Painful lower extremity syndrome
   1. Acute pain, tenderness, and swelling
   2. Particularly involves the heels and ankles
   3. Occurs in many patients
   4. Appears to be due to the development of stress fractures

      5. Probably related to rapid bone turnover
      6. Treatment
         a. Discontinue the medication
         b. Rest and analgesia
         c. Resolution usually in 6–8 weeks
      7. Tends not to recur if later re-instituted
   iii. Slow release preparation
      1. Lower incidence of all side effects

17. Androgens
  a. Anabolic agents that stimulate osteoblastic bone formation
  b. Methyltestosterone
     i. Given at 2.5 mg/day in combination with estrogens
    ii. For postmenopausal women
   iii. Increases bone mass significantly more than estrogens alone
   iv. Improved anti-fracture efficacy not demonstrated
    v. Side effects
      1. Hirsutism
      2. Acne
      3. Temporal balding
      4. Dose related
         a. Mild or absent with lower doses
  c. Testosterone replacement therapy
     i. Significantly increases skeletal mass in hypogonadal males
    ii. Not been shown to have a beneficial effect in eugonadal males

18. Growth Hormone (GH)
  a. An anabolic agent that promotes bone formation
  b. Clearly beneficial in children and adults with GH deficiency
  c. Moderate effects in women with postmenopausal and senile osteoporosis
  d. Costly
  e. Side effects
     i. Arthralgias
    ii. Acral enlargement
   iii. Hyperglycemia
   iv. Hypertension
  f. Insulin-like growth factor-1
     i. Beneficial effects on bone remodeling

19. Vertebroplasty and Kyphoplasty
  a. For patients with painful or deforming vertebral fractures
  b. Vertebroplasty
     i. Percutaneous injection of bone cement (polymethylmethacrylate-PMMA) under radiologic guidance
    ii. Successful for pain relief
   iii. Does not restore vertebral height
   iv. High rates of cement leakage

   c. Kyphoplasty
      i. Percutaneous placement of an inflatable balloon into the fractured vertebral body
      ii. Results in the elevation of depressed vertebral body endplates
      iii. Restores vertebral body height
      iv. Balloon is removed and PMMA injected under low pressure
      v. Less cement extravasation
   d. For select patients
      i. Patient with a recent vertebral fracture is the ideal candidate
      ii. Older vertebral fractures with no evidence of bone marrow edema on MRI less likely to respond
   e. Should be performed by experienced operators

Metabolic Bone Disorders

24

1. Osteomalacia
   a. Word means "soft bones"
   b. Impaired mineralization (deposition of hydroxyapatite) in **mature** bone
   c. Pathogenesis
      i. Inadequate concentration of extracellular fluid phosphate and/or calcium
      ii. A circulating inhibitor of mineralization
   d. Major causes
      i. Vitamin D deficiency
         1. Low oral intake plus inadequate sunlight exposure
         2. Intestinal malabsorption
      ii. Abnormal vitamin D metabolism
         1. Liver disease
         2. Renal disease
         3. Drugs
            a. Anticonvulsants
            b. Antituberculous drugs
            c. Ketoconazole
      iii. Hypophosphatemia
         1. Low oral phosphate intake
         2. Phosphate-binding antacids
         3. Excess renal phophate loss
      iv. Inhibitors of mineralization
         1. Aluminum
         2. Bisphosphonates
         3. Fluoride
      v. Hypophosphatasia
         1. A rare congenital disorder
         2. Caused by mutations in the gene that codes for the alkaline phosphatase isoform found in cartilage and bone
         3. Affected patients present with
            a. Osteomalacia

N.T. Colburn, *Review of Rheumatology*,
DOI 10.1007/978-1-84882-093-7_24, © Springer-Verlag London Limited 2012

  b. Rickets
     i. Low serum alkaline phosphatase levels
     ii. Mineralization defect
     iii. Inability to break down inorganic pyrophosphate
          1. A known inhibitor of mineralization
  4. Frequently severe and often fatal
  5. Milder forms may be asymptomatic until adulthood
  6. No known effective treatment
e. Clinical manifestations
   i. Pain and deformity
      1. Particularly in the long bones and pelvis
   ii. "Waddling gait"
f. Radiographs
   i. Characteristic pseudofractures
      1. Located at points where large arteries cross bones
   ii. "Milkman's fractures"
   iii. "Looser's zones"
        1. Fractures on the compression side of bone
g. Laboratory abnormalities
   i. **Low** serum calcium and/or phosphorous
   ii. **Elevated** serum alkaline phosphatase
   iii. **Low** serum 25-hydroxyvitamin D levels

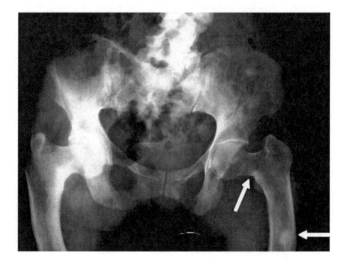

Fig. 24.1 Radiographs demonstrate diminished bone density with cortical thinning, bilateral coxa vara, Looser zones of the left femoral neck, and body of the left femur (*arrows*), all of which establish the diagnosis of osteomalacia (Reproduced with permission from Systematic approach to metabolic diseases of bone.*Diagnostic Imaging of Musculoskeletal Diseases.* DOI:10.1007/978-1-59745-355-4_2. Springer; 2009-01-01)

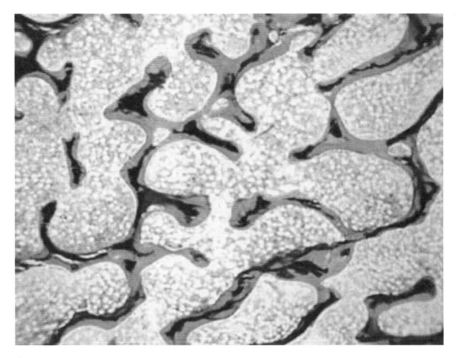

Fig. 24.2 Features of osteomalacia demonstrated in this photomicrograph with toluidine blue stain. The mineralized bone stains dark blue and the thickened osteoid is in light blue. (40x magnification enhanced) (Reproduced with permission from Bone histomorphometry and undecalcified sections.*Bone Pathology.* DOI:10.1007/978-1-59745-347-9_8. Springer; 2009-01-01)

      iv. **Low** urinary calcium excretion
         1. Any patient with a 24-hour urine calcium less than 50 mg/total volume should be investigated for vitamin D deficiency
      v. **Elevated** PTH levels
      vi. **Low** serum phosphorous and **elevated** urinary phosphorus excretion
         1. Osteomalacia due to phosphate wasting
   h. Histology
      i. Increased amount of osteoid
      ii. Deficient hydroxyapatite deposition
 2. Rickets
   a. Impaired mineralization of the skeleton during childhood
   b. Result from the same conditions that cause osteomalacia in adults as above
   c. Three congenital disorders
      i. Hypophosphatemic rickets
         1. An inherited disorder
            a. Most commonly X-linked

        2. Excessive renal tubular phosphate losses
          a. Serum phosphorus levels too low to allow normal bone mineralization
          b. Normal bone mineralization requires a calcium times phosphorus product of 24
     ii. Congenital 1-alpha-hydroxylase deficiency
        1. Caused by a genetic mutation in the 1-alpha-hydroxylase (renal enzyme) gene
        2. Results in the inability to form 1,25 dihydroxyvitamin D
        3. Inadequate intestinal calcium and phosphate absorption
    iii. Congenital resistance to 1,25 dihydroxyvitamin D
        1. Caused by a genetic mutation in the vitamin D receptor gene
          a. Leads to a defective or absent vitamin D receptor
        2. Results in deficient 1,25 dihydroxyvitamin D–mediated intestinal absorption of calcium and phosphorus
  d. Clinical Manifestations
     i. Bone pain
     ii. Fractures
    iii. Muscle weakness
    iv. Growth retardation
     v. Deformities (differ depending on the time of onset)
        1. First year of life
          a. Widened cranial sutures
          b. Frontal bossing
          c. Craniotabes
          d. Rachitic rosary
          e. Harrison's groove
          f. Flared wrists
        2. After first year of life
          a. Flared ends of long bones
          b. Bowing of long bones
          c. Sabre shins
          d. Coxa vara
          e. Genu varum
          f. Genu valgum
  e. Laboratory abnormalities
     i. Similar to those seen in osteomalacia
  f. X-ray findings
     i. Delayed opacification of the epiphyses
     ii. Widened growth plates
    iii. Widened and irregular metaphyses
    iv. Thin cortices
     v. Sparse and coarse trabeculae in the diaphyses
  g. Histology
     i. Increased osteoid
     ii. Deficient mineralization

Fig. 24.3 Clinical
manifestations of rickets
(Reproduced with permission
from Nephrology. *Atlas of
Pediatrics.* ImagesMD;
2006-01-20)

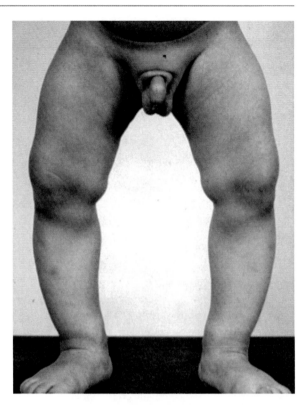

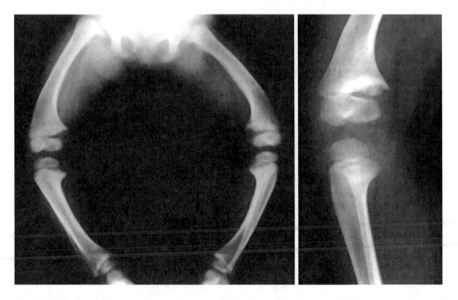

Fig. 24.4 Radiographic appearance of rickets with bowing of the femora and tibiae and metaphyseal
flaring (Reproduced with permission from Metabolic and endocrine disorders of the skeleton. *Children's
Orthopaedics and Fractures.* DOI:10.1007/978-1-84882-611-3_8. Springer; 2009-01-01)

3. Treatment of Bone Deposition Disorders Based on Etiology
    a. Simple nutritional vitamin D deficiency
        i. Vitamin D 5,000 U/day until healing
        ii. Maintain 400 U/day
    b. Malabsorption
        i. Vitamin D 50,000–100,000 U/day
    c. Renal disease
        i. Vitamin D 50,000–100,000 U/day
        ii. Calcitriol 0.25–1.0 µg/day
    d. Hypophosphatemic rickets
        i. Calcitriol 0.25–1.0 µg/day and
        ii. Oral phosphate
    e. Alpha-hydroxylase deficiency
        i. Calcitriol 0.25–1.0 µg/day and
        ii. Oral phosphate
    f. Resistance to 1,25 dihydroxyvitamin D
        i. Vitamin D 100,000–200,00 U/day
        ii. Calcitriol 5–60 µg/day
        iii. IV calcium infusions
    g. Severe liver disease or medications that interfere with 25 hydroxylation of vitamin D
        i. Calderol (25 OH vitamin D)
            1. Usual dose 20 µg three times a week
                a. Can be advanced to daily
        ii. Follow serum calcium levels
    h. Patients with malabsorption
        i. Calciferol in oil
            1. 500,000 IU/ml IM
    i. Patients with malabsorption and renal disease
        i. Calcijex (1,25 OH vitamin D)
            1. Subcutaneous 1–2 µg three times per week
        ii. Follow calcium levels
    j. **Do not** let 1,25 OH vitamin D level get above the upper limit of normal
        i. Upregulates RANK ligand on osteoblasts
        ii. Stimulates RANK on osteoclasts
        iii. Results in increased osteoclastogenesis
4. Idiopathic Hypercalciuria
    a. Patients with osteopenia excreting excessive calcium in their 24-h urine of unknown etiology
        i. Normal value
            1. 100–300 mg/24 h
        ii. Upper limit
            1. 3.5 mg/kg (women) and 4 mg/kg (men)

    b. Major causes
       i. Gut hyperabsorption
         1. Place on a low-calcium diet for 3 days
           a. Will markedly decrease urinary calcium
      ii. Renal calcium wasting
         1. Place on a low-calcium diet for 3 days
           a. Will **NOT** decrease urinary calcium
         2. High normal or elevated PTH
           a. To maintain a normal serum calcium
           b. Leads to osteoporosis
         3. Treat with thiazide diuretics
           a. HCTZ 25 mg qd (**NOT** furosemide)
           b. Increases distal renal tubular calcium absorption
           c. Lowers PTH levels
           d. Maintains **normal** serum calcium levels
           e. If serum calcium increases
             i. Evaluate for mild primary hyperparathyroidism

5. Osteogenesis Imperfecta
    a. Results from mutations in one of the two genes that code for type I procollagen
    b. Osteoblasts produce abnormal osteoid which results in
       i. Osteopenia
      ii. Fragile bones
    c. Subtypes vary in severity ranging from
       i. Fatal infantile form
      ii. Mild adult form
    d. Associated abnormalities
       i. Blue sclerae
      ii. Dentinogenesis imperfecta
     iii. Deafness
    e. Diagnosis made on clinical grounds
    f. Treatment
       i. Bisphosphonates
         1. Significantly improve bone mass
      ii. Management measures
         1. Supportive
         2. Orthopedic
         3. Rehabilitation

6. Osteopetrosis
    a. "Marble bone disease"
    b. Caused by defective osteoclast unable to resorb bone
    c. Abnormalities in bone and bone marrow
       i. Bone appearance
         1. Dense

Type	Clinical severity	Typical features	Typical molecular mechanism
I	Mild	Stature normal or slightly short; little or no limb deformity; blue sclera; ligamentous laxity; hearing loss; dentinogenesis imperfecta	Autosomal dominant; haploid insufficiency; nonfunctional COL1A1 allele; usually due to premature stop codon
II	Perinatal, lethal	Pronounced deformities; multiple fractures at birth; micromelia; broad long bones; beading of the ribs; undermineralized skull; dark sclera	Autosomal dominant; glycine substitution in COL1A1 or COL1A2
III	Severely deforming	Very short stature; severe scoliosis; cystic change at epiphyses; characteristic triangular facies; gray sclera; dentinogenesis imperfecta; dental malocclusion	Autosomal dominant; glycine substitution in COL1A1 or COL1A2
IV	Moderately deforming	Marked heterogeneity; moderate short stature; variable degree of scoliosis; white or gray sclera; dentinogenesis imperfecta	Autosomal dominant; glycine substitution in COL1A1 or COL1A2
V	Moderately deforming	Mild to moderate short stature; mineralized interosseous membrane of forearm; limited supination/pronation; dislocation of radial head; hyperplastic callous; no dentinogenesis imperfecta; "mesh-like" pattern of bone lamellation	Autosomal dominant; no abnormality of type 1 collagen, COL1A1 or COL1A2
VI	Moderately to severely deforming	Moderate short stature; scoliosis; white sclera; no dentinogenesis imperfecta; "fish-scale" pattern of bone lamellation; accumulation of osteoid	No abnormality of type 1 collagen, COL1A1 or COL1A2

Fig. 24.5 Classification of osteogenesis imperfecta (Reproduced with permission from Osteogenesis imperfecta. *Bone and Development.* DOI:10.1007/978-1-84882-822-3_13. Springer; 2010-01-01)

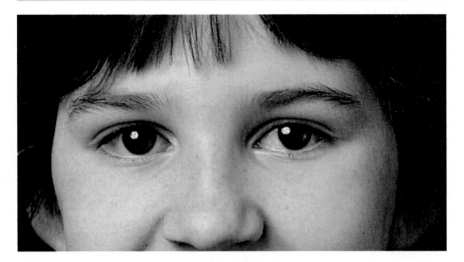

Fig. 24.6 Blue sclera in osteogenesis imperfecta (Reproduced with permission from Osteoporosis associated with systemic illness and medications. *Atlas of Clinical Endocrinology.* ImagesMD; 2002-01-28)

       2. Chalky
       3. Fragile
    ii. Marrow appearance
       1. Replaced with pancytopenia
  d. Several subsets
    i. Mutations in the gene for carbonic anhydrase II (CA II)
       1. Results in CA II deficiency
       2. Osteoclasts unable to generate the hydrogen ions (acidification) necessary for bone resorption
    ii. RANK-RANK ligand deficiencies or excessive osteoprotegrin
       1. Leads to ineffective differentiation of osteoclast
  e. Radiographs
    i. See osteosclerosis
  f. Several clinical forms
    i. A severe, usually fatal, infantile form
    ii. A more benign form that allows survival into adulthood
  g. Treatment
    i. Bone marrow transplantation
       1. For the severe infantile type
       2. Provides normal osteoclasts
    ii. High-dose calcitriol

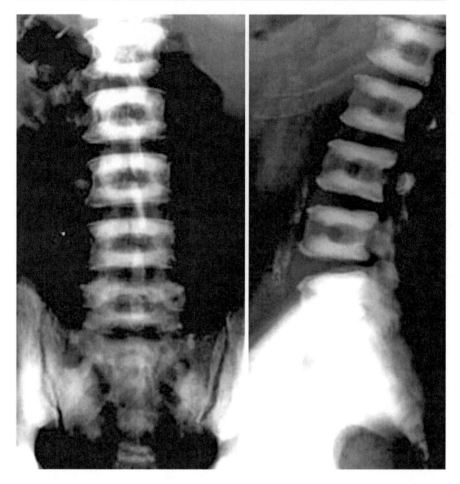

Fig. 24.7 "Rugger-jersey appearance" of the spine in a 61-year-old man with autosomal dominant osteopetrosis showing a sandwich-like sclerosis of the vertebral endplates (Reproduced with
permission from A clinical and molecular overview of the human osteopetroses. *Calcified Tissue
International.* DOI:10.1007/s00223-005-0027-6. Springer; 2005-11-01)

Paget's Disease of Bone

25

1. First described in 1877 by the British physician Sir James Paget
   a. Used the term *osteitis deformans*
   b. Evidence supports its existence in prehistoric times
2. A localized disorder of hyperactive bone remodeling
   a. Abnormal osteoclasts accelerate the process of normal bone turnover
      i. Large numbers of highly multinucleated osteoclasts
      ii. Result in extensive bone resorption
   b. Followed by recruitment of osteoblasts and increased bone formation
      i. Osteoblasts appear normal
3. Hyperactive remodeling of bone
   a. Disorganized and thickened
   b. A mosaic pattern of woven and lamellar bone
   c. Mechanically weakened
      i. Microarchitectural abnormalities prone to fracture

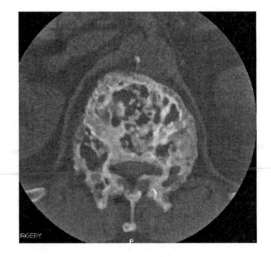

Fig. 25.1 Axial CT image of the L1 vertebral body demonstrates the characteristic appearance of Paget's disease with thickened, coarsened trabeculae and overall enlargement of the bone (Reproduced with permission from Paget's disease of the spine and secondary osteosarcoma. *HSS Journal.* DOI: 10.1007/s11420-006-9007-2. Springer; 2006-08-31)

N.T. Colburn, *Review of Rheumatology,*
DOI 10.1007/978-1-84882-093-7_25, © Springer-Verlag London Limited 2012

Fig. 25.2 Clinical features of Paget's
disease (Reproduced with permission
from Diseases of bone and connective
tissue. *Atlas of Rheumatology.*
ImagesMD; 2002-03-07)

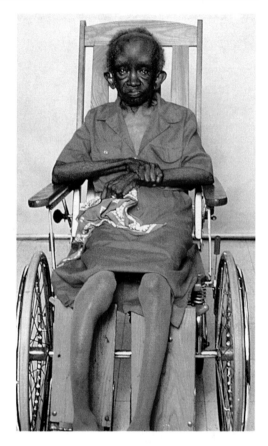

  d. Often hypervascular
      i. Excessive bleeding (i.e., during surgery)
      ii. Vascular steal syndromes
  e. Can cause marrow fibrosis
4. Clinical sequelae
  a. Bony pain
  b. Deformity
  c. Fracture
  d. Neurological symptoms from
      i. Nerve impingement
      ii. Vascular steal from hypervascular bone
  e. Secondary joint disorders from primary bony deformities
5. Epidemiology
  a. Prevalence in a British study of 30,000 abdominal radiographs
      i. 6.2% among men over the age of 55
      ii. 3.9% among women over the age of 55
      iii. 5% overall
      iv. Increased in an age-dependent manner
          1. 20% among men older than 85

    b. Overall incidence increases with age

        i. 3–3.7% of patients over age 40

        ii. 90% after the eighth decade of life

    c. Prevalence in the USA

        i. Overall 2%

        ii. More common in the northern states

        iii. Men have slightly higher risk than women (3:2)

    d. More common in

        i. Britain

        ii. Caucasians of British and northern European descent

    e. Less common in

        i. Blacks

        ii. Asians

        iii. Far East

        iv. India

        v. Africa

        vi. Middle East

    f. Prevalence appears to be declining

6. Etiology

    a. Viral infections

        i. Paramyxovirus infection implicated

            1. Pagetic osteoclasts shown to contain intracellular particles

            2. Particles resemble nucleocapsids of the Paramyxoviridae family of RNA viruses

            3. Controversial

        ii. Measles virus and canine distemper virus found in Pagetic bone

            1. Three-fold higher incidence noted in owners of unvaccinated dogs compared with owners of vaccinated dogs

            2. Results not replicated universally

    b. A lack of animal models

        i. Difficult to apply Koch's postulates

    c. Genetic susceptibility

        i. 15–30% report a positive family history

        ii. Seven times more often in relatives of patients than in controls

            1. Risk further increased if the affected relative has

                a. Severe disease

                b. Diagnosis at an early age

        iii. HLA DQw1 and DR antigens

            1. Found with increased frequency

7. Clinical Features

    a. Polyostotic (80%)

    b. Monostotic (20%) most common in

        i. Tibia

        ii. Iliac bones

    c. Noted to occur in every bone in the skeleton

        i. More common in the axial skeleton

Fig. 25.3 Late phase of Paget's disease with sclerosis, expansion, and bowing (sabre deformity) of the tibia (Reproduced with permission from Paget disease. *Encyclopedia of Diagnostic Imaging*. DOI: 10.1007/978-3-540-35280-8_1849. Springer; 2008-01-01)

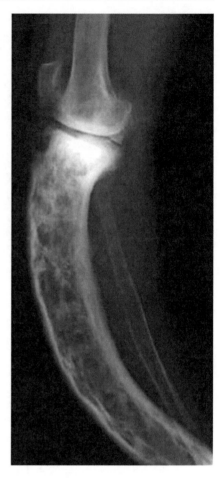

    d. Sites affected most frequently (in descending order)
       i. Pelvis
      ii. Lumbar spine
     iii. Femur
     iv. Thoracic spine
      v. Sacrum
     vi. Skull
    vii. Tibia
   viii. Humerus
    e. Frequently asymptomatic
    f. Diagnosis often made as an incidental finding
       i. Pagetic findings on routine radiographic studies
      ii. Elevated levels of alkaline phosphatase
         1. In the absence of liver dysfunction

Fig. 25.4 Pathologic fractures in Paget's disease (Reproduced with permission from Diseases of bone and connective tissue. *Atlas of Rheumatology*. ImagesMD)

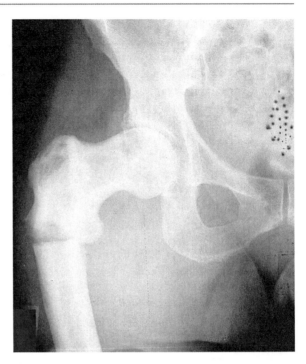

g. Complications
  i. Bone pain
  ii. Bone and joint deformities
    1. Bowing
    2. Frontal bossing
  iii. Fractures
    1. 7% of patients
  iv. Neurologic
    1. Deafness
      a. Auditory nerve entrapment (13%)
    2. Nerve entrapment
      a. Cranial nerves
      b. Spinal nerve roots
    3. Spinal stenosis
    4. Basilar invagination
    5. Headaches
    6. Stroke
      a. Blood vessel compression
  v. Vascular
    1. Hyperthermia
    2. Vascular steal syndrome
      a. External carotid blood flow to the skull at the expense of the brain

      vi. Metabolic
        1. Hypercalcemia
        2. Hypercalciuria
        3. Nephrocalcinosis
  h. Symptomatic Paget's
     i. Only one-third of patients
    ii. Usually presents with
      1. Pain
        a. The most common symptom (80%)
        b. Joint pain (50%) involving the
          i. Knee
          ii. Hip
         iii. Spine
      2. Bony deformity
      3. Neurologic manifestations
  i. Pain etiologies
     i. Hypervascularity
      1. Associated with warmth over the area
    ii. Periosteal distortion
      1. Due to thickened bone
    iii. Fractures
      1. Most commonly in the
        a. Femur
        b. Tibia
        c. Humerus
        d. Forearm
      2. Stress
      3. Full
  j. Periarticular disease
     i. Due to Pagetic involvement in the adjacent bones
    ii. Classically spares the joints
    iii. Pain at the hip, knees, and spine
      1. Hip pain from involvement of the proximal femur or pelvis near the acetabulum
  k. Etiologies of back pain in Paget's
     i. Vertebral enlargement
      1. Loss of lumbar lordosis
    ii. Vertebral fracture
    iii. Nerve-root impingement
    iv. Gait changes
      1. Secondary to Paget's disease at other sites
     v. Spinal artery steal syndrome
      1. Hypervascular vertebral bone
    vi. Coexistence with OA

l. Bony deformities
    i. Less common but highly specific for Paget's
    ii. Changes typically asymmetric
    iii. Of the femur and tibia
        1. Classical bowed leg
    iv. Of the skull
        1. Skull thickening in advanced cases
        2. Frontal bossing
        3. Enlarged maxilla
        4. Neurologic sequelae
            a. Hearing loss
                i. Most common
                ii. Multifactorial etiologies
                    1. Cochlear dysfunction
                        a. Secondary to temporal bone involvement
                    2. Compression of cranial nerve VIII
        5. Involvement of the basilar skull
            a. Pressure on the brain stem
                i. Obstructive hydrocephalus
                ii. Long tract signs
m. Serious complications
    i. Cardiac
        1. High-output congestive heart failure
            a. Due to increased pagetic bone vascularity
        2. Hypertension
        3. Cardiomegaly
        4. Angina
    ii. Excessive bleeding
        1. Fractures through hypervascular pagetic bone
            a. Spontaneous
            b. During orthopedic procedures
                i. Internal fixation
                ii. Joint replacement
        2. Preparation before surgery
            a. Elective
                i. Disease should be well-controlled with bisphosphonate therapy
            b. Urgent or emergent surgery
                i. Prior use of IV pamidronate
    iii. Development of bony malignancy
        1. Rare
            a. Fewer than 1% of people with Paget's disease
        2. Types
            a. Osteogenic sarcomas (0.2–1.0%)
            b. Fibrosarcomas
            c. Benign giant cell tumors

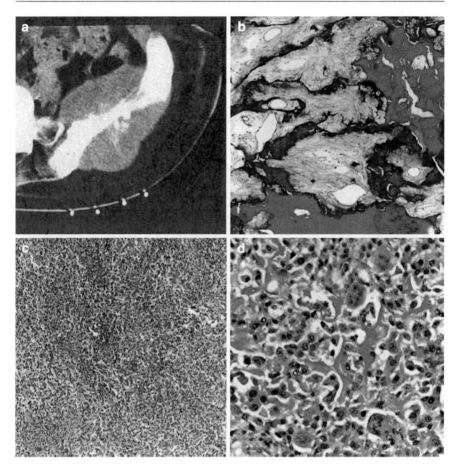

Fig. 25.5 Osteosarcoma arising in Paget's disease. (**a**) Left ileum with expansile mass in a patient
with Paget's disease. (**b**) Area of Paget's disease uninvolved by sarcoma. (**c**, **d**) Osteogenic sarcoma corresponding to iliac lesion with abundant hyperchromatic, pleomorphic cells and lace-like
osteoid (Reproduced with permission from Premalignant conditions of bone. *Journal of
Orthopaedic Science*. DOI: 10.1007/s00776-006-1037-6. Springer; 2006-08-07)

       3. Typical presentations
          a. Severe and rapid worsening of pain in an area of long-standing
            pagetic bone
          b. Follow-up with radiographic studies of the area
          c. Pathologic fractures may occur
    8. Differential Diagnosis of Paget's
      a. Diagnosis made by
        i. Radiographs
       ii. Routine laboratory testing
      iii. Both

   b. Pagetic vertebrae
      i. May resemble lymphoma and metastatic cancers
         1. Especially adenocarcinoma of the prostate
      ii. Usually enlarged
   c. Distinguish Paget's in other affected bones by
      i. Characteristic cortical thickening
      ii. Adjacent thickened trabeculae
   d. Paget's progresses through different stages
      i. Lytic to sclerotic
      ii. Helps differentiate from osteoblastic metastatic lesions
   e. Focal increased uptake on scintigraphy
      i. Seen in many conditions besides Paget's
         1. Osteomyelitis
         2. Arthritis
         3. Metastases
         4. Fractures
9. Radiographic Features
   a. Evaluated by both
      i. Plain radiography
      ii. Technetium bone scanning (^{99m}Tc-bisposphonate)
   b. Discordance between radiographic and scintigraphic findings
      i. 12% of lesions seen on bone scan will not be seen on radiographs
      ii. 6% of radiographic abnormalities absent on bone scan
   c. Paget's does not spread to adjacent bones or "metastasize" to distant regions
   d. Classic radiographic finding
      i. Mixed areas of bony lysis (reflecting osteoclast activity) and sclerosis
         (reflecting osteoblast activity)
   e. Findings highly characteristic of Paget's
      i. Flame-shaped lytic lesions in long bone
         1. Edge of lytic fronts gives a "blade of grass" appearance
      ii. Cortical thickening along with adjacent trabecular thickening
      iii. Trabecular thickening of the iliopubic and ilioischial lines along the
         inner aspect of the pelvis
         1. "Brim sign"
         2. "Pelvic ring"
      iv. Skull lesions
         1. Extensive lytic involvement in the skull
            a. "Osteoporosis circumscripta"
         2. Thickened cranium with regions of dense sclerosis and osteopenia
            a. "Cotton-wool" appearance
   f. Lytic lesions can progress
      i. Usually at a rate of less than 1 cm/year
   g. Bone scans
      i. Classically see regions of focal increased uptake
      ii. Help determine the extent of bony involvement

Fig. 25.6 AP radiograph of left
proximal femur showing the
advancing ("blade of grass") lytic
phase of Paget's in the shaft and the
more mature osteoblastic phase in
the femoral head with trabecular
thickening (Reproduced with
permission from Paget's disease of
bone. *Rheumatology and
Immunology Therapy*. DOI:
10.1007/3-540-29662-X_2082.
Springer; 2004-01-01)

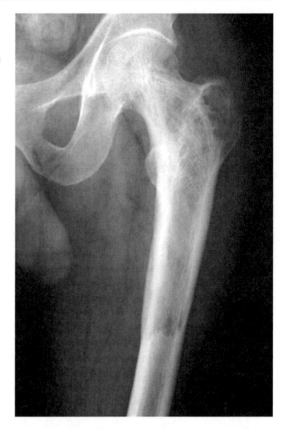

Fig. 25.7 Pelvic radiographic
in late Paget's disease with
marked bone remodeling,
thickened cortices, coarsened
trabeculae and deformed bone
(Reproduced with permission
from Paget's disease of bone.
*A Clinician's Pearls and
Myths in Rheumatology*. DOI:
10.1007/978-1-84800-934-
9_41. Springer; 2009-01-01)

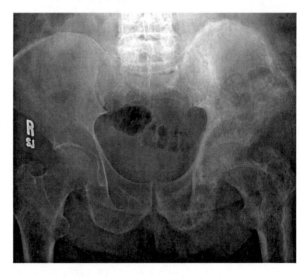

Fig. 25.8 Osteolytic phase of Paget's disease affecting the frontal bones of the skull (osteoporosis circumscripta) (Reproduced with permission from Paget disease. *Encyclopedia of Diagnostic Imaging.* DOI: 10.1007/978-3-540-35280-8_1849. Springer; 2008-01-01)

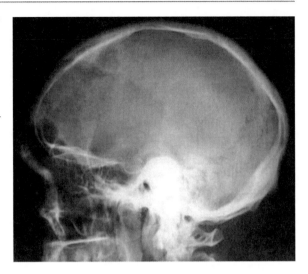

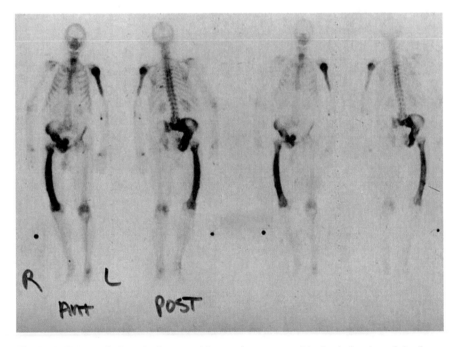

Fig. 25.9 Polyostotic Paget's disease evident on bone scan, with classic bowing of the femur (Reproduced with permission from Paget's disease of bone. *A Clinician's Pearls and Myths in Rheumatology.* DOI: 10.1007/978-1-84800-934-9_41. Springer; 2009-01-01)

     iii. Should **not** be used to make the diagnosis of Paget's
     iv. Presence of monostotic disease
        1. Seen in 20% of people with Paget's
        2. Should raise suspicion for other lesions such as
          a. Fracture
          b. Infection
          c. Malignancy
     v. Initial scans helpful in
        1. Evaluating the extent of disease
        2. Long-term follow-up
        3. Detecting relapses following treatment
        4. Assessing new symptoms
10. Laboratory Features
   a. Paget's characterized by accelerated bone turnover
     i. Bone resorption and formation occur simultaneously
        1. Markers of these processes typically elevated
     ii. Markers of bone resorption
        1. Urinary hydroxyproline
        2. Collagen cross-links
          a. N-telopeptides
          b. C-telopeptides
        3. Pyridinoline cross-links
     iii. Markers of bone formation
        1. Total alkaline phosphatase
          a. The most reproducible biochemical marker
          b. Interpretation may be complicated in liver disease
          c. Elevated levels present in 86% of Paget's
          d. Levels greater than ten times normal associated with
            i. Skull involvement
            ii. High cardiac input
          e. Lower levels associated with other bony involvement
            i. Pelvis
            ii. Sacrum
            iii. Lumbar spine
            iv. Femoral head
          f. The most effective method for
            i. Monitoring disease activity
               1. Levels correlate
            ii. Assessing the effectiveness of anti-pagetic therapy
          g. Often identified in asymptomatic patients on routine chemistries
        2. Fractionated bone alkaline phosphatase
        3. Osteocalcin
          a. A less reliable index of the disease process
   b. Biochemical testing useful in the diagnosis
     i. Rules out other causes of metabolic bone disease
     ii. Determines the effectiveness of medical therapy

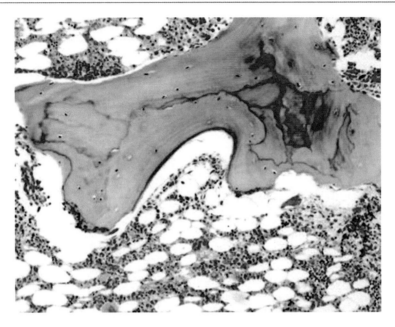

Fig. 25.10 In Paget's disease, bone histology shows thickened bone trabeculae with irregular scalloping and haphazard cement lines (Reproduced with permission from The bone marrow in normal and disease states. *Neoplastic Hematopathology.* DOI: 10.1007/978-1-60761-384-8_5. Springer; 2010-01-01)

    c. Tests commonly used to evaluate metabolic bone disease typically normal in Paget's
       i. Serum calcium
         1. If elevated consider
           a. Malignancy
           b. Primary hyperparathyroidism
           c. Presence of fracture
           d. Immobilization
      ii. Phosphorous
      iii. Parathyroid hormone (PTH)
         1. Secondary hyperparathyoidism seen in active Paget's
           a. Elevated PTH in the setting of normal calcium levels
      iv. Vitamin D
      v. Osteocalcin levels
11. Histopathologic Features
    a. Initial increased bone resorption
      i. Mediated by giant multinucleated osteoclasts
    b. Followed by compensatory increase in bone formation
    c. Accelerated lamellar and woven bone deposition in a disorganized fashion
    d. Characteristic mosaic pattern
    e. Areas of resorbed bone replaced with fibrous tissue
    f. Vascular hypertrophy occurs

12. Treatment
  a. Safe and effective
  b. Only withheld in asymptomatic patients
      i. Disease located in areas with no risk of complications
  c. NSAIDS
      i. Pain associated with OA when Paget's occurs near joints
  d. Calcitonin
      i. First successful therapy for Paget's
      ii. Alternative agent typically used when
          1. Extensive lytic disease
          2. Severe pain
          3. Rapid response desired
              a. Neurologic symptoms
              b. High-output heart failure
          4. Bisphosphonates do not work or are poorly tolerated
      iii. Human and salmon parenteral preparations
          1. Administered subcutaneously at 100 IU daily
              a. Until clinical and biochemical improvements seen
          2. Dose then reduced to 50–100 IU every other day or three times per week
      iv. Nasal sprays
          1. Low bioavailability
          2. Not approved for Paget's
      v. Symptoms usually diminish within a few weeks
          1. Return when therapy discontinued
      vi. Plateau phenomenon
          1. Results from neutralizing antibodies to salmon calcitonin
          2. 25% of patients
          3. Human calcitonin usually benefits these patients
      vii. Side effects
          1. Flushing
          2. Nausea
          3. Transient hypocalcemia
          4. Up to 20%
          5. Minimized by
              a. Starting at lower doses (25–50 IU)
              b. Gradually increasing every 1–2 weeks
  e. Bisphosphonates
      i. First-line therapy for Paget's disease
      ii. Etidronate was the first bisphosphonate to be approved
          1. Associated with osteomalacia
      iii. Newer generations more effective
      iv. Replaced the use of calcitonin and etidronate due to
          1. Excellent effectiveness in reducing disease activity
          2. Prolonged duration of response
          3. Short courses of therapy

        4. Relatively inexpensive
        5. Well-tolerated
     v. Works by inhibiting osteoclastic activity
    vi. Results in significant and prolonged inhibition of bone resorption
   vii. Vast majority of patients experience a rapid reduction in symptoms
        1. Also improvement in biochemical markers
  viii. Approved for treatment of Paget's in the USA
        1. Alendronate
           a. 40 mg/day for 6 months
        2. Pamidronate
           a. Given IV
           b. 30 mg weekly for 6 weeks
           c. 60 mg every 2 weeks for three doses
        3. Risedronate
           a. 30 mg/day for 2 months
        4. Tiludronate
           a. 400 mg/day for 3 months
    ix. Other bisphosphonates
        1. Zoledronate
        2. Ibandronate
        3. Neridronate
        4. Olpadronate
     x. Side effects
        1. Tend to be poorly absorbed
        2. Erosive disease of the upper GI tract
           a. Take on an empty stomach with 8 oz of water
           b. Ingest no other food, beverage, or medication for the next 30 min
           c. Maintain an upright position during the 30 min
        3. Other GI side effects
           a. Esophagitis
           b. Dyspepsia
         4. Reduce serum calcium levels
           a. Unusual in Paget's
           b. Patients must receive adequate amounts of calcium and vitamin D
             to prevent secondary hyperparathyoidism
        5. Etidronate
           a. Mineralization defects
         6. Pamidronate
           a. Low-grade fever
           b. Transient leukopenia
           c. Flu-like symptoms
  f. Plicamycin (mithramycin)
     i. Unacceptable toxicity profile
  g. Gallium nitrate

h. Surgery
   i. To relieve nerve compression
   ii. Increase joint mobility
i. Indications for treatment
   i. Symptomatic disease
      1. Bone or joint pain
         a. Bone pain will respond to bisphosphonate therapy
            i. Especially IV pamidronte
         b. Secondary pain from OA will **not** respond
      2. Bone deformity
   ii. Risk for complications
      1. Bone, joint, or neurologic
      2. Preparation for orthopedic surgery
      3. Sites at high risk for complications
         a. Skull
            i. Hearing loss
            ii. Other neurologic
         b. Spine
            i. Neurologic
         c. Lower extremity long bones and areas adjacent to major joints
            i. Fracture
            ii. Osteoarthritis
            iii. Markedly elevated levels of alkaline phosphatase
               1. Will normalize alkaline phosphatase in one-half to two-thirds of affected patients
            iv. Immobilization hypercalcemia
            v. Young patients
j. Monitoring
   i. Disease activity effectively monitored by measurement of
      1. Serum alkaline phosphatase
      2. Urinary N-telopeptide
   ii. Therapy aimed at normalizing these biochemical markers
      1. Usually occurs several months after the end of therapy
      2. Failure to normalize results in
         a. Development of new complications in 60–70%
         b. Despite a favorable effect on pain
      3. Indication for retreatment
         a. Recurrence of markers 20–30% above ULN
   iii. Alkaline phosphatase levels
      1. During therapy
      2. At 3–6 month intervals
      3. If levels rise
         a. Additional course often effective in reducing activity
   iv. Symptomatic patients monitored every 3–6 months for changes

Osteonecrosis

26

1. Osteonecrosis (ON)
   a. A generic term used to describe the death of all cellular elements of bone and contiguous bone marrow resulting from ischemia
   b. Occurs in a variety of clinical settings
      i. Defined disease
         1. Gaucher's
      ii. Medications
         1. Corticosteroids
      iii. Physiologic processes
         1. Pregnancy
      iv. Pathologic processes
         1. Thromboembolism
      v. No apparent predisposing factors
         1. Idiopathic
2. Other Terms
   a. Ischemic bone necrosis
   b. Avascular necrosis
   c. Aseptic necrosis
3. Epidemiology
   a. Estimated 15,000 new cases develop each year in the USA
   b. Affects both genders
      i. Males more frequently than females (8:1)
      ii. Reflects higher incidence of trauma in males
   c. Age groups
      i. Majority of cases
         1. Develop in the <50 year olds
      ii. Exceptional cases
         1. Women over 50 predisposed to ON of the knee
   d. Spontaneous osteonecrosis of the knee (SONK)
      i. Affects the femoral condyles and proximal tibia

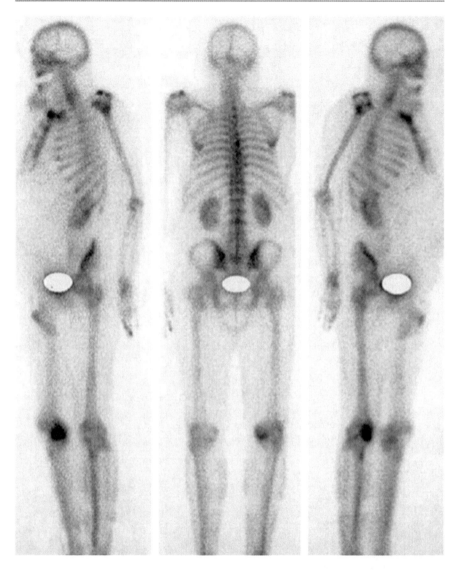

Fig. 26.1 Three-phase bone scintigraphy (99mTC-MDP) in an elderly patient with early-stage spontaneous osteonecrosis of the knee showing a typical distribution pattern of radionuclide uptake in the right medial femoral condyle (Reproduced with permission from Postoperative osteonecrosis of the condyle: diagnosis and management. *The Meniscus*. DOI:10.1007/978-3-642-02450-4_36. Springer; 2010-01-01)

     ii. MRI shows small lesions on the medial more often than the lateral femoral condyle

     iii. F:M about 3:1

  e. Cases of nontraumatic ON

     i. 50% due to

Fig. 26.2 Plain radiograph of osteonecrosis of the femoral head. The infarct shows segmental collapse and compression into the lower part of the femoral head (Reproduced with permission from Common problems in orthopedic pathology including trauma, reactive conditions and necrosis of bone. *Essentials in Bone and Soft-Tissue Pathology.* DOI:10.1007/978-0-387-89845-2_2. Springer; 010-01-01)

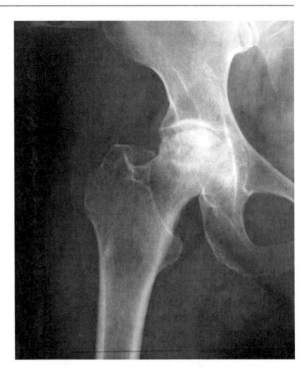

        1. Steroid use
        2. Alcohol abuse
     ii. Up to 40%
        1. No identifiable risk factor (idiopathic)
  4. Skeletal Regions Predisposed to ON
    a. Most vulnerable areas
       i. Limited vascular supply
      ii. Restricted collateral circulation
     iii. Covered by articular cartilage
    b. Epiphyses of long bones
       i. Femoral and humeral heads
        1. Femoral head most frequent
      ii. Capitulum of humerus (Panner's disease)
     iii. Femoral condyles
     iv. Proximal tibia
    c. Other bones
       i. Phalanges (Thiemann's disease)
      ii. Carpal
        1. Scaphoid
        2. Lunate (Kienbock's disease)
     iii. Tarsal
        1. Navicular (Preiser's disease)

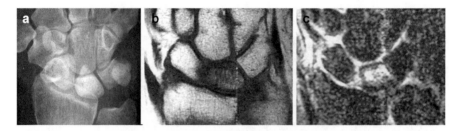

Fig. 26.3 A patient with early Kienbock's disease of the lunate. (**a**) Radiograph shows patchy sclerosis of the lunate. Coronal (**b**) T1-W and (**c**) TIRM MR images show T1-hypointense and T2-hyperintense signal within the marrow of the lunate (Reproduced with permission from Circulatory diseases of bone and adjacent soft tissues. *Diagnostic Imaging of Musculoskeletal Diseases.* DOI:10.1007/978-1-59745-355-4_4. Springer; 2009-01-01)

      iv. Metatarsals

         1. Second metatarsal (Freiberg's disease)

      v. Talus

      vi. Vertebral body (Calve's disease)

  5. Involvement of More than One Bone

    a. Sequentially and simultaneously

    b. 50% with symptomatic hip ON have asymptomatic disease in the contralateral hip at the time of initial presentation

    c. Two-thirds of asymptomatic hips will progress to late-stage disease

    d. Recommend bilateral hip MRI at time of presentation

    e. Similar frequencies expected in ON of the humeral head and knee

  6. Pathogenesis

    a. Bone death is the result of diminished arterial blood supply

      i. Reproduced in experimental animals

      ii. Most obvious and best understood in posttraumatic cases

      iii. Various pathologic processes capable of inducing ischemia

    b. Final outcome depends on

      i. The size of the affected area

      ii. The success of reparative processes

      iii. Viable bone cells ability to replace necrotic or nonviable bone

    c. Failure to revitalize large involved areas leads to

      i. Bone collapse

      ii. Osseous microfractures

      iii. Joint incongruity

      iv. Secondary OA

    d. Final common pathway for various inciting factors

      i. Local intravascular coagulation

      ii. Resultant tissue ischemia

    e. Characteristic histopathologic findings

      i. Marrow fibrosis

      ii. Fat-cell necrosis

      iii. Necrotic and dead bone
         1. Subchondral cancellous bone death
         2. Collapse of the articular structure
      iv. Bone marrow death
      v. Evidence for attempts at repair
  f. Well-recognized causes of ischemia
      i. Small-vessel vasculitis
      ii. Arteriolar thrombosis
      iii. Venous occlusion
      iv. Microembolism
         1. Fat/lipid (etiologic factor common to several conditions)
           a. Fatty liver
           b. Hyperlipidemia
              i. Particularly types II and IV
           c. Disruption of fatty bone marrow
              i. Long-bone fracture
           d. Alcohol abuse
           e. Carbon tetrachloride poisoning
           f. Diabetes
           g. Hypercortisolism
           h. Decompression illness
           i. Pregnancy
           j. Oral contraceptive use
           k. Hemoglobinopathies
         2. Thrombi
         3. Sickle cells
         4. Nitrogen gas
      v. External vascular compression
         1. Marrow hypertrophy/infiltration
         2. Infiltration alters vascular supply by compressing the sinusoids
           a. Gaucher's
  g. Cytotoxic factors
      i. Direct toxic effect of substances on different bone cell populations
      ii. Moderate amounts of alcohol
         1. Toxic to osteocytes
      iii. Corticosteroids
         1. Toxic to lipocytes
  h. Elevated intraosseous pressure (IOP)
      i. Postulated as the common pathway of ON
      ii. Increased pressure in bone leads to ischemia and cell damage
      iii. Used as a tool for early diagnosis
      iv. Not the *sine qua non* of ON
         1. Also occurs in other pathologic processes
         2. Not found in experimentally induced ON in rabbits

7. Clinical Features
   a. Nonspecific signs and symptoms
   b. Morning stiffness
      i. Typically absent or of short duration (<1 h)
      ii. Allows differentiation from inflammatory monoarticular arthritis
   c. Relatively abrupt onset of pain
      i. First clinical manifestation of ON
      ii. Occurs in the early stages of involvement
      iii. Occurs before any radiographic changes noted
      iv. Possibly due to elevated intraosseous pressure (IOP)
         1. Can be relieved by decompression
      v. Initially elicited only with movement and weight-bearing activities

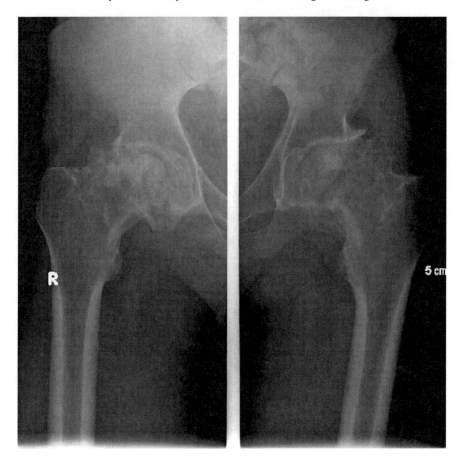

Fig. 26.4 Radiographic Anteroposterior view of both hip joints showing bilateral osteonecrosis of both femoral heads complicated with secondary osteoarthritic changes, narrowing of joint spaces and multiple marginal osteophytes (Reproduced with permission from Osteonecrosis in kidney recipients: has hypocalcaemia a role? *Rheumatology International.* DOI:10.1007/s00296-009-0918-3. Springer; 2009-11-14)

d. Hip pain
  i. The most common joint involved
  ii. Unilateral pain at onset
  iii. Sometimes the only complaint with late ON
  iv. Localizes to the
    1. Groin
    2. Buttock
    3. Medial thigh
    4. Medial aspect of the hip
    5. Knee pain
e. Sign and symptoms of progressive disease
  i. Pain at rest
  ii. Severe pain
  iii. Late onset pain
  iv. Comparatively asymptomatic
    1. Usually seen in a small infarction area with no collapse
    2. Radiographs reveal sclerotic areas
      a. "Bone islands"
      b. "Bone infarcts"
  v. Loss of range of motion
  vi. Articular surface collapse
  vii. Secondary degenerative changes
  viii. Bone remodeling
    1. Allows some patients to remain functional
f. End-stage disease
  i. Persistent and worsening pain
  ii. Progressive loss of ROM
  iii. Significant loss of function
  iv. Time to end stage varies widely
    1. Months to years
8. Conditions Associated with ON
  a. Typical clinical scenario
    i. Young woman with SLE develops ON
    ii. History of prolonged corticosteroid use
  b. Corticosteroid use
    i. The greater the use, the higher the likelihood
    ii. Especially seen with rapidly developing profound cushingoid features
    iii. Renal transplantation
    iv. Significant variation in drug administration and ON association
      1. Average dose
      2. Cumulative dosage
        a. Estimate of risk 20 mg of prednisone for over 30 days
        b. Risk increases by 5% for every 20 mg increase

Fig. 26.5 Legg–Calvé–
Perthes disease (Reproduced
with permission from Legg
Calvé Perthes disease. *Current
Orthopedic Diagnosis and
Treatment.* ImagesMD;
2002-06-04)

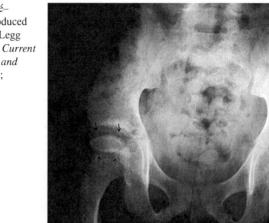

c. High-dose pulse corticosteroids
     i. Does not add to risk
    ii. Controversial
    iii. 1 g Medrol daily for 3 days
  3. Duration of use
  4. Route of administration
c. Other medications
     i. Oral contraceptive use
    ii. Protease inhibitors
      1. Used to treat HIV
      2. Side effects
        a. Lipodystrophy
        b. Diabetes
             i. Hyperlipidemia
            ii. Hypercoagulability
      3. Hyperlipidemia and hypercoagulability may lead to ON
d. Trauma
     i. Hip dislocation
    ii. Hip fracture
    iii. Hip trauma without fracture or dislocation
    iv. Hip surgery
e. Juvenile
     i. Slipped capital femoral epiphysis
    ii. Legg–Calve–Perthes disease
f. Connective tissue disease
     i. SLE
    ii. RA
    iii. Systemic vasculitis
    iv. APS

    g. Hematologic disorders
       i. Sickle cell disease
      ii. Clotting disorder
     iii. Hemoglobinopathies
    h. Infiltrative diseases
       i. Gaucher's
      ii. Solid tumors
    i. Metabolic disorders
       i. Gout
      ii. Cushings
     iii. Diabetes
    j. Disorders associated with fat necrosis
       i. Pancreatitis
    k. Hyperlipidemia
    l. Arteriosclerosis
   m. Embolism
       i. Decompression sickness (Caisson disease)
    n. GI disorders
       i. IBD
    o. Cytotoxic agents
       i. Vinblastin
      ii. Cyclophsophamide
     iii. MTX
     iv. Carbon tetrachloride poisoning
    p. Alcohol
    q. Radiation
    r. Pregnancy
    s. Idiopathic
       i. Accounts for 30–40% of all cases
      ii. Many have a hypercoagulable state as evidenced by
         1. Elevated lipoprotein (a)
         2. Low tissue plasminogen activator activity
         3. High plasminogen activator inhibitor levels
         4. High homocysteine levels
         5. Elevated antiphospholipid-lipid antibodies
         6. Low protein C or S levels
         7. The presence of Factor V Leiden
9. Diagnosis Procedures in ON
    a. "Gold standard" of diagnosis
       i. Histologically proven dead bone
    b. MRI
       i. Highest sensitivity and best diagnostic accuracy (> 95%)
      ii. Diagnostic tool of choice for detecting early disease
     iii. Helps predict patient outcomes

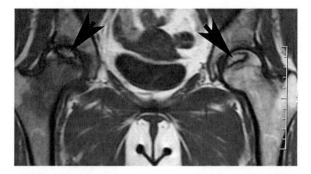

Fig. 26.6 A T1-weighted coronal MRI image shows a patient with osteonecrosis of the left femoral head. The arrow is pointing to the characteristic serpiginous border between nonviable and viable bone (Reproduced with permission from Magnetic resonance imaging criteria of successful core decompression in avascular necrosis of the hip. *Skeletal Radiology*. DOI:10.1007/s00256-004-0811-9. Springer; 2004-09-01)

    iv. Obviates invasive diagnostic procedures
        1. Biopsy
        2. Bone marrow pressure determinations
    v. Demonstrates extent of bone involvement with distinctions between
        1. Normal bone and marrow
        2. Unrepaired, dead bone and marrow
        3. Unrepaired, dead bone and marrow replaced by debris
        4. Zones of repair
    vi. Bone marrow produces high-signal intensity in both T1 and T2
    vii. Subchondral bone appears as dark striations
    viii. **Line of decreased signal** on both T1 and T2 images
        1. Demarcation between live regenerating bone and necrotic tissue
    ix. Characteristic **serpiginous pattern** with combined signals
  c. Radionuclide bone scan
    i. Much more sensitive than plain radiography
    ii. Capable of detecting ON at earlier and potentially treatable stages
    iii. Used less frequently
        1. Better specificity and sensitivity of MRI
    iv. "Hot spot"
        1. Nonspecific
    v. "Cold area"
        1. Represents necrotic tissue
        2. Seen with an area of enhanced uptake
    vi. "Cold-hot" lesion
        1. Highly specific for ON
  d. Plain radiographs
    i. Detect advanced disease
    ii. Do not detect early disease
        1. Usually normal initially

Fig. 26.7 AP hip radiograph shows an increased subchondral radiolucency (*arrow*) known as the "crescent sign" (Reproduced with permission from Magnetic resonance imaging criteria of successful core decompression in avascular necrosis of the hip. *Skeletal Radiology*. DOI:10.1007/s00256-004-0811-9. Springer; 2004-09-01)

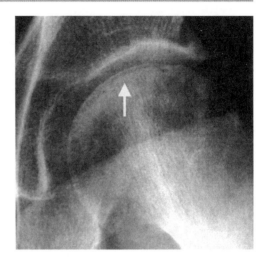

     iii. Later detects a region of generalized osteopenia
       1. Nonspecific
     iv. Radiographic findings
       1. Occurs after bone repair mechanisms
       2. Mottled appearance develops in the affected area
       3. Presence of "cysts"
         a. Regions of dead bone resorption
       4. Contiguous sclerosis
         a. Regions of bone repair
     v. "Crescent sign"
       1. A pathognomonic radiolucent line
       2. Represents the earliest irreversible lesion of ON
       3. Early collapse of cancellous bone beneath subchondral plate
         a. Articular surface collapses and flattens
         b. Further collapse almost inevitable once in this stage
       4. Secondary degenerative changes develop
         a. Joint space narrowing
         b. Secondary involvement of other bones within the articulation
     vi. AP and frog views useful for detecting hip disease
10. Bone Marrow Edema Syndrome (BMES)
   a. "Transient osteoporosis of the hip"
   b. Bone marrow edema without other findings
   c. Self-limited and transitory
   d. Clinical presentation
     i. Hip pain
     ii. Osteopenia on radiographs
     iii. Bone marrow edema of femoral head and neck on MRI
     iv. Usually one hip involved
     v. Symptoms last an average of 6 months
     vi. 40% have recurrence or involvement of other joints

vii. Differs from ON on MRI
1. **Both** femoral head **and** neck abnormalities
2. ON has **only** femoral head involvement
e. Typically affects
i. Women in the third trimester of pregnancy
ii. Middle-aged men
f. Treatment
i. Analgesics
ii. Protective weight-bearing
iii. A reversible condition
iv. Surgical interventions contraindicated
1. Such as core decompression
11. Staging in ON (Steinberg Staging of ON of the Femoral Head)
a. Seven stages of disease in the hip most commonly used
b. Stage 0
i. "At risk" asymptomatic, uninvolved hip
ii. Seen in an individual with ON on the contralateral side
iii. Clinical manifestations absent
iv. Normal radiographs
c. Stage 1
i. Clinical manifestations present
ii. Normal radiographs
iii. Abnormal MRI
d. Stage 2
i. Radiographs with areas of osteopenia, osteosclerosis, and bony cysts
ii. Abnormal MRI
e. Stage 3
i. Early subchondral bone collapse
1. Manifested as the "crescent sign"
2. Translucent subcortical bone delineates the area of dead bone
3. Without articular surface flattening
ii. Abnormal MRI
f. Stage 4
i. Late bone collapse
1. Manifested as flattening of the femoral head
2. Without joint incongruity
ii. Abnormal MRI
g. Stage 5
i. Flattening of the articular surface
1. With joint space narrowing
2. And/or acetabular involvement
ii. Abnormal MRI
h. Stage 6
i. Advanced degenerative changes
ii. Abnormal MRI

Fig. 26.8 Core decompression in early femoral head AVN. Radiograph shows the core compression track and patchy sclerosis in the left femoral head (Reproduced with permission from Circulatory diseases of bone and adjacent soft tissues. *Diagnostic Imaging of Musculoskeletal Diseases.* DOI:10.1007/978-1-59745-355-4_4. Springer; 2009-01-01)

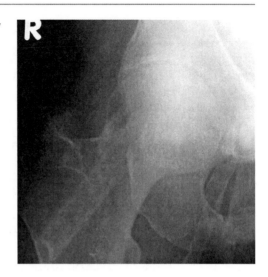

12. Treatment
    a. Goals
        i. To prevent bony collapse
        ii. To prevent deformity
        iii. Contingent upon diagnosis in the early stages
            1. Stage 2 or less
    b. Stages 0, 1, and 2
        i. Conservative medical measures
            1. Judicious use of analgesics
            2. Physical therapy
                a. Maintain muscle strength
                b. Prevent contractures
            3. Assistive devices
                a. To facilitate ambulation
                b. Discontinue weight-bearing on the affected side for 4–8 weeks
            4. Hip survival with nonoperative management
                a. 13–35% for stage 1–4 disease
                b. Femoral head involvement ≤15%
                    i. Prognosis more favorable
            5. Pulsed electromagnetic field therapy (PEMF)
                a. Some reports of safety and efficacy
        ii. Core decompression
            1. For **early, reversible** stages
                a. Particularly Stage 1
            2. Rationale
                a. Reduce intraosseous pressure (IOP)
                b. Reestablish blood supply
                c. Living bone adjacent to dead bone contributes to the reparative process
                d. Prevent progression of the lesion

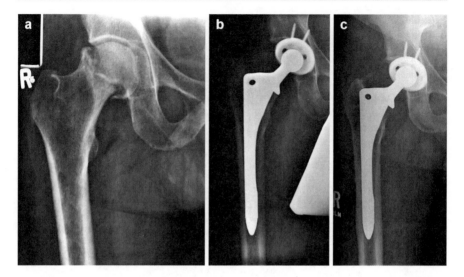

Fig. 26.9 Total hip arthroplasty (THA) for osteonecrosis. (**a**) Preoperative radiograph shows collapse of the femoral head. (**b**) Postoperative radiograph shows the THA. (**c**) Radiograph at 10 years demonstrating bony ingrowth (Reproduced with permission from Durability of second-generation extensively porous-coated stems in patients age 50 and younger. *Clinical Orthopaedics and Related Research*®. DOI:10.1007/s11999-009-1062-9. Springer; 2010-01-14)

3. Evidence for efficacy
   a. Several studies with success rates in the range of 47–84% for stage 1–4 disease
   b. One randomized controlled study of 50 hips from 31 patients
      i. ON staged 1–3 randomized to conservative or surgical treatment
      ii. Decompression reduced pain more reliably and led to less hip surgery (90%)
   c. Hips with clinical failure (defined as the need for more surgery)
      i. 16% in Stage 1
      ii. 53% in Stage 2A
      iii. 80% in Stage 2 B
      iv. 100% in Stage 4
   d. Bone grafting
      i. Alternative for treatment of **early, reversible** stages of ON
      ii. In advanced disease can delay the need for arthroplasty
         1. Allow the patient to remain functional
         2. Especially important in relatively young patients
      iii. Study of 89 patients
         1. Included idiopathic, corticosteroid use, alcohol use, and trauma
         2. All improved significantly by the standardized Harris questionnaire
         3. Probability of failure
            a. Defined as the need for arthroplasty
            b. Within 5 years varied from

   i. 11% for patients with early-stage disease

   ii. 30% for those with advanced disease

  c. Low incidence for stage 2–4 disease

 e. Nonreversible stages of ON (particularly stages 5 and 6)

  i. Indications for arthroplasty

   1. Persistent, intractable pain

   2. Progressive functional loss

   3. Radiographic progression PLUS worsening pain and incapacitation

  ii. Before total collapse of the femoral head

  iii. Young patients experience higher rates of mechanical failure than older patients

 f. Patients with ON of non-weight joints

  i. May not require any intervention

  ii. May have only mild to moderate pain

  iii. May have limited, tolerable functional losses

13. Prognosis

 a. Better outcomes with diagnosis of very early ON using MRI

 b. Manipulating modifiable risk factors

  i. Steroid dose

   1. Equivalent of ≥ 20 mg prednisone/day

    a. Attributed to a vast majority of corticosteroid-related ON

    b. Especially taken for prolonged periods

   2. ON rare in RA patients

    a. Prednisone rarely exceeds 10–15 mg/day

   3. 30–50% incidence in SLE

    a. Higher doses of steroids frequently used

  ii. Alcohol intake

  iii. Speed of decompression

   1. Divers

   2. Caisson workers

  iv. Control of diabetes and hyperlipidemia

 c. Factors which contribute to lower success rates for arthroplasty in ON as compared with other diseases such as OA

  i. Size of the necrotic area

  ii. Degree of bone collapse

  iii. Presence of an underlying condition

Hypertrophic Osteoarthropathy

27

1. Hypertrophic Osteoarthropathy (HO) (*acropachy*)
   a. A syndrome characterized by excessive proliferation of skin and bone at the distal parts of the extremities seen in many diverse diseases
2. Connective-tissue abnormalities of HO
   a. "Clubbing" of fingers and toes
      i. Most conspicuous feature
      ii. A bulbous deformity of the tips of the digits
      iii. Subungual proliferation diminishes the normal nail angle
         1. Usually 20° or more with the projected line of the digit
   b. Periostitis of long tubular bones
      i. Periosteal proliferation
      ii. Synovial effusions with advanced stages
      iii. Radiographic appearance
         1. New bone separated from old cortex by a thin radiolucent line
   c. Arthritis

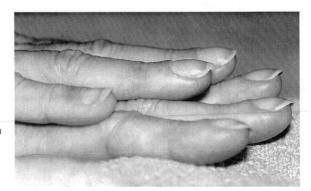

Fig. 27.1 Clubbing in Hypertrophic osteoarthropathy (Reproduced with permission from Arthritis and systemic disease. *Atlas of Rheumatology*. ImagesMD; 2005-01-18)

N.T. Colburn, *Review of Rheumatology*,
DOI 10.1007/978-1-84882-093-7_27, © Springer-Verlag London Limited 2012

Fig. 27.2 Periostitis of the femur in hypertrophic osteoarthropathy secondary to pulmonary metastatic osteogenic sarcoma (Reproduced with permission from Arthritis and systemic disease. *Atlas of Rheumatology.* ImagesMD; 2002-03-07)

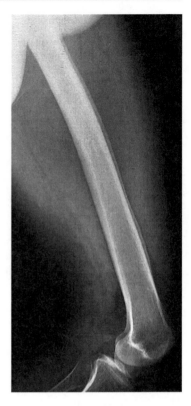

3. Classification
   a. Primary
      i. Hereditary
      ii. Appears during childhood
      iii. Usually self-limited
   b. Secondary (associated conditions)
      i. Subdivided into
         1. Generalized
            a. Neoplasms or infectious diseases
               i. Most common
            b. Congenital heart disease
            c. Inflammatory bowel disease
            d. Cirrhosis
            e. Graves' disease
         2. Localized
            a. Hemiplegia
            b. Aneurysms
            c. Infective arteritis
            d. Patent ductus arteriosus

4. Epidemiology
   a. A high male-to-female ratio (9:1)
   b. A familial predisposition
      i. One-third report a close relative with the same illness
5. Pathology and Pathogenesis
   a. Bulbous deformities develop from
      i. Edema
      ii. Excessive collagen deposition
   b. Other prominent features
      i. Vascular hyperplasia
         1. Associated with periosteal layer proliferation at the tubular bone level
      ii. Endothelial cell activation
      iii. Enhanced activation of platelets
         1. Central to HO
         2. Platelet-endothelial interaction produces
            a. von Willebrand factor antigen
            b. Vascular thrombi
            c. Antiphospholipid antibodies
   c. Cyanotic heart disease
      i. An excellent model for the pathogenesis of HO
      ii. Nearly all have lifelong clubbing
      iii. More than one-third display the fully developed syndrome
      iv. Frequent circulating macrothrombocytes
         1. Associated with distorted volume-distribution curves
      v. Large platelets
         1. Seen in patients with right-to-left shunts
         2. Direct access to the systemic circulation
         3. Reach distal sites on axial streams
         4. Interact with endothelial cells
            a. Subsequently release growth factor
         5. Elevated von Willebrand factor antigen
   d. Vascular endothelial growth factor (VEGF)
      i. A potent angiogenic stimulus and osteoblast-differentiation agent
      ii. Contributes to the pathogenesis of HO
      iii. Derived from platelets
      iv. Induced by hypoxia
      v. Produced by a variety of malignant tumors
         1. Fosters uncontrolled growth
         2. Elevated plasma levels in patients with lung CA and HO
6. Clinical Features
   a. Clinical course of secondary HO
      i. Relates to the nature and activity of the primary disease
      ii. Many are asymptomatic
         1. Unaware of digit deformities

    iii. Others suffer incapacitating bone pain
        1. Especially those with pulmonary malignancies
        2. Characteristically deep-seated
        3. Most prominent in the legs
  b. Diagnosis
    i. Based primarily on physical exam
        1. Bulbous deformity of the digits unique to HO
        2. Increased volume of digit soft tissue
          a. Molds the nail into a "watch-crystal" convexity
          b. Nail bed rocks when palpated
        3. Toes can also be affected
    ii. Digital index
        1. A practical bedside method using a string to measure clubbing
        2. Measure the circumference of each finger at the nail bed (NB) and the DIP
        3. Clubbing present if the sum of the 10 NB/DIP ratios is more than 10

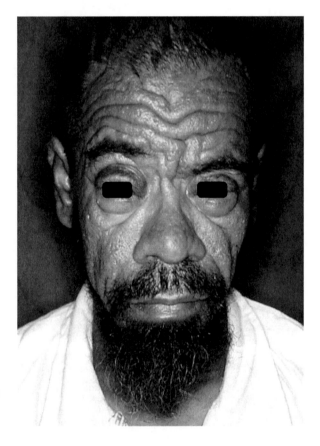

Fig. 27.3 The face of the patient with pachydermo-periostosis shows thickened and furrowed skin of forehead and thickened eyelids (Reproduced with permission from Primary hypertrophic osteoarthropathy with myelo-fibrosis.*Rheumatology International.* DOI:10.1007/s00296-007-0477-4. Springer; 2008-04-01)

     iii. Bone thickening
        1. Detected in ankles and wrists
        2. Tender to palpation
     iv. Effusions of the large joints
        1. Common
        2. A sympathetic reaction to adjacent periostosis
     v. Decreased ROM of the joint
     vi. Not an inflammatory or proliferative synovial disease
        1. No detectable synovial hypertrophy
        2. Arthrocentesis results
           a. Clear viscous fluid
           b. Few inflammatory cells
           c. Leukocyte count less than 1,000 cells/mm^3

c. *Pachydermoperiostosis*
     i. Seen in primary HO
     ii. A generalized skin hypertrophy
        1. Roughens the facial features
        2. Misdiagnosed as acromegaly

d. *Cutis vertices gyrata*
     i. Most advanced stage of skin hypertrophy
     ii. Associated glandular dysfunction
        1. Hyperhidrosis
        2. Seborrhea
        3. Acne

e. Types of HO with distinctive clinical findings
     i. Thyroid acropachy
        1. Distinguished by an exuberant periosteal proliferation
        2. Primarily involves small tubular bones of the hands and feet
        3. Clubbing coexist with
           a. Exophthalmos
           b. Pretibial myxedema
     ii. HO localized to one or two extremities
        1. Variant forms
        2. Response to prominent endothelial injury to the involved limb
        3. Associated with
           a. Aneurysms
           b. Infective endarteritis
           c. Patent ductus arteriosus and reversal of blood flow

7. Laboratory Features
  a. No distinctive clinical laboratory test abnormality
  b. Reflects the underlying illness
     i. Array of biochemical alterations

8. Imaging Features
   a. Plain radiographs of the extremities
      i. Reveal abnormalities in asymptomatic patients
   b. Radionuclide bone scanning
      i. A sensitive method for demonstrating periosteal involvement
   c. Prominent bone remodeling of the distal phalanx
      i. Seen with long standing clubbing
   d. Joint space typically preserved
   e. No erosions or periarticular osteopenia
   f. Periostosis
      i. Symmetrical bone changes in an orderly manner
      ii. Initially affects the distal parts of the lower extremities
      iii. Evolves in a centripetal fashion
      iv. Mild disease
          1. Involves only a few bones
             a. Tibia
             b. Fibula
          2. Periosteal apposition limited to the diaphysis
          3. A monolayer configuration
      v. Severe disease
          1. Affects all tubular bones
          2. Spreads to the metaphyses and epiphyses
          3. Generates irregular configurations
9. Diagnosis
   a. Combined requirement
      i. Clubbing
      ii. Periostosis of the tubular bones
   b. Synovial effusion
      i. Not essential for the diagnosis
   c. Features that distinguish HO from inflammatory types of arthritis
      i. Pain involves the joint **and** the adjacent bones
      ii. Non-inflammatory synovial fluid
      iii. Absent serum rheumatoid factor
   d. Previously healthy person develops HO manifestations
      i. Undertake a thorough search for underlying illness
   e. Primary HO diagnosed only after secondary HO ruled out
   f. Patient presents with clubbing
      i. A poor prognostic sign with a previous diagnosis of
          1. Pulmonary fibrosis
          2. Cystic fibrosis
          3. Liver cirrhosis
      ii. Indicate infective endocarditis with known rheumatic heart disease
      iii. POEMS syndrome with polyneuropathy of recent onset
          1. *P*olyneuropathy
          2. *O*rganomegaly

   3. *E*ndocrinopathy
   4. *M*-protein
   5. *S*kin changes
10. Treatment
 a. Painful osteoarthropathy responds to
   i. Analgesics
   ii. NSAIDs
 b. Rapid regression achieved with
   i. Correction of a heart defect
  ii. Removal of a lung tumor
  iii. Successful treatment of endocarditis

Storage and Deposition Diseases

28

1. Diseases characterized by deposition of normal metal ions
   a. Hemochromatosis = iron
   b. Ochronosis = calcium
   c. Wilson's = copper
2. Diseases characterized by cellular storage of abnormal lipids
   a. Gaucher's
      i. Glucocerebroside
   b. Fabry's
      i. Glycosphingolipids
   c. Farber's
      i. Ceramide
      ii. Usually die before age 4
   d. Multicentric reticulohistiocytosis
      i. Glycolipid-laden histiocytes
      ii. Multinucleated giant cells in skin and joints
      iii. Arthritis is a prominent feature
3. Hemochromatosis
   a. Common inherited autosomal recessive disorder
   b. Characterized by excessive body-iron stores
      i. Increased intestinal iron absorption and visceral deposition
      ii. Deposition of hemosiderin
      iii. Causes tissue damage and organ dysfunction
   c. Epidemiology
      i. Affects as many as 5 per 1,000 Caucasians of European extraction
      ii. Rarely appears before age 40 unless a family history
      iii. Men affected ten times more frequently than women
         1. Men have onset of symptoms at an earlier age
         2. Women protected by menstruation
   d. Phenotypic features
      i. Hepatic cirrhosis
      ii. Cardiomyopathy

    iii. Diabetes mellitus

    iv. Pituitary dysfunction

       1. Hypogonadism

    v. Sicca syndrome

    vi. Abnormal skin pigmentation

       1. Mostly melanin

e. Survey of 2,852 patients with hemochromatosis

    i. Symptoms present for an average of 10 years before diagnosis made

    ii. Arthralgia the most common and troublesome complaints (44%)

f. HFE gene (*HFE*, *HLA-H*)

    i. Gene for hemochromatosis

    ii. Discovered in 1996 by positional cloning

    iii. Near the HLA-A locus on chromosome 6

    iv. Accounts for 80% of cases in the USA and 100% of cases in Australia

    v. Mainly expressed in crypt enterocytes

    vi. Encodes for a protein that regulates brush border iron transport from the gut lumen

    vii. Occurs in 5% of whites

       1. Gives a carrier (heterozygote) frequency of approximately 1:10

       2. Gives a disease (homozygote) frequency of 1:400

    viii. A wide variation in gene frequency

       1. Highest mutation frequency

          a. Individuals of northwestern European descent

       2. Less common frequency

          a. Southern and eastern Europe population

       3. Rare mutation frequency

          a. Africa

          b. Americans

          c. Asia

          d. Pacific Islands

       4. Scandinavian families

          a. Frequency of homozygosity as high as 1%

    ix. Global prevalence of the gene mutation

       1. 1.9%

       2. One of the most commonly inherited metabolic diseases

    x. C282Y mutation

       1. More than 90% of patients

       2. A single G-to-A mutation

       3. A cysteine-to-tyrosine single amino acid substitution at position 282

       4. Defective protein causes crypt cells to misread the body's iron stores

          a. Iron absorption inappropriately increased

       5. Odds ratio 2,300 for disease if homozygous mutation

    xi. H63D mutation

       1. Less common

       2. An aspartate substitution for histidine at position 63

3. Not associated with iron overload
4. Odds ratio 6 for disease if homozygous mutation
5. May act synergistically with C3824 in a small percentage

   xii. Iron overload in the **absence** of the C282Y mutation
1. Reported in some European population

   xiii. Homozygous and heterozygous genotypes
1. Correlate with major and minor disease expression
2. Homozygotes
   a. Arthritis more common
   b. Heaviest iron overload

g. Normal human iron stores
   i. Contain 3–4 g of iron
   ii. Two thirds contained in
1. Hemoglobin
2. Myoglobin
3. A variety of enzymes
   iii. One third contained as storage iron
1. In ferritin and hemosiderin
2. Hepatocytes and macrophages of the liver
3. Bone marrow
4. Spleen
5. Muscle
   iv. Typical Western diet
1. Contains 10–20 mg of iron a day
2. Only 1–2 mg absorbed daily by the duodenal mucosa
   a. To balance iron loss from
     i. Exfoliated GI epithelial cells
     ii. Desquamation of the skin

h. Iron stores in hemochromatosis
   i. Excess GI iron absorption ranges from 3 to 4 mg per day
   ii. An accumulation of 15–35 g of iron over a 35–60 year period

i. Secondary hemochromatosis
   i. Chronic hypoproliferative anemia and thalassemia
1. Tissue damage occurs as a result of iron overload
2. Prolonged excessive iron ingestion
3. Repeated blood transfusions
   ii. *Hemosiderosis*
1. Iron overload without tissue damage
2. Iron deposition in macrophages
   a. Less tissue damage and end-organ dysfunction

j. Clinical features
   i. Variable disease severity
1. Manifestations usually between the ages of 40 and 60 years
2. A few develop full clinical expression by age 20
3. 30% of homozygotes never develop clinical symptoms

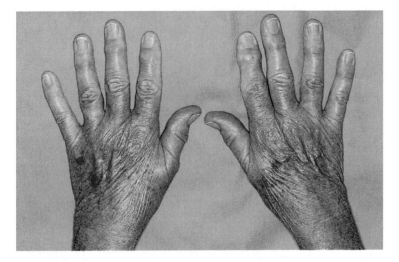

Fig. 28.1 The hands in hereditary hemochromatosis demonstrate characteristic skin pigmentation (Reproduced with permission from Hemochromatosis and Wilson disease. *Gastroenterology and Hepatology.* ImagesMD; 2006-06-27)

   ii. Asymptomatic abnormal liver function tests
      1. Typical presentation
      2. 95% have hepatomegaly
      3. Usually progresses to hepatic cirrhosis in untreated cases
  iii. Skin
      1. Slate-gray appearance
        a. Due to iron in eccrine sweat glands
      2. Brown skin pigmentation
        a. Due to melanin deposition (50%)
  iv. Diabetes mellitus
   v. Hypogonadism
      1. Decreased libido (20–40%)
      2. Impotence
      3. Amenorrhea
      4. Sparse body hair
  vi. Constitutional symptoms (80%)
      1. Weakness or lethargy
      2. Cardiac involvement
        a. CHF (30%)
        b. Principle cause of death in untreated patients
 vii. Arthritis
      1. Characteristic arthropathy
        a. Occurs in 20–50% of patients
        b. Chronic and progressive

Fig. 28.2 Characteristic
arthropathy associated with
hemochromatosis
(Reproduced with permission
from Arthritis and systemic
disease. *Atlas of
Rheumatology.* ImagesMD;
2005-01-18)

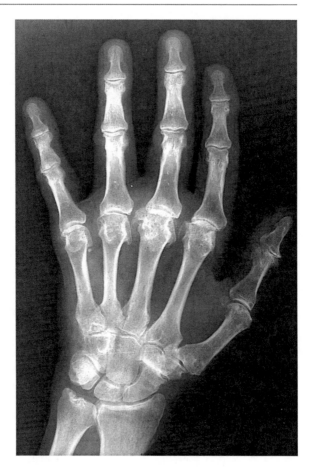

    c. Presenting feature in about one-half of cases
    d. May develop after treatment initiated
  2. Predominantly affects the second and third MCP and PIP joints
    a. MCP involvement more common in about one-half of cases
    b. Dominant hand solely or more severely affected
    c. Finger joints and wrists mildly tender and limited in motion
  3. Larger joints affected
    a. Shoulders, hips, and knees
    b. Hips and shoulders may be rapidly progressive
  4. True morning stiffness is not a feature
  5. Physical exam
    a. Firm swelling with mild tenderness
    b. Warmth and effusion absent
      i. Distinguishes from RA
  6. Suspicious for hemochromatosis
    a. An OA-like disease that involves MCP and wrist joints

Fig. 28.3 Oblique radiograph of the left hand in a patient with hemochromatosis shows large characteristic hook-like osteophytes arising from the radial aspect of the second and third metacarpal heads (Reproduced with permission from Arthropathies. *Bone Pathology*. DOI: 10.1007/978-1-59745-347-9_12. Springer; 2009-01-01)

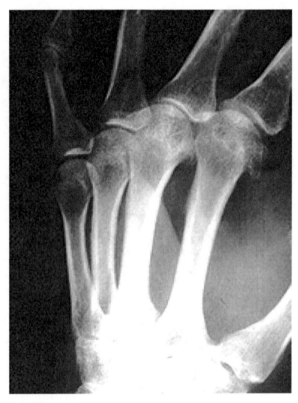

      b. Particularly in men during the fourth and fifth decade

      c. Reported in individuals as young as 26 years

    7. Pathogenesis of arthritis unknown

      a. Degenerative changes not necessarily in relation to synovial iron

      b. Ionic iron inhibits pyrophosphatase activity

      c. Calcium pyrophosphate concentrates locally in the joint

      d. Deposition of calcium in cartilage

      e. Predisposes to inflammatory and degenerative disease

  k. Radiographic features of hemochromatosis

    i. Radiologic changes resemble OA

      1. Sclerotic margins

      2. Joint space narrowing

      3. Osteophyte formation

        a. Less osteophytosis in hemochromatosis

        b. Osteophytes characteristically hook-like in hemochromatosis

      4. DIP joints may be affected

      5. CMC joint changes of generalized OA **not** a feature

    ii. Degrees of diffuse osteoporosis

      1. Due to hypogonadism

       a. Pituitary iron infiltration decreases gonadotropin levels

       b. Hepatic cirrhosis leads to testicular atrophy

       c. Poor conversion of vitamin D to 25-OH vitamin D

   2. Direct effects of iron on bone

       a. Increased synovial iron compared with serum levels

       b. Directly inhibits bone formation

l. Infections in hemochromatosis

   i. *Yersinia* septic arthritis or septicemia

      1. Unusual complication

      2. Microbe requires an iron-rich environment

   ii. Hepatitis B and C viral infections

      1. Accelerates liver damage

m. Chondrocalcinosis

   i. Characteristic of hemochromatosis arthropathy

   ii. Superimposed attacks of CPPD crystal synovitis

   iii. A late complication (about 50%)

   iv. Occurs as the sole abnormality

      1. Without the degenerative arthropathy

   v. Areas affected

      1. Hyaline cartilage

         a. Shoulder

         b. Wrist

         c. Hip

         d. Knee

      2. Fibrocartilage

         a. Triangular ligament of the wrist

         b. Symphysis pubis

n. Diagnosis

   i. Transferrin saturation (iron/total iron binding capacity (TIBC) × 100)

      1. Transferrin (a plasma iron-binding protein)

      2. Greater than 60% in men or 50% in women

      3. With an elevated ferritin greater than two times normal

         a. Serum ferritin levels

            i. Accurate measure of peripheral iron stores

            ii. Also increased in the setting of

               1. Acute liver injury

               2. Systemic inflammation

               3. Neoplasia (lymphoma)

      4. Obtained in the fasting state

      5. 95% sensitive and 85% specific

      6. Cornerstone test for diagnosis

   ii. Liver biopsy

      1. Provides definitive evidence of iron overload

      2. Direct measurement of iron

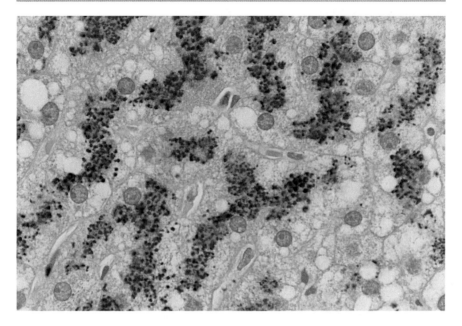

Fig. 28.4 Liver biopsy in hereditary hemochromatosis provides definitive evidence of iron over-load (Reproduced with permission from Arthritis and systemic disease. *Atlas of Rheumatology.* ImagesMD; 2002-03-07)

3. Reserved for cases in diagnostic doubt
   a. Persons heterozygous for the C282Y mutation with abnormal iron indices or liver function tests
4. Assess the severity of liver damage
   a. Fibrosis
      i. Serum ferritin >1,000 ng/l
   b. Cirrhosis
   c. Hepatoma
5. Primary (idiopathic) hemochromatosis
   a. Iron deposits affect parenchymal hepatic cells
6. Secondary hemochromatosis
   a. Reticuloendothelial cells most affected
      iii. Synovial biopsy
         1. Iron deposition in **type B** synovial lining cells
      iv. Direct noninvasive magnetic measurements of hepatic iron stores
         1. Quantitative method
         2. Early detection of iron overload
         3. Rapid evaluation of treatment
      v. Patient with abnormal iron studies homozygous for the C282Y gene
         1. Biopsies may not be necessary

 o. Laboratory features

  i. Synovial fluid (SF)

   1. Good viscosity

   2. Leukocyte counts below 1,000 cells/mm^3

   3. During acute episodes of pseudogout

    a. Leukocytosis

    b. CPPD crystals

  ii. ESR usually normal

  iii. Rheumatoid factor may be positive

   1. Patients with chronic liver disease

  iv. Unbound iron binding capacity (UIBC)

   1. Population screening

   2. Higher sensitivity

   3. Fewer false-positives

  v. Urine

   1. May see evidence of iron in sediment

   2. The amount of iron excreted in the urine after administration of the iron-chelating agent deferoxamine

    a. Correlates with the presence of parenchymal hepatic iron

  vi. Biopsies

   1. Synovium

    a. Diagnostic with iron deposits in **type B** synthetic lining cells

    b. Iron deposits in phagocyte **type A** lining cells

     i. RA

     ii. Traumatic hemarthrosis

     iii. Hemophilia

     iv. Villonodular synovitis

   2. Cartilage

    a. Chondrocytes with hemosiderin deposits

   3. Other tissues with evidence of iron deposits

    a. Skin

    b. Intestinal mucosa

    c. Bone marrow

 p. Treatment

  i. Obtain biochemical screening of all first-degree relatives

   1. For medical prevention

   2. Homozygotes diagnosed and treated before cirrhosis

    a. Life expectancy same as that of the general population

  ii. Screening

   1. Measure serum iron-binding transferrin

   2. Perform the UIBC test

   3. May defer until the second decade

   4. Perform iron studies in **all** men by age 40

    a. Given disease frequency in the general population

    iii. Genotyping
       1. C282Y (and H63D) mutations of the *HFE* gene
       2. Useful diagnostic aid
       3. Helpful in healthy relatives
          a. Counseling
          b. Predicting disease risk
       4. Does **not** indicate
          a. Iron stores
          b. Prognosis
   iv. Aggressive phlebotomy therapy
       1. Promotes longevity with increased life expectancy
          a. 90% 5-year survival
          b. 33% survival **without** therapy
       2. Prevents or reverses organ damage
          a. Definite improvements in
             i. Hepatomegaly
            ii. Liver function studies
           iii. Pigmentation
          b. Cardiac function stabilizes or improves
          c. Diabetes mellitus improves by 50%
          d. Hepatic fibrosis may improve
             i. Cirrhosis irreversible
          e. Hepatocellular carcinoma **not** diminished
             i. A late sequelae
            ii. One-third of those who develop hepatic cirrhosis
               1. 200× increased risk
           iii. Major cause of death in treated individuals
               1. 30–45%
          f. Arthritis
             i. Little effect on arthritis usually
            ii. Does not prevent progression of arthritis
       3. Weekly phlebotomies
          a. Twice weekly until
             i. Transferrin saturation <50%
            ii. Ferritin level <50 ng/ml
          b. Iron depletion
          c. Mild anemia may be present
       4. Phlebotomies continued as required
          a. Up to 2–3 years
          b. Usually every 3–4 months
          c. Maintain normal serum iron levels
       5. Prophylactic phlebotomy
          a. Considered on the basis of genetic predisposition
    v. Iron chelating therapy
       1. Intravenous (IV) deferoxamine
       2. Generally effective

        3. Impractical
          a. Expensive
          b. Requires IV administration
     vi. Control arthritis symptoms
        1. NSAIDs
        2. Avoid agents requiring hepatic metabolism
          a. Diclofenac
          b. Nabumetone
    vii. Total joint replacements
        1. As indicated

4. Alkaptonuria (Ochronosis)
  a. Rare autosomal recessive disorder
  b. Human *HGO* gene
    i. Cloned
    ii. Loss of function mutations
    iii. Mapped to chromosome 3q2 in 6 reported pedigrees
  c. Disorder of tyrosine catabolism
    i. Complete deficiency of the enzyme homogentisic acid oxidase (HGO)
    ii. Defect causes accumulation of homogentisic acid
        1. Normal intermediate in phenylalanine and tyrosine metabolism
        2. Large amounts of homogentisic acid excretion in the urine
          a. Alkalization and oxidation causes urine to turn black
        3. Retained in the body as an oxidized pigmented polymer
          a. Cartilage
            i. Deeper layers of articular cartilage
            ii. Bound to collagen fibers
            iii. Loses its normal resiliency
            iv. Becomes brittle and fibrillated
            v. Erosions
               1. Denuded subchondral bone
               2. Synovium
               3. Joint cavity
            vi. Osteochondral bodies can form
          b. Skin
          c. Sclerae
  d. Clinical features
    i. Progressive degenerative arthropathy
    ii. Symptoms begin between the second and third decade
    iii. Arthritis of the spine (ochronotic spondylosis)
        1. Initially affects the spinal column
          a. First sign may be an acute disc syndrome
        2. Pigment in the intervertebral disc
          a. Annulus fibrosus
          b. Nucleus pulposus
          c. Predisposes to herniation

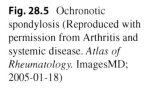

Fig. 28.5 Ochronotic
spondylosis (Reproduced with
permission from Arthritis and
systemic disease. *Atlas of
Rheumatology.* ImagesMD;
2005-01-18)

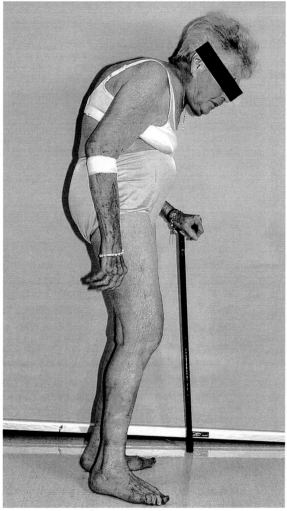

3. Eventually resembles ankylosing spondylitis
   a. Progressive lumbar rigidity
   b. Loss of stature
   c. Forward stoop
   d. Loss of lumbar lordosis
   e. Loss of height
   f. Flexed hips and knees
   g. Wide-based stance
   h. Contrast to AS
      i. SI and apophyseal joints **not** affected
iv. Arthritis of larger peripheral joints
   1. Usually seen later
   2. Less frequent than spinal disease

Fig. 28.6 Bluish discoloration of the ear pinnae in ochronosis (alkaptonuria) (Reproduced with permission from Arthritis and systemic disease. *Atlas of Rheumatology.* ImagesMD; 2005-01-18)

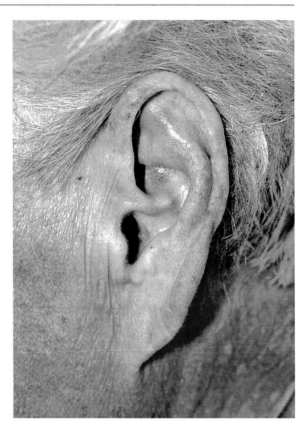

     3. Involvement of
       a. Knees
       b. Shoulders
       c. Hips
     4. **Sparing** of small peripheral joints
       a. Hands
       b. Wrists
       c. Feet
   v. Associations
     1. Chondrocalcinosis
     2. Osteochondral bodies
     3. Synovial effusions
       a. Ochronotic peripheral arthropathy
  vi. Predominant complaints
     1. Stiffness
     2. Loss of joint mobility
     3. Knee effusions and crepitus
     4. Flexion contractures
     5. Pain less prominent
     6. Lacking other signs of articular inflammation

Fig. 28.7 Triangular pigmentation of the sclera in ochronosis (alkaptonuria) (Reproduced with permission from Arthritis and systemic disease. *Atlas of Rheumatology*. ImagesMD; 2005-01-18)

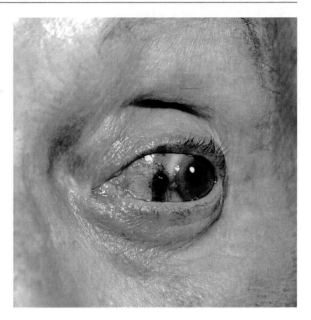

    vii. Nonarticular features
        1. Bluish discoloration and calcification of the ear pinnae
        2. Other ear involvement
           a. Concha
           b. Antihelix
           c. Cerumen
        3. Triangular pigmentation of the sclera
        4. Pigmentation over the nose, axillae, and groin
        5. Prostatic calculi common
        6. Cardiac murmurs from valvular pigment deposits
        7. Deposits in arterial walls
    viii. Depositions can lead clinically to
        1. Aortic stenosis
        2. Conduction hearing loss
        3. Prostatic calculi
        4. Ochronotic arthropathy
        5. Chondral calcification
        6. Osteochondral loose bodies
  e. Radiographic features
      i. Multiple vacuum discs of the spine
        1. Earliest visible feature
      ii. Ossification of the discs
        1. Dense calcification of the intervertebral discs
        2. Narrowing of the intervertebral spaces
        3. Progressive collapse and fusion

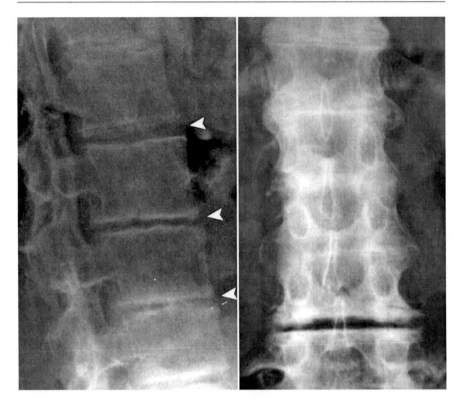

Fig. 28.8 Anteroposterior and lateral plain radiograph of the lower thoracic vertebrae shows severe intervertebral disc space narrowing (*arrowheads*) in a patient with ochronosis (Reproduced with permission from Ochronosis. *Internal Medicine.* DOI: 10.1007/978-3-642-03709-2_69. Springer; 2010-01-01)

      4. Eventually the entire spine involved
      5. Premature degenerative changes
  iii. Differential diagnosis
      1. Hemochromatosis
      2. Hyperparathyroidism
      3. Calcium pyrophosphate deposition
      4. Paralytic poliomyelitis
      5. Amyloidosis
  iv. Chondrocalcinosis affects
      1. Symphysis pubis
      2. Costal cartilage
      3. Ear helix
   v. Peripheral joint findings resemble OA
      1. Loss of cartilage space
      2. Marginal osteophytes
      3. Eburnation of the subchondral bone

      vi. Contrast to OA
        1. Shoulder and hip degeneration more severe
        2. Osteochondral bodies
  f. Laboratory features
      i. Diagnosis suspected when
        1. Patient gives a history of passing dark urine
        2. When fresh urine turns black on standing
        3. When fresh urine turns black on alkalinization
        4. A false-positive test for diabetes mellitus
        5. Arthritis onsets
      ii. Darkly pigmented synovium seen on arthroscopy
      iii. Quantitation of homogentisic acid in urine and blood
        1. A specific enzymatic method
      iv. Molecular cloning of the HGO gene
        1. Enables detection of heterozygotic carriers
      v. Synovial fluid
        1. Clear, yellow, and viscous
        2. Does **not** darken with alkalinization
        3. Speckled with particles of debris resembling ground pepper
        4. Leukocyte counts of a few hundred cells
          a. Predominantly mononuclear
          b. Cytoplasm contains dark inclusions of phagocytosed ochronotic pigment
        5. Centrifugation and microscopic examination of sediment
          a. Fragments of pigmented cartilage
        6. Effusions may contain CPPD crystals
          a. No inflammation
      vi. Synovium
        1. Embedded pigmented cartilage fragments
        2. Often surrounded by giant cells
  g. Treatment
      i. Nothing effective available
      ii. Deposition may be prevented by
        1. Large amounts of ascorbic acid
        2. Diets low in
          a. Protein
          b. Phenylalanine
          c. Tyrosine
      iii. Symptomatic measures most practical
      iv. Surgery
        1. Removal of osteochondral bodies
        2. Prosthetic joint replacements
5. Wilson's Disease
  a. Rare metabolic disorder (hepatolenticular degeneration)
  b. Deposition of copper leads to organ dysfunction
      i. Liver

      ii. Brain

      iii. Kidneys

  c. Genetics

      i. Inherited as an autosomal recessive trait

      ii. Affects about 1 in 30,000 persons in most populations

      iii. Symptomatic for individuals aged 6–40

      iv. Defective gene *ATP7B*

         1. Related mutations produce a wide phenotypic variation

         2. Localized to human chromosome 13

         3. Codes for an abnormal P-type adenosine triphosphatase

            a. Membrane copper transport protein

            b. Normally transports hepatocellular copper into bile

            c. Defect allows copper to build up in hepatocytes

         4. More than 60 mutations identified

      v. Genetic testing

         1. Uses polymorphic DNA markers

         2. Helpful for testing presymptomatic siblings

         3. Recommended before treatment initiated

  d. Clinical features

      i. Hepatocytes capacity to store copper exceeded

      ii. Excessive copper deposition

         1. Liver

         2. Extrahepatic sites

             a. Brain

            b. Kidneys

            c. Urine

            d. Serum

      iii. Increased total body copper accumulation leads to

         1. Cirrhosis in the liver

         2. Kayser–Fleischer rings in the cornea

             a. Characteristic green or brown deposits of copper in Descemet's membrane

            b. Do not interfere with vision

            c. Present in 95% of cases with neurologic or psychiatric manifestations

            d. Also seen in other causes of hepatic cirrhosis and nonhepatic diseases

         3. Lenticular degeneration

             a. Movement disorders in the basal ganglia

            b. Rigid dystonia

         4. Psychiatric disorders

             a. Mood disturbances

            b. Neurosis

            c. Hypophonia

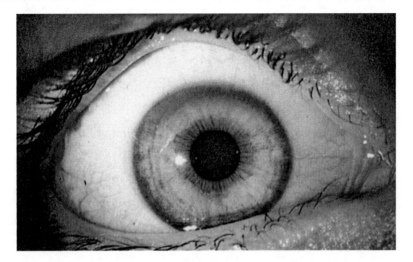

Fig. 28.9 Kayser–Fleischer ring in a patient with Wilson's disease (Reproduced with permission from Movement disorders. *Atlas of Clinical Neurology.* ImagesMD; 2002-01-24)

5. Gynecologic manifestations
   a. Infertility
   b. Amenorrhea
6. Kidney renal tubular damage
   a. Renal tubule acidosis
   b. Fanconi's syndrome
      i. Generalized osteopenia or osteomalacia
7. Arthritis
   a. Develops in up to 50% of adults
   b. Rare in children
   c. Pathogenesis unclear
   d. Characterized by mild premature OA
      i. Involves the
         1. Wrists
         2. MCPJ
         3. Knees
         4. Spine
      ii. Involvement of the hip uncommon
      iii. Presents with pain and swelling
   e. Ossified bodies of the wrists
      i. Associated with subchondral cyst
   f. Knee involvement
      i. Chondromalacia patellae
      ii. Osteochondritis dissecans

          iii. Chondrocalcinosis
             1. No crystals isolated
          iv. Mild knee effusions
      g. Asymptomatic radiographic changes also seen
      h. Joint hypermobility
      i. Presence does not correlate with neurologic, hepatic, or renal disease
      j. Copper found in articular cartilage by elemental analysis
    iv. Hepatic or neurologic symptoms
      1. Develop in childhood or adolescence
      2. Liver disease
        a. The most common presentation between ages 8 and 16
        b. Symptoms
          i. Nausea
          ii. Vomiting
          iii. Jaundice
        c. Transient hepatitis
        d. Fulminant hepatitis
        e. Chronic active hepatitis
        f. Cirrhosis
        g. Presentation of fulminant hepatic failure with
          i. Disproportionately low amino transferases
            1. Usually <1,500 u/l
          ii. Markedly increased bilirubin
            1. Due to associated hemolysis
      3. Neurologic symptoms
        a. Rare before age 12
    v. Other presenting symptoms
      1. Acute hemolytic anemia
      2. Arthralgia
      3. Renal stones
  e. Radiographic features
    i. Subchondral cysts
    ii. Cortical fragmentation
    iii. Joint space narrowing
    iv. Sclerosis helps to distinguish from primary OA
      1. Marginal
      2. Subchondral
      3. Central
    v. Marked osteophyte formation
    vi. Multiple calcified loose bodies
      1. Especially at the wrist
    vii. Periostitis
      1. At the femoral trochanter
      2. Other tendinous insertions
    viii. Periarticular calcifications

Fig. 28.10 Several MCP joints are surrounded by small ossicles, characteristic radiographic feature of Wilson's disease (Reproduced with permission from Arthritis and systemic disease. *Atlas of Rheumatology.* ImagesMD; 2002-03-07)

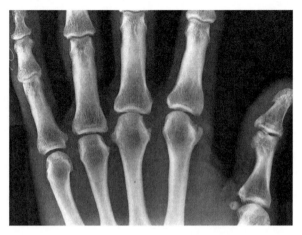

 ix. Chondrocalcinosis
  x. Changes in the lumbar areas
      1. Squaring of the vertebral bodies
      2. Intervertebral joint space narrowing
      3. Osteophytes
      4. Osteochondritis
 xi. Osteoporosis (up to 50%) and osteomalacia
      1. As a result of Fanconi's syndrome
      2. Secondary to renal tubular acidosis
 f. Laboratory features
    i. Establish the diagnosis
   ii. Low serum copper and decreased serum ceruloplasmin
      1. Copper levels <70 μg/dl
      2. Serum ceruloplasmin <100 μg/day
  iii. Urinary copper excretion
      1. Increased in symptomatic patients
   iv. Biliary excretion of copper
      1. Decreased markedly
    v. Needle biopsy of the liver
      1. Microchemical evidence of copper deposition
      2. Elevated hepatic copper concentration
         a. >250 μg Cu/g dry weight
         b. Most reliable test early in the course
   vi. Specialized studies with radioactive copper
  vii. Synovial biopsies
      1. Hyperplasia of synovial lining cells
      2. Mild chronic inflammation
      3. Microvilli formation
      4. Vascular changes

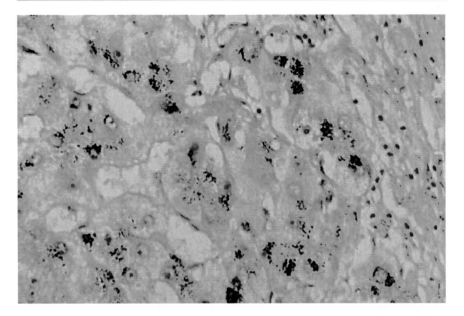

Fig. 28.11 Liver histology in Wilson's disease. Deposition of copper as golden-brown granules is shown in the rhodanine-stained section (×400 magnification) (Reproduced with permission from Wilson's disease. *Clinical Hepatology.* DOI: 10.1007/978-3-642-04519-6_27. Springer; 2010-01-01)

       viii. Joint fluid
          1. Low leukocyte counts
      ix. Screen first-degree relatives older than 6 years
          1. Physical exam
          2. Liver functions
          3. Serum copper
          4. Ceruloplasmin
          5. 24-h urine copper
          6. Slit-lamp examination
  g. Treatment
      i. Penicillamine
          1. Life long copper chelation
          2. In conjunction with dietary copper restriction
          3. Prevents or improves every disease manifestation
             a. Unclear regarding arthropathy control
          4. Most patients live normal and healthy lives
     ii. Side effects of penicillamine
          1. Acute polyarthritis
          2. Polymyositis
          3. Syndrome resembling SLE

     iii. Trientine
        1. Chelating agent
        2. For patients intolerant of penicillamine
     iv. Other treatment options
        1. Zinc
        2. Ammonium tetrathiomolybdate
     v. Avoid foods rich in copper
        1. Organ meats
        2. Nuts
        3. Chocolate
        4. Mushrooms
     vi. Liver transplant
        1. Acute hepatic failure
        2. Long-standing cirrhosis
           a. Where penicillamine or trientine are not options

6. Gaucher's Disease
  a. Lysosomal glycolipid storage disease
  b. Glucocerebrosidase
     i. Hydrolytic enzyme
     ii. Subnormal activity
     iii. Accounts for the disease's non-neurologic features
     iv. Affects all cells
     v. Glycolipid-engorged macrophages
     vi. Accumulates in reticuloendothelial cells
        1. Spleen
        2. Liver
        3. Bone marrow
  c. Autosomal recessive
     i. Gene located on chromosome 1q21
     ii. Mild forms seen frequently in the Jewish population
  d. Classified into clinical subdivisions
     i. Type 1
        1. Most common form
           a. 99% of cases
        2. Adult or chronic type
        3. Best prognosis
        4. Primarily in Ashkenazi Jews
        5. Defined by the **lack** of neurologic involvement
        6. Affected adults with glucocerebroside in the RE system
           a. Organomegaly
           b. Hypersplenism
           c. Conjunctival pingueculae
           d. Skin pigmentation
           e. Osteoarticular disease
        7. Typical presentation

   a. Lymphadenopathy
   b. Hepatosplenomegaly
   c. Signs or symptoms of hypersplenism
   d. Rheumatic complaints
      i. May be mistaken for juvenile RA
      ii. Appears early in the disease course
      iii. Pain in the hip, knee, or shoulder
      iv. Caused by disease of the adjacent bone
      v. Chronic aching around the hip or proximal tibia
         1. Young adults
         2. May last only a few days
         3. Usually recurrent
   8. Patients with few or no clinical manifestations
      a. Discovered when bone marrow examined for some other reason
      b. Discovered through an investigation of mild thrombocytopenia
   9. Bone crisis of the femur or tibia
      a. Excruciating pain
         i. Tenderness
         ii. Swelling
         iii. Erythema
      b. Unexplained polyarthritis
      c. Bone pain tends to lessen with age
  10. Other skeletal features
      a. Pathologic long-bone fractures
      b. Vertebral compression
      c. Osteonecrosis
         i. Femoral or humeral heads or proximal tibia
         ii. Develops slowly or rapidly with bone crisis
         iii. Usually affects only one bone area at a time
         iv. Positive acute phase reactants and bone scans
            1. Mimics a pseudo-osteomyelitis
            2. Conservative management recommended
            3. Surgical drainage leads to infection
  11. Radiographic features
      a. Common
         i. Asymptomatic areas of rarefaction
         ii. Patchy sclerosis
         iii. Cortical thickening
      b. Serious and deforming features
         i. ON of the hips
         ii. Pathologic fractures of the femur and vertebrae
      c. Flaring or widening of the distal portion of bones
         i. Radiologic appearance of an Erlenmeyer flask
         ii. Femur most commonly involved
         iii. Also involves the tibia and humerus

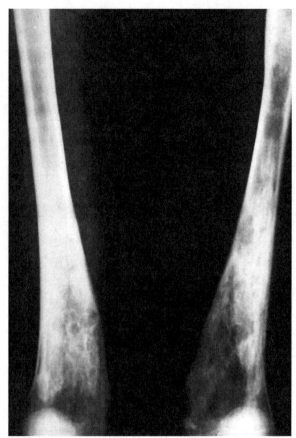

Fig. 28.12 Bone lesions in Gaucher disease with the radiographic appearance of an "Erlenmeyer flask" (Reproduced with permission from Metabolic genetics. *Atlas of Pediatrics*. ImagesMD; 2006-01-20)

12. Laboratory features
    a. Elevated serum acid phosphatase and ACE
       i. Especially with bone pain or articular symptoms
    b. Reliable method of diagnosis
       i. Determination of leukocyte B-glucosidase
       ii. Bone marrow aspirate for the Gaucher cell
          1. A large lipid-storage histiocyte
          2. Differentiate from the globoid cells of Krabbe's disease (galactocerebrosidosis)
    c. Biopsies for glucocerebroside testing
       i. Histologic diagnosis unnecessary
       ii. Needle biopsy of the liver
       iii. Washed leukocytes
       iv. Extracts of cultured skin fibroblasts
       v. Assays used to detect heterozygous carriers
    d. Amniocentesis
       i. Prenatal detection of diseased fetuses

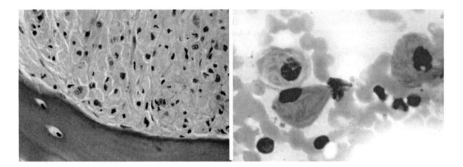

Fig. 28.13 Gaucher disease. (**a**) Bone marrow biopsy shows sheets of histiocytes with cytoplasm distended by striated tubular inclusions. (**b**) Bone marrow aspirate shows characteristic wrinkled tissue paper–like appearance of storage histiocytes (Reproduced with permission from The bone marrow in normal and disease states. *Neoplastic Hematopathology*. DOI: 10.1007/978-1-60761-384-8_5. Springer; 2010-01-01)

        ii. PCR
           1. Most useful genetic screening
        iii. Genetic counseling
           1. Family members
           2. Prospective parents
    ii. Type 2
        1. Infantile Gaucher's disease
        2. Fulminating disorder with severe brain involvement
        3. Death occurs within the first 18 months of life
    iii. Type 3
        1. Intermediate or juvenile form
        2. Begins in early childhood
        3. Many features of the chronic form
        4. With or without CNS involvement
        5. Skeletal involvement to a lesser extent
  e. Treatment
    i. Mostly symptomatic
    ii. Aimed at controlling pain and infection
    iii. Bisphosphonates
        1. Used to treat bone disease
        2. Intermittent IV pamidronate
           a. With oral calcium
    iv. Splenectomy
        1. Used in adults
        2. To control hypersplenism
        3. May accelerate bone disease
        4. Partial splenectomy protective against
           a. Infection
           b. Hepatic effects
           c. Bone effects

     v. TJR

       1. For advanced osteoarticular disease

       2. Prosthetic loosening

         a. Occurs more often than in other disorders

       3. Bleeding can be an operative problem

    vi. Replacement enzyme

       1. Modified form of glucocerebroside (Ceredase)

       2. Periodic IV infusions

         a. Over many months

         b. Results in regression of symptoms

       3. N-butyldoxynojirimycin

         a. Oral treatment

         b. Decreases glucocerebroside substrate

         c. Reduced visceromegaly

         d. Used as a monotherapy

         e. Used combination with IV enzyme replacement

       4. Allogeneic bone marrow transplantation

         a. An option

         b. With an HLA-identical donor

       5. Gene-transfer therapy

         a. Retroviral vector constructs

         b. Codes the gene for glucocerebrosidase into hematopoietic progenitors

7. Fabry's Disease

  a. Lysosomal lipid-storage disease

  b. Glycosphingolipids accumulate widely in

    i. Nerves

    ii. Viscera

    iii. Skin

    iv. Osteoarticular tissues

  c. Slowly progressive disorder predominantly affecting males

    i. Sex-linked inherited disease

    ii. Caused by a deficiency of the enzyme alpha galactosidase A

    iii. Gene and mutations

      1. Localized to middle of the long arm of the X chromosome

  d. Clinical features

    i. Widespread and nonspecific

    ii. Diagnosis often missed or delayed

    iii. Children

      1. Deposition marked in and around blood vessels

      2. Characteristic rash

        a. Dark blue or red angiokeratomas or angiectases

        b. Located around the buttocks, thighs, and lower abdomen

        c. *Angiokeratoma corporis diffusum*

          i. Term used when rash is diffuse

        d. Almost always associated with hypohydrosis

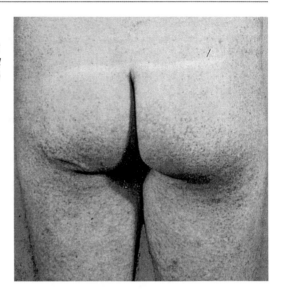

Fig. 28.14 Characteristic rash of Fabry's disease (Reproduced with permission from Genetic diseases of the nervous system. *Atlas of Clinical Neurology.* ImagesMD; 2002-01-24)

   iv. Renal involvement
      1. Main target organs
      2. Proteinuria
         a. Gradually develops in childhood or adolescence
      3. Abnormal urinary sediments
         a. Birefringent lipid crystals
         b. Maltese crosses
      4. Usually requires dialysis or transplantation
      5. Most affected males succumb to renal failure before age 50
   v. Cardiovascular and cerebrovascular deposition of sphingolipid
      1. Parallels the renal disease
      2. Vascular insufficiencies
      3. Sudden death
  vi. Ocular changes
      1. Severe
      2. Characteristic corneal opacity
         a. Seen by slip-lamp
      3. Occurs early
      4. Helpful in diagnosis
         a. Even in heterozygous women
 vii. Musculoskeletal
      1. Insidious development of polyarthritis
      2. Degenerative changes
      3. Flexion contractures of the fingers
         a. Particularly the DIPJ
      4. Foam cells seen in synovial vessels and connective tissue

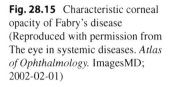

Fig. 28.15 Characteristic corneal opacity of Fabry's disease (Reproduced with permission from The eye in systemic diseases. *Atlas of Ophthalmology*. ImagesMD; 2002-02-01)

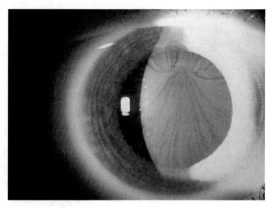

      viii. Pain crisis
         1. 80% of children
         2. Burning paresthesias of the hands and feet
           a. Later the whole extremities may be involved
         3. Associated with fever and elevations of the ESR
    e. Radiographs
      i. Infarct-like opacities of bone
      ii. Osteoporosis of the spine
      iii. ON of the hip and talus
    f. Diagnosis
      i. Genetic counseling to affected families
      ii. Discriminate carriers and noncarriers
      iii. Measure alpha galactosidase activity ratios in leukocytes and fibroblasts
      iv. DNA studies
    g. Treatment
      i. Not satisfactory
      ii. Gene therapy
         1. Recombinant adenovirus AxCAGα-gal
         2. To provide enzyme replacement
      iii. Antiplatelet medication
         1. Suppresses vascular damage
      iv. Carbamazepine or phenytoin
         1. Benefits burning paresthesias
  8. Multicentric Reticulohistiocytosis (MRH)
    a. Rare dermatoarthritis
    b. Unknown cause or familial association
    c. Cellular accumulation in the skin and joints
      i. Glycolipid-laden histiocytes
      ii. Multinucleated giant cells

    d. Most common presentation
       i. Painful destructive polyarthritis resembling RA
      ii. Joint presentation precedes the appearance of skin lesions
         1. Months to years
         2. Two-thirds of patients
      iii. Skin nodules not entirely characteristic of RA
         1. Differ in appearance and location
    e. Sex and ages affected
       i. Predominantly affects middle-age women
      ii. Self-limited form seen in childhood
    f. Clinical features
       i. Insidious disease onset
      ii. Polyarthritis
         1. Inflammatory
         2. Usually chronic
         3. Symmetric
         4. Can be destructive
         5. Resembles RA when PIPJ affected
         6. Resembles psoriatic arthritis when DIPJ affected
           a. Severely deforming arthritis mutilans occurs
           b. One half of patients
         7. Can involve the cervical spine
         8. Remission after many years of progressive disease
      iii. Tenosynovial involvement
      iv. Skin nodules
         1. Classic finding
         2. Firm yellowish or purple papulonodules
         3. Characteristic lesions
           a. Small papules and "coral bead-like" clusters
           b. Occurs around the nail folds
         4. Sites of skin nodulation
           a. Face
           b. Hands
           c. Elbows
           d. Neck
           e. Chest
           f. Ears
         5. Vary in size
         6. Wax and wane or disappear completely
       v. Xanthelasma
      vi. Oral, nasal, and pharyngeal mucosa involvement
         1. Sometimes with ulcerations
         2. One-fourth of patients
      vii. Various visceral sites may be affected

g. Radiographs
   i. "Punched out" bony lesions
      1. Resembles gouty tophi
   ii. Widened joint spaces
   iii. Absent or disproportionately mild periarticular osteopenia
   iv. Severe joint destruction
      1. Later disease
   v. Spinal involvement
      1. Erosions and subluxations
      2. Atlantoaxial damage
h. Laboratory features
   i. No specific abnormality demonstrated
   ii. Biopsies of affected tissue
      1. Establishes the diagnosis
      2. Large, multinucleated giant cells
         a. Infiltrate skin and synovium
      3. Cytoplasm
         a. Granular, ground glass appearance
         b. PAS-positive
            i. Periodic acid-Schiff stain
            ii. For lipids and glycoproteins
            iii. Possible histiocytic granulomatous reaction
               1. Unidentified stimulus
         c. Positive fat stains
            i. Sudan black
      4. Histologically different from RA
         a. RA with myofibroblast cells in a collagen matrix
   iii. Form of lipid storage disease or histiocytes stimulated to produce
      1. Triglycerides
      2. Cholesterol
      3. Phosphate esters
      4. No consistent lipid abnormality
   iv. Multicentric reticulocytosis cells
      1. Lymphocytic origin proposed
         a. Presence of T-cell markers
      2. Monocyte/macrophage origin proposed
         a. Stain for macrophage markers
         b. Macrophage-activated cytokines
            i. IL-1 beta
            ii. IL-12
            iii. TNF-alpha
               1. Similar to RA synovial cell distribution
   v. Synovial fluid
      1. Leukocyte counts range from 220 to 79,000 cells/mm^3
      2. Mononuclear cells predominate
      3. Giant cells or large, bizarre macrophages

   i. Pathogenesis
      i. Hidden malignancy and TB implicated
      ii. Rheumatoid factor does **NOT** occur
      iii. Some patients develop positive reactions to TB
         1. PPD-positive
         2. About 50%
         3. Only a few patients reported to have active TB
      iv. Associations
         1. Sjogren's
         2. Polymyositis
         3. Variety of malignancies (25%)
            a. Precede, concurrent, or follow the development of MRH
            b. Treatment of the malignancy led to improvement of MRH
         4. Xanthelasma
            a. Occurs in one-third of patients
      v. Death due to the disease rare
j. Treatment
      i. No treatment consistently shown benefit
      ii. Rare disease
         1. Precludes a good prospective study
      iii. Spontaneous remission of skin disease and arthritis
         1. Occurs especially in childhood
      iv. Symptomatic treatment
         1. For mild disease
         2. NSAIDs
         3. Nonnarcotic analgesics
      v. Glucocorticoid therapy
         1. Essentially no effect on arthritis
      vi. Corticosteroids or topical nitrogen mustard
         1. May improve skin lesions
      vii. Cytotoxic therapy
         1. Reported to achieve partial and complete remissions
      viii. Combination therapy for severe skin and joint disease
         1. Corticosteroids
         2. Methotrexate
            a. Alone shown prolonged effect
            b. Plus hydroxychloroquine beneficial
         3. Cyclophosphamide
         4. Cyclosporine
         5. TNF blockade
            a. Presence of synovial TNF

Amyloidoses

29

1. Insoluble proteinaceous material deposited in tissue extracellular matrix
   a. Local or systemic
   b. Subclinical or a variety of manifestations
2. Amyloid term
   a. Coined in 1854 by Rudolph Virchow
   b. Material reacted with iodine and sulfuric acid
3. Amyloid deposits
   a. Encroach on parenchymal tissues
   b. Organ function compromised
   c. Amount of compromise related to
      i. Location
      ii. Quantity
      iii. Rate of deposition
4. Three forms associated with arthropathy
   a. AL
      i. Associated with immunoglobulin L-chain deposition
   b. $A\beta_2m$
      i. Derived from β_2-microglobulin in chronic renal failure
   c. ATTR
      i. Transthyretin (TTR) associated with familial disease
5. Pathology
   a. Histology
      i. All amyloid material on H&E staining
         1. Homogeneous
         2. Hyaline
         3. Eosinophilic
      ii. Positive Congo red
         1. Apple-green birefringence
         2. Under polarized light
      iii. Fibrillar structure on electron microscopy
      iv. Positive antibody specific for P-component

N.T. Colburn, *Review of Rheumatology*,
DOI 10.1007/978-1-84882-093-7_29, © Springer-Verlag London Limited 2012

Fig. 29.1 Amyloid material on H&E
staining (Reproduced with permission from
Pathology of the colon and rectum. *Gastroenterology
and Hepatology.* ImagesMD; 2002-01-28)

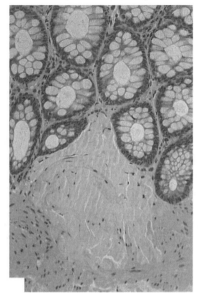

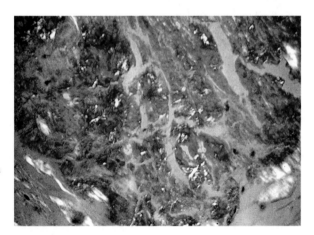

Fig. 29.2 Congo red stain
shows green birefringence
in cardiac amyloidosis
(Reproduced with permission
from The etiologic basis of
congestive heart failure.
Atlas of Heart Diseases.
ImagesMD; 2008-04-23)

    b. Structure
        i. All amyloid material by electron microscopy
           1. Share a unique ultrastructure
        ii. Protein fibrils
           1. Thin, nonbranching
           2. Constitute about 90% of amyloid deposits
           3. Tend to aggregate laterally to form fibers
           4. All display a crossed, beta-pleated sheet structure

     iii. Protein P-component
       1. Composed of two pentagonal subunits
       2. Form a doughnut-like structure
       3. Constitute about 5%
       4. Associated with all types of amyloid
       5. Not essential for fibril formation
       6. A salt-soluble molecule
       7. Identical to serum amyloid P (SAP)
        a. A normal serum component
        b. 50% homology with CRP
        c. SAP is **NOT** an acute phase reactant
       8. Undefined role in the pathogenesis of amyloid deposition
        a. IV injected purified radiolabeled P-component binds to deposited fibrils in tissues
        b. Used in gamma scanning
         i. Detects presence and extent of deposits
    iv. Apolipoprotein E (Apo-E)
       1. Second molecule common to all amyloids
       2. Role unclear
       3. ApoE4 allele
        a. Linkage dysequilibrium with Alzheimer cases
     v. Heparan sulfate proteoglycan (HSPG) perlecan
       1. Third common component of amyloids
       2. Normal constituent of basement membranes
       3. Unknown role in fibrillogenesis or amyloid deposition
       4. Low-molecular-weight analogs inhibit development of experimental murine SAA
     vi. Small amounts of carbohydrate and mucopolysaccharides
       1. Composes the remainder
  c. Classification of amyloidoses
     i. By the major protein component of the fibril

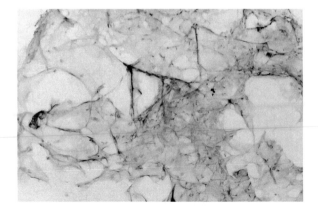

Fig. 29.3 Abdominal fat aspirate in primary amyloidosis (Reproduced with permission from Arthritis and systemic disease. *Atlas of Rheumatology*. ImagesMD; 2002-03-07)

  d. Diagnosis
     i. Characteristic biopsy staining from clinically affected organs
     ii. Accessible tissues
        1. Rectum
        2. Other regions of the GI tract
        3. Subcutaneous fat
6. Pathogenesis
  a. Amyloid protein A
     i. Increased production of a precursor
     ii. Result of prolonged stimulus to the synthesizing cell
  b. Amyloid protein AL
     i. Monoclonal cellular proliferation
     ii. Produces the amyloidogenic protein
  c. Aβ2m
     i. Decreased excretion of the precursor
  d. AβPP, AA
     i. Aberrant, inappropriate, or incomplete proteolytic cleavage
     ii. Increased amounts of profibrillogenic precursor
  e. Amyloid protein TTR
     i. Structural abnormalities of a normal protein
     ii. Germline mutations predispose to fibril formation
7. Clinical Features
  a. AL disease
     i. Presents as either primary amyloidosis or multiple myeloma
     ii. Nephropathy with proteinuria or renal failure
        1. Usual presentation
        2. Nephropathic proteinuria
        3. Excretion of large amounts of free monoclonal L-chains
        4. Massive tubular casts
           a. Resultant renal failure
           b. Myeloma kidney
        5. Renal tubular defect
           a. Concentration
           b. Acidification
        6. Hypertension
  b. Cardiomyopathy
     i. Second most common presentation
     ii. Diastolic dysfunction
        1. Earliest echocardiographic abnormality
        2. Atrial component to ventricular filling
     iii. Noncompliant hemodynamics
     iv. Thickening of the interventricular septum and valve leaflets
     v. Restriction

vi. Diagnostic measures
   1. Endomyocardial biopsy followed by staining
   2. Radioactive technetium scanning
      a. Screen for cardiac amyloid deposits
   3. Cardiac AL > AA
vii. Digoxin and nifedipine
   1. Toxic in the setting of cardiac amyloid depositions
   2. Bind to fibrils
   3. Effective concentrations disproportionately increased
c. Neuropathic presentation
   i. Seen in 20%
   ii. Carpal tunnel syndrome (CTS)
      1. Frequently the first manifestation
      2. May precede others by a significant time period
      3. TTR amyloid
         a. Most common form of isolated carpal tunnel deposition
         b. In absence of other significant organ involvement
      4. 2–3% of CTS requires carpal tunnel release
   iii. Sensorimotor symptoms
   iv. Biopsies of involved areas may reveal amyloid
   v. Asymptomatic sural nerve biopsy low yield
d. Periarticular amyloid deposition
   i. Presents as pseudoarthritis
   ii. Joint effusions
      1. Amyloid fibrils found in the fluid
   iii. Soft tissue "shoulder pad sign"
      1. Major physical finding
e. Hematologic
   i. Acquired deficiency of clotting factor X
   ii. Factor bound to fibrils
   iii. Potentially fatal complication

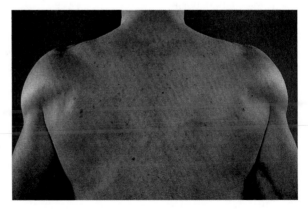

Fig. 29.4 Shoulder pad sign in primary amyloidosis (Reproduced with permission from Arthritis and systemic disease. *Atlas of Rheumatology.* ImagesMD; 2002-03-07)

8. Treatment
   a. Organ failure
      i. Treated with supportive measures
   b. Dialysis and renal transplantation
      i. For ESRD
      ii. Recurrent disease in transplanted organ
         1. Can occur within 4 years
         2. Precursor synthesis should be controlled
   c. Melphalan and prednisone
      i. Randomized prospective trials show enhanced survival
      ii. Colchicine alone or added had no effect
   d. Chemotherapy
      i. Good results but high toxicity
      ii. Those with cardiac involvement do not tolerate this regimen
      iii. Anthracycline compounds
         1. Inhibit the process of fibrillogenesis
         2. Do **not** affect proliferative capacity of Ig-producing cells
9. Pathogenesis
   a. SPEP or UPEP reveal a monoclonal Ig precursor
      i. Lamba light chains
         1. Precursors more than twice as frequent as kappa chains
      ii. $V\lambda6$ and $V\kappa1$ subclasses
         1. Statistically significant increase in their proportion
   b. Most deposits contain L-chain fragments that begin with a normal amino terminus
      i. Fewer than 10% contain only intact L-chains
      ii. 25% contain both intact chains and one or more fragments
      iii. 10% contain fragments 12 kDa or smaller
   c. A form of proteolysis or synthesis of abnormal chains may be responsible
      i. Marrow cells from all patients can synthesize excess, free L-chains
      ii. Certain substitutions at particular positions may result in more amyloidogenic structures
10. Light chain deposition disease
   a. Shares many of the clinical features of AL
   b. Cardiac and renal deposition of Ig-L or L- and H-chain related molecules
      i. 5% with multiple myeloma do not bind Congo red
   c. Diagnosis
      i. By immunofluorescence or immunohistochemistry
      ii. Demonstrate monoclonal deposits
      iii. Accompanied by characteristic electron microscopic appearance
11. Amyloid beta-2-Microglobulin Disease
   a. Seen in patients with chronic renal disease
   b. Usually on dialysis for periods longer than 7 years

Fig. 29.5 Erosive cystic
arthritis of A β₂M
amyloidosis. *Arrows* point
to areas of cystic destruction
(Reproduced with
permission from Arthritis and
systemic disease. *Atlas of
Rheumatology*.
ImagesMD; 2002-03-07)

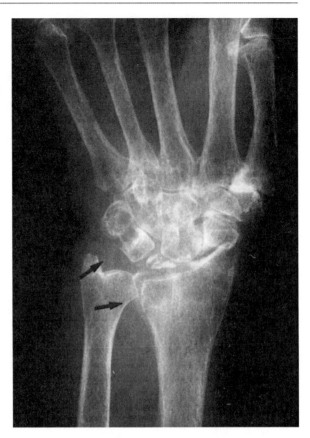

c. Patients present with
   i. Joint pain
   ii. Carpal tunnel syndrome
   iii. Osteonecrosis
d. Beta2-microglobulin
   i. Deposited fibril protein
   ii. 12.5 kDa polypeptide component of class I proteins of the MHC
   iii. Intact polypeptide with a normal amino-acid sequence
   iv. Deposited as either a monomer or dimer
   v. Evidence of nonenzyme glycation
e. Pathogenesis
   i. Monocyte/macrophage participation in deposition
   ii. Not clearly a result of decreased renal clearance
12. Amyloid A (AA) Disease
   a. Found in patients with
      i. Chronic infectious diseases
         1. Tuberculosis
         2. Osteomyelitis
         3. Leprosy

    ii. Chronic noninfectious inflammatory diseases
        1. RA
        2. FMF
        3. Every form of inflammatory arthropathy except SLE
        4. JRA
            a. Frequency higher in Europe (5–10%) than in the USA (1%)
  b. Serum amyloid A (SAA)
      i. Fibril serum precursor
     ii. Circulates as an apoprotein of HDL
        1. Molecular complex of about 250 kDa
    iii. Role in cholesterol metabolism during the inflammatory process
     iv. Behaves as an acute phase reactant
      v. Synthesized primarily in the liver
        1. Response to elevated levels of the cytokine IL-6
     vi. Fibril subunit has a normal sequence and molecular size of 7.5 kDa
  c. Worldwide AA the most common form of amyloidosis
      i. Related to the frequency of chronic infectious diseases
     ii. 25% of RA patients have amyloid deposits at autopsy
    iii. 5% of RA patients in the USA and the UK have detectable deposits
  d. Genetic predisposition
      i. Polymorphisms in the SAA gene
        1. Associated with the propensity to develop SAA
     ii. Found in groups of patients with genetic disease
    iii. FMF
        1. Daily colchicine aborts development of amyloid
13. Aging and Amyloid
  a. Five different anatomic sites of amyloid deposition associated with aging
      i. Brain
        1. Beta protein of Alzheimer's
     ii. Pancreas
        1. Islet-associated polypeptide of type II DM
    iii. Cardiac
        1. Isolated atrial amyloid with atrial natriuretic factor
        2. Senile systemic amyloid with transthyretin
     iv. Aorta
        1. Medin
            a. Fragment of the milk-fat lobule protein lactadherin
            b. Precursor of aortic medial amyloid
            c. Associates with atherosclerotic plaques (APO A1)
      v. Muscle
        1. Abeta protein identified in rimmed vacuoles in muscles
        2. Patients with inclusion body myositis

14. Mutant TTR
    a. Severe sensorimotor and autonomic neuropathy
    b. Vitreopathy
    c. Cardiomyopathy
    d. Nephropathy
15. Familial Amyloidosis
    a. Three forms
        i. Rare
        ii. Familial
        iii. AD
    b. Deposition of mutant form of gelsolin
        i. An actin binding protein
    c. Associated with
        i. Finnish form of amyloidotic neuropathy
        ii. Lattice corneal dystrophy
        iii. Mutation in the gene encoding cystatin C
            1. A lysosomal proteinase inhibitor
        iv. Icelandic kindreds with hereditary cerebral hemorrhage
            1. Deposited in cerebral blood vessels
    d. Three nephropathic familial forms
        i. Mutation in the A-alpha chain of fibrinogen
        ii. Mutant APO A1
        iii. Mutations in lysozyme
        iv. Ostertag form of renal amyloidosis

The Autoinflammatory Diseases

30

Section A: Familial Mediterranean Fever (FMF)

1. Epidemiology
    a. A recessively inherited disorder most frequent in the following ancestries
        i. Armenian
        ii. Arab
        iii. Turks
        iv. Iraqi
        v. Italian
        vi. Greek
        vii. Sephardic Jewish from northern Africa and Turkey
            1. Jewish population that left Spain after the Inquisition in 1,492
        viii. Ashkenazi (east European) Jewish
    b. Male:female ratio of 1.5–2.0:1
        i. Females may be under diagnosed because of
            1. Misdiagnosis of abdominal attacks as gynecological disease
            2. Possible hormonal effects on FMF symptoms
                a. Some symptoms begin at menarche
                b. Pregnancy may be associated with a remission of attacks
            3. Underreporting of females for social/cultural reasons
    c. Up to 90% of first episodes occurs before the age of 20 years
        i. Small minority with onset after age 40
    d. Only ½ of cases have a positive family history
    e. Earliest recognizable description of FMF in medical literature was 1908, and first case series in 1945
    f. Synonymous terms for FMF in older literature are
        i. Recurrent polyserositis
        ii. Recurrent hereditary polyserositis
        iii. Familial paroxysmal polyserositis
        iv. Periodic peritonitis

N.T. Colburn, *Review of Rheumatology*,
DOI 10.1007/978-1-84882-093-7_30, © Springer-Verlag London Limited 2012

2. Genetics and Pathophysiology
   a. Single-gene recessive disorder with incomplete penetrance
      i. A history of consanguinity may be elicited
         1. Seen with families of the Middle East
   b. Pseudodominance
      i. Parent to child transmission
      ii. One parent is affected and the other is an asymptomatic carrier
   c. Identical twins are concordant for FMF
   d. Carrier frequencies
      i. Estimated between 1:3 and 1:16
         1. Based on certain population estimates and family studies
            a. 20% rate among north African, Iraqi, Ashkenazi Jews, Arabs, Turks, and Armenian
            b. Incidence of FMF is less than half of estimated population frequency
               i. Suggest incomplete penetrance
         2. High frequencies suggest an advantage for heterozygotes
   e. *MEFV* is the FMF gene
      i. Mapped to the short arm of chromosome 16 in 1992
         1. Located on chromosome 16p13.3
      ii. Identified by positional cloning in 1997
      iii. A 10-exon gene spanning approximately 15 kb
      iv. Protein is a 781 amino acid product denoted pyrin or marenostrin
      v. Expressed predominantly in granulocytes
         1. As well as monocytes, dendritic cells, and synovial fibroblasts
         2. Not expressed at significant levels in lymphocytes
   f. Pyrin (marenostrin) is the FMF protein
      i. The N-terminal portion
         1. First 92 amino acids known as the pyrin domain (PYD)
            a. A six α-helix configuration
            b. Member of a superfamily of death domains, death effector domains and caspase recruitment domains
            c. PYD of pyrin binds to an adaptor protein called ASC (apoptosis-associated specklike protein with a caspase recruitment domain)
               i. Involved in protein-protein interactions in the regulation of
                  1. Cytokine activation
                     a. IL-1β
                     b. IL-18
                  2. Apoptosis
                  3. NF-κB activation
      ii. The C-terminal portion contains
         1. A B-box zinc finger (residues 375–407)
         2. α-helical (coiled-coil) domain (residues 408–594)
         3. B30.2 (ret finger protein) domain (residues 598–774)
            a. Where the majority of disease associated mutations are located

      b. Associates with p20 and p10 subunits of caspase-1 to prevent conversion of pro-IL-1 beta to its active form

         i. M694V and M680I mutations prevent this binding

   iii. Endogenous pyrin localizes in the nucleus of

      1. Synovial fibroblasts

      2. Neutrophils

      3. Dendritic cells

   iv. Full-length pyrin shown to associate with the cytoskeleton

    v. Precise biochemical function remains unknown

      1. Thought to be a negative regulator of inflammation

        a. The net effect of FMF mutations is an **autoinflammatory** state

      2. Only subtle structural changes are expected in the protein since the majority of mutations are missense

        a. Manifested as an easily perturbed equilibrium predisposed to intermittent exacerbations

g. Four major disease-associated mutations in *MEFV*

    i. All are single nucleotide substitutions in exon 10

   ii. All cause conservative amino acid substitution in the B30.2 domain of pyrin

   iii. Two mutations affect residue 694

      1. Substitution of valine or isoleucine for the normal methionine

        a. M694V

           i. The predominant mutation in North African Jews

          ii. Probably descended from a common ancient founder over 2,000 years ago

         iii. Homozygotes are associated with

            1. An increased risk of amyloidosis

              a. Especially Jewish, Armenian, and Arab patients

            2. Earlier onset of disease

            3. Greater frequency of attacks

            4. Arthritis

            5. Erysipelas-like erythema

        b. M694I

           i. Allele may confer increased risk for amyloidosis

          ii. Common among Arabs

   iv. Substitution of isoleucine for methionine at codon 680

      1. M680I

    v. Substitution of alanine for valine at position 726

      1. V726A

        a. Broadly distributed

           i. More common in Italians and Ashkenazi Jews

        b. Associated with a single ancestral haplotype, suggestive of a common founder

h. Other disease associated mutations in *MEFV*

    i. Second major cluster of mutations is in exon 2

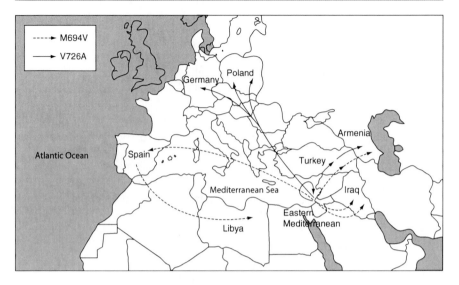

Fig. 30.1 Map showing the spread of M694V and V726A from the Middle East (Reproduced with permission from Familial Mediterranean fever. *Pediatric Nephrology.* DOI: 10.1007/s00467-003-1185-2. Springer; 2003-09-01)

1. One variant seen in a substantial numbers of patient is described at codon 148
   a. Substitution of glutamine for glutamic acid (E148Q)
      i. Regarded as being a less penetrant milder mutation
      ii. Usually found in patients who are compound heterozygotes for E148Q and an exon 10 mutation
         1. These patients may have moderate to severe disease
         2. The V726A-E148Q complex allele may confer an increased risk for amyloidosis
      iii. Can also be seen as a complex allele in *cis* with an exon 10 mutation
      iv. Seen in high frequency among Indians and Chinese
      v. Haplotype data suggest a third major ancient founder
   ii. Mutations common among certain ethnic groups
      1. M694I in Arabs
      2. R761H in Iranians and Armenians
      3. F479L in Greeks
   iii. Mutations in exon 1, encoding the PYD, are very rare
   iv. Single *MEFV* mutations
      1. May manifest as a biochemical and/or clinical inflammatory phenotype
         a. May exhibit an increased acute-phase response
         b. Seen in up to 30% with clinical FMF

     v. Dominant transmission
       1. Seen with certain *MEFV* rare variants
         a. The deletion of codon 694 (ΔM694)
         b. The M694I-E148Q complex allele

3. Diagnosis
  a. Two major tools for diagnosing FMF
    i. Clinical criteria
    ii. Genetic testing
  b. Clinical criteria
    i. Four sets of diagnostic criteria concur on the following cardinal features:
      1. Short, recurrent episodes of fever
        a. Rectal temperature $> 38°$
        b. Last from 12 h to 3 days
        c. Recurrent of three or more
      2. Pain in the absence of other causative factors in the following locations
        a. Abdomen
        b. Chest
        c. Joints
        d. Skin
    ii. Tel-Hashomer criteria
      1. Most frequently used
      2. Includes major, minor and supportive criteria
      3. Minor criteria
        a. Milder attacks
        b. Exertional leg pain
        c. Favorable response to colchicine
      4. Supportive criteria
        a. Positive family history
        b. Age of onset < 20 years
        c. Appropriate ethnicity
        d. Parental consanguinity
        e. An acute phase response during attacks
        f. Episodic proteinuria/hematuria
        g. Unproductive laparotomy
      5. Performs well in Middle Eastern populations
        a. Sensitivities and specificities $> 95\%$
  c. Genetic testing
    i. Plays an adjunctive role
      1. Deemed unnecessary for people from high-risk ethnic groups who experience typical attacks and respond therapeutically to colchicine
    ii. Does not make the diagnosis alone
      1. As many as one-third of patients meeting clinical criteria many have only one demonstrable mutation

Fig. 30.2 Erysipelas-like
erythema of FMF
(Reproduced with permission
from Familial Mediterranean
fever: revisiting an ancient
disease. *European Journal of
Pediatrics.* DOI: 10.1007/
s00431-003-1223-x.
Springer; 2003-07-01)

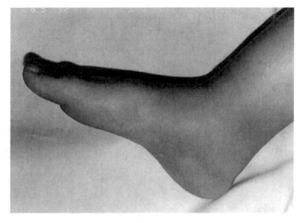

2. A small number of patients with clinical FMF may have no demonstrable mutation
3. Clinically asymptomatic people may have two classic *MEFV* mutations
   iii. Complicated by
   1. Presence of *MEFV* mutations that are currently not screened
   2. The existence of complex and heterozygotic alleles
   3. Low-penetrant polymorphic mutations
   4. Possibility of a second FMF locus not currently identified
   d. With clinical uncertainty and negative genetic testing consider
      i. A therapeutic trial of colchicine
      ii. The evaluation of other hereditary periodic fever syndromes
4. Clinical Features
   a. Acute attacks manifested by
      i. Fever
      ii. Localized inflammation of
         1. Peritoneum
         2. Pleura
         3. Joints
         4. Skin
      iii. Last 12–72 h
         1. Longer if involving the joints
   b. Atypical presentations
      i. Fever and myalgia alone
         1. Can be seen as the only presenting signs in children
5. Treatment
   a. Colchicine
      i. Prophylactic daily oral doses
         1. 1–2 mg per day
      ii. Preventive and therapeutic

        1. Acute inflammatory attacks
        2. Development of systemic amyloidosis
        3. Progression of amyloid nephropathy
     iii. Toxicities
        1. Gastrointestinal
          a. A major limitation to dosing
          b. Diarrhea
          c. Bloating
        2. Bone marrow suppression (rare)
        3. Myoneuropathy
          a. Seen in elderly adults with renal insufficiency
          b. Proximal muscle weakness
          c. Elevated CK
          d. EMG consistent with polymyositis
  b. Colchicine non-responders
     i. Limited alternatives
     ii. Corticosteroids
        1. Ineffective
        2. May accelerate amyloidosis (anecdotal)
        3. Used with certain manifestations of FMF
          a. Protracted febrile myalgia
          b. Henoch Schönlein purpura
     iii. Interferon-alpha
        1. May abort attacks if given early
        2. 3 million units subcutaneously
        3. Induces a transient fever and flu-like syndrome
        4. No significant therapeutic effect by a double-blind study
        5. No data on effectiveness in amyloidosis
     iv. Anakinra (IL-1 blockade)
        1. Targets known dysfunctional pathways in FMF
        2. Symptomatic responses shown in case reports
     v. Anti-TNF blockade
        1. Inflixamab
        2. Etanercept
        3. Symptomatic responses shown in case reports

Section B: Tumor Necrosis Factor Receptor-Associated Periodic Syndrome (TRAPS)

1. Epidemiology
  a. A dominantly inherited disorder described in the following family cohorts
     i. Irish/Scottish
        1. First large pedigree reported by Williamson in 1982
        2. Termed familial Hibernian (Irish) fever (FHF)

　　　　ii. Australian family of Scottish ancestry
　　　　　　1. Termed benign autosomal dominant familial periodic fever (FPF)
　　　iii. Swedish
　　　iv. Spanish
　　　　v. German
　　　vi. Finnish
　　　vii. Dutch
　　viii. Austrian
　　　ix. Mixed Irish/English/German ancestry
　　　　x. Puerto Rican
　　b. Disease mutations seen in several ethnic populations
　　　　i. African-American
　　　ii. French
　　　iii. Belgian
　　　iv. Portuguese
　　　　v. Italian
　　　vi. Arabic
　　　vii. Czech
　　viii. Mexican
　　　ix. Jewish
2. Genetics and Pathophysiology
　　a. Disease caused by mutations in the gene *TNFRSF1A*
　　　　i. Found on the short arm of chromosome 12
　　　ii. Encodes the p55 receptor for TNF
　　　iii. Over 50 mutations described
　　　　　1. Catalogued on the INFEVERS website

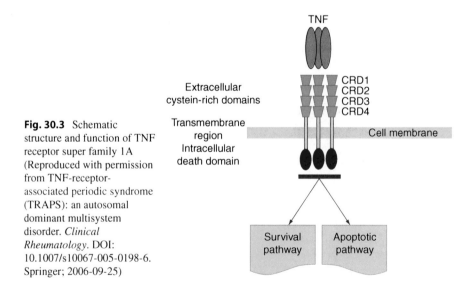

Fig. 30.3 Schematic structure and function of TNF receptor super family 1A (Reproduced with permission from TNF-receptor-associated periodic syndrome (TRAPS): an autosomal dominant multisystem disorder. *Clinical Rheumatology.* DOI: 10.1007/s10067-005-0198-6. Springer; 2006-09-25)

b. TNFRSF1A protein (p55 TNF receptor)
   i. Four highly conserved extracellular cysteine-rich domains (CRD)
      1. Each a loop structure constrained by three disulfide bonds
      2. Location of nearly all of the mutations
   ii. Transmembrane domain
      1. No mutations identified within this domain
   iii. Intracellular carboxy-terminal death domain
      1. No mutations identified within this domain
      2. Similar to the pyrin domain
      3. A cognate interaction motif
c. Major disease associated mutations
   i. Nearly all in CRD1 and CRD2 at the amino terminus
   ii. C30R (substitution of arginine for cysteine)
   iii. C33Y (substitution of tyrosine for cysteine)
   iv. C52F (substitution of phenylalanine for cysteine)
   v. C88R, C88Y (substitution of either arginine or tyrosine for cysteine)
   vi. Cysteine substitutions disrupt disulfide bonds
   vii. T50M (substitution of methionine for threonine)
      1. Disrupts a conserved hydrogen bond on CRD1
d. Variant mutations
   i. Broad spectrum of clinical findings
   ii. Controversial pathologic significance
   iii. Defined as polymorphisms
   iv. R92Q (glutamine for arginine)
      1. Seen in about 1% of Caucasian control chromosomes
      2. Increased frequency in non-TRAPS entities
         a. Early arthritis
         b. Atherosclerosis
         c. Systemic amyloidosis in juvenile idiopathic arthritis
      3. No documented in vitro functional abnormality
   v. P46L (leucine for proline)
      1. Found in about 2% of African-American control chromosomes
      2. High frequency in some sub-Saharan African populations
      3. In vitro abnormalities seen in activation-induced receptor cleavage
e. Mechanistic studies of mutant receptors
   i. "Shedding hypothesis"
      1. Reduced activation-induced ectodomain receptor cleavage
         a. Shed receptors normally
            i. Bind soluble ligand
            ii. Act as competitive antagonists
      2. Impaired homeostatic effect on inflammation
         a. Higher levels of membrane p55
         b. Lower levels of soluble p55
      3. Demonstrated in some mutations but not all
   ii. Reduced binding to TNF

        iii. Decreased signaling for apoptosis

        iv. Abnormal intracellular trafficking

           1. Mutant receptors retained in the endoplasmic reticulum (ER)

           2. May trigger a ligand-independent cellular activation

              a. Constitutive activation of NFκB

              b. ER stress response

           3. May account for the dominant inheritance

3. Diagnosis

    a. Mutation in *TNFRSF1A* in a patient with unexplained periodic fever

        i. Family history of TRAPS not necessary

           1. Reduced genetic penetrance

           2. Reports of de novo mutations

    b. Genomic DNA sequencing is the preferred method

    c. Consider *TNFRSF1A* screening for patients who test negative for *MEFV* mutations

4. Prognosis

    a. Dependent upon the development of amyloidosis

5. Clinical and Laboratory Feature

    a. Acute attacks

        i. Fever

           1. Sometimes a sole manifestation

              a. Especially in children

        ii. Prolonged duration usually greater than 7 days

        iii. Characteristic migratory myalgia and rash

           1. Localized area of muscle warmth and tenderness

           2. Overlying macular erythematous blanchable rash

              a. Torso

              b. Extremities

                  i. Migrates centrifugally over several days

                  ii. Associated with synovitis and effusion across a joint

           3. MRI demonstrates inflammatory changes into the muscle compartments

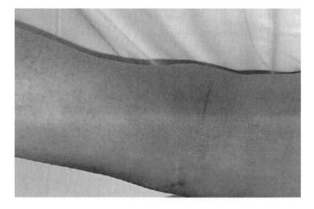

Fig. 30.4 Characteristic erythematous migratory rash of TRAPS (Reproduced with permission from Hereditäres periodisches Fieber. *Der Internist.* DOI: 10.1007/s00108-004-1254-z. Springer; 2004-08-01)

      4. No elevation in muscle enzymes
      5. Biopsy of the involved area reveals
        a. Panniculitis
        b. Fasciitis
        c. Perivascular inflammation
        d. No myofibrilar involvement
   iv. Pleuritic chest pain
    v. Severe abdominal pain
      1. With or without peritoneal signs
      2. May develop peritoneal adhesions
   vi. Arthralgia
      1. More frequent than arthritis
  vii. Arthritis
      1. Uncommon
      2. Non-erosive
      3. Monoarticular
      4. Areas most frequently involved
        a. Hips
        b. Knees
        c. Ankles
      5. Non-chronic
 viii. Ocular involvement
      1. Distinguishing feature from FMF
      2. Seen in 80% of patients
      3. Conjunctivitis
      4. Periorbital edema
      5. Periorbital pain
      6. Rarely iritis or uveitis
b. Systemic AA amyloidosis
    i. May develop in about 15% of TRAPS patients
   ii. Secondary to the deposition of the cleaved product of SAA
  iii. Tissue deposition similar to FMF
      1. Renal failure (most common)
      2. Hepatic failure
   iv. Common among families studied with these cysteine mutations
      1. C30R
      2. C52F
      3. C88Y
    v. Rare or not observed in families with these mutations
      1. C33Y
      2. T50M
      3. C88R
c. Laboratory findings
    i. Neutrophilia
   ii. Thrombocytosis
      1. Especially in children

      iii. Accelerated ESR

      iv. Elevated CRP

      v. Elevated SAA

      vi. Elevated haptoglobin and fibrinogen

      vii. Anemia of chronic disease

      viii. Polyclonal hypergammaglobulinemia

      ix. Low titer IgM and IgG anticardiolipin antibodies

      x. Negative autoantibodies

         1. ANA

         2. RF

         3. ANCA

      xi. Soluble 55 kDa TNF receptors

         1. Subnormal between attacks

         2. Contrast to other inflammatory diseases

6. Treatment

  a. Colchicine

      i. Ineffective

      ii. Does not prevent attacks

      iii. Does not prevent the development of amyloidosis

  b. NSAIDS

      i. Used with mild attacks

  c. Corticosteroids

      i. Used to treat acute severe attacks

      ii. May require escalating doses with time

      iii. Often see diminishing efficacy

      iv. Associated with serious toxicity

  d. Etanercept

      i. Reduces the frequency and severity of attacks

         1. Open label study

      ii. Reverses or slows progression of renal amyloidosis

         1. Shown in case reports

         2. Dose modification to normalize SAA levels

  e. Anakinra

      i. Used in select patients intolerant to etanercept

      ii. Anecdotal data for effectiveness

         1. Controls symptoms

         2. Reduction of acute phase reactants

Suggested Reading

The Musculoskeletal System

Ala-Kokko L, Prockop DJ. Collagen elastin. In: Ruddy S, Harris ED, Sledge CB, eds. *Kelley's Textbook of Rheumatology*. 6th ed. Philadelphia: WB Saunders; 2001.

Heinegard D, Lorenzo P, Saxne T. Matrix glycoproteins, proteoglycans, and cartilage. In: Ruddy S, Harris ED, Sledge CB, eds. *Kelley's Textbook of Rheumatology*. 6th ed. Philadelphia: WB Saunders; 2001.

Okada Y. Proteinases and matrix degradation. In: Ruddy S, Harris ED, Sledge CB, eds. *Kelley's Textbook of Rheumatology*. 6th ed. Philadelphia: WB Saunders; 2001.

The musculoskeletal system. In: Klippel JH, ed. *Primer on the Rheumatic Diseases*. 11th ed. Atlanta: Arthritis Foundation; 1997.

Mediators of Rheumatic Pathology

Aurier RB. Prostaglandins, leukotrienes, and related compounds. In: Ruddy S, Harris ED, Sledge CB, eds. *Kelley's Textbook of Rheumatology*. 6th ed. Philadelphia: WB Saunders; 2001.

Gabay C, Kushner I. Acute-phase proteins and other systemic responses to inflammation. *N Engl J Med*. 1999;340(6):448-454.

Green DR. Apoptotic pathways: the roads to ruin. *Cell*. 1998;94(6):695-698.

Johnston RB Jr. The complement system in host defense and inflammation: the cutting edges of a double-edged sword. *Pediatr Infect Dis J*. 1993;12(11):933-941.

Medzhitov R, Janeway C Jr. Innate immunity. *N Engl J Med*. 2000;343(5):338-344.

Immunity

Abbas AK, Lichtman AH, Bell E, Bird L, eds. *Cellular and Molecular Immunology*. 5th ed. Philadelphia: Saunders; *Nature*. 2005;435:583-627.

Diamond B, Davidson A. Autoimmune diseases. *N Engl J Med*. 2001;345:340-350.

Janeway C. *Immunobiology: The Immune System in Health and Disease*. 6th ed. New York: Garland Science; 2005.

N.T. Colburn, *Review of Rheumatology*,
DOI 10.1007/978-1-84882-093-7, © Springer-Verlag London Limited 2012

Genetics

Daly AK, Day CP. Candidate gene case-control association studies: advantages and potential pitfalls. *Br J Clin Pharmacol.* 2001;52(5):489-499.

Gregersen PK. Genetics of rheumatic diseases. In: Ruddy S, Harris ED, Sledge CB, eds. *Kelley's Textbook of Rheumatology.* 6th ed. Philadelphia: WB Saunders; 2001.

Hunter DJ. Gene-environment interactions in human diseases. *Nat Rev Genet.* 2005;6(4): 287-298.

Kelley J, Trowsdale J. Features of MHC and NK gene clusters. *Transpl Immunol.* 2005;14 (3–4):129-134.

Rheumatoid Arthritis

Arend WP. Physiology of cytokine pathways in rheumatoid arthritis. *Arthritis Rheum.* 2001;45(1):101-106.

Bathon JM, Martin RW, Fleischmann RM, et al. A comparison of etanercept and methotrexate in patients with early rheumatoid arthritis. *N Engl J Med.* 2000;343(22):1586-1593.

Boers M, Verhoeven AC, Markusse HM, et al. Randomized comparison of combined step-down prednisolone, methotrexate and sulphasalazine with sulphasalazine alone in early rheumatoid arthritis. *Lancet.* 1997;350(9074):309-318.

Bresnihan B, Newmark R, Robbins S, Genant HK. Effects of anakinra monotherapy on joint damage in patients with rheumatoid arthritis. Extension of a 24-week randomized, placebo-controlled trial. *J Rheumatol.* 2004;31(6):1103-1111.

Dorner T, Egerer K, Feist E, Burmester GR. Rheumatoid factor revisited. *Curr Opin Rheumatol.* 2004;16(3):246-253.

Drosos AA. Epidemiology of rheumatoid arthritis. *Autoimmun Rev.* 2004;3(Suppl 1):S20-S22.

Edwards JC, Szczepanski L, Szechinski J, et al. Efficacy of B-cell-targeted therapy with rituximab in patients with rheumatoid arthritis. *N Engl J Med.* 2004;350(25):2572-2581.

Firestein GS. Evolving concepts of rheumatoid arthritis. *Nature.* 2003;423(6937):356-361.

Genovese MC, Becker JC, Schiff M, et al. Abatacept for rheumatoid arthritis refractory to tumor necrosis factor alpha inhibition. *N Engl J Med.* 2005;353(11):1114-1123.

Gregersen PK. Pathways to gene identification in rheumatoid arthritis: PTPN22 and beyond. *Immunol Rev.* 2005;204:74-86.

Gregersen PK, Silver J, Winchester RJ. The shared epitope hypothesis. An approach to understanding the molecular genetics of susceptibility to rheumatoid arthritis. *Arthritis Rheum.* 1987;30(11):1205-1213.

Hochberg MC, Spector TD. Epidemiology of rheumatoid arthritis: update. *Epidemiol Rev.* 1990;12:247-252.

Moreland LW, Weinblatt ME, Keystone EC, et al. Etanercept treatment in adults with established rheumatoid arthritis: 7 years of clinical experience. *J Rheumatol.* 2006;33(5):854-861.

O'Dell JR, Haire CE, Erikson N, et al. Treatment of rheumatoid arthritis with methotrexate alone, sulfasalazine and hydroxychloroquine, or a combination of all three medications. *N Engl J Med.* 1996;334(20):1287-1291.

Smolen JS, Kalden JR, Scott DL, et al. Efficacy and safety of leflunomide compared with placebo and sulphasalazine in active rheumatoid arthritis: a double-blind, randomized, multicentre trial. European Leflunomide Study Group. *Lancet.* 1999;353(9149):259-266.

Symmons DP, Barrett EM, Bankhead CR, Scott DG, Silman AJ. The incidence of rheumatoid arthritis in the United Kingdom: results from the Norfolk Arthritis Register. *Br J Rheumatol.* 1994;33(8):735-739.

Psoriatic Arthritis

Gladman DD, Brockbank J. Psoriatic arthritis. *Expert Opin Investig Drugs.* 2000;9(7): 1511-1522.

Jones G, Crotty M, Brooks P. Interventions for psoriatic arthritis. *Cochrane Database Syst Rev.* 2000;3:CD000212.

McGonagle D, Conaghan PG, Emery P. Psoriatic arthritis: a unified concept twenty years on. *Arthritis Rheum.* 1999;42(6):1080-1086.

Mease PJ, Goffe BS, Metz J, VanderStoep A, Finck B, Burge DJ. Etanercept in the treatment of psoriatic arthritis and psoriasis: a randomised trial. *Lancet.* 2000;356(9227):385-390.

Systemic Lupus Erythematosus (SLE)

Austin HA 3rd, Boumpas DT, Vaughan EM, Balow JE. Predicting renal outcomes in severe lupus nephritis: contributions of clinical and histologic data. *Kidney Int.* 1994;45(2):544-550.

Boumpas DT, Austin HA 3rd, Fessler BJ, Balow JE, Klippel JH, Lockshin MD. Systemic lupus erythematosus: emerging concepts. Part 1: renal, neuropsychiatric, cardiovascular, pulmonary, and hematologic disease. *Ann Intern Med.* 1995;122(12):940-950.

Buyon JP, Hiebert R, Copel J, et al. Autoimmune-associated congenital heart block: demographics, mortality, morbidity and recurrence rates obtained from a national neonatal lupus registry. *J Am Coll Cardiol.* 1998;31(7):1658-1666.

Chan TM, Li FK, Tang CS, et al. Efficacy of mycophenolate mofetil in patients with diffuse proliferative lupus nephritis. Hong Kong-Guangzhou Nephrology Study Group. *N Engl J Med.* 2000;343(16):1156-1162.

Gladman DD. Systemic lupus erythematosus: clinical features. In: Klippel JH, Weyand CM, Wortmann RL, eds. *Primer on the Rheumatic Diseases.* 11th ed. Atlanta: Arthritis Foundation; 1997:267-272.

Manderson AP, Botto M, Walport MJ. The role of complement in the development of systemic lupus erythematosus. *Annu Rev Immunol.* 2004;22:431-456.

Petri M. Detection of coronary artery disease and the role of traditional risk factors in the Hopkins Lupus Cohort. *Lupus.* 2000;9(3):170-175.

Rosner S, Ginzler EM, Diamond HS, et al. A multicenter study of outcome in systemic lupus erythematosus. II. Causes of death. *Arthritis Rheum.* 1982;25(6):612-617.

Rubin RL, Kretz-Rommel A. Initiation of autoimmunity by a reactive metabolite of a lupus-inducing drug in the thymus. *Environ Health Perspect.* 1999;107(Suppl 5):803-806.

Ruiz-Irastorza G, Khamashta MA, Hughes GR. Therapy of systemic lupus erythematosus: new agents and new evidence. *Expert Opin Investig Drugs.* 2000;9(7):1581-1593.

Ruiz-Irastorza G, Khamashta MA, Castellino G, Hughes GR. Systemic lupus erythematosus. *Lancet.* 2001;357(9261):1027-1032.

Tan EM. Antinuclear antibodies: diagnostic markers for autoimmune diseases and probes for cell biology. *Adv Immunol.* 1989;44:93-151.

Traynor AE, Schroeder J, Rosa RM, et al. Treatment of severe systemic lupus erythematosus with high-dose chemotherapy and haemopoietic stem-cell transplantation: a phase I study. *Lancet.* 2000;356(9231):701-707.

Wallace DJ, Hahn B, eds. *Dubois' Lupus Erythematosus.* 5th ed. Baltimore: Williams & Wilkins; 1997.

Ward MM, Pyun E, Studenski S. Long-term survival in systemic lupus erythematosus. Patient characteristics associated with poorer outcomes. *Arthritis Rheum.* 1995;38(2):274-283.

West SG. Neuropsychiatric lupus. *Rheum Dis Clin North Am.* 1994;20(1):129-158.

Arthritis Associated with Calcium-Containing Crystals

Doherty M, Dieppe P. Clinical aspects of calcium pyrophosphate dihydrate crystal deposition. *Rheum Dis Clin North Am.* 1988;14(2):395-414.

O'Shea FD, McCarthy GM. Basic calcium phosphate deposition in the joint: a potential therapeutic target in osteoarthritis. *Curr Opin Rheumatol.* 2004;16(3):273-278.

Rosenthal AK. Calcium crystal-associated arthritides. *Curr Opin Rheumatol.* 1998;10(3): 273-277.

Rosenthal AK, Mandel N. Identification of crystals in synovial fluids and joint tissues. *Curr Rheumatol Rep.* 2001;3(1):11-16.

Rull M. Calcium crystal-associated diseases and miscellaneous crystals. *Curr Opin Rheumatol.* 1997;9(3):274-279.

Gout

Campion EW, Glynn RJ, DeLabry LO. Asymptomatic hyperuricemia. Risks and consequences in the Normative Aging Study. *Am J Med.* 1987;82(3):421-426.

Emmerson BT. The management of gout. *N Engl J Med.* 1996;334(7):445-451.

McGill NW, Dieppe PA. The role of serum and synovial fluid components in the promotion of urate crystal formation. *J Rheumatol.* 1991;18(7):1042-1045.

Nakayama DA, Barthelemy C, Carrera G, Lightfoot RW Jr, Wortmann RL. Tophaceous gout: a clinical and radiographic assessment. *Arthritis Rheum.* 1984;27(4):468-471.

Palmer DG, Highton J, Hessian PA. Development of the gout tophus. An hypothesis. *Am J Clin Pathol.* 1989;91(2):190-195.

Pittman JR, Bross MH. Diagnosis and management of gout. *Am Fam Physician.* 1999;59(7): 1799-1806, 1810.

Simkin PA. Gout and hyperuricemia. *Curr Opin Rheumatol.* 1997;9(3):268-273.

Vasculitides

Arend WP, Michel BA, Bloch DA, et al. The American College of Rheumatology 1990 criteria for the classification of Takayasu arteritis. *Arthritis Rheum.* 1990;33(8):1129-1134.

Barilla-LaBarca ML, Lenschow DJ, Brasington RD Jr. Polymyalgia rheumatica/temporal arteritis: recent advances. *Curr Rheumatol Rep.* 2002;4(1):39-46.

Barron KS, Shulman ST, Rowley A, et al. Report of the national institutes of health workshop on Kawasaki disease. *J Rheumatol.* 1999;26(1):170-190.

Dajani AS, Taubert KA, Takahashi M, et al. Guidelines for long-term management of patients with Kawasaki disease. Report from the Committee on Rheumatic Fever, Endocarditis, and Kawasaki Disease, Council on Cardiovascular Disease in the Young, American Heart Association. *Circulation.* 1994;89(2):916-922.

Ferri C, Mascia MT. Cryoglobulinemic vasculitis. *Curr Opin Rheumatol.* 2006;18(1):54-63.

Gayraud M, Guillevin L, le Toumelin P, et al. Long-term followup of polyarteritis nodosa, microscopic polyangiitis, and Churg-Strauss syndrome: analysis of four prospective trials including 278 patients. *Arthritis Rheum.* 2001;44(3):666-675.

Gravanis MB. Giant cell arteritis and Takayasu aortitis: morphologic, pathogenetic and etiologic factors. *Int J Cardiol.* 2000;75(Suppl 1):S21-S33; discussion S35-S36.

Guillevin L, Lhote F, Amouroux J, Gherardi R, Callard P, Casassus P. Antineutrophil cytoplasmic antibodies, abnormal angiograms and pathological findings in polyarteritis nodosa and Churg-Strauss syndrome: indications for the classification of vasculitides of the polyarteritis Nodosa Group. *Br J Rheumatol.* 1996;35(10):958-964.

Guillevin L, Lhote F, Gherardi R. Polyarteritis nodosa, microscopic polyangiitis, and Churg-Strauss syndrome: clinical aspects, neurologic manifestations, and treatment. *Neurol Clin.* 1997; 15(4):865-886.

Hunder GG. Giant cell arteritis and polymyalgia rheumatica. *Med Clin North Am.* 1997;81(1): 195-219.

Hunder GG, Bloch DA, Michel BA, et al. The American College of Rheumatology 1990 criteria for the classification of giant cell arteritis. *Arthritis Rheum.* 1990;33(8):1122-1128.

Jennette JC, Falk RJ, Andrassy K, et al. Nomenclature of systemic vasculitides. Proposal of an international consensus conference. *Arthritis Rheum.* 1994;37(2):187-192.

Kawasaki T, Kosaki F, Okawa S, Shigematsu I, Yanagawa H. A new infantile acute febrile mucocutaneous lymph node syndrome (MLNS) prevailing in Japan. *Pediatrics.* 1974;54(3):271-276.

Kerr GS. Takayasu's arteritis. *Rheum Dis Clin North Am.* 1995;21(4):1041-1058.

Langford CA, Sneller MC. Update on the diagnosis and treatment of Wegener's granulomatosis. *Adv Intern Med.* 2001;46:177-206.

Leavitt RY, Fauci AS, Bloch DA, et al. The American College of Rheumatology 1990 criteria for the classification of Wegener's granulomatosis. *Arthritis Rheum.* 1990;33(8):1101-1107.

Lhote F, Guillevin L. Polyarteritis nodosa, microscopic polyangiitis, and Churg-Strauss syndrome. Clinical aspects and treatment. *Rheum Dis Clin North Am.* 1995;21(4):911-947.

Lightfoot RW Jr, Michel BA, Bloch DA, et al. The American College of Rheumatology 1990 criteria for the classification of polyarteritis nodosa. *Arthritis Rheum.* 1990;33(8): 1088-1093.

Masi AT, Hunder GG, Lie JT, et al. The American College of Rheumatology 1990 criteria for the classification of Churg-Strauss syndrome (allergic granulomatosis and angiitis). *Arthritis Rheum.* 1990;33(8):1094-1100.

Newburger JW, Takahashi M, Gerber MA, et al. Diagnosis, treatment, and long-term management of Kawasaki disease: a statement for health professionals from the Committee on Rheumatic Fever, Endocarditis and Kawasaki Disease, Council on Cardiovascular Disease in the Young, American Heart Association. *Circulation.* 2004;110(17):2747-2771.

Numano F. Differences in clinical presentation and outcome in different countries for Takayasu's arteritis. *Curr Opin Rheumatol.* 1997;9(1):12-15.

Olin JW. Thromboangiitis obliterans (Buerger's disease). *N Engl J Med.* 2000;343(12):864-869.

Stone JH, Nousari HC. "Essential" cutaneous vasculitis: what every rheumatologist should know about vasculitis of the skin. *Curr Opin Rheumatol.* 2001;13(1):23-34.

Weyand CM. The Dunlop-Dottridge Lecture: the pathogenesis of giant cell arteritis. *J Rheumatol.* 2000;27(2):517-522.

Wung PK, Stone JH. Therapeutics of Wegener's granulomatosis. *Nat Clin Pract Rheumatol.* 2006;2(4):192-200.

Systemic Sclerosis and Related Syndromes

Abraham DJ, Varga J. Scleroderma: from cell and molecular mechanisms to disease models. *Trends Immunol.* 2005;26(11):587-595.

Badesch DB, Tapson VF, McGoon MD, et al. Continuous intravenous epoprostenol for pulmonary hypertension due to the scleroderma spectrum of disease. A randomized, controlled trial. *Ann Intern Med.* 2000;132(6):425-434.

Clements PJ, Furst DE, eds. *Systemic Sclerosis.* Philadelphia: Lippincott Williams & Wilkins; 2004:29-37.

Furst DE. Rational therapy in the treatment of systemic sclerosis. *Curr Opin Rheumatol.* 2000;12(6):540-544.

Korn JH. Pathogenesis of systemic sclerosis. In: Koopman WJ, Moreland LW, eds. *Arthritis and Allied Conditions.* Philadelphia: Lippincott Williams & Wilkins; 2005:1621-1632.

LeRoy EC, Black C, Fleischmajer R, et al. Scleroderma (systemic sclerosis): classification, subsets and pathogenesis. *J Rheumatol*. 1988;15(2):202-205.

Preliminary criteria for the classification of systemic sclerosis (scleroderma). Subcommittee for scleroderma criteria of the American Rheumatism Association Diagnostic and Therapeutic Criteria Committee. *Arthritis Rheum*. 1980;23(5):581-590.

Tashkin DP, Elashoff R, Clements PJ, et al. Cyclophosphamide versus placebo in scleroderma lung disease. *N Engl J Med*. 2006;354(25):2655-2666.

Sjogren's Syndrome

Daniels TE. Labial salivary gland biopsy in Sjogren's syndrome. Assessment as a diagnostic criterion in 362 suspected cases. *Arthritis Rheum*. 1984;27(2):147-156.

Fox RI, Stern M, Michelson P. Update in Sjogren syndrome. *Curr Opin Rheumatol*. 2000;12(5): 391-398.

Gottenberg JE, Busson M, Loiseau P, et al. In primary Sjogren's syndrome, HLA class II is associated exclusively with autoantibody production and spreading of the autoimmune response. *Arthritis Rheum*. 2003;48(8):2240-2245.

Ramos-Casals M, Font J, Garcia-Carrasco M, et al. Primary Sjogren syndrome: hematologic patterns of disease expression. *Medicine (Baltimore)*. 2002;81(4):281-292.

Vitali C. Classification criteria for Sjogren's syndrome. *Ann Rheum Dis*. 2003;62(1):94-95; author reply 95.

Behcet's Disease

Borhani Haghighi A, Pourmand R, Nikseresht AR. Neuro-Behcet disease. A review. *Neurologist*. 2005;11(2):80-89.

Calamia KT, Schirmer M, Melikoglu M. Major vessel involvement in Behcet disease. *Curr Opin Rheumatol*. 2005;17(1):1-8.

Criteria for diagnosis of Behcet's disease. International Study Group for Behcet's disease. *Lancet*. 1990;335(8697):1078-1080.

Kaklamani VG, Vaiopoulos G, Kaklamanis PG. Behcet's disease. *Semin Arthritis Rheum*. 1998;27(4):197-217.

Sakane T, Takeno M, Suzuki N, Inaba G. Behcet's disease. *N Engl J Med*. 1999;341(17): 1284-1291.

Yurdakul S, Mat C, Tuzun Y, et al. A double-blind trial of colchicine in Behcet's syndrome. *Arthritis Rheum*. 2001;44(11):2686-2692.

Relapsing Polychondritis

Foidart JM, Abe S, Martin GR, et al. Antibodies to type II collagen in relapsing polychondritis. *N Engl J Med*. 1978;299(22):1203-1207.

Kent PD, Michet CJ Jr, Luthra HS. Relapsing polychondritis. *Curr Opin Rheumatol*. 2004;16(1):56-61.

McAdam LP, O'Hanlan MA, Bluestone R, Pearson CM. Relapsing polychondritis: prospective study of 23 patients and a review of the literature. *Medicine (Baltimore)*. 1976;55(3):193-215.

Park J, Gowin KM, Schumacher HR Jr. Steroid sparing effect of methotrexate in relapsing polychondritis. *J Rheumatol*. 1996;23(5):937-938.

Trentham DE, Le CH. Relapsing polychondritis. *Ann Intern Med*. 1998;129(2):114-122.

Antiphospholipid Syndrome

Crowther MA, Ginsberg JS, Julian J, et al. A comparison of two intensities of warfarin for the prevention of recurrent thrombosis in patients with the antiphospholipid antibody syndrome. *N Engl J Med.* 2003;349(12):1133-1138.

Khamashta MA, Hughes GR. Antiphospholipid antibodies and antiphospholipid syndrome. *Curr Opin Rheumatol.* 1995;7(5):389-394.

Khamashta MA, Cuadrado MJ, Mujic F, Taub NA, Hunt BJ, Hughes GR. The management of thrombosis in the antiphospholipid-antibody syndrome. *N Engl J Med.* 1995;332(15): 993-997.

Levine JS, Branch DW, Rauch J. The antiphospholipid syndrome. *N Engl J Med.* 2002;346(10): 752-763.

Miyakis S, Lockshin MD, Atsumi T, et al. International consensus statement on an update of the classification criteria for definite antiphospholipid syndrome (APS). *J Thromb Haemost.* 2006;4(2):295-306.

Myones BL, McCurdy D. The antiphospholipid syndrome: immunologic and clinical aspects. Clinical spectrum and treatment. *J Rheumatol Suppl.* 2000;58:20-28.

Petri M. Pathogenesis and treatment of the antiphospholipid antibody syndrome. *Med Clin North Am.* 1997;81(1):151-177.

Triplett DA. Many faces of lupus anticoagulants. *Lupus.* 1998;7(Suppl 2):S18-S22.

Adult Still's Disease

Efthimiou P, Georgy S. Pathogenesis and management of adult-onset Still's disease. *Semin Arthritis Rheum.* 2006;36(3):144-152.

Efthimiou P, Paik PK, Bielory L. Diagnosis and management of adult onset Still's disease. *Ann Rheum Dis.* 2006;65(5):564-572.

Fautrel B, Borget C, Rozenberg S, et al. Corticosteroid sparing effect of low dose methotrexate treatment in adult Still's disease. *J Rheumatol.* 1999;26(2):373-378.

Fautrel B, Le Moel G, Saint-Marcoux B, et al. Diagnostic value of ferritin and glycosylated ferritin in adult onset Still's disease. *J Rheumatol.* 2001;28(2):322-329.

Fitzgerald AA, Leclercq SA, Yan A, Homik JE, Dinarello CA. Rapid responses to anakinra in patients with refractory adult-onset Still's disease. *Arthritis Rheum.* 2005;52(6): 1794-1803.

Husni ME, Maier AL, Mease PJ, et al. Etanercept in the treatment of adult patients with Still's disease. *Arthritis Rheum.* 2002;46(5):1171-1176.

Rheumatic Drug Therapies

Dipiro JT, Talbert RL, Yee G, Matzke G, Wells B, Posey LM, eds. *Pharmacotherapy: A Patho-Physiologic Approach.* 7th ed. New York: McGraw-Hill Medical; 2008.

Drug Facts and Comparisons. 7th ed. St Louis, MO: *Facts and Comparisons,* 2011.

Dunkin MA. Drug Guide. *Arthritis Today.* 2001;15(suppl 7):40-45.

Guidelines for monitoring drug therapy in rheumatoid arthritis. American College of Rheumatology Ad Hoc Committee on Clinical Guidelines. *Arthritis Rheum.* 1996;39(5):723-731.

Jones KW, Patel SR. A family physician's guide to monitoring methotrexate. *Am Fam Physician.* 2000;62(7):1607-1612, 1614.

Lacy CF, Armstrong LL, Goldman MP, Lance LL. *Drug Information Handbook.* 16th ed. Hudson: Lexi-Comp; 2008.

Osteoporosis

Cooper C, Campion G, Melton LJ 3rd. Hip fractures in the elderly: a world-wide projection. *Osteoporos Int.* 1992;2(6):285-289.

Eastell R. Treatment of postmenopausal osteoporosis. *N Engl J Med.* 1998;338(11):736-746.

Holick MF, Siris ES, Binkley N, et al. Prevalence of Vitamin D inadequacy among postmenopausal North American women receiving osteoporosis therapy. *J Clin Endocrinol Metab.* 2005;90(6):3215-3224.

McClung MR, Geusens P, Miller PD, et al. Effect of risedronate on the risk of hip fracture in elderly women. Hip Intervention Program Study Group. *N Engl J Med.* 2001;344(5):333-340.

Naganathan V, Macgregor A, Snieder H, Nguyen T, Spector T, Sambrook P. Gender differences in the genetic factors responsible for variation in bone density and ultrasound. *J Bone Miner Res.* 2002;17(4):725-733.

NIH Consensus Development Panel on Osteoporosis Prevention. Diagnosis, and therapy, March 7–29, 2000: highlights of the conference. *South Med J.* 2001;94(6):569-573.

Osteoporosis: review of the evidence for prevention, diagnosis and treatment and cost-effectiveness analysis. Executive summary. *Osteoporos Int.* 1998;8(suppl 4):S3-S6.

Recommendations for the prevention and treatment of glucocorticoid-induced osteoporosis: 2001 update. American College of Rheumatology Ad Hoc Committee on Glucocorticoid-Induced Osteoporosis. *Arthritis Rheum.* 2001;44(7):1496-1503.

Reginster J, Minne HW, Sorensen OH, et al. Randomized trial of the effects of risedronate on vertebral fractures in women with established postmenopausal osteoporosis. Vertebral Efficacy with Risedronate Therapy (VERT) Study Group. *Osteoporos Int.* 2000;11(1):83-91.

Reid DM, Hughes RA, Laan RF, et al. Efficacy and safety of daily risedronate in the treatment of corticosteroid-induced osteoporosis in men and women: a randomized trial. European Corticosteroid-Induced Osteoporosis Treatment Study. *J Bone Miner Res.* 2000;15(6):1006-1013.

Ross PD. Osteoporosis. Frequency, consequences, and risk factors. *Arch Intern Med.* 1996;156(13):1399-1411.

Saag KG, Emkey R, Schnitzer TJ, et al. Alendronate for the prevention and treatment of glucocorticoid-induced osteoporosis. Glucocorticoid-Induced Osteoporosis Intervention Study Group. *N Engl J Med.* 1998;339(5):292-299.

Sambrook P, Birmingham J, Kelly P, et al. Prevention of corticosteroid osteoporosis. A comparison of calcium, calcitriol, and calcitonin. *N Engl J Med.* 1993;328(24):1747-1752.

Watts NB. Fundamentals and pitfalls of bone densitometry using dual-energy X-ray absorptiometry (DXA). *Osteoporos Int.* 2004;15(11):847-854.

Metabolic Bone Disorders

Favus MJ, ed. *Primer on the Metabolic Bone Diseases and Disorders of Mineral Metabolism.* 4th ed. Philadelphia: Lippincott Williams & Wilkins; 1999.

Sillence D. Osteogenesis imperfecta. In: Rimoin DL, Connor JM, Pyeritz RE, Korf B, eds. *Principles and Practice of Medical Genetics.* 5th ed. New York: Elsevier; 2007, Chapter 149.

Paget's Disease of Bone

Altman RD. Musculoskeletal manifestations of Paget's disease of bone. *Arthritis Rheum.* 1980;23(10):1121-1127.

Altman RD, Johnston CC, Khairi MR, Wellman H, Serafini AN, Sankey RR. Influence of disodium etidronate on clinical and laboratory manifestations of Paget's disease of bone (osteitis deformans). *N Engl J Med.* 1973;289(26):1379-1384.

Altman RD, Bloch DA, Hochberg MC, Murphy WA. Prevalence of pelvic Paget's disease of bone in the United States. *J Bone Miner Res.* 2000;15(3):461-465.

Burckhardt P. Biochemical and scintigraphic assessment of Paget's disease. *Semin Arthritis Rheum.* 1994;23(4):237-239.

Delmas PD, Meunier PJ. The management of Paget's disease of bone. *N Engl J Med.* 1997;336(8):558-566.

Hadjipavlou A, Lander P, Srolovitz H, Enker IP. Malignant transformation in Paget disease of bone. *Cancer.* 1992;70(12):2802-2808.

Michou L, Collet C, Laplanche JL, Orcel P, Cornelis F. Genetics of Paget's disease of bone. *Joint Bone Spine.* 2006;73(3):243-248.

Singer FR. Paget's disease of bone: classical pathology and electron microscopy. *Semin Arthritis Rheum.* 1994;23(4):217-218.

Siris ES. Epidemiological aspects of Paget's disease: family history and relationship to other medical conditions. *Semin Arthritis Rheum.* 1994;23(4):222-225.

Tiegs RD. Paget's disease of bone: indications for treatment and goals of therapy. *Clin Ther.* 1997;19(6):1309-1329; discussion 1523–1524.

Walsh JP, Ward LC, Stewart GO, et al. A randomized clinical trial comparing oral alendronate and intravenous pamidronate for the treatment of Paget's disease of bone. *Bone.* 2004;34(4):747-754.

Osteonecrosis

Assouline-Dayan Y, Chang C, Greenspan A, Shoenfeld Y, Gershwin ME. Pathogenesis and natural history of osteonecrosis. *Semin Arthritis Rheum.* 2002;32(2):94-124.

Felson DT, Anderson JJ. Across-study evaluation of association between steroid dose and bolus steroids and avascular necrosis of bone. *Lancet.* 1987;1(8538):902-906.

Frankel ES, Urbaniak JR. Osteonecrosis. In: Ruddy S, Harris ED, Sledge CB, eds. *Kelley's Textbook of Rheumatology.* 6th ed. Philadelphia: WB Saunders; 2001:1653-1665.

Glueck CJ, Freiberg R, Tracy T, Stroop D, Wang P. Thrombophilia and hypofibrinolysis: pathophysiologies of osteonecrosis. *Clin Orthop Relat Res.* 1997;334:43-56.

Jones LC, Hungerford DS. Osteonecrosis: etiology, diagnosis, and treatment. *Curr Opin Rheumatol.* 2004;16(4):443-449.

Koo KH, Kim R, Kim YS, et al. Risk period for developing osteonecrosis of the femoral head in patients on steroid treatment. *Clin Rheumatol.* 2002;21(4):299-303.

Mont MA, Carbone JJ, Fairbank AC. Core decompression versus nonoperative management for osteonecrosis of the hip. *Clin Orthop Relat Res.* 1996;324:169-178.

Mont MA, Marulanda GA, Jones LC, et al. Systematic analysis of classification systems for osteonecrosis of the femoral head. *J Bone Joint Surg Am.* 2006;88(suppl 3):16-26.

Urbaniak JR, Harvey EJ. Revascularization of the femoral head in osteonecrosis. *J Am Acad Orthop Surg.* 1998;6(1):44-54.

Hypertrophic Osteoarthropathy

Guyot-Drouot MH, Solau-Gervais E, Cortet B, et al. Rheumatologic manifestations of pachydermoperiostosis and preliminary experience with bisphosphonates. *J Rheumatol.* 2000;27(10):2418-2423.

Martinez-Lavin M, Matucci-Cerinic M, Jajic I, Pineda C. Hypertrophic osteoarthropathy: consensus on its definition, classification, assessment and diagnostic criteria. *J Rheumatol.* 1993;20(8):1386-1387.

Martinez-Lavin M, Pineda C, Valdez T, et al. Primary hypertrophic osteoarthropathy. *Semin Arthritis Rheum.* 1988;17(3):156-162.

Pineda C, Fonseca C, Martinez-Lavin M. The spectrum of soft tissue and skeletal abnormalities of hypertrophic osteoarthropathy. *J Rheumatol*. 1990;17(5):626-632.

Silveira LH, Martinez-Lavin M, Pineda C, Fonseca MC, Navarro C, Nava A. Vascular endothelial growth factor and hypertrophic osteoarthropathy. *Clin Exp Rheumatol*. 2000;18(1):57-62.

Vazquez-Abad D, Pineda C, Martinez-Lavin M. Digital clubbing: a numerical assessment of the deformity. *J Rheumatol*. 1989;16(4):518-520.

Storage and Depostion Diseases

Chanoki M, Ishii M, Fukai K, et al. Farber's lipogranulomatosis in siblings: light and electron microscopic studies. *Br J Dermatol*. 1989;121(6):779-785.

Gaines JJ Jr, Tom GD, Khankhanian N. An ultrastructural and light microscopic study of the synovium in ochronotic arthropathy. *Hum Pathol*. 1987;18(11):1160-1164.

Gorman JD, Danning C, Schumacher HR, Klippel JH, Davis JC Jr. Multicentric reticulohistiocytosis: case report with immunohistochemical analysis and literature review. *Arthritis Rheum*. 2000;43(4):930-938.

Gow PJ, Smallwood RA, Angus PW, Smith AL, Wall AJ, Sewell RB. Diagnosis of Wilson's disease: an experience over three decades. *Gut*. 2000;46(3):415-419.

Mathews JL, Williams HJ. Arthritis in hereditary hemochromatosis. *Arthritis Rheum*. 1987;30(10): 1137-1141.

Menerey KA, Eider W, Brewer GJ, Braunstein EM, Schumacher HR, Fox IH. The arthropathy of Wilson's disease: clinical and pathologic features. *J Rheumatol*. 1988;15(2):331-337.

Pastores GM, Meere PA. Musculoskeletal complications associated with lysosomal storage disorders: Gaucher disease and Hurler-Scheie syndrome (mucopolysaccharidosis type I). *Curr Opin Rheumatol*. 2005;17(1):70-78.

Perry MB, Suwannarat P, Furst GP, Gahl WA, Gerber LH. Musculoskeletal findings and disability in alkaptonuria. *J Rheumatol*. 2006;33(11):2280-2285.

Pietrangelo A. Hereditary hemochromatosis–a new look at an old disease. *N Engl J Med*. 2004;350(23):2383-2397.

Rooney PJ. Hyperlipidemias, lipid storage disorders, metal storage disorders, and ochronosis. *Curr Opin Rheumatol*. 1991;3(1):166-171.

Ross JM, Kowalchuk RM, Shaulinsky J, Ross L, Ryan D, Phatak PD. Association of heterozygous hemochromatosis C282Y gene mutation with hand osteoarthritis. *J Rheumatol*. 2003;30(1): 121-125.

Amyloidoses

Falk RH, Comenzo RL, Skinner M. The systemic amyloidoses. *N Engl J Med*. 1997;337(13): 898-909.

Hawkins PN, Lavender JP, Pepys MB. Evaluation of systemic amyloidosis by scintigraphy with 123I-labeled serum amyloid P component. *N Engl J Med*. 1990;323(8):508-513.

Kyle RA, Gertz MA, Greipp PR, et al. A trial of three regimens for primary amyloidosis: colchicine alone, melphalan and prednisone, and melphalan, prednisone, and colchicine. *N Engl J Med*. 1997;336(17):1202-1207.

Merlini G, Bellotti V. Molecular mechanisms of amyloidosis. *N Engl J Med*. 2003;349(6): 583-596.

Miyata T, Inagi R, Iida Y, et al. Involvement of beta 2-microglobulin modified with advanced glycation end products in the pathogenesis of hemodialysis-associated amyloidosis. Induction of human monocyte chemotaxis and macrophage secretion of tumor necrosis factor-alpha and interleukin-1. *J Clin Invest.* 1994;93(2):521-528.

Pepys MB. Amyloidosis. *Annu Rev Med.* 2006;57:223-241.

Sipe JD, Cohen AS. Review: history of the amyloid fibril. *J Struct Biol.* 2000;130(2–3):88-98.

The Autoinflammatory Diseases

Ancient missense mutations in a new member of the RoRet gene family are likely to cause familial Mediterranean fever. The International FMF Consortium. *Cell.* 1997;90(4):797-807.

Chae JJ, Komarow HD, Cheng J, et al. Targeted disruption of pyrin, the FMF protein, causes heightened sensitivity to endotoxin and a defect in macrophage apoptosis. *Mol Cell.* 2003;11(3): 591-604.

French FMF Consortium. A candidate gene for familial Mediterranean fever. *Nat Genet.* 1997;17(1):25-31.

Hull KM, Wong K, Wood GM, Chu WS, Kastner DL. Monocytic fasciitis: a newly recognized clinical feature of tumor necrosis factor receptor dysfunction. *Arthritis Rheum.* 2002a;46(8): 2189-2194.

Hull KM, Drewe E, Aksentijevich I, et al. The TNF receptor-associated periodic syndrome (TRAPS): emerging concepts of an autoinflammatory disorder. *Medicine (Baltimore).* 2002b; 81(5):349-368.

Kim PW, Aksentijevich I, Colburn NT, Kastner DL. Hereditary recurrent fevers. In: Hochberg MC, Silman AJ, Smolen JS, Weinblatt ME, Weisman MH, eds. *Rheumatology.* 5th ed. Philadelphia: Mosby Elsevier; 2011:1637-1658.

McDermott EM, Smillie DM, Powell RJ. Clinical spectrum of familial Hibernian fever: a 14-year follow-up study of the index case and extended family. *Mayo Clin Proc.* 1997;72(9):806-817.

McDermott MF, Aksentijevich I, Galon J, et al. Germline mutations in the extracellular domains of the 55 kDa TNF receptor, TNFR1, define a family of dominantly inherited autoinflammatory syndromes. *Cell.* 1999;97(1):133-144.

Index

A

Abatacept, 162–163
Abdominal fat aspirate, in primary
     amyloidosis, 673
Adalimumab, 548
ADAMs, 72
Adaptive immune response, 85–86, 108
Adenosine, 82
Adrenal insufficiency, corticosteroids,
     502–503
Adrenocorticotropic hormone (ACTH),
     gout, 269
Adult Still's disease
     clinical features and epidemiology, 455
     clinical findings
          arthritis, 457
          fever, 456–457
          rash in, 458–459
          wrist involvement, 458
     diagnosis, 460–461
     differential diagnosis, 461–462
     disease course and outcome, 462–463
     laboratory findings, 459
     pathogenesis, 455
     radiographic findings, 459–460
     treatment
          acute, 463
          chronic, 463–464
Affected sibling pair (ASP) method, 121
Age related changes, in articular cartilage, 13
Aggrecan core protein, 8–10
     degradation, 13
Aggressive phlebotomy therapy,
     hemochromatosis, 648
Alendronate, 579–580
Alkaptonuria (ochronosis)
     clinical features, 649–652
     radiographic features, 652–654
     treatment, 654
     tyrosine catabolism, disorder of, 649

Allopurinol, for gout
     dosing, 272
     hypersensitivity syndrome, 273
     indications for, 271–272
     mechanism of action, 271
     side effects, 272–273
Alopecia, in SLE, 192–193
Alveolar hemorrhage, in microscopic
     polyangiitis, 292
American College of Rheumatology (ACR)
     giant cell arteritis, 321
     systemic sclerosis, 368
     Takayasu's arteritis, 321
Amniocentesis, 662–663
Amsler grid, 516
Amyloid A (AA) disease, 677–678
Amyloid beta-2-microglobulin disease,
     676–677
Amyloidoses
     aging and amyloid, 678
     amyloid
          beta-2-microglobulin disease, 676–677
          deposition, 671
     amyloid A disease, 677–678
     arthropathy, forms associated with, 671
     clinical features
          AL disease, 674
          cardiomyopathy, 674–675
          hematologic and neuropathic
               presentation, 675
     description, 671
     familial amyloidosis, 679
     light chain deposition disease, 676
     mutant TTR, 679
     pathogenesis, 676
     pathology, 671–674
     treatment, 676
Anakinra, TRAPS, 692
Anchoring-fibril-forming collagen, 35–36
Androgens, osteoporosis, 586

N.T. Colburn, *Review of Rheumatology*,
DOI 10.1007/978-1-84882-093-7, © Springer-Verlag London Limited 2012